Bedside Clinics in PEDIATRICS Ready Reckoner

Bedside Clinics in PEDIATRICS Ready Reckoner

Editor

Sudip Saha

MD (Pediatrics)

Associate Professor

Department of Pediatric Medicine

Chittaranjan Seva Sadan

College of Obstetrics, Gynecology and Child Health

Kolkata, West Bengal, India

Foreword

Sutapa Ganguly

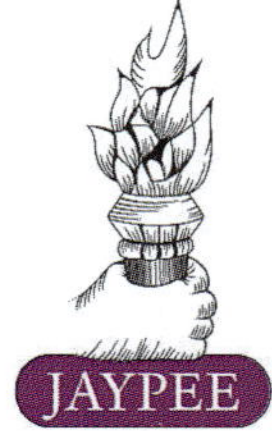

JAYPEE BROTHERS MEDICAL PUBLISHERS

The Health Sciences Publisher

New Delhi | London

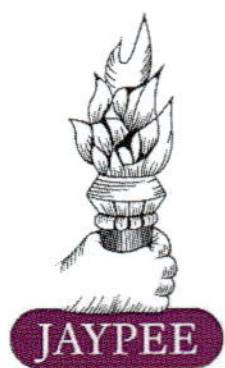

Jaypee Brothers Medical Publishers (P) Ltd

Headquarters
EMCA House, 23/23-B
Ansari Road, Daryaganj
New Delhi 110 002, India
Landline: +91-11-23272143, +91-11-23272703
+91-11-23282021, +91-11-23245672
e-mail: jaypee@jaypeebrothers.com

Corporate Office
4838/24, Ansari Road, Daryaganj
New Delhi 110 002, India
Phone: +91-11-43574357
Fax: +91-11-43574314
e-mail: jaypee@jaypeebrothers.com

Overseas Office
JP Medical Ltd.
83, Victoria Street, London
SW1H 0HW (UK)
Phone: +44-20 3170 8910
e-mail: info@jpmedpub.com

EU GPSR Authorised Representative
Logos Europe, 9 rue Nicolas Poussin
17000, La Rochelle, France
Phone: +33 (0) 6 67 93 73 78
e-mail: contact@logoseurope.eu

Website: www.jaypeebrothers.com
Website: www.jaypeedigital.com

Inquiries for bulk sales may be solicited at: jaypee@jaypeebrothers.com

Bedside Clinics in Pediatrics: Ready Reckoner

First Edition: **2026**

ISBN: 978-93-6616-465-6

Printed at: Samrat Offset Pvt. Ltd.

Dedicated to

Lord Jagannath and my grandfather and father

Contributors

Agnik Chattopadhyay
MBBS DNB (Ped) MNAMS
Medical Officer
Department of Neonatal unit
Chittaranjan Seva Sadan
College of Obstetrics, Gynecology
and Child Health
Kolkata West Bengal, India

Ira Das MBBS DCH MD (Pediatrics)
Assistant Professor
Department of Pediatrics Medicine
Chittaranjan Seva Sadan
College of Obstetrics, Gynecology
and Child Health
Kolkata, West Bengal, India

Joydeep Das
DNB (Pediatrics) MRCPCH (UK) BMCP MNAMS
Fellowship in HIV Medicine
Professor and Head
Department of Pediatrics
Jaganath Gupta Institute of Medical
Science and Hospital
Kolkata, West Bengal, India

Kalapana Datta MD (Pediatrics)
Professor and Head
Department of Pediatrics
Medical College Kolkata
Kolkata, West Bengal, India

Lopamudra Mishra
MD (Pediatrics) DM (Pediatric Cardiology) AIIMS
Assistant Professor
Department of Pediatric Cardiology
Institute of Postgraduate Medical
Education and Research (SSKM Hospital)
Kolkata, West Bengal, India

Madhumita Nandi
MD (Pediatrics) FIAP
Professor and Head
Department of Pediatrics
North Bengal Medical College
Darjeeling, West Bengal, India

Mousumi Das
MD (Pediatrics)
Assistant Professor
Department of Pediatrics Medicine
Chittaranjan Seva Sadan
College of Obstetrics, Gynecology
and Child Health
Kolkata, West Bengal, India

Mrigank Choube
MD (Pediatrics) DM (Pediatric Cardiology)
Associate Professor
Department of Pediatrics
Command Hospital Eastern Command
Kolkata, West Bengal, India

Pradip Prava Paria
MBBS DPM MD (Ped) DM (Neurology)
Assistant Professor
Department of Pediatrics
Government Medical College
and Hospital
Raiganj, West Bengal, India

Rajasree Sinha MD
Senior Resident
Department of Pediatrics
Government Medical College
Kolkata, West Bengal, India

Samik Basu
MBBS (Gold Medalist) DCh DNB (Pediatrics)
MNAMS
Consultant Pediatrician
Department of Pediatrics
Fortis Hospital and Iris Hospital
Kolkata, West Bengal, India

Sanjana Samanta
MD (Ped) DCH MD (Pediatrics)
Assistant Professor
Department of Pediatrics Medicine
Chittaranjan Seva Sadan
College of Obstetrics, Gynecology
and Child Health
Kolkata, West Bengal, India

Saugata Chaudhuri
MBBS DNB (Ped) DM (Neonatology)
Assistant Professor
Department of Neonatology
Institute of Postgraduate Medical
Education and Research (SSKM Hospital)
Kolkata, West Bengal, India

Sayan Chatterjee
MD (Pediatrics Medicine)
Associate Professor
Department of Pediatrics Medicine
Prafulla Chandra Sen Government
Medical College and Hospital
Hooghly, West Bengal, India

Shatanik Sarkar
MD (Pediatrics) DM (Pediatric Cardiology)
Assistant Professor
Department of Pediatrics and
Pediatric Cardiology
Institute of Postgraduate Medical
Education and Research (SSKM Hospital)
Kolkata, West Bengal, India

Shayamajit Samaddar
MD (Pediatrics) DM (Pediatric Cardiology)
Consultant Pediatric Cardiologist
Department of Pediatric Cardiology
BM Birla Heart Hospital
Kolkata, West Bengal, India

Sneha Dasgupta
MD (Ped) PDCC (Ped Gastro)
Assistant Professor
Department of Pediatrics
Institute of Child Health
Kolkata, West Bengal, India

Subhamoy Das
MBBS MD (Ped) DM (Ped Gastro, PGI Chandigarh)
Senior Consultant
Department of Pediatric
Gastroenterology
Institute of Gastrosciences
Apollo Multispecialty Hospitals
Kolkata, West Bengal, India

Subhasish Bhattacharyya
MBBS DCH MD (Ped) DNB (Ped) MNAMS FIAP
Professor and Head
Department of Pediatric Medicine
Chittaranjan Seva Sadan
College of Obstetrics, Gynecology
and Child Health
Kolkata, West Bengal, India

Sudip Saha MD (Pediatrics)
Associate Professor
Department of Pediatrics Medicine
Chittaranjan Seva Sadan
College of Obstetrics, Gynecology
and Child Health
Kolkata, West Bengal, India

Sumana Kundagrami
MD (Pediatrics) MRCPCH (UK)
Associate Professor
Department of Pediatrics
KPC Medical College and Hospital
Kolkata, West Bengal, India

Sumantra Kumar Raut
MD (Ped) DM (Nephrology)
Associate Professor
Department of Pediatric Nephrology
North Bengal Medical College
Siliguri, West Bengal, India

Swapan Ray
MBBS DCH DNB (Ped) MNAMS FIAP
Professor
Department of Pediatrics
MGM Medical College and LSK Hospital
Kishanganj, Bihar, India

Foreword

It gives me immense pleasure to write the foreword for the book *Bedside Clinics in Pediatrics* by Dr Sudip Saha who has been associated with undergraduate and postgraduate teaching for more than 20 years.

The book explains the clinical aspects of pediatrics in a lucid manner so that it becomes easy to understand by the students.

The recent advances, clinical photographs, illustrations, and flowcharts enrich the contents of the book and help the students to understand the clinical problems in a better manner.

It is important for the clinicians to know the normal milestones applicable to children so that any deviation from normal can be identified and the cause can be treated.

Important aspects of nutrition including breastfeeding and infant feeding are also emphasized in the chapter on nutrition.

The detailed examination of different systems including the common disorders related to individual system, e.g., cardiovascular system, respiratory system, gastrointestinal system, central and peripheral nervous systems, genitourinary system, hemopoietic system, endocrine system, muscular and rheumatological disorders, and chromosomal disorders, is a treasure of the book.

Due importance has been given to neonatology, neonatal resuscitation examination of term and preterm babies, common neonatal problems like neonatal jaundice, sepsis, etc.—these have been dealt with great care. Chapters on OSCE, Instruments, and Asthma Devices with their proper use and updates on vaccines will not only help the undergraduate students but also benefit the postgraduate students and clinicians.

Sutapa Ganguly
MD (Pediatrics) FIAP
Former Principal
Chittaranjan Seva Sadan
College of Obstetrics, Gynecology and Child Health
Kolkata, West Bengal, India
Former President
West Bengal Academy of Pediatrics (WBAP)

Preface

It gives me immense pleasure to be able to present the first edition of *Bedside Clinics in Pediatrics* published by Jaypee Brothers Medical Publishers.

Pediatric medicine has become a mainstream subject which is a part of 3rd professional MBBS and has also evolved as a sole subject for Masters' degree.

My long experience as an undergraduate and postgraduate examiner and teacher in pediatrics helped me to understand the difficulties faced by the students in answering during practical examinations. Also, the curriculum has changed with OSCE being introduced in both undergraduate and postgraduate examinations.

This book will be helpful for all students to know the questions that can be asked in practical examination system-wise.

However, my request is to learn clinical methods from standard textbooks.

This book also deals with oral examinations which is a part of practical examination. It includes X-rays, vaccines, and instruments.

I welcome suggestions and comments from the readers, critics, and my teachers of pediatric medicine which will be gratefully acknowledged and will make the book more useful and valuable for the students in future.

Sudip Saha

Acknowledgments

Writing a book is rarely a solitary pursuit. It is a journey interwoven with the support, encouragement, and expertise of many. I extend my heartfelt gratitude to the Almighty for giving me the opportunity.

I thank my family, especially my wife and daughter, for their support and for pushing me to make it better for students.

I take this opportunity to thank my teachers, Professors Sibarjun Ghosh, Maitreyi Basu, and Gautam De, for teaching pediatrics to me.

I thank all those who have contributed to this book and my patients who have helped me to learn pediatrics. I also thank my department and Head of my department, Professor Subhasish Bhattacharyya, for his support. I thank my principal Professor Ashis Mukhopadhyay and Medical Superintendent Professor Gita Basu Banarjee.

I extend my thanks to the team of M/s Jaypee Brothers Medical Publishers (P) Ltd, New Delhi, India, comprising Mr Sabyasachi Hazra (Director—PG and PNR Content), Bikram Sardar (Commissioning Editor), and Aarti Kushwah (Development Editor), for their keen eye, insightful suggestions, and commitment to making this manuscript the best it could be.

Finally, I thank you—the reader—for picking up this book. I hope you find your answers within the pages.

I hope to come up with further modifications in future editions.

Contents

CHAPTER 1

History Taking

Sudip Saha

In pediatrics, usually parents or grandparents are informant. Children above 6 years can tell us their problems.

- *Name:* Name is asked to get confidence of patient/ informant and also as an identity for future communication.
- *Age:* If date of birth is available, it will give the correct age. Many a time, parents cannot tell exactly the age. Age is a clue for many cut-offs for diseases, example, usually a typhoid fever will manifest after 1 year. Urinary tract infection investigations are age specific and also 3 years is the cut off for differentiating nephrotic syndrome from nephritic syndrome. Age also varies for precocious puberty and delayed puberty.
- *Sex:* Please write male or female and not boy or girl but while stating in summary one can write boy or girl. Very rarely, you could come across an indeterminate sex and should plan for endocrinology workup. Do not forget to ask the informant the sex as by name and look it is not always possible as the children are sometimes dressed like a boy though she is a girl.
- *Address:* Usually tells us about some diseases which are prevalent in some states like Japanese Encephalitis in Assam, Bengal, or Kala-azar in Bihar or scrub from northern India. If coming from outside India, many diseases are to be ruled out. Never forget to ask if their parents are working with a transferable policy.
- *Religion:* Each religion has some characteristics like dress sense, toilet habits, and food habits. Even the consanguinity in marriage is prevalent in Muslims. Jains or Vegans have vitamin B_{12} deficiency. Also, dress sense, i.e., covered clothing from childhood causes less sun exposure and many have vitamin D deficiency.
- Date of admission and date of examination to be mentioned for calculating duration of illness.
- *Chief complaints:* Write the specific problems, i.e., fever, cough, vomiting, pain abdomen, headache, and its duration in chronological order.
- *History of present illness (HOPI):* Elaborating the chief complaints in details. Usually stated, that the child was apparently well, say 6 month or 1 year ago.

But some diseases may have started since birth like cerebral palsy, down's syndrome or other syndromes, cystic fibrosis or malnutrition or developmental delays.

Details of every complaint in easy lucid language both for examiners and the doctor himself/herself is important. Say fever its character (continuous/intermittent/ remittent), responding to medications or any associations like chill, rigor, and abnormal movement. Vomiting is of projectile or nonprojectile, associated symptoms like headache, pain abdomen, with or without food particles or blood. Headache, its character, and site sometimes guide us to identify the etiology. Pain abdomen area can sometimes help us for etiology like epigastric or right hypochondriac or right iliac or any radiation of pain.

- *History of past illness:* History of similar episode or different episode but having some relevance. Mention the duration of the treatment of previous illness. Example, nephrotic syndrome or urinary tract infection guides us to the present treatment. Past history of any malignancy or tuberculosis is important. Recurrence in respiratory or gastrointestinal symptoms will give clue to various diseases like bronchiectasis, interstitial lung disease, foreign body, or sequestration.
- *Birth history:* It comprises three parts antenatal, natal, and postnatal. In antenatal, important events are mother's age, booked or nonbooked, and serious maternal illness which can lead to difficult labor like short stature, diabetes, congenital infection, twins/triplets, polyhydramnios, intrauterine growth retardation—symmetric/asymmetric, congenital anomalies, premature rupture of membranes, antepartum hemorrhage.

In natal, ask about Cesarean section/normal delivery/ forceps, birth weight of baby, liquor, presentation, and cry at birth.

In postnatal, enquire of initiation of breastfeeding, passage of stool, and whether there was any admission and for what reason or what duration and special events during admission such as seizures or hypoglycemia.

- *Development history:* It has four phases, i.e., gross motor, fine motor, social, and language. A chart for the milestones achieved, and their age at which the child was able to do and the delay if any **(Table 1)**.

  It is important to show the development quotient.

Immunization history: Enquire whether the child is vaccinated till date or has skipped any vaccinations. If vaccine card is available, it is the best way to understand the vaccination status **(Table 2)**. Always look for BCG scar.

- *Nutritional history or diet history:* Very important to find out the cause of growth failure. It starts from birth with exclusive breastfeeding done or not (prelacteals given or not). Duration of exclusive breastfeeding and when was weaning started.

  You must enquire about the diet chart by recall method.

The various calorie and protein of cooked and uncooked items **(Table 3)** should be ready reckoner.

TABLE 1 : Developmental milestones in children from birth to six years.

Physical	*Cognitive*	*Emotional and social*	*Language*
Birth to 6 months			
Gross (Large) motor skills • Lifts head and chest when on stomach • Rolls from back to side or side to back • Rolls completely over from back or stomach • Sits with support • Holds head erect *Fine (small) motor skills* • Reaches for objects • Holds objects for short periods of time before dropping them Touches and pats bottle	*Recognizes and responds to own name* • Discriminates between familiar and unfamiliar faces • Demonstrates happiness and unhappiness with sounds • Demonstrates memory by waiting while feeding is prepared and stopping crying when person enters room Looks forward to feeding by sight	*Expresses affection* • Shows interest in human faces • Has sense of humor • Becomes excited when played with • Stares at strangers • Smiles at familiar faces • Develops attachment to primary caregiver • Becomes trusting when needs are met; fretful when needs are not met • Shows displeasure when loses contact with person Smiles and babbles at people and toys	• Uses crying to signal distress and pain • Responds to human voice • Turns head and moves eyes toward noise and sound • Startles to loud noise • Coos, chuckles, laughs and squeals • Babbles and repeats sounds • May fix his gaze on a person's mouth as the person talks • Likes musical sounds and squeaky toys Laughs out loud
6–12 Months			
Gross (large) motor skills • Progresses from sitting steady when supported to sitting without support • Crawls on hands and knees • Pulls to standing position • Walks with help • Stands alone *Fine (small) motor skills* • Reaches for small objects • Places objects in a container • Picks up medium and large objects • Changes objects from one hand to another • Plays with two toys; one in each hand Points with fingers	• Follows simple directions • Searches for object that has disappeared • Pours objects out of container and put each back in • Imitates actions of others • Understands basic cause and effect relationships (touching hot stove burns hand) • Enjoys repetition of events • Enjoys picture book for short period of time Assembles simple nesting toys	• Becomes more emotionally attached to caregiver • Protests at separation from mother • Shows some negative reaction to strangers • Seeks approval; doesn't want disapproval • Plays simple games with adults • Enjoys being center of attention • Enjoys communicating with others • Smiles, pats and plays with image in mirror Expresses pleasure and displeasure	• Babbles intentionally to get others to respond • Responds to name when it is used • Understands a few words such as no and bye • Says mama and dada • Begins to babble in sentence-like sounds • Responds correctly to a few words • Uses gestures in an intentional manner to express wants • Can wave bye-bye • Enjoys simple rhymes and songs Makes two-syllable words like dada and bye bye

Contd...

Contd...

Physical	*Cognitive*	*Emotional and social*	*Language*
12–18 months			
• Stands alone • Walks without support; starting and stopping with control • Walks backward with pull toy • Squats down to pick up object and stands up • Climbs upstairs; creeps down backwards one at a time • Climbs out of crib and play pen fine (small) motor skills • Turns several pages of book at one time • Scribbles on paper with crayon • Releases ball with slight thrust • Picks up small objects between thumb and forefinger • Can open small box • Holds spoon with fist • Feeds self with fingers Holds and drinks from cup	• Learns by exploring • Responds to simple directions • Points to familiar objects upon request • Identifies family members in photos • Remembers where things are in different areas of house (room) • Hunts for hidden toy • Shows brief interest in picture book • Gives mechanical toy to caregiver to activate Places a large round shape in a formboard	• Is self-centered, demanding, stubborn and self-assertive • Imitates adults • Is inconsistent in expressing emotions • May become upset when adults place limitations on activities • Expresses anger • Engages in parallel play • Rolls ball to adult • Likes to show off for audience • Shows fear of strangers • Is unable to share • Responds to simple instructions • Takes pride in accomplishments • Increases negativism • May show fear of storms and animals Is easily distracted	• Uses one word at a time as a sentence, such as go, see and milk" • Experiences rapid gain in learning and understanding new words • Knows at least three words other than mama and dada • Uses several words that can beunderstood • Says hi or bye if asked • Points to a few body parts if asked • Listens to simple stories, songs and rhymes Uses words that resemble real words such as ba-ba for bottle
18–24 months			
• Runs stiffly • Jumps off ground with both feet • Bends at waist to pick up object • Walks up and down steps, one step at a time • Throws objects overhead • Kicks large ball • Climbs onto low objects fine (small) motor skills • Manages spoon • Makes vertical marks and circles with crayon (pencil) • Turns doorknobs • Pulls down zippers • Shows hand preference, but switches hands often Assists in dressing and undressing self	• Points to body parts upon request • Acknowledges absence of familiar persons (points to door, says gone) • Points to and names objects in book • Begins to recognize shapes • Enjoys cause-and-effect relationships (banging drum, turning on TV) • Follows simple instructions • Asks names of objects Identifies more objects with names	• Expresses love and affection openly • Seeks approval and praise • Is outgoing, friendly and less self-centered • Continues to be easily distracted • May show need for security object • Expresses pride and jealousy • Continues parallel play • Is possessive; refuses to share • Shows strong positive and negative actions • Shows strong desire for own way • May exhibit aggressive actions (hitting, biting, pushing)	• Uses one to two words to make a sentence, for example, "Me," and "Me shoe" • Names pictures of common objects (cat, dog, man, house) • Knows and uses approximately 50 words • Makes 25–50% of her words understood • Follows simple, one-step directions ("Bring the book to me") • Uses word no often • Takes part in simple conversations • Likes singing and rhymes • Tries to talk about experiences Uses words to make wants known
2 to 3 years			
Gross (large) motor skills • Is constantly in motion • Jumps off low objects • Pushes self on wheeled toys	• Follows simple directions • Enjoys reciting finger plays, nursery rhymes and songs	• Becomes less easily distracted • Is self-centered, aggressive and temperamental	• Uses a vocabulary of between 50 and 300 words by age three • Understands most of what is said to them

Contd...

Contd...

Physical	*Cognitive*	*Emotional and social*	*Language*
2 to 3 years			
• Runs but has difficulty stopping • Seats self in small chairs • Alternates feet going upstairs, but not downstairs • Kicks ball • Throws ball overhand; no aim • Catches objects with arms extended and elbows stiff *Fine (small) motor skills* • Turns individual pages of book • Screws lids on and off • Builds crude towers of six or more blocks • Scribbles circles and horizontal and vertical lines • Takes simple objects apart and puts back together • Uses spoon; spills a lot	• Repeats radio and TV commercials • Responds to rhythms • Learns simple relationships such as big and small • Invents simple sentences to express thoughts • Uses names of familiar people and objects • Asks names of objects	• Views situations in terms of own needs • See-saws between independence and dependence • Wants to do things for self • Desires consistency • Desires approval; feels hurt when disciplined for actions • Is unable to share • Wants to be accepted by others • Likes to play with adults and older children • Is difficult to understand and control • May continue to express negativism • Has temper tantrums • Resists naps but needs rest	• Uses the word no often • Has understandable speech at least 65–70% of the time • Follows two-step directions • Uses own name when referring to self before using me or I • Uses two to four word sentences, regularly Grammar may be incorrect, such as "Me do it" • Uses plurals • Recognizes that language is effective inexpressing needs • Asks questions frequently such as, "What's that?" • Understands many more words than uses when talking • Wants to participate when being read to by turning the pages of the book, pointing or making sounds • Enjoys books, singing and rhymes • Speaks loudly, at times, before learning voice control • Knows first and last name
3 to 4 Years			
Gross (large) motor skills • Hops, skips, jumps and runs • Makes sudden stops and starts • Walks on tiptoes • Hops on one foot • Marches to rhythm • Alternates steps when climbing stairs; comes down one step at a time • Throws ball by thrusting with arm and shoulder; catches with arms held out straight • Swings on a swing • Walks a low balance beam • Rides tricycle *Fine (small) motor skills* • Builds block towers of about 9 or 10 blocks • Holds pencils and crayons with control	• Is curious about how things work • Begins to understand reasoning of caregivers • Interested in size and shape • Identifies colors • Counts from one to ten • Counts two or more objects • Asks why questions • Responds to how questions • Learns name, address, phone number, sex, age and parents names • Holds up fingers to indicate age • Uses bathroom words and laughs	• Becomes less self-centered • Is sunny and agreeable most of time • Displays feelings in more acceptable manner • Learns to take turns and share • Shows new fears (animals, storms, dark and monsters) • Makes friends easily and may prefer one over another • Engages in cooperative play • Tries to please caregivers; desires praise and approval • Usually follows requests and can be reasoned with • Has strong likes and dislikes • Is pleased with self • Expresses anger physically (hitting, biting and pushing) • Seeks comfort from parents and caregivers	• Says full name • Knows an average of 900 words • Shows rapid language development • Uses sentences that are three to four words long • Mispronounces 40% of speech sounds • Enjoys listening to stories • Understands more words than able to use • Asks simple who and what questions • Tells simple events in sequence • Demonstrates beginning phonological awareness (hearing and recognizing the sounds of language) • Uses words to express ideas and feelings

Contd...

Contd...

Physical	*Cognitive*	*Emotional and social*	*Language*
3 to 4 years			
• Draws straight lines and copies circles • Draws three-part person • Cuts with scissors • Unbuttons clothes • Pulls up large zippers Uses spoon and fork	• Enjoys doing things for self • Develops better understanding of cause and effect Distinguishes between fact and fiction	• Engages in imaginative play • Has imaginary friend Enjoys assisting in simple housekeeping and mealtime tasks	• Usually follows requests and can be reasoned with Draws circles and lines in artwork
4 to 5 years			
Gross (large) motor skills • Whirls around, turns, somersaults and hangs on bars • Hops several times in a row • Climbs large play equipment • Jumps forward using a forward arm action • Jumps up and down • Throws ball overhead with less body movement • Bounces ball and catches ball with elbows in front of body *Fine (small) motor skills* • Builds straight block towers • Draws a house and person • Prints name • Forms crude shapes with clay • Cuts on lines with scissors • Brushes teeth, combs hair and washes hands • Dresses self except for tying shoes Develops hand preference	• Improves ability to reason • Knows birthday • Identifies coins such as penny, nickel and dime • Understands seasons • Begins to understand need for rules • Understands concept of texture, size, distance and temperature • Forms logical conclusions • Enjoys games that test abilities • Improves ability to remember past events Has difficulty understanding time	• Struggles for independence • Is moody • Doesn't want to be told what to do • Accuses adults of being bossy and unfair • Feels strong attachment to family and home • Desires approval from parents and caregivers • Brags on parents and home • Enjoys cooperative play and simple competitive games • Is often bossy and inconsiderate • Increases interest in friends • Shares personal belongings • Has difficulty in taking turns • Resents being treated like a baby • Accepts changes in routine • Shows concern and sympathy for others	• Has vocabulary of 1500 words • Uses sentences of five to six words • Mispronounces 20 percent of speech sounds • Listens attentively to stories • Tells stories • Uses puppets, flannel board and pictures • Names months and days of week • Notices signs and prints in the environment • Asks who, what, where and why questions Responds to open-ended questions
5 to 6 years			
Gross (large) motor skills • Runs, swerves and turns corners faster and smoother • Walks a straight line • Climbs and tumbles • Races with others • Skips and jumps rope • Beats rhythm instruments to beat of music • Rides bicycle with training wheels • Draws arm back and uses body weight to project ball • Catches ball; elbows at sides	• Learns right from wrong • Accepts rules; but doesn't always understand reason • Enjoys routines • Exhibits increased attention span and concentration • Follows instructions concerning numbers • Understands terms like more than and less than • Uses many words without understanding definitions	• Is more cooperative and conscientious • Desires support and approval • Asks permission and follows instructions • Likes to work and play with others • Prefers friends own age; usually own sex • Has strong desire to please • Is proud of and likes to assist parents • May voluntarily help with younger siblings	• Vocabulary increases to over 2200 words • Mispronounces ten percent of speech sounds • Pretends and fantasizes (tells tall tales, has imaginary Playmates, associates with story characters) • Uses many words without understanding definitions • Names or describes people, places, things, locations, sizes, colors, shapes, numbers and actions • Gives simple one-step directions

Contd...

Contd...

Physical	*Cognitive*	*Emotional and social*	*Language*
5 to 6 years			
Fine (small) motor skills • Builds towers, bridges and houses with blocks • Makes simple drawings • Draws recognizable person • Makes alphabet letters • Buttons, snaps and zips clothes • Ties shoelaces • Pours from small pitcher Uses fork, spoon and knife	• Understands simple classifications such as groups of trees and animals • Places blocks and nesting toys in order(small to large) Asks a lot of questions, especially, "Why?"	• Forms sex-role identity (what it means to be male or female) • Respects other's property • Expresses anger more verbally than physically • Boys quarrel more and use more physical force than girls Engages in elaborate and imaginative roleplay situations	• Uses pictures to orally retell a story with a beginning, middle, and end, with or without prompts • Demonstrates active listening behaviors such as facing the speaker, making eye contact, and maintaining attention Writes simple sentences around known words, repetitive phrases, and sentence beginnings

TABLE 2: National Immunization Schedule (NIS) for infants, children.

Vaccine	*When to give*	*Dose*	*Route*	*Site*
For infants				
BCG	At birth or as early as possible till 1 year of age	0.1 mL (0.05 mL until 1 month age)	Intradermal	Left upper arm
Hepatitis B—birth dose	At birth or as early as possible within 24 hours	0.5 mL	Intramuscular	Anterolateral Side of mid-thigh
OPV-0	At birth or as early as possible within the first 15 days	2 drops	Oral	Oral
OPV 1, 2, and 3	At 6 weeks, 10 weeks, and 14 weeks (OPV can be given till 5 years of age)	2 drops	Oral	Oral
Pentavalent 1, 2, and 3	At 6 weeks, 10 weeks, and 14 weeks (can be given till 1 year of age)	0.5 mL	Intramuscular	Anterolateral Side of mid-thigh
Rotavirus	At 6 weeks, 10 weeks, and 14 weeks (can be given till 1 year of age)	5 drops	Oral	Oral
IPV	Two fractional dose at 6 and 14 weeks of age	0.1 mL	Intradermal two fractional dose	Intradermal: Right upper arm
Measles/MR 1st dose$	9 completed months to 12 months (can be given till 5 years of age)	0.5 mL	Subcutaneous	Right upper arm
JE 1	9 completed months to 12 months	0.5 mL	Subcutaneous	Left upper arm
Vitamin A (1st dose)	At 9 completed months with measles-rubella	1 mL (1 lakh IU)	Oral	Oral
For children				
DPT booster-1	16–24 months	0.5 mL	Intramuscular	Anterolateral Side of mid-thigh
Measles/MR 2nd dose$	16–24 months	0.5 mL	Subcutaneous	Right upper arm
OPV booster	16–24 months	2 drops	Oral	Oral
JE-2	16–24 months	0.5 mL	Subcutaneous	Left upper arm
Vitamin A (2nd to 9th dose)	16–18 months. Then one dose every 6 months up to the age of 5 years	2 mL (2 lakh IU)	Oral	Oral
DPT booster-2	5–6 years	0.5 mL	Intramuscular	Upper arm
TT	10 years and 16 years	0.5 mL	Intramuscular	Upper arm

(BCG: Bacillus Calmette–Guérin; DPT: diphtheria, pertussis, tetanus; JE: Japanese encephalitis; IPV: inactivated polio vaccine; OPV: oral polio vaccine; TT: tetanus toxoid)

TABLE 3: Calorie and protein values of various food ingredients and food preparations.

Item	Amount/quantity	Calorie	Protein
Indian dals			
Arhar dal	100	53	2.8
Chana dal	100	99	4.5
Dal makhani	100	117	6.8
Maa ki dal	100	92	20.2
Moong dal	100	211	12.8
Masoor dal	100	165	10.8
Urad dal	100	107	6.0
Sambhar	100	5	15
Dal Dhokli	100	238	7.0
Indian rice			
Boiled rice	100	111	2.2
Pulao	100	119	3.2
Khichri	100	215	4.3
Indian milk items			
Milk (Buffalo)	100	117	4.3
Milk (cow)	100	67	3.2
Curd	100	60	3.1
Butter milk	100	15	0.8
Skimmed milk	100	29	2.5
Paneer	100	265	18.3
Khoa	100	421	20
Cheese	100	69	24.1
Lassi	100	69	5.7
North Indian foods			
Paratha	1(6")	180	5.1
Puri	1(6")	150	4.5
Roti	1(6")	85	7.85
Missi roti	1(6")	90	7.3
Dal with tadka	100	101	12
Rajma/chana	100	101	8.7
Dahi	100	60	11
Lassi			6.4
Mixed vegetable	100	184	3.3
Chicken tikka	100	182	21
Chicken curry	100	216	6
Meat curry	100	364	18
Halwa	100	220	12
Gulab jamun	1 pc	140	2.3

Contd…

Contd…

Item	Amount/quantity	Calorie	Protein
Common Indian food			
Eggs	100	143	13.0
Apple	100	45	0.6
Oranges	100	35	0.94
Grapes	100	65	0.6
Banana	100	80	1.09
Peanuts	100	570	25.8
Breads	100	230	3.1
Rice whole boiled	100	120	2.69
Cornflakes with milk	100	250	7.0
Horlicks, milk, and sugar	100	120	9.3
Chocolate biscuits	100	520	6.3
Wheat bran	100	200	16.0
Beans	100	20	9.0
Cabbage	100	10	1.3
Carrot	100	20	0.8
Potatoes	100	80	2.2
Cauliflower	100	10	1.92
Peas	100	50	4.9
Cucumber	100	20	0.65
Other Indian food			
Aloo Baingan mixed vegetable	100	103	1.3
Aloo beans mixed vegetable	100	134	2.3
Aloo curry	100	105	1.4
Baigan	100	70	5.7
Bhindi	100	161	12.1
Chole	100	74	3.3
Gatte ki Sabji	148	275	11.6
Mattar paneer	100	147	10.7
Kaddu	100	67	6.7
Shahi paneer	95	263	10.7
Shimla mirch aloo	100	93	12.8
Stuffed tomato	100	65	11.0
Turai (ridge gourd)	100	147	4.0
Vegetable kofta curry	100	85	13.3
South Indian food			
Idli	100	100	6.0
Dosa plain	100	120	3.9
Masala dosa	100	250	3.9
Sambhar	100	150	11.63

Family history: Enquire about the family members including maternal and paternal origin. Enquire of any diseases running in families. Enquire about communicable and sexually transmitted diseases, example, measles, mumps, chickenpox, malaria, dengue, enteric fever, human immunodeficiency virus, syphilis, gonorrhea, and leprosy. Do not forget to ask of tuberculosis and whether treatment started or completed.

Age of parents and consanguinity should be enquired. Diseases with autosomal recessive pattern of inheritance are common in the children born to the parents with consanguineous marriage. The degree of consanguinity and its effects in expression of autosomal recessive condition are detailed in **Figure 1 and Table 4**. Drawing of family tree or pedigree chart **(Fig. 2)** helps in better understanding. This is a pictorial depiction of the members of the family using standard symbols.

Socioeconomic history: Find out the number of family members and their income per day/month. Calculate the per capita income, i.e., total income of family divided by total number of family members. Enquire about their education level. You have to enquire how many rooms are there in their house. Whether there is separate bathroom and kitchen and whether their house gets waterlogged in rainy season or floods. Though people nowadays cook in gas ovens still enquire the mode of cooking.

The socioeconomic history helps us to understand the reason for diseases as for if the per capita income is less, chances of undernutrition and malnutrition increase. Too many people in small rooms help in spread of many diseases specially droplet infection.

Ask about the water source to rule out water-borne diseases. If you can remember then you can use the Kuppuswamy scale **(Table 5)**.

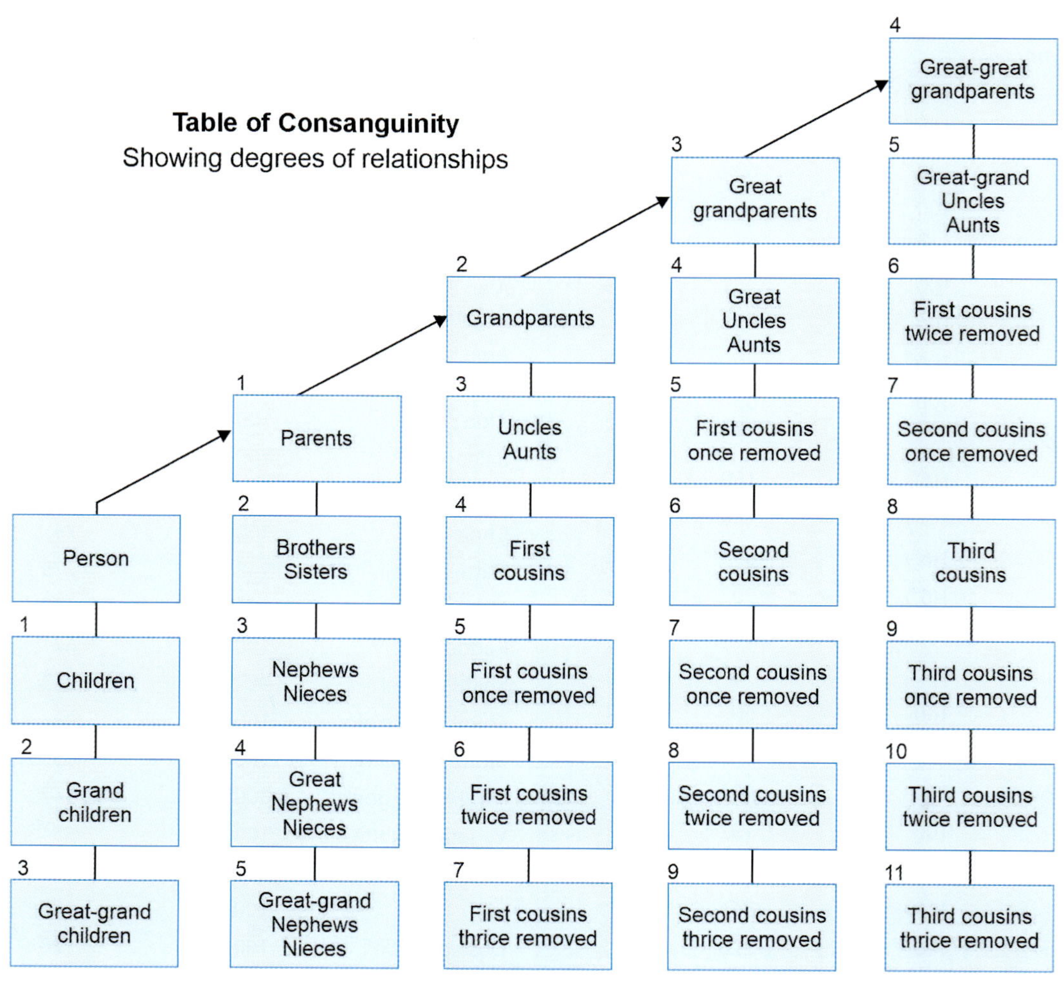

Fig. 1: Table of consanguinity.

TABLE 4: Degree of relationship.

Biological relationship	*Genetic relationships*	*Coefficient of relationship (r)*	*Coefficient of inbreeding (F)*
• Incest • Parent–child • Sibling	First degree	0.5	0.25
• Half-sibling • Uncle–niece • Double first cousin	Second degree	0.25	0.125
First cousin	Third degree	0.125	0.0625
• First cousin once removed • Double second cousin	Fourth degree	0.0625	0.0313
Second cousin	Fifth degree	0.0313	0.0156
• Second cousin once removed • Double third cousin	Sixth degree	0.0156	0.0078
Third cousin	Seventh degree	0.0078	0.0039

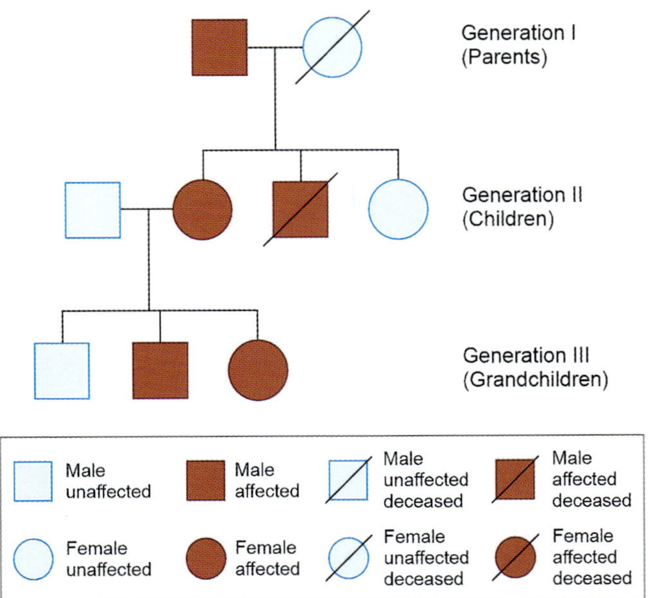

Fig. 2: Family tree depicting disease affection.

TABLE 5: Kuppuswamy scale.

Education of head of family	*Score*
Profession or honors	7
Graduate or postgraduate	6
Intermediate or posthigh school diploma	5
High school certificate	4
Middle school certificate	3

Contd...

Contd...

Education of head of family	*Score*
Primary school certificate	2
Literate	1
Occupation of head of family	
Profession	10
Semi-profession	6
Clerical, shop-owner	5
Skilled worker	4
Semiskilled worker	3
Unskilled worker	2
Unemployed	1
Monthly income of family (2017)	
>14,130	12
20,715–14,129	10
15,536–20,714	6
10,357–15,535	4
6,214–10,356	3
2,092–6,213	2
<2,091	1
Socioeconomic status classification	*Total score*
I—Upper	26–29
II—Upper middle	16–25
III—Lower middle	11–15
IV—Upper lower	5–10
V—Lower	<5

Personal history: It is very relevant for a schoolgoing child. This tells us about the child's mental condition, i.e., his/her areas of interest, television, and mobile usage. Also, enquire about food habits to understand the cause of obesity or vitamin deficiencies.

SUGGESTED READING

1. Douglas G, Nicol F, Robertson C, editors. Macleod's clinical examination. 15th ed. London: Elsevier; 2023.
2. Gupta P. Clinical methods in pediatrics. 6th ed. New Delhi: CBS Publishers & Distributors; 2025
3. Lakshmanaswamy, A. 2026, Clinical pediatrics: history taking and case discussion, 6th edn, Wolters Kluwer India Pvt Ltd, New Delhi.
4. Munro JF, Campbell IW, McCuish AC. Hutchison's Clinical Methods. 24th ed. Edinburgh: Elsevier; 2018.
5. Singh M. Pediatric clinical methods. 7th ed. New Delhi: CBS Publishers & Distributors; 2023.

CHAPTER 2

Examination of Children

Sudip Saha

GENERAL SURVEY

After taking history it is the general survey which gives further clue to reach the diagnosis. It is supportive to the history taking stating the condition of patient.

What are the essential tools to carry to examination hall:

- Stethoscope
- Torch
- Percussion hammer
- Fiber glass tape
- Sphygmomanometer—sometime. It is provided.
- Developmental assessment tools.

Things provided in examination hall:

- Weight machine
- Height chart/infantometer

Proper position, exposure, and good elimination are the keys to good physical examination.

Please try and provide chocolates and soft toys.

Position for Patient

Younger the age the more difficult to examine, except when they are sleeping. If you are examining a sleepy child, be gentle to not awake and do most of the examination after running through a short history.

- *0-3 months:* Examination bed
- *3 months-1 year:* Mother's lap
- *1-3 years:* Sitting on bed
- *Adolescent girl:* Mother or female attendant

Always follow the sequence of examination

- Higher function
- Decubitus
- Built and nutrition
- Anthropometry
- Vitals
- Faces
- Anemia
- Lymphadenopathy
- Jaundice
- Cyanosis
- Edema
- Clubbing
- Neck veins and neck glands
- Skin and appendages

Decubitus: Posture of patient in bed, the different types of posture are:

- Of choice
- Propped up not very commonly seen in pediatric patients
  15-30°,
  - *45°:* Mild dyspnea
  - *60°:* Moderate dyspnea
  - *90°:* Severe dyspnea

Cause of propped up decubitus

15-30° raised intracranial tension management,
45-90° cardiac problem such as heart failure, respiratory problem, asthma, pleural effusion, and huge ascites

- In pleural effusion—sometimes patient/child feels better on side of pleural effusion.
- Curled up decubitus—acute renal colic, acute biliary colic, and pancreatitis.
- Opisthotonus—tetanus (rare), meningitis (spinal or tubercular), maple syrup urine disease, and hysterical
- Listless attitude—unconscious patient, hysterical

Build: Skeletal structure in relation to age and sex of the individual as compared to normal person. Build is short in those below the 3rd percentile of a normal population of age and sex and tall when the height is above, the 97th percentile. This will be discussed in endocrinology section.

Nutrition—in pediatrics for build and nutrition anthropometry is done.

1. *Weight*
   - *Method:* Up to 10 kg or those who are unable to stand as in sick child—use a beam type weighing scale or an electronic weighing scale. Above 10 kg

or if the child can stand alone, a bathroom type scale or an electronic weighing scale.

- *Method:* First switch on the machine if it is an electronic one and then place a thin piece of paper or cloth to avoid the metal or plastic transporting cold to the baby, then adjust/tare the machine to 0. Then place the baby after exposing the baby or infant on the machine **(Figs. 1 and 2)**.
- *Method:* For standing weight, make the child stand without shoes and dress and only under garments.

2. *Height:* Up to 2 years of age, recumbent length is measured with the help of infantometer while for older child, standing height is measured with stadiometer
    - *Method:* The child is placed supine on infantometer with one person holding the head in midline and the upper plank should be touching the head. Another person or attendant/mother will hold the leg straight over the knee. The 90°, the movable petal plank of the meter is snuggled opposed against the soles and length is read from the scale **(Figs. 3 and 4)**.

In children who can stand, height, can be measured with stadiometer or a rod attached to the lever type machine.

But for examination purpose make the child stand bare feet against the wall with buttock and shoulder and occiput touching the wall, the head should be held erect

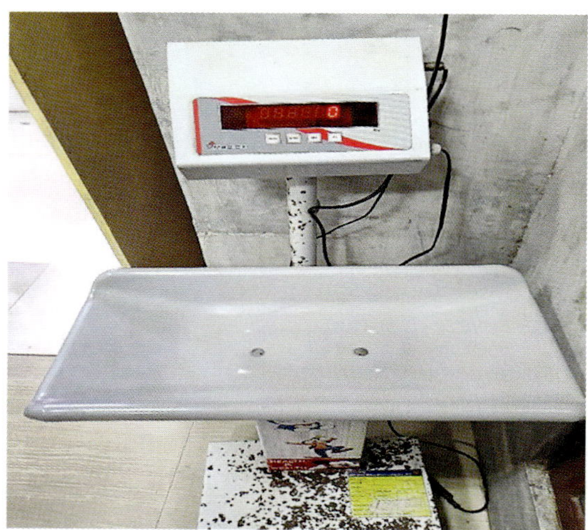

Fig. 1: Infant weighing machine.

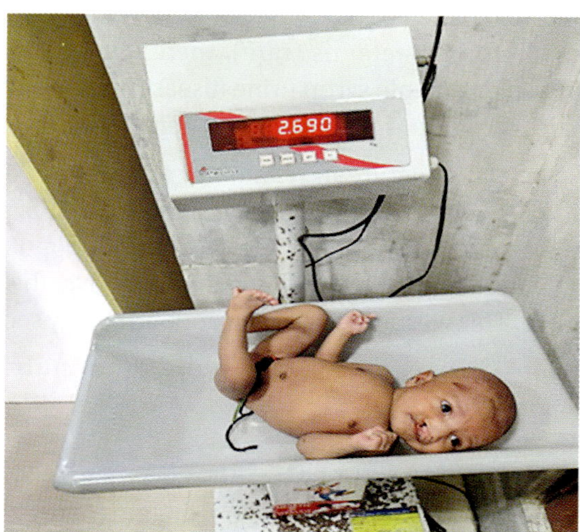

Fig. 2: Baby being weighed.

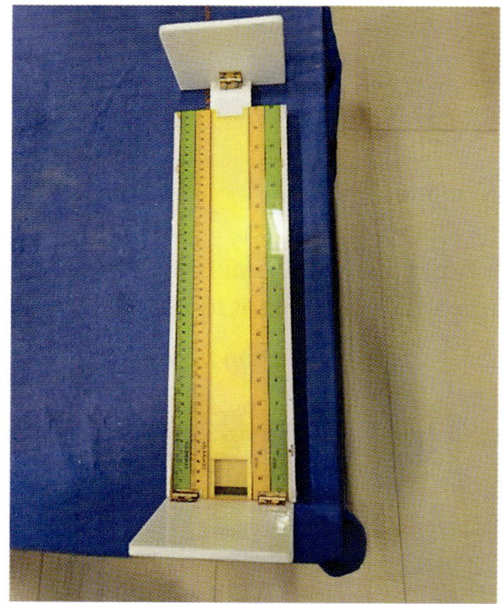

Fig. 3: Infantometer.

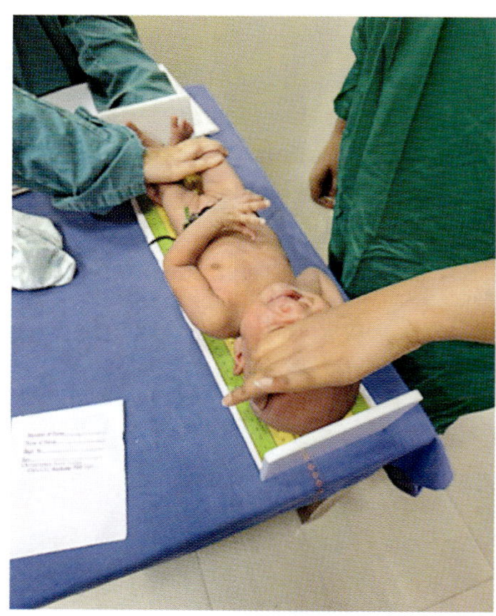

Fig. 4: Length measurement of baby.

with eyes aligned horizontally and ears vertically without any tilt. Use a plastic ruler, the highest point of vertex is identified on wall, using a tape measure the point to floor if the height is >150–155 cm, a single tape has to be used twice by making two points.

Approx height with age:

- *At birth or 40 weeks:* 50 cm
- *At 1 year:* 75 cm
- *At 2 years:* 87 cm
- *At 3 years:* 94 cm
- *At 4 years:* 100 cm
- *5 years:* 107 cm
- *Post 6 years:* Age × 6 + 77

3. *Head circumference:* Asked to demonstrate in examination.
    - *Method:* Use a fiberoptic tape or a plastic tape. The tape should encircle the occiput and supraorbital frontal area. Use the one which gives the maximum.

Head circumference with age:

- *At birth or 40 weeks:* 35 cm
- *Next 3 months:* 2 cm/month
- *Next 3 months:* 1 cm/month
- *6–12 months:* 0.5 cm/month
- *12–60 months:* 0.5 cm/6 months

Size of head: Any deviation in the size and proportion of the head should be noted.

Macrocephaly: Defined as head circumference more than two standard deviation above the mean or beyond 97th percentile for normal population of same age, sex, and religion.

Causes of macrocephaly **(Table 1)**

TABLE 1: Causes of macrocephaly.

Structures affected	*Disease/condition*
Skull/cranium	Osteopetrosis, achondroplasia. Hemolytic anemia
Subdural space	Subdural effusion/hematoma
Subarachnoid space	Hydrocephalus
Brain parenchyma	Alexanders. Canavan's, Sotos syndrome
Vessels	Vein of Galen malformation
Ventricles	Hydrocephalus
Miscellaneous	Intracranial tumor, infiltrations—mucopolysaccharidosis (Hurlers syndrome, Tay Sachs)

What is megalencephaly?:

It is a condition where the weight and size of the brain are more than average for the age and sex of the child.

Megalencephaly is seen in following conditions:

- Normal children
- Cerebral gigantism like Sotos syndrome
- Neuro cutaneous syndrome like tuberous sclerosis, Sturge Weber syndrome,
- Metabolic disorders such as leukodystrophy, lipidosis, histiocytosis, and mucopolysaccharidosis.

Microcephaly: Head circumference less than three standard deviations of mean for the age, sex, race, and religion.

Types of microcephaly:

Primary: Present since birth, inherited, chromosomal anomalies—autosomal recessive and autosomal dominant such as Down syndrome, Edwards, Cri-Du-Chat, Cornelia De Lange Syndrome, Rubenstein-Tavi syndrome

Secondary causes:

- Radiation
- Infection (TORCH)
- Drugs such as fetal alcohol and fetal hydantoin
- Metabolic such as hypoglycemia and phenylketonuria
- Hyperthermia
- Hypothyroidism and hypopituitarism
- Birth asphyxia and birth injuries

How many fontanelles?

- Anterior
- Posterior
- Two anterolateral—pair of sphenoids
- Two posterolateral—pair of mastoids

Shape of anterior fontanelle: It is rhomboid shape.

How to measure anterior fontanelle?

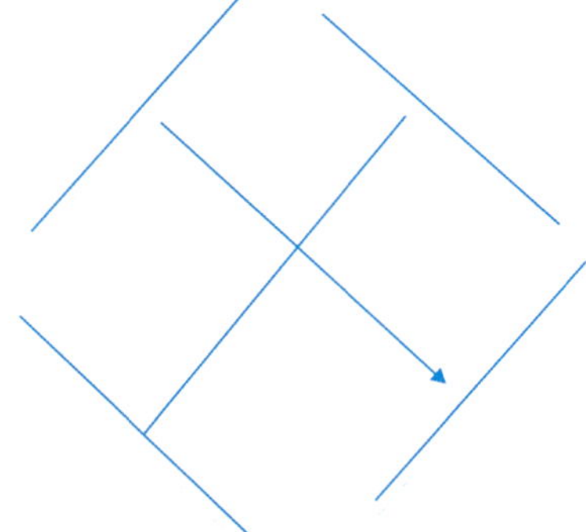

What is the usual time of closure of anterior fontanelle—7–19 months of age.

Causes of early closer of anterior fontanelle

- Craniosynostosis
- Primary microcephaly

Causes of delayed closer of anterior fontanelle

- Achondroplasia
- Apert syndrome
- Congenital hypothyroidism
- Congenital rubella syndrome
- Cutis laxa
- Down syndrome
- Rickets

How to examine anterior fontanelle?

Gently and lightly touch the spot on the top middle of your baby's head with flat pads of your fingers **(Flowchart 1)**.

4. *Mid upper arm circumference* (MUAC)—6 months to 5 years.

- *Method:*
    - Non-dominant hand that is left hand.
    - Hanging position to avoid getting increased bulk of muscle in flexed position.
        - Find out acromion process—the lateral end of the clavicle **(Fig. 5)**.
        - Find out olecranon process—flex the elbow-lower most hard point of forearm.
        - Find the midpoint of two parts points **(Fig. 6)**.
        - Use a Shakir's tape/fiber glass/steel tape or a tailor tape.

Shakir tape **(Fig. 7)** is a fiber glass tape with red (<11.5 cm), yellow (11.5-13.5 cm) and green (>13.5 cm). This is for assessment of nutritional status.

Assessment of malnutrition:

- *<11.5 cm:* Severe acute malnutrition
- *11.5-12.5 cm:* Moderate malnutrition
- *>13.5 cm:* Normal

5. *Arm span*
    - *Method:* Make the child stand straight against a wall with both hands and fingers outstretched. Mark two points at outstretched middle fingers of both hands.

Importance

- *<5 years:* 1-2 cm, smaller than body length
- *10-12 years:* Equal to height
- *Adults:* Plus 2 cm more than height.

Flowchart 1: Assessment of the anterior fontanelle.

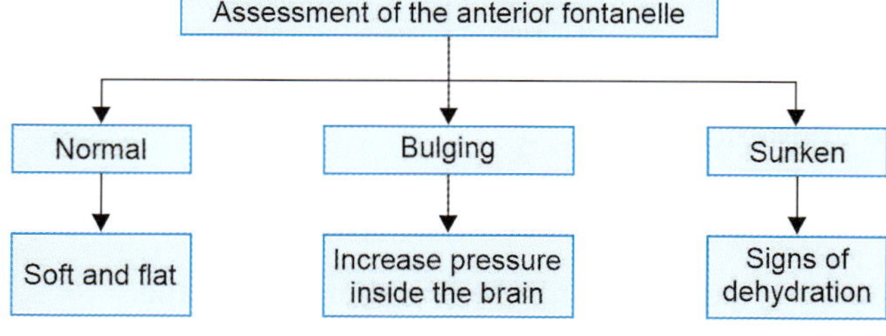

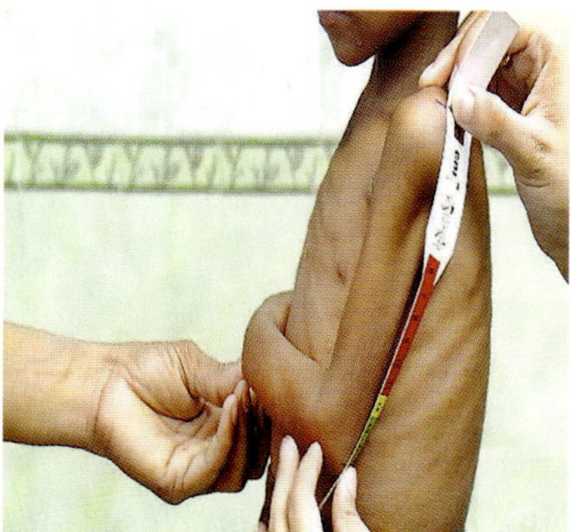

Fig. 5: MUAC measurement.

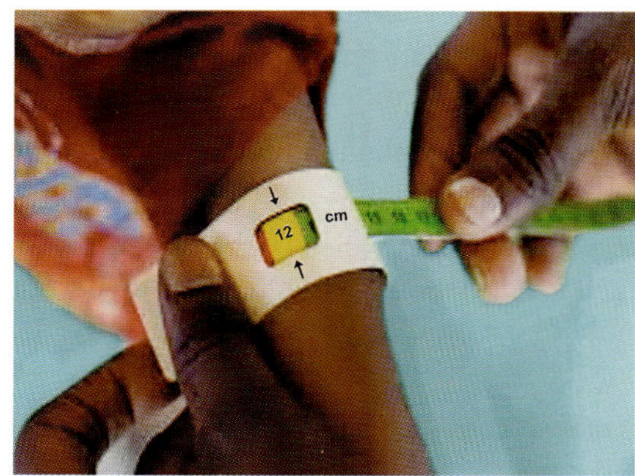

Fig. 6: Zone finding.

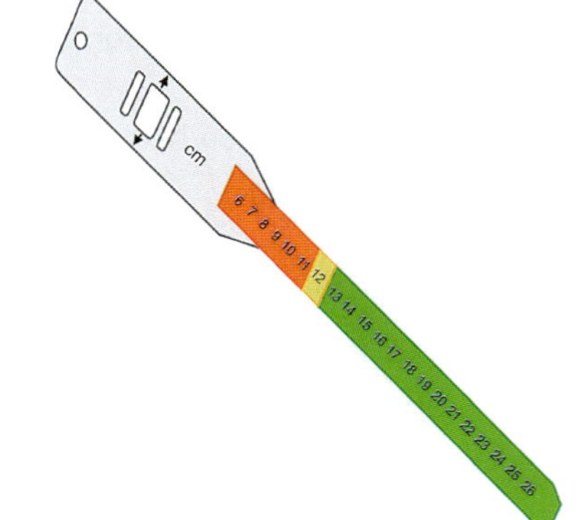

Fig. 7: Shakir's tape.

6. *Body mass index* (BMI) =

$$\frac{\text{Weight in kilograms}}{\text{Height in m}^2}$$

Importance

- *BMI, >85th percentile:* Overweight
- *BMI, >95th percentile:* Obesity

VITALS

1. *Pulse*
    - *Definition:* Rhythmic expansion of the arterial wall imparted by the column of arterial blood due to contraction of the left ventricle.
    - *Method:* To check the rate rhythm and delay.

Radial pulse in both upper limbs and arteria dorsalis pedis in both lower limbs.

To see volume and character check carotid pulse **(Table 2)**.

Pulse is examined under following heads:

- Rate
- Rhythm
- Character
- Volume
- Radio femoral and radio radial delay
- Condition of the vessel wall

2. *Respiration*
    - *Method:* Place the infant on mother's lap or bed, expose the baby till mid chest and count the rate for 60 seconds. Also, look for accessory muscle involvement at suprasternal area, intercostal area, and subcoastal area **(Tables 3 and 4)**.

3. *Blood pressure*

It should ideally be recorded in all four limbs.

- *Method*: Cuff size—appropriate size covers 2/3rd of the length of the arm on which it is tied with the inflatable bladder covering the entire circumference of the arm with no overlapping.

TABLE 2: Normal pulse rate at various ages.

Age	*Pulse/minute*
<6 months	120–160
6–12 months	110–120
1–5 years	95–110
6–12 years	80–110
>12 years	60–100

- *Technique*:
    - Auscultatory method (by using a sphygmomanometer)

      Upper limb
      - The cuff is tied about 2.5 cm above the cubital fossa.
      - It is inflated rapidly to about 20–30 mm Hg above the level at which the radial pulse cannot be felt.
      - The cuff is then deflated gradually.
      - The Korotkoff sounds are auscultated over the brachial artery in the cubital fossa.

      Lower limb
      - The cuff is tied on the thigh and the stethoscope is placed over the popliteal artery.
      - The point at which the first Korotkoff sounds are heard is the systolic pressure.
      - On deflation the Korotkoff sounds get muffled and then disappear.
      - The point at which the sounds start muffling and not disappearing is the diastolic pressure.

TABLE 3: Normal respiratory rate at various ages.

Age	*Normal rate*	*Tachypnea*
Up to 2 months	30–50	>60
2–12 months	20–40	>50
12 months – 5 years	20–30	>40
5–10 years	15–20	>30
>10 year	15–18	>30

TABLE 4: Etiology of abnormal respiratory problems.

Tachypnea (increased rate)	*Bradypnea (decreased rate)*	*Hyperpnea (increased depth of breathing)*
Anxiety/exertion	Alkalosis	Acidosis
Fever	Hypothyroidism	Hysterical
Hypoxia	Raised intracranial pressure	Brainstem lesion
Acidosis		
Pneumonia		
Pulmonary edema		
Hysterical/ hyperventilation		

If you are unable to record the blood pressure with sphygmomanometer, you can use the palpatory method.

- *Palpatory method.*
  - The radial pulse is felt while deflating the cuff.
  - The point at which the radial pulse appears is the systolic pressure.

Normal blood pressure in children

The blood pressure is lower in newborn and infants and increases as the age grows. Also, the lower limb has more pressure than upper limb. It is always better to do in left upper limb in supine and sitting posture.

Formula to calculate the expected blood pressure in children (50th percentile of blood pressure)

- *Systolic blood pressure: 90 + (2 × age in year)*
- *Diastolic blood pressure: 55 + (2 × age in year)*

It is always better to use charts and marking the 50-percentile blood pressure **(Fig. 8)**.

4. *Temperature*
   - *Method:* Use a digital thermometer. The thermometer is started by pressing the switch and waiting for it to indicate low on 94°F and then placed in axilla after cleaning the area. Place it till the alarm beeps. Note the temperature on the digital screen.
   - *Other sites:*
     - Groin
     - Ear canal
     - Skin over the forehead
5. *Facies **(Table 5)***

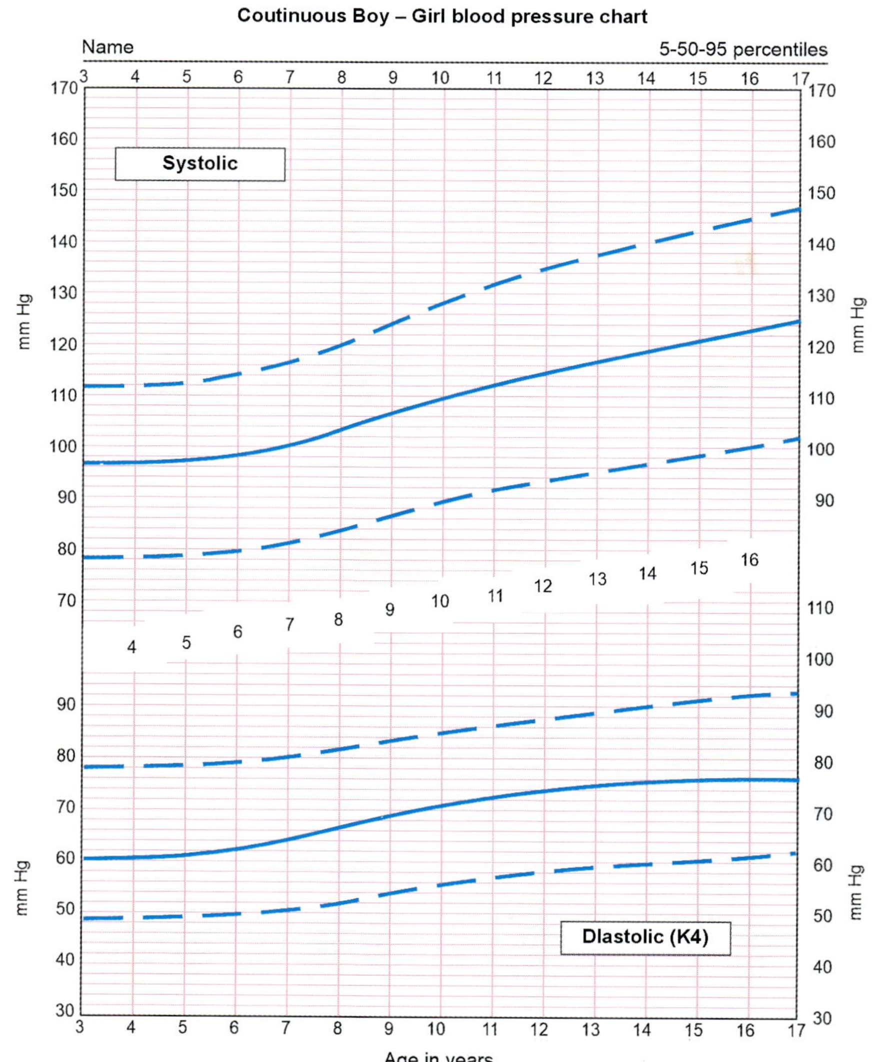

Fig. 8: Blood pressure chart.

TABLE 5: Types of facies and their disease.

1.	Round face and head with flat occiput, mongoloid slant of the eyes with epicanthic folds and thick large and protruding tongue	Mongoloid facies	Down syndrome **(Fig. 9)**
2.	Expression less space		BL facial palsy **(Fig. 10)** Parkinsonism
3.	Moon face with fish mouth, prominent flushed cheeks, double chin, and buffalo hump	Cushingoid facies **(Fig. 11)**	Cushing syndrome, obesity
4.	Puffy face with frontal and parietal bossing with teeth malocclusion	Hemolytic facies	Hemolytic anemia
5.	Appearance of a sardonic grin due to down and out pull on the corners of the mouth with the upper lips stretched across eyes, are slit like and puckered up	Risus sardonicus	Tetanus
6.	Coarse face, thick lips, low set ears, depressed nasal bridge, and enlarged tongue with peg-like teeth that are widely separate	Gargoylism	Mucopolysaccharidosis
7.	Heavy face with a dull look, thick eyebrows, and a thick protruding tongue	Cretinoid facies **(Fig. 12)**	Hypothyroidism

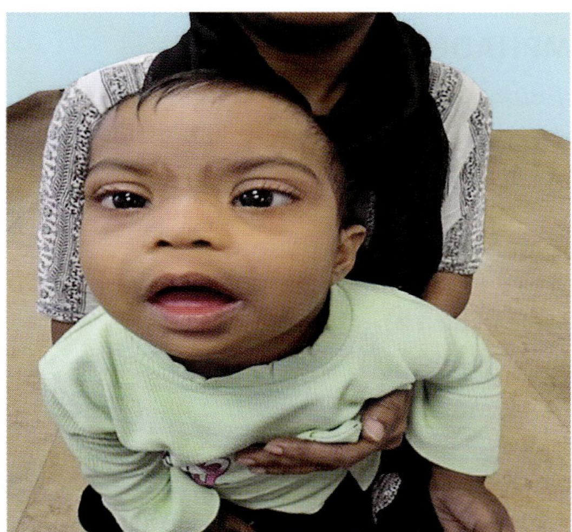

Fig. 9: Downs syndrome.

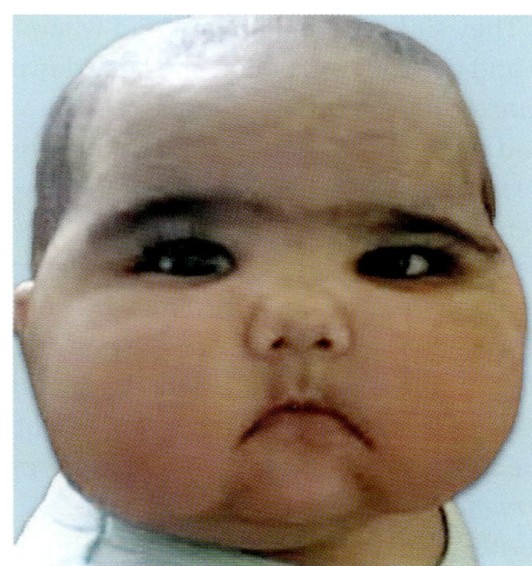

Fig. 11: Cushingoid syndrome.

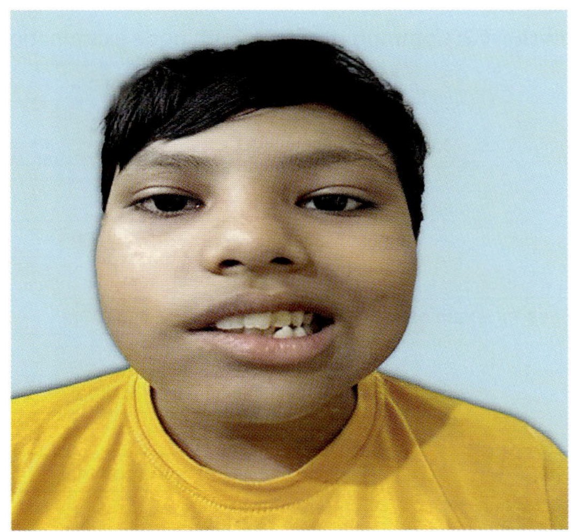

Fig. 10: Bell's palsy.

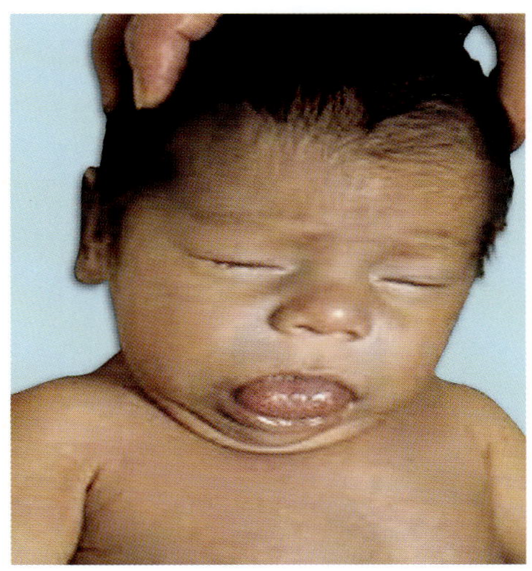

Fig. 12: Cretinoid facies.

NECK VEINS

Internal jugular veins reflect most reliable the hemodynamic of the right atrium.

- *Method* ***(Fig. 13)****:*
  - *Position the patient:* The patient should lie down with their head and torso elevated at a 30–45° angle, but they may need to be adjusted to 90° or lying flat to get the best view of the pulsations. Remove pillows to allow the neck to be straight.
  - *Locate the veins:* Find the internal jugular vein, which is typically just above the sternoclavicular joint. The pulsations are often visible just above the medial head of the clavicle.
  - *Identify venous pulsations:* Look for a "bifid" or "flicking" pulsation that is not palpable, unlike an arterial pulse. Key signs of venous pulsations are:
    - They sink with inspiration and when in sitting and rise with exhalation and lying down.
- *Measure the jugular venous pressure (JVP):*
  - Find the highest point of the venous pulsation in the neck.
  - Mentally draw a horizontal line from this point to the sternal angle (also known as the angle of Louis).
  - Measure the vertical distance in centimeters between the sternal angle and the horizontal line.
  - Add 5 cm to this measurement to account for the distance from the sternal angle to the right atrium.
  - The sum is the estimated central venous pressure.
- *Perform the abdominojugular reflux test:*
  - Gently press on the patient's abdomen for 10–15 seconds while observing their neck veins.
  - A positive result occurs if the JVP rises by >3 cm for at least 15 seconds after the pressure is released, indicating increased right atrial pressure.
- *Interpreting the findings*
  - *Normal JVP:* A normal JVP is generally <8 cm of water.
  - *Increased JVP:* A high JVP can indicate conditions such as right-sided heart failure, left-sided heart failure, or other fluid overload states.
  - *Abdominojugular reflux:* A positive test suggests the heart is unable to handle the added fluid volume and is a sign of heart failure.
  - *Note:* The internal jugular vein pulsations are not always visible, especially in obese individuals or those with a beard, making ultrasound a valuable alternative in some cases.

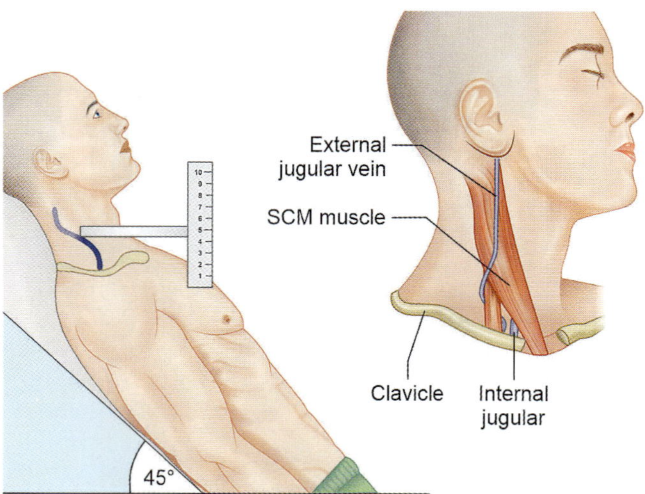

Fig. 13: Jugular venous pressure measurement.

LYMPHADENOPATHY

- *Definition:* Enlargement of nodes in significant size due to inflammatory or non-inflammatory causes.
- *Types of lymphadenopathies:*
  - Generalized—involvement of more than two non-contagious lymph node areas.
  - Localized involvement of one lymph node areas **(Flowchart 2)**.

What is the significance of lymphadenopathy?

- *It is considered significant. If any of the factors are present*:
  - Size inguinal lymph node >1.5 cm diameter, cervical **(Figs. 14 and 15)** and axillary lymph node >1 cm diameter **(Fig. 16)**, epitrochlear and supra clavicular any size—multiple sites

Flowchart 2: Common sites for lymph node examination.

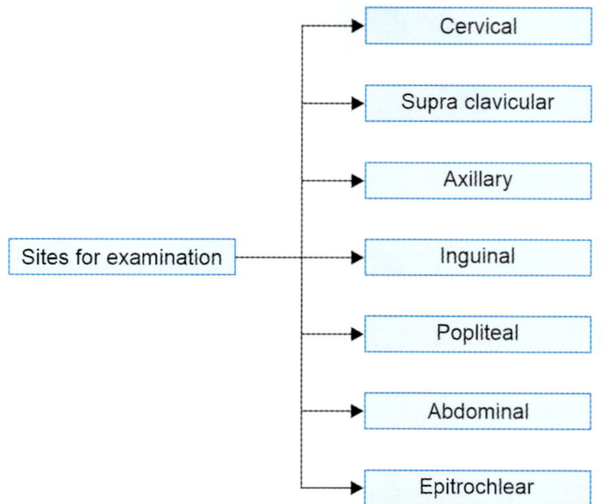

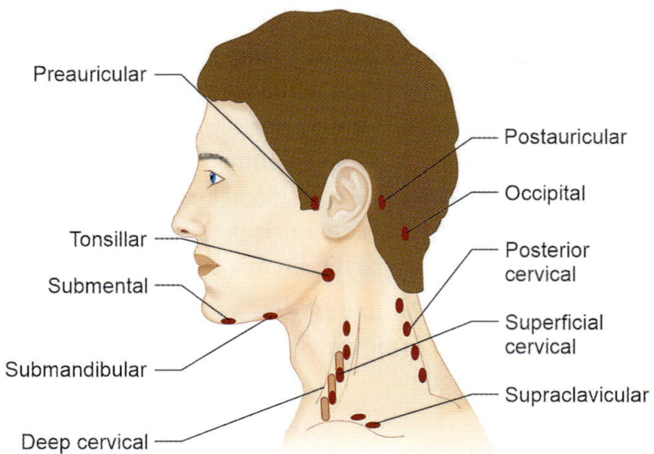

Fig. 14: Sites of cervical lymph nodes.
Courtesy: Clinical Skills Resource Centre, University of Liverpool, UK.

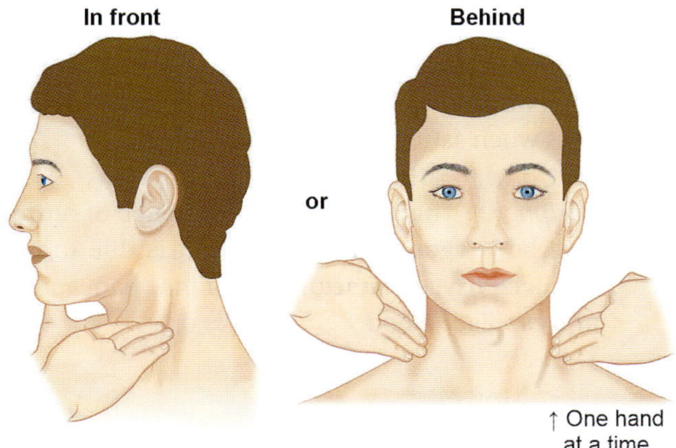

Fig. 15: Method of cervical lymph node examination.
Courtesy: Clinical Skills Resource Centre, University of Liverpool, UK.

- Matted notes
- Tender and ulcerated
- Associated with systemic signs and symptoms.

- *Method of examination*
  - *Patient positioning:* The patient should be in a comfortable position, and their muscles should be relaxed, often by slightly tilting their head down for a neck examination.
  - *Palpation technique:* Use the soft pads of two or three fingers, not the fingertips, to apply gentle pressure. Move your fingers in a circular motion to feel the lymph nodes under the skin.
- *What is being assessed?*
  - *Size:* Are the nodes enlarged?
  - *Consistency:* Are the nodes soft (often from infection) or hard (sometimes associated with malignancy)?

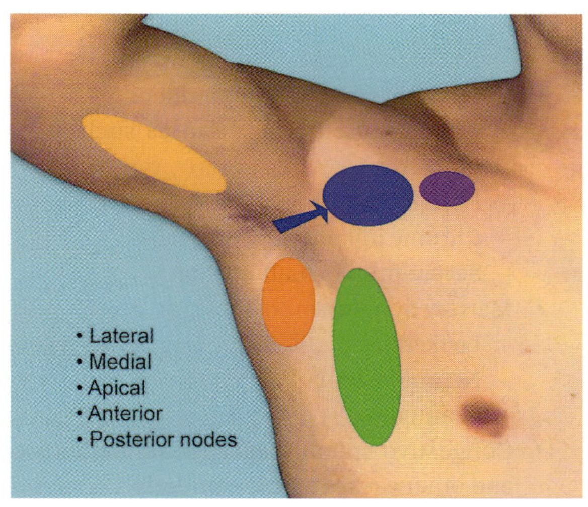

Fig. 16: Sites of axillary lymph nodes.

Flowchart 3: Causes of anemia.

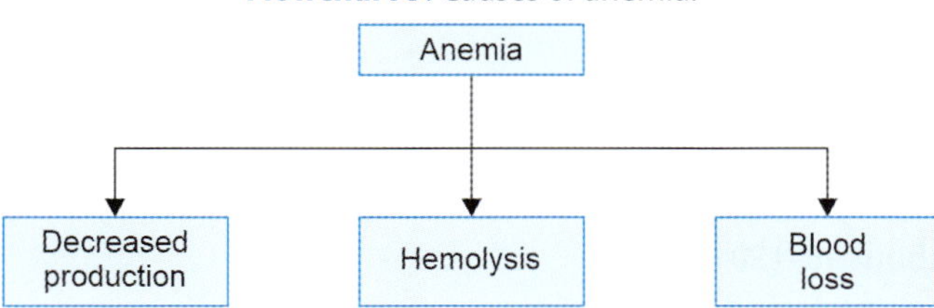

  - *Tenderness:* Are they painful or tender to the touch?
  - *Mobility:* Do they move freely, or are they fixed to the surrounding tissue?
  - *Matted:* Do they feel connected and move as a unit?

ANEMIA

- *Definition:* It refers to reduction in the RBC volume. It is said to be present peripheral blood is below the normal range of values for that age and sex.
- *Etiology:* Anemia occurs due to decreased production of erythrocytes, hemolysis or blood loss **(Flowchart 3)**.

Decrease production of erythrocytes

- *Physiologic anemia of infancy*
- *Hyperplastic and aplastic anemia*
  - Congenital hypoplastic anemia
  - Transient erythroblastopenia of childhood
  - Fanconi anemia.
  - Osteopetrosis, Marble bone disease
  - Aplastic crisis in hemolytic anemia
  - Aplastic anemia.
    - Deficiency specific factors
      - Iron deficiency dentification
      - Copper deficiency

- Megaloblastic anemia,
- B12 or folic acid

- Impaired erythropoietin production
  - Anemia in chronic diseases such as renal problems
  - Hypothyroidism
  - Chronic inflammatory diseases
  - Severe protein malnutrition
- Marrow dysplasia
  - Leukemia
  - Neuroblastoma
  - Granuloma
- Congestive splenomegaly, Gaucher's disease and other causes of splenomegaly.
- Lead poisoning
- Acute infection and inflammation
- Sideroblastic anemia

Hemolysis:

Hemolytic anemia occurs due to increase destruction or shorten lifespan of

Erythrocytes. The normal lifespan of erythrocytes is about 90–120 days.

- *Intrinsic defects*
  - *Erythrocyte membrane defects*
    - Hereditary spherocytosis
    - Hereditary elliptocytosis
    - Infantile poikilocytosis
    - Hereditary stomatocytosis
    - Paroxysmal nocturnal hemoglobinuria
    - Erythropoietic porphyria
    - Abetalipoproteinemia
  - *Haemoglobinopathies*
    - Sickle cell disorders
    - Thalassemia syndromes
    - Unstable Hbs
    - Hereditary persistence of fetal hemoglobin.
  - *Enzyme defects can be hereditary or acquired. Acquired defects can be* drug induced or due to ingestion of Fava beans. Hereditary defects include
- *Defects of the Embden-Meyerhof or anaerobic pathway:*
  - Pyruvate kinase deficiency, glucose phosphatase isomerase, hexokinase, and phosphofructokinase
  - Defects of oxidative hexose monophosphate pathways, example, G6PD deficiency and deducts non enzyme deficiencies, example, abnormalities of cycle metabolism, extra corporate mechanisms, immune Harit anemia; auto immune, I assume immune Harit. This is a new bond due to Rcom ability or AB and captivity; drug-induced secondary immune media disease such as sarcoidosis ID, non-immune anemia, drugs antibiotics, poisons like snake venom, mechanical injury, disease, believer, disease by Wilson disease, blood loss, it may be acute chronic. Classification, microcytic, anemia, sciatic, anemia, and microcytic anemia.

Sites of anemia examination ***(Fig. 17)****:*

- Lower palpebral conjunctiva
- Dorsum of tongue
- Nail beds
- Palms and sole
- Face

CYANOSIS

- *Definition:* Bluish discoloration of the skin and mucus membranes due to excessive amount of reduce hemoglobin in the blood (>5 g/dL). Clinically cyanosis appears when saturation is <85%.
- *Types:*
  - *Peripheral:* This occurs in the presence of normal arterial oxygen saturation, and it is due to pronounced oxygen unsaturation of the venocapillary and capillary blood.
    - *Sites:*
      - Nose
      - Fingers and toes
      - Ear lobules
      - Palms and soles
    - *Mechanism:*
      - Vaso-construction exposure to cold
      - Low cardiac output-left ventricular failure
      - Sluggish circulation in extremities due to shock from severe burns and hemorrhage
  - Central cyanosis—due to excessive unsaturation of the arterial blood
    - *Sites:*
      - Tongue.
      - Inner surface of lips
    - *Causes:*
      - Heart cause—like congenital cyanotic heart disease. Eisenmenger complex and syndrome
      - Lung causes—respiratory failure, pneumothorax, cystic fibrosis, pneumonia, interstitial lung disease.
      - Others—methemoglobinemia, carbon monoxide poisoning.

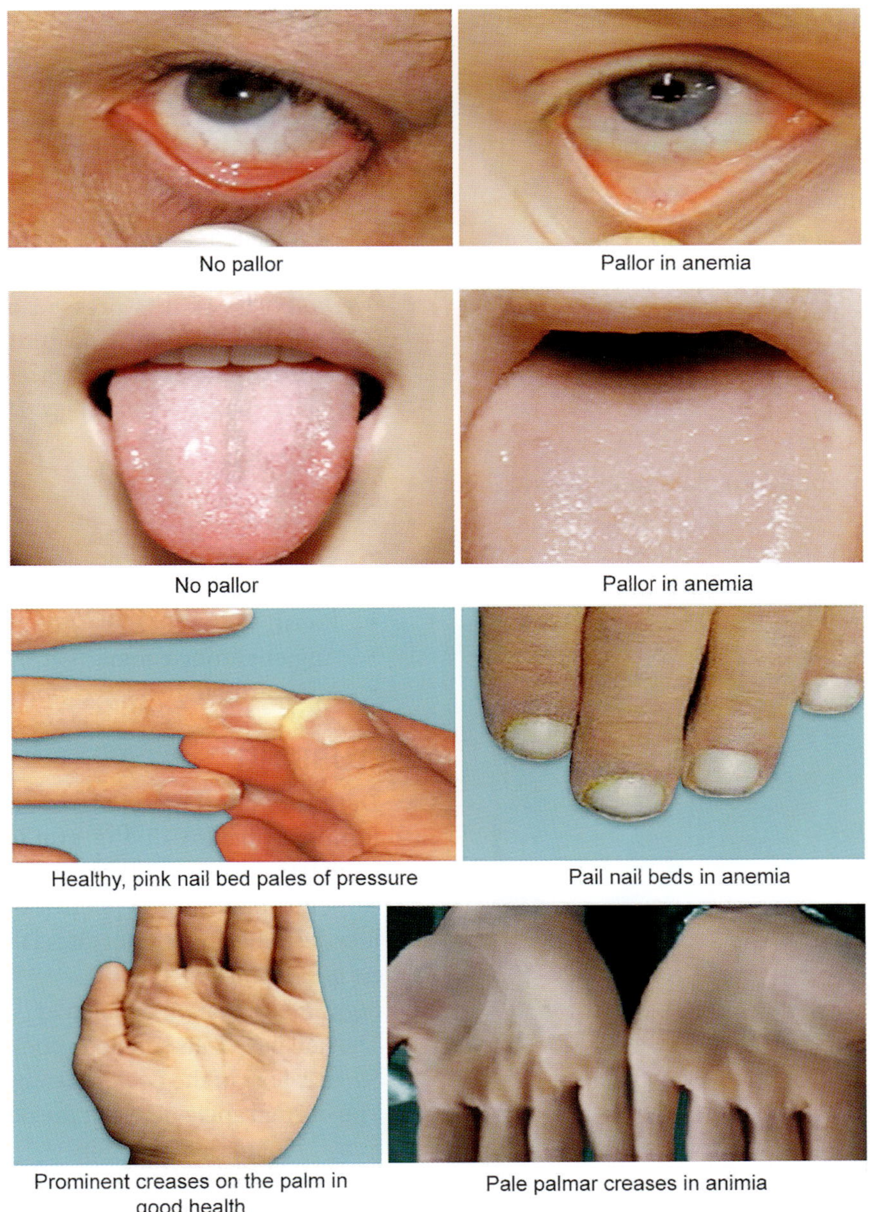

No pallor

Pallor in anemia

No pallor

Pallor in anemia

Healthy, pink nail bed pales of pressure

Pail nail beds in anemia

Prominent creases on the palm in good health

Pale palmar creases in animia

Fig. 17: Sites of anemia detection.

What is differential cyanosis?

It is present when the preductal (right upper extremity) oxygen saturation is higher than the post ductal (lower extremity) saturation.

Causes:

- PDA with reversal of shunt—cyanosis in seen in lower limbs only.
- Persistent pulmonary hypertension of the newborn (PPHN).

JAUNDICE

- *Definition:* Yellow discoloration of the skin mucus membranes due to excessive bilirubin (pigments of blood) in the blood.
- *Sites **(Fig. 18)**:*
  - Skin
  - Nail bed,
  - Under surface of tongue
  - Palms and sauces
  - Soft palate

Earliest detection of jaundice—sclera, as it contains more elastic tissue and has more affinity for bilirubin.

Types of jaundice ***(Table 6)***

- Obstructive or posthepatic
- Hemolytic or prehepatic
- Hepatocellular jaundice

Enumerate, some causes of hepatocellular jaundice:

- Viral hepatitis—hepatitis A, B, C, D, E, cytomegalovirus Epstein-Barr virus and yellow fever
- Spirochetal—leptospirosis
- Protozoal—toxoplasmosis, malaria,
- Rickettsial—*Coxiella burnetii*
- *Toxic:*
  - Drugs such as antitubercular, antiepileptic, and paracetamol,
  - Poisoning such as yellow phosphorus carbon tetrachloride, copper sulphate, and parathion amantoide phyllodes

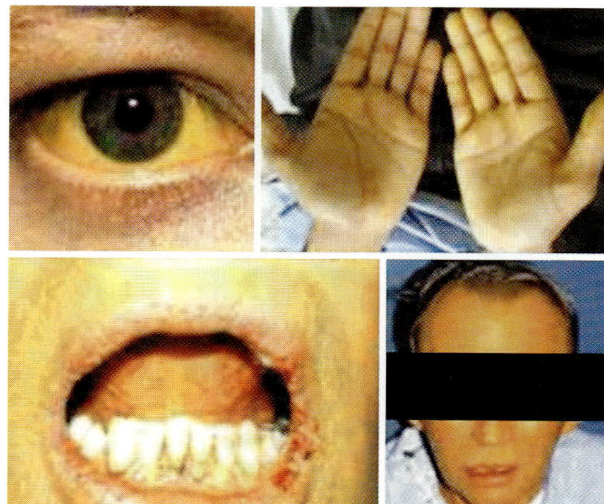

Fig. 18: Sites of yellowish discoloration.

EDEMA

- *Definition:* Swelling of the tissue due to accumulation of fluid
- *Sites:*
  - Ankle
  - Dorsum of the feet
  - Sacral edema—confined to bed
  - Eyelids
- *Method:* The skin is pressed over a bony area for 30 seconds. If there is no pitting, it is non-pitting edema. If pitting persists after removal of the pressure, it is called pitting edema **(Figs. 19 and 20)**.

Types:

- *Localized:*
- *Generalized:*
  - Cardiac
  - Hepatic
  - Renal
  - Angioneurotic edema
  - Malnutrition

CLUBBING

- *Definition:* Enlargement of the distal portion of terminal phalanx due to proliferation of subungual connective tissue. Clubbed fingers are frequently call serpents, hands, or hypocritical fingers as they were first described by Hippocrates **(Fig. 21)**.

Stages of clubbing:

- *Stage 1:* Fluctuation of nail bed
  The nail base feels soft and spongy when pressed.
- *Stage 2:* Loss of the Lovibond angle
  The normal angle between the nail and skin (>180°).
- *Stage 3:* Increased convexity
  Nail becomes more curved and shinier.

TABLE 6: Differentiation of types of jaundice.

	Obstructive	*Hepatocellular*	*Hemolytic*
Sclera	Greenish yellow		Lemon yellow
Pruritus	Intense	Mild	Absent
Splenomegaly	-	=/-	+
Hepatomegaly	+	++	-
Liver function test	Deranged with high GGT and alkaline phosphatase	Deranged with high enzymes	Mild deranged with normal enzymes
Reticulocyte count	Normal	Normal	Raised
Stool	Clay colored	Clay colored	Yellow
Urine	High colored	High colored	Straw colored

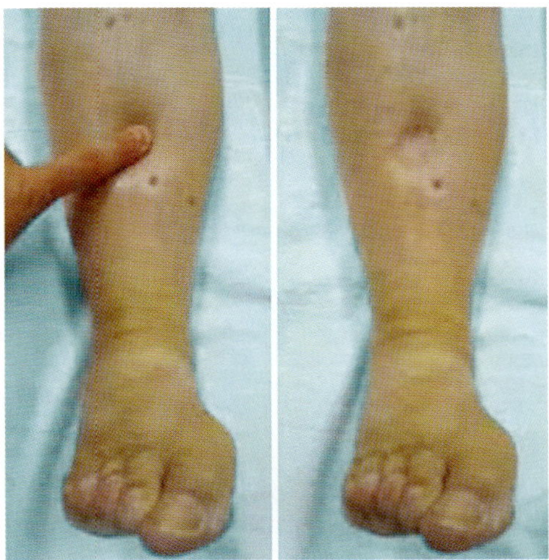

Fig. 19: Shin bone edema.

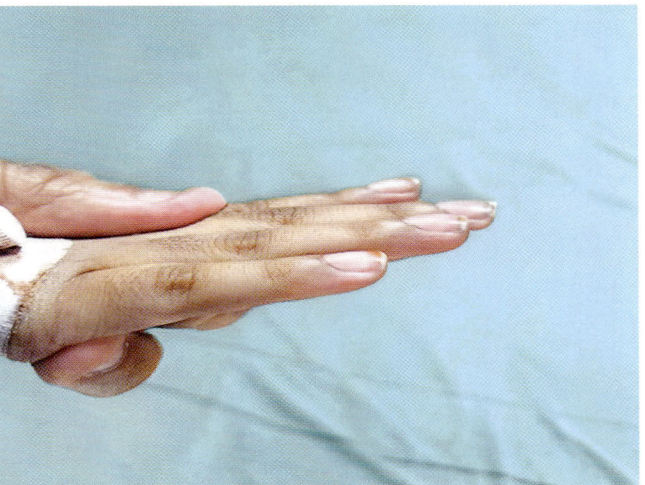

Fig. 21: Clubbing in fingers.

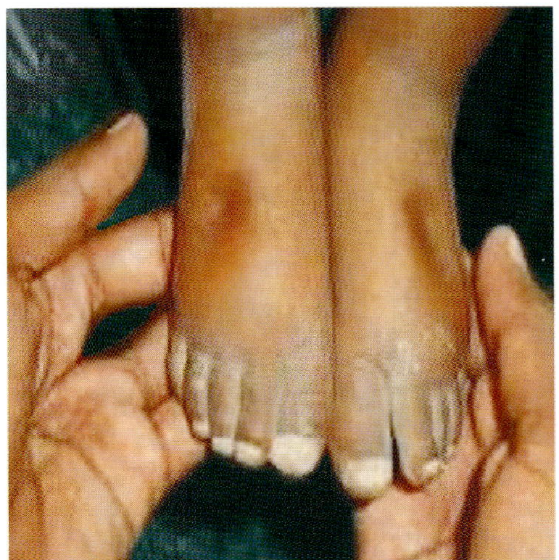

Fig. 20: Pedal edema.

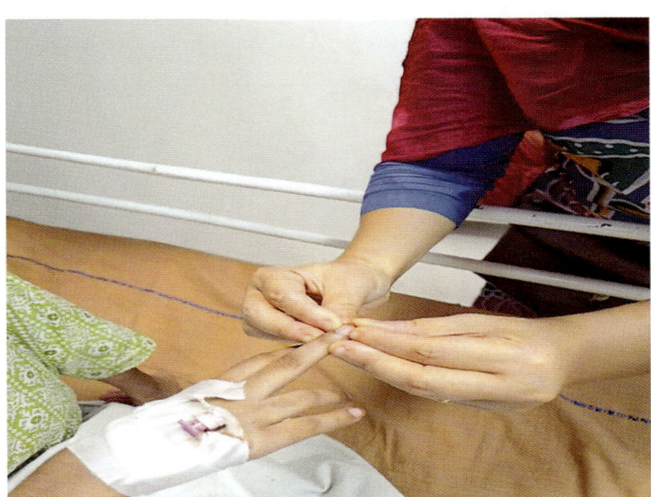

Fig. 22: Method of clubbing examination.

- *Stage 4:* Drumstick appearance
  The tip of the finger looks bulbous like a drumstick.
- *Stage 5:* Hypertrophic osteoarthropathy
  Painful swelling of joints and long bones (advanced stage).

How to elicit—place the hands both at the level of eye. Also examine the feet. The patient's fore finger is held with both the thumbs. The examiner then places both the index finger on either side near the base of the patient's nail. Pressure is then applied with one index finger, and the movement is felt by the other finger **(Figs. 22 and 23)**.

Result: If fluctuation is present. It is positive.

Pathophysiology:

- Toxic like infective inquiries
- Anoxia like congenital cyanotic heart disease
- Reflex phenomena like bronchogenic carcinoma
- Metabolic like thyrotoxicosis
- Alteration of pressure gradient

Types of clubbing:

- *Acute clubbing develops within 2–3 weeks*
  - Infective endocarditis
  - Lung abscess
  - Mesothelioma
- *Chronic clubbing developing in about 6 months*
  - Cyanotic heart disease
  - Bronchiectasis

Causes of clubbing:

- *C:* Cyanotic heart disease, congestive, cardiac failure, Crohn's disease
- *L:* Bronchogenic carcinoma (adult) and lung abscess

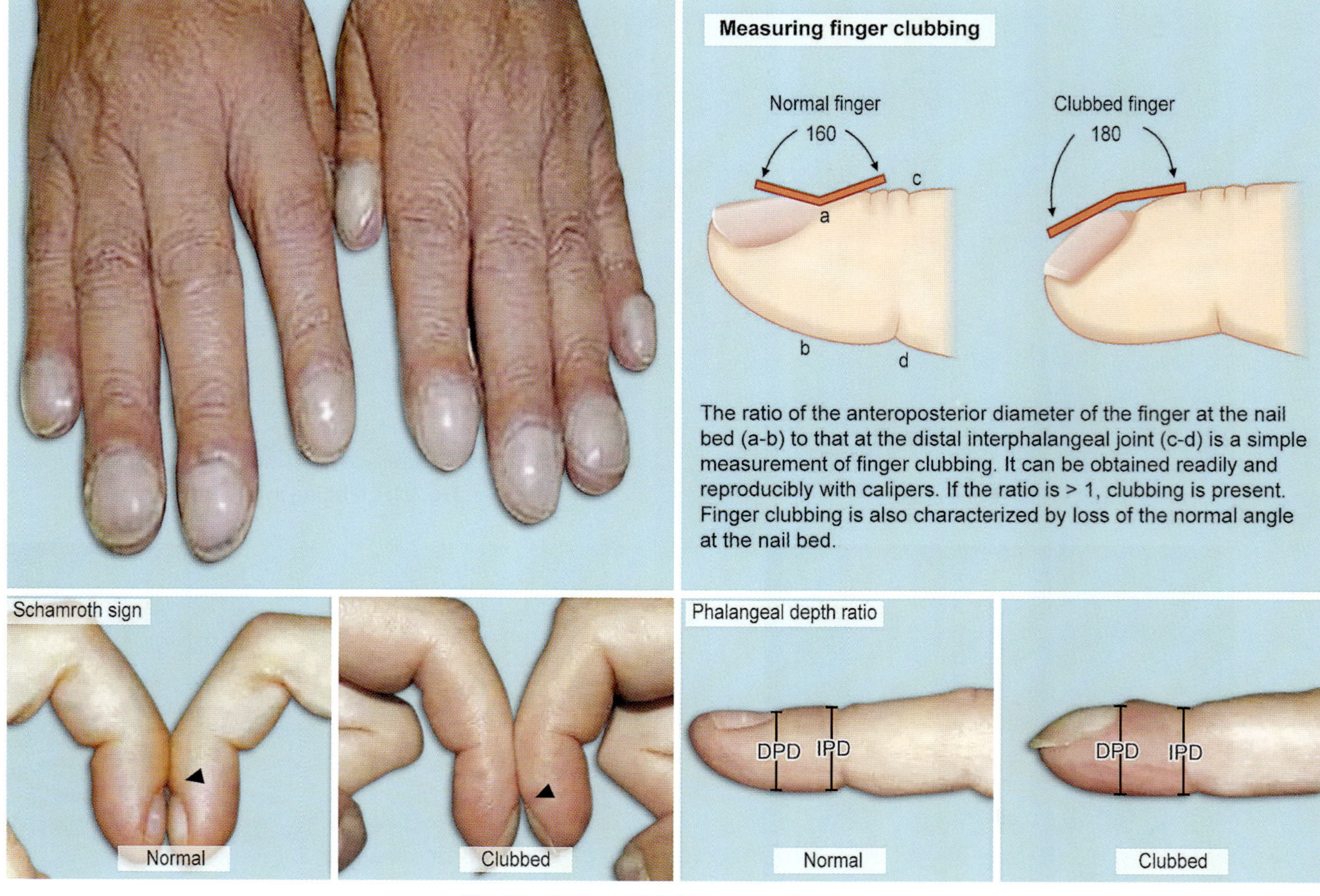

Fig. 23: Method of clubbing examination.

- *U:* Ulcerative colitis
- *B:* Biliary cirrhosis
- *B:* Bronchiectasis
- *I:* Idiopathic
- *N:* Normal
- *G:* Genetic

Pseudo clubbing: It refers to the appearance of clubbing without being present.

- Hyperparathyroidism due to excessive resorption of the distant phalanx
- Hansen's disease—damage to the finger due to sensory neuropathy
- Leukemia with sensory deposits in the bone results in destruction of bones

SKIN AND ITS APPENDAGES

Examination of skin must be conducted in a well-limited room.

Magnifying glass should be used to study the morphology of skin lesion **(Tables 7 and 8)**. It is desirable to completely expose the young child, while older children can have a loose-fitting gown. All areas of skin, including palm, sole creases, scalp, and anogenital skin should be scrutinized. Because of external origin of skin and CNS many genetic and developmental defects of skin are associated with CNS malformation or hamartomas **(Fig. 24)**.

APPENDAGES OF SKIN

Hairs and nails provide protection of the skin and have common biological origin.

- *Neck veins:* Internal jugular veins reflect most reliable the hemodynamic of the right atrium.
- *Method:* Patient reclining at a suitable angle (say 45°) and the neck muscles are relationship with respiration. Examine the internal jugular vein and not external jugular one.

TABLE 7: Primary lesions.

Macules	Flat non-palpable area of color changes of skin may be hypopigmented or hyperpigmented
	Example: Café-au-lait spots vitiligo, Mongolian spots
Papules	Circumscribed ray skin lesions of <0.5 cm in diameter
	Example: Molluscum contagiosum, warts
Nodules	Elevated skin lessons <0.5 cm in diameter located in epidermis dermis or subcutaneous tissue
	Example: Epidermolysis bullosa, fibromas
Tumors	Large nodules generally >2 cm in diameter, they may be benign or malignant
Papule	Well circumscribed broad-based lesions often formed by coalescence of a number of papules. The diameter or size of the lesion is greater than its height or elevation
	Example: Psoriasis
Wheal	Transient raised edematous skin lesions with irregular edges. The lesions are erythematous with the central pallor. Intense itching is usually present
	Example: Urticaria, insect bite
Vesicles	Elevated fluid containing skin lesions of <1 cm diameter
	Example: Chickenpox, herpes simplex, contact dermatitis
Bulla	Vesicles larger than 1 cm diameter, they may be intradermal or sub epidermal
	Example: Epidermolysis bullosa staphylococcal scalded skin syndrome
Cysts	Circumscribed tumors containing semisolid or fluid contents
	Example: Epidermal cysts occur after puberty
Pustules	Elevated well, circumscribed skin lesions containing purulent material or pus
	Example: Folliculitis or pyoderma
Come domes	• Characteristic skin lesions of acne distributed in the face and upper back • Opens comedones or blackhead 2–5 mm fluid colored papules with black center • Closed comedones or white heads 1–3 mm flesh-colored papules with a pinpoint opening
Purpura	Leakage of blood in the skin, it cannot be blanched by pressure with a finger or glass slide
Burrows	Linear skin lesions produced by adult female mites as she tunnels into the stratum corneum

TABLE 8: Secondary lesion.

Crusts	Formed by drying of blood serum and exudate overlying the disease skin
	Example: Impetigo
Excoriation	Develops as a result of linear losses of skin secondary to self-induced scratching and rubbing
	Example: Contact dermatitis atopic dermatitis
Ulcers	Occur due to deeper loss of the skin involving both epidemic and a variable depth of dermis or subcutaneous, tissue
	Example: Infection, vascular insufficiency burns
Fissures	Linear clefts deep through the epidermal layer in thickened or chronically inflamed skin
Lichenification	Exaggeration of skin markings due to chronic rubbing
	Example: Allergic or infective skin lesions
Atrophy	Loss or thinking of the epidemic or dermis
Eczematous skin lesions	Inflammatory skin lesions, which have distinct margins with erythema and vesiculations in the acute phase
Hyperkeratosis	Histologic term to describe the thickening of stratum corneum.

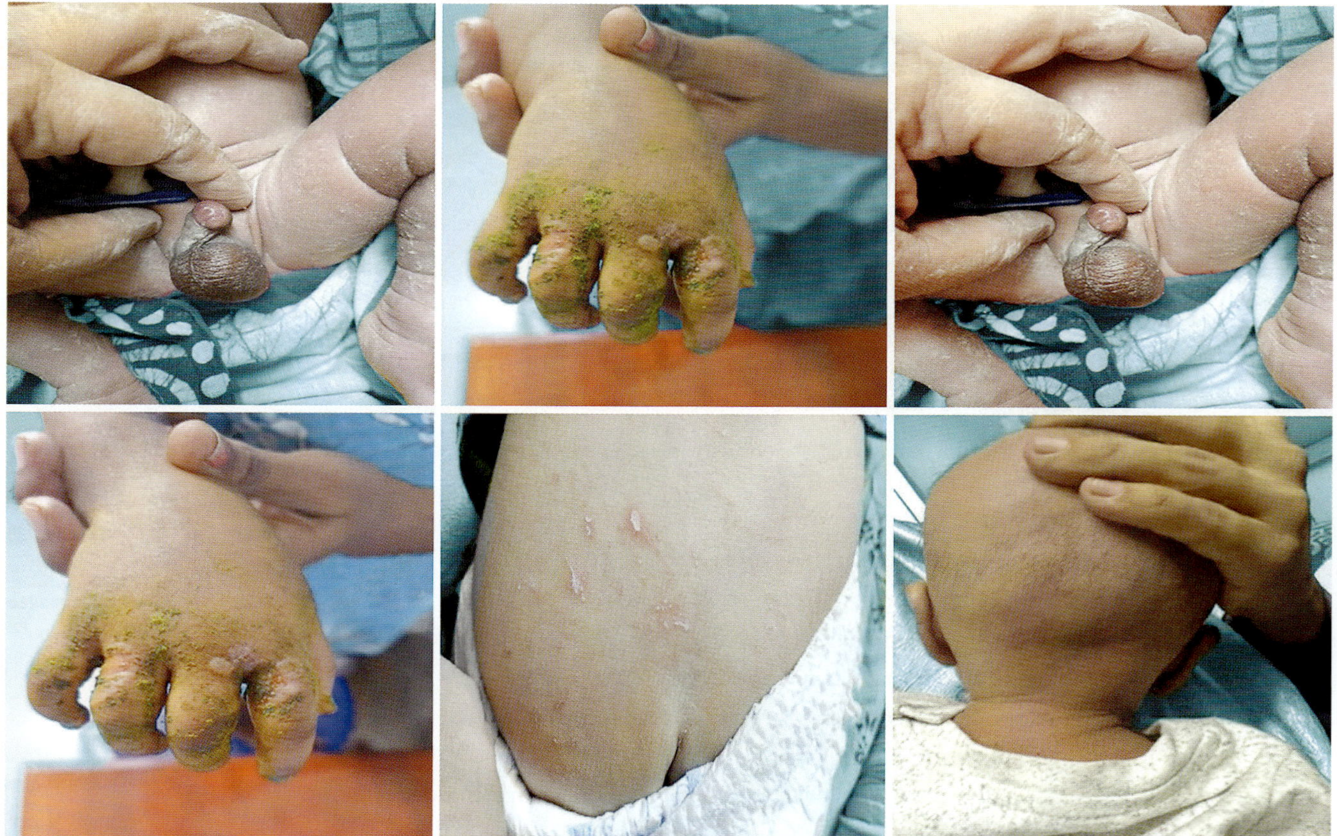

Fig. 24: Various skin lesions.

- *Internal jugular vein between two heads of sterno-cleidomastoid:* Note the vertical height (from the sternal angle) of the pulsation, its character, the waves refraction is relationship with respiration and heart sounds pulse rate.

FURTHER READING

1. Douglas G, Nicol F, Robertson C, editors. Macleod's clinical examination. 15th ed. London: Elsevier; 2023.
2. Gupta P. Clinical methods in pediatrics. 6th ed. New Delhi: CBS Publishers & Distributors; 2025.
3. Lakshmanaswamy, A. 2026, Clinical pediatrics: history taking and case discussion, 6th edn, Wolters Kluwer India Pvt Ltd, New Delhi.
4. Munro JF, Campbell IW, McCuish AC. Hutchison's Clinical Methods. 24th ed. Edinburgh: Elsevier; 2018.
5. Singh M. Pediatric clinical methods. 7th ed. New Delhi: CBS Publishers & Distributors; 2023.

CHAPTER 3

Growth and Development and Nutrition

Kalapana Datta, Rajasree Sinha

PART A: SEVERE ACUTE MALNUTRITION

Q1. What is malnutrition?

Ans. Malnutrition is defined as undernutrition resulting from inadequate consumption, poor absorption or excessive loss of nutrients but the term also encompasses overnutrition, resulting from excessive intake of specific nutrients.

Q2. How to measure undernutrition?

Ans. Anthropometry is widely used to access the general nutritional status of an individual or a population group. The three commonly used anthropometric indices are:

- Weight-for-age (WFA)
- Height/length-for-age (HFA)
- *Weight-for-height/length (WFH):* It is an age independent criterion, if the child can stand but 2 years add 0.7 cm to the height or if the child cannot stand and supine length is taken subtract 0.7 cm from length.

Q3. What are the types of undernutrition?

Ans. Underweight: Weight-for-age Z score that is at least two standard deviations (-2SD) below the median in the World Health Organization (WHO) child growth standards.

Stunting: Height-for-age Z score that is at least two standard deviations (-2 SD) below the median for the WHO child growth standards.

Wasting: Weight-for-height Z score that is at least two standard deviations (-2SD) below the median for the WHO child growth standards.

Severe acute malnutrition:

- *Above 6 months up to 5 years:* Weight-for-height/length (Z-score below -3 SD of the median WHO child growth standards), or a mid-upper arm circumference <11.5 cm, or by the presence of nutritional edema or severe wasting.
- *Below 6 months:* Weight-for/length (Z-score below -3 SD of the median WHO child growth standards), or by the presence of nutritional edema or severe wasting (consider length to be >50 cm).
- *Moderate acute malnutrition:* Weight-for- height (Z score of <-3SD to <-2 SD), or a mid-upper arm circumference of 11.5–12.5 cm and no edema. In addition, the child should have appetite, be alert and clinically well.

Q4. How to look for signs of severe malnutrition?

(A) Severe wasting

Ans. Look at the front view of the child:

- The child's ribs easily seen.
- The skin of the upper arms and thighs will appear loose.

Look at the posterior view of the child:

- The ribs and shoulder bones easily seen.
- Wasting seen on buttock.

(When wasting is extreme, there are folds of skin on the buttocks and thighs. It looks as if the child is wearing "baggy pants")

(B) How to look for edema?

Ans. Grasp the foot so that it rests in your hand with your thumb on dorsum of the foot. Press your thumb gently for approximately 10 seconds. Edema is present if a pit (dent) remains in the foot when the thumb is lifted. To be considered a sign of severe acute malnutrition, edema must appear in both feet. If the swelling is only in one foot, it may just be a sore or infected foot.

The extent of edema is commonly rated in the following way:

- + *mild:* Both feet
- + + *moderate:* Both feet, plus lower legs, hands, or lower arms

- + + + *severe:* Generalized edema including feet, legs, hands, arms, and face

Note: Edema is a characteristic of kwashiorkor, which is a form of severe acute malnutrition.

Q5. How to measure length/height of child?

Ans. To measure length, use a measuring board like infantometer with a headboard and sliding foot piece.

To measure height, use a stadiometer with a vertical backboard, a fixed base board, and a movable headboard.

- If a child is >2 years and cannot stand or <87 cm if the age is not available, measure recumbent length.
- If the child is aged 2 years or older or not willing to lie down or 87 cm or more if the age is not available and able to stand, measure standing height.
- If a child who is <2 years old and not willing to lie down for measurement of length, measure standing height and add 0.7 cm to convert it to length. If a child aged 2 years or older cannot stand, measure recumbent length and subtract 0.7 cm to convert it to height.

Q6. How to weigh the child?

Ans. It is recommended to weigh children using a scale with the following features: Electronic (digital reading) and measures to a precision of 0.01 kg (10 g).

Allows tared weighing ["tared weighing" means that the scale can be re-set to zero ("tared")] with the person just weighed still on it. Thus, a mother can stand on the scale, be weighed, and the scale tared. While remaining on the scale, if she is given her child to hold, the child's weight alone appears on the scale).

Q7. How to measure MUAC?

Ans. Arm circumference is measured preferably on the upper left arm or non-dominant hand >2 years. To locate the correct point for measurement, the child's elbow is flexed to 90°. A measuring tape is used to find the midpoint between the end of the shoulder (acromion) and the tip of the elbow (olecranon); this midpoint should be marked in flexed condition. The arm is then allowed to hang freely, palm toward the thigh, and the measuring tape is placed snugly around the arm at the midpoint mark. The tape should not be pulled too tight just to allow the little finger.

Q8. What is reductive adaptation?

Ans. The systems of the body begin to "shut down" with severe malnutrition. The systems slow down and do less in order to allow survival on limited calories. This slowing down is known as reductive adaptation. This is more prevalent in a marasmic child, i.e., a child with SAM but no edema.

Q9. Criteria for SAM.

Ans. Recommended criteria for identifying SAM in infants >6 months of age:

Any child who has following features are treated as severe acute malnutrition:

- Weight-for-height less than -3 SD and/or
- Visible severe wasting and/or
- Mid arm circumference (MUAC) <11.5 cm and/or
- Edema of both feet

Recommended criteria for identifying SAM in infants <6 months of age

Any infant >49 cm** in length who has following features are treated as severe acute malnutrition:

- Weight-for-height less than -3 SD and/or
- Visible severe wasting and/or
- Edema of both feet

***For children with length <49 cm in length, visible severe wasting can be used as criteria to identify SAM.*

Q10. Criteria for hospitalization in SAM.

Ans. Children with following complications should be admitted to a nutrition rehabilitation center or a health facility based:

Presence of any of emergency signs like:

- Persistent vomiting
- Generalized weakness
- Presence of documented fever
- Respiratory distress
- Extensive skin lesions, eye lesions, post-measles states
- Diarrhea with dehydration
- Severe anemia
- Hypothermia

In addition to above criteria, if the caregiver is unable to take care of the child at home and poor appetite, the child should be admitted.

Q11. What are the steps of routine care in SAM?

Ans. The steps of routine care in SAM are given below in **Table 1**.

TABLE 1: Management steps for stabilization and rehabilitation.

Management steps	Stabilization		Rehabilitation
	Day 1–2	Day 3–7	Week 2–6
1. Treat/prevent hypoglycemia			
2. Treat/prevent hypothermia			
3. Treat/prevent dehydration			
4. Correct imbalance of electrolytes			
5. Treat infections			
6. Correct deficiencies of micronutrients	noniron		With iron
7. Start cautious feeding			
8. Rebuild wasted tissues (catch-up growth)			
9. Provide loving care and play			
10. Prepare for follow-up			

Q12. Vitamin A supplementation in SAM.

Ans. **Table 2**

Same dose given on days 1, 2, and 14 if there is clinical evidence of vitamin A deficiency otherwise single dose.

TABLE 2: Vitamin A oral dose according to child's age.

Age	Vitamin A dose
3 months to 6 months	50000 IU
6 months to 12 months	100000 IU
12 months to 5 years	200000 IU

Q13. What nutrient supplementation is required?

Ans. Multivitamin supplement (should contain vitamin A, C, D, E, and B12 and not just vitamin B-complex):

- *Dosage:* Twice recommended daily allowance (use any multivitamin syrup containing vitamin A and D).
- *Folic acid:* 5 mg on day 1, then 1 mg/day.
- *Elemental zinc:* 2 mg/kg/day.
- *Copper:* 0.3 mg/kg/day (if separate preparation not available use commercial preparation containing copper).
- *Iron:* Start daily iron supplementation after two days of the child being on catch up diet. Give elemental iron in the dose of 3 mg/kg/day in two divided doses, preferably between meals. (Do not give iron in stabilization phase.)

Q14. Feeding in SAM.

Ans. The child is stabilized by feeding with starter diet. It is low in protein and sodium and high in carbohydrate, which is more easily handled by the child and provides much-needed glucose. Starter diet contains 75 kcal and 0.9 g protein per 100 mL. Starter feed to be given 130 mL/kg every 2 hourly by oral/NG route. Breastfeeding to be encouraged.

After stabilization (usually after 2–7 days), catch-up diet is used to rebuild wasted tissues. Catch-up diet contains more calories and protein—100 kcal and 2.9 g protein per 100 mL.

Q15. When to switch from starter to catch-up diet?

Ans. It may take up to 7 days, or even longer, for the child to stabilize on starter diet. After stabilization begin to offer catch-up diet, the higher calorie, higher protein "catch-up" feed intended to rebuild wasted tissues.

How will you know Readiness for transition?

Return of appetite (easily finishes 4-hourly feeds of starter diet).

- Reduced edema or minimal edema.
- The child may also smile at this stage.

Transition usually takes 3 days. After transition, the child is in the "rehabilitation" phase and can feed freely on Catch-up diet to an upper limit of 220 kcal/kg/day.

Q16. Sensory stimulation.

Ans. During rehabilitation provide:

- Tender loving care (smiling, laughing, patting, touching, talking, etc.).
- A cheerful stimulating environment.
- Structured play therapy for 15–30 minutes a day.
- Use locally available discarded materials to make toys for play sessions.
- Start physical activity as soon as child is stable and playful.
- Ensure maternal involvement as much as possible (e.g., comforting, feeding, play) so that the special care is continued at home.

Q17. What are the criteria for discharge?

Ans.

- Weight gain of >15% or has satisfactory weight gain for three consecutive days of admission weight (>5 g/kg/day)
- Edema has resolved
- Adequate eating of nutritious food preparable at home
- All infections and medical complications have resolved.

- Micronutrient supplementation started
- Age appropriate vaccines are given.

Q18. Definition of rickets.

Ans. Rickets is a generalized metabolic bone disorder, characterized by a failure of, or delay in mineralization of growing bones, occurring in children before fusion of the epiphysis. The disease usually results from an inadequate supply of calcium (calcipenic rickets) or phosphate (phosphopenic rickets) to the zone of provisional calcification at the growth plate, and at the newly formed osteoid surface.

Q19. Classification of rickets.

Ans. **Table 3.**

TABLE 3: Etiological classification of rickets—calcipenic and phosphopenic causes.

Calcipenic	*Phosphopenic*
Nutritional calcipenic rickets *(a) Vitamin D deficiency:* • Maternal and/or nutritional vitamin D deficiency • Reduced skin synthesis of vitamin D—sunlight deprivation, sunscreen use, increased skin pigmentation • Malabsorption—celiac disease, hepatobiliary disease, inflammatory bowel disease, etc. • Drugs—anticonvulsants, glucocorticoids, etc. *(b) Calcium deficiency:* • Nutritional deficiency *Non-nutritional calcipenic rickets* • Inborn errors of vitamin D metabolism— deficiency of 1α-hydroxylase (VDDR type 1), loss of function mutation of vitamin D receptor (VDDR type 2)	*Renal tubular disorders* *(a) Increased renal phosphate wasting (FGF-23 dependent):* • *Hereditary hypophosphatemic rickets* • *Acquired:* McCune–Albright syndrome, tumor-induced osteomalacia, linear nevus sebaceous syndrome *(b) Primary defect in renal phosphate absorption (FGF-23 independent):* • Proximal tubular dysfunction—Fanconi syndrome, cystinosis, tyrosinemia, and galactosemia • Hereditary hypophosphatemic rickets with hypercalciuria (HHRH) *Dietary phosphate deficiency* • Prematurity, antacids (aluminum containing)

Q20. Symptoms of rickets.

Ans. Neonates and young infants usually present with hypocalcemic seizures. Skeletal signs are seen in latter half of infancy and toddlers. Muscle cramps and tetany occur more frequently in adolescent age group. Short stature, deformities of lower limbs and pelvis may develop in long-standing cases.

Q21. Signs of rickets.

Ans. **Table 4.**

TABLE 4: Clinical skeletal manifestations of rickets across different body regions.

Region	*Clinical features*
Skull	Craniotabes (early sign), frontal bossing, caput quadratum, and delayed closure of anterior fontanelle
Teeth	Delayed eruption and enamel hypoplasia
Thorax	Rachitic rosary, pigeon chest/pectus carinatum, and Harrison groove
Extremities	• Arms—wrist widening • Leg—genu varum, genu valgum, saber shin deformity, green stick fractures, and wind-swept deformity • Ankle—double malleolus
Ligaments and muscles	Laxity and decreased tone, myopathy
Spine	Kyphoscoliosis (>2 years vertebral softening)

Q22. Approach to a child with rickets.

Ans.

History taking:

- Dietary history especially milk and dairy products, and sun exposure
- Anticonvulsants/drugs history
- Any hepatic/renal disease/malabsorption
- History of prematurity
- History of polyuria, polydipsia, failure to thrive with muscular weakness—RTA
- Parental consanguinity, similar involvement in siblings: inherited disorders
- Previous administration of calcium/vitamin D

Examination:

- Anthropometry (weight and height)
- Signs of vitamin deficiency, rachitic deformities
- Trousseau sign (carpopedal spasm)
- Milia, epidermal cysts, and alopecia—VDDR type 2
- Anemia, hypertension, short stature—chronic renal disease
- Jaundice, edema, hepatosplenomegaly—chronic liver disease
- Systemic examination including muscle power

Biochemical investigations:

- Serum (Sr) calcium, phosphorus, alkaline phosphatase, creatinine, albumin
- Venous blood gas
- Serum PTH, 25(OH)D, 1,25$(OH)_2$ D
- Urine calcium creatinine ratio

Radiology: X-ray wrist and or knee joint—widening of growth plate, metaphysis shows cupping, splaying, fraying

Q23. Biochemical features in different forms of rickets.

Ans. **Table 5**

TABLE 5: Summary of the biochemical features in different forms of rickets.

Disorder	*Ca*	*Pi*	*ALP*	*PTH*	*25(OH)D*	*1,25(OH)$_2$D*	*Urine Ca*	*Urine Pi*
Vitamin D deficiency	N, ↓	↓	↑	↑	↓	↓, N, ↑	↓	↑
Dietary Ca deficiency	N, ↓	↓	↑	↑	N, ↓	↑	↓	↑
VDDR, type 1	N, ↓	↓	↑	↑	N	↓	↓	↑
VDDR, type 2	N, ↓	↓	↑	↑	N	↑↑	↓	↑
Chronic renal failure	N, ↓	↑	↑	↑	N	↓	N, ↓	↓
XLH, ADHR	N	↓	↑	N	N	↓, N	↓	↑
HHRH	N	↓	↑	N	N	N, ↑	↑	↑
Fanconi syndrome	N	↓	↑	N	N	N, ↑	↓ or ↑	↑

(ADHR: autosomal dominant hypophosphatemic rickets; ALP: alkaline phosphatase; Ca: calcium; HHRH: hereditary hypophosphatemic rickets with hypercalciuria; Pi: phosphorus; PTH: parathyroid hormone; VDDR: vitamin D-dependent rickets; XLH: X-linked hypophosphatemic rickets; 25(OH)D: 25-hydroxyvitamin D; 1,25(OH)$_2$D: 1,25-dihydroxyvitamin D; N: normal; ↓: decreased; ↑: increased)

Q24. Management of nutritional rickets (hypovitaminosis D).

Ans. Symptomatic hypocalcemia including seizure: iv calcium gluconate 1–2 mL/kg

Normal calcium/asymptomatic:

- *Age <6 months*: Vitamin D 2000 IU for 90 days + 50–75 mg/kg/day oral calcium (maximum 500 mg/day)
- *Age 6 months to 1 year*: Vitamin D 2000 IU for 90 days or 30,000 IU fortnightly for 6 weeks or 60,000 IU monthly dose for 3 months + 50–75 mg/kg/day oral calcium (maximum 500 mg/day)
- *Age >1 year:* Vitamin D 3000 IU for 90 days or 60,000 IU fortnightly for 5 doses + 50–75 mg/kg/day oral calcium (maximum 500 mg/day)

Q25. Management of non-nutritional rickets.

Ans. **Table 6.**

TABLE 6: Management strategies for different types of non-nutritional rickets.

Type of rickets	*Treatment*
Hypophosphatemic rickets	Oral phosphorous 35–75 mg/kg/day and oral calcitriol 20–40 ng/kg/day
Vitamin D-dependent rickets type 1 (VDDR 1)	Calcitriol 150–200 ng/kg/day and oral calcium (30–75 mg/kg/day)
Vitamin D-dependent rickets type 2 (VDDR 2)	Very high doses of calcitriol (1–6 µg per day) and intravenous calcium or high dose calcium (150–200 mg/kg/day)

Q26. Prevention of rickets.

Ans.

- All children from birth till 1 year should receive 400 IU vitamin D daily
- After 1-year routine supplementation not required except in high-risk cases (cerebral palsy, malabsorption, renal disease, on steroids, etc.)
- Recent IAP guidelines recommend a sunlight exposure of 17–30 minutes (infants) and 30–45 minutes (older children). The ideal time of exposure is 11 am to 3 pm and the frequency of exposure advised is 5 times a week.

PART B: RICKETS

Q27. Define rickets.

Ans. Rickets is a disorder of the growing skeleton in which mineral deposition at the growth plate and newly formed osteoid is inadequate or delayed, occurring before epiphyseal fusion. Functionally, the problem reflects insufficient calcium-phosphate availability at the zone of provisional calcification. Clinically and biochemically, this is most often due to either deficiency of vitamin D or calcium (calcipenic rickets) or to chronic phosphate deficiency from renal or hereditary causes (phosphopenic rickets).

Q28. Classification of rickets.

Ans.

- *Calcipenic rickets*
  - *Nutritional forms:*
    - *Vitamin D deficiency:* Maternal or infant dietary deficiency; limited cutaneous synthesis (inadequate sunlight exposure, extensive sunscreen use, darker skin pigmentation); malabsorption (e.g., celiac disease, hepatobiliary disease, inflammatory bowel disease); and medication effects (notably anticonvulsants, glucocorticoids).
    - *Dietary calcium deficiency.*
      - *Non-nutritional calcipenic rickets:* Inborn errors of vitamin D metabolism such as 1α-hydroxylase deficiency [vitamin D-dependent rickets (VDDR) type 1] and vitamin D receptor loss-of-function (VDDR type 2).
- *Phosphopenic rickets*
  - *FGF-23-dependent renal phosphate wasting:*
    - Hereditary hypophosphatemic rickets
    - Acquired causes including tumor-induced osteomalacia, McCune-Albright syndrome, and linear nevus sebaceous syndrome.
  - *FGF-23-independent renal phosphate loss:*
    - Proximal tubular dysfunction (Fanconi syndrome, cystinosis, tyrosinemia, galactosemia)
    - Hereditary hypophosphatemic rickets with hypercalciuria (HHRH).
  - Nutritional/iatrogenic phosphate deficiency (e.g., severe prematurity, prolonged use of aluminum-containing antacids)

Q29. Symptoms of rickets.

Ans. Presentation varies with age. Neonates and young infants may first come to attention with hypocalcemic seizures. In late infancy and toddlerhood, skeletal manifestations become apparent. Adolescents may report muscle cramps and tetany. Long-standing disease can lead to short stature, pelvic and lower-limb deformities, and delayed motor milestones.

Q30. Signs of rickets.

Ans.

- *Skull:* Craniotabes (often an early clue), frontal bossing, caput quadratum, delayed anterior fontanelle closure.
- *Teeth:* Delayed eruption, enamel hypoplasia
- *Chest:* Rachitic rosary, pectus carinatum (pigeon chest), Harrison sulcus
- *Extremities:* Wrist widening, genu varum or valgum, Saber-Shin deformity; greenstick fractures, wind-swept deformity, ankle "double malleolus" appearance.
- *Ligaments and muscles:* Generalized ligamentous laxity, hypotonia, and proximal myopathy.
- *Spine:* Kyphoscoliosis (vertebral softening visceroptosis becomes relevant after ~2 years).

Q31. Approach to a child with rickets.

Ans.

- *History:* Detailed dietary intake (milk/dairy, calcium); sunlight exposure pattern; medication history (especially anticonvulsants, glucocorticoids); prior illnesses suggesting malabsorption or chronic liver/kidney disease; prematurity; polyuria/polydipsia, failure to thrive with muscle weakness suggesting renal tubular acidosis; consanguinity and similar illness in siblings (inherited disorders); prior vitamin D or calcium supplements.
- *Examination:* Anthropometry (weight, length/height); signs of micronutrient deficiency and classic rachitic deformities; Trousseau sign (carpopedal spasm); cutaneous clues such as milia/epidermal cysts and alopecia (supporting VDDR type 2); anemia, hypertension, and growth failure (chronic kidney disease); stigmata of chronic liver disease; full systemic exam including muscle power.
- *Biochemistry:* Serum total or albumin-corrected calcium, inorganic phosphate, alkaline phosphatase (ALP), creatinine, albumin; venous blood gas;

CHAPTER 4

Examination of Cardiovascular System and its Disorders

Lopamudra Mishra, Shatanik Sarkar, Shayamajit Samaddar, Mrigank Choube

SYMPTOMS OF CARDIOVASCULAR DISORDERS

- *Feeding difficulty and "suck–rest–suck cycle":* Infants often face feeding difficulty in suck–rest–suck cycle as a result of respiratory muscle fatigue due to increased energy consumption—similar to exertional dyspnea in older children. It is seen more commonly in children with congestive heart failure (CHF), e.g., significant left-to-right shunt and low ejection fraction.
- *Shortness of breath (breathing difficulty/dyspnea):* Mostly exertional, due to increased energy consumption and respiratory muscles fatigue equivalent to feeding difficulty in infants; lung congestion may also contribute in it.
- *Fast breathing (tachypnea):* It occurs as a result of stimulation of pulmonary interstitial receptor.
- *Feeding diaphoresis is usually manifested as excessive forehead sweating:* It occurs due to increased adrenergic output required to meet increased cardiac output.
- *Cyanosis:* Bluish discoloration of nail beds, tongue, and oral cavity noticed at rest or exertion; it occurs as a result of increased deoxygenated hemoglobin.
- *Cyanotic spell:* Episodic excessive bluish discoloration on with continuous crying; common after waking up in the morning, defecation, and during fever; proposed mechanisms are increased chemoreceptor sensitivity, cry-induced infundibular spasm (D/D from breath-holding spell by deep and troubled breathing than holding of breath).
- *Squatting:* It is observed in older children aged 2 years or more with congenital cyanotic heart disease with decreased Qp [tetralogy of Fallot (TOF) physiology].
- *Recurrent lower respiratory tract infection:* Predisposing factors are lung congestion due to left-to-right shunt, genetic predisposition for immunodeficiency (Catch 22), airways compression by *dilated* bronchial vessel and pulmonary vessel (remember: Frequent upper respiratory tract infection is not sign of cardiovascular involvement; vascular ring may present with choking or stridor).
- *Easy fatigability or exercise intolerance:* Impaired perfusion to the various organs cyanotic; acyanotic heart disease with increased or decreased flow, stenotic or regurgitant lesion
- *Poor weight gain and failure to thrive—due to demand supply mismatch:* Increased calorie demand and decreased intake; weight gain suffer more than stunting
- Increased precordial activity, feeling of abnormal pulsations on touching as a result of hyperdynamic circulation (sympathetic overactivity)
- Precordial bulge and chest wall deformity may present in severe and chronic cardiac problem because of pliable chest.
- *Edema:* Swelling of eyelids and feet, abdominal distension—swelling increases at the end of the day (D/D—from renal cause where it occurs most in the morning after lying down). CHF leading to third space retention of water leading to activation of the renin–angiotensin pathway → renal salt and water retention. Sacral edema rather than ankle edema is found in infants.

CHEST PAIN

Causes

Noncardiac causes are most common in children.

- *Cardiac:* Ischemic noncoronary (supply–demand mismatch) → aortic stenosis (AS), hypertrophic obstructive cardiomyopathy (HOCM), aortic regurgitation (AR), patent ductus arteriosus (PDA), hypertension (HTN)/pulmonary HTN and pulmonary stenosis (PS) (right ventricular ischemia), and severe anemia
  - *Ischemic:* Coronary artery disease (dyslipidemia, homocystinuria, Kawasaki disease, and other vasculitis—congenital or acquired coronary artery stenosis, and coronary artery abnormalities

- *Nonischemic:* Myocarditis, pericarditis, mitral valve prolapse (MVP), aortic dissection, and pulmonary embolism (PE)

- *Respiratory:* Pleuritis, bronchitis, pneumonia, and pneumothorax
  Gastrointestinal (GI) cause: Gastroesophageal reflux disease (GERD), peptic ulcer, pancreatitis, cholecystitis, esophageal spasm
- *Local:* Musculoskeletal syndrome—Tietze syndrome (costochondritis), herpes zoster, rib fracture, trauma, and osteoarthritis
- Psychogenic cause

Important History in Chest Pain

- *Onset:* Relation with activity—cardiac causes are usually exercise-induced and get relieved with rest.
- *Positional chest pain:* Likely due to trauma or muscle spasm
- *Relation with deep breathing and cough:* Except pericarditis other cardiac causes are not usually precipitated.
- *Reproducibility:* Local compression may reproduce pain due to costochondritis or muscle spasm.
- *Character:* Ischemic cardiac pain—deep pressure compressing or squeezing, not sharp; pain due to pericarditis—sharp, pin-pricking sensation
- *Associated palpitation:* May indicate MVP
- *History of bereavement:* Psychogenic
- *Syncope:* Transient loss of consciousness and loss of muscle tone due to generalized cerebral hypoperfusion with rapid and complete recovery

Syncopal episodes may occur suddenly or with presyncope (preceding signs or symptoms dizziness, lightheadedness, diaphoresis, nausea, visual disturbances, etc.).

Approximately 15% of children experience at least one episode of syncope. However, in fewer than 5% of cases important cardiac pathology is found. Girls are affected more than boys and the peak incidence was between 15 and 19 years of age. Most common cause is benign vasovagal/neurocardiogenic syncope. Abrupt onset, with negligible prodrome that occurred *during* exercise or during an acute auditory trigger may indicate presence of predisposing cardiac cause.

DEFINITION OF SYNCOPE

Syncope is a transient loss of consciousness and postural tone followed by spontaneous recovery.

CAUSES OF SYNCOPE

- *Disorders of blood flow and vascular tone (M/C) (reflex-mediated):*
  - Vasovagal (neurocardiogenic) (common faint)
  - Orthostatic hypotension (medications, autonomic failure, peripheral neuropathy, and decreased blood flow)
  - Situational (cough, laugh, micturition, defecation, postprandial, deglutition, and sneeze)
  - Carotid sinus syncope
- Cerebrovascular causes (vertebrobasilar insufficiency)
- *Cardiovascular disorders:*
  - Cardiac arrhythmias (both tachy- and brady-arrhythmias)
  - Structural and obstructive disorders [valvular obstruction like AS, PS, mitral stenosis (MS), HOCM, myocardial infarction (MI), PE, pulmonary HTN]
- *Others that mimic syncope:*
  - Seizures
  - Metabolic (hypoglycemia, hypoxia, symptomatic anemia)
  - Psychogenic (panic attacks)

The Evaluation of Guidelines in Syncope Study (EGSYS) scores can be used to predict cardiac cause of syncope in children. A score ≥3 indicates high risk of cardiac syncope. Neurally mediated syncope (NMS) is mostly triggered by prolonged standing, postural change, dehydration, urination, coughing, emotional surges, and stuffy or crowded environments **(Table 1)**. Prodromes, such as dizziness, visual blurring, nausea, abdominal discomfort, hyperventilation, sweating, and pallor, appear either singularly or in combination before the onset of syncope.

TABLE 1: The Evaluation of Guidelines in Syncope Study (EGSYS) scores.

Predictors	*Point*
Abnormal ECG and/or structural heart disease	+3
Palpitations	+4
Syncope during effort	+3
Syncope in supine position	+2
Precipitating and/or predisposing factors	–1
Autonomic neurovegetative prodromes	–1

(ECG: electrocardiogram)

DEFINITION OF DYSPNOEA

Dyspnea (breathlessness/short of breath) is the subjective sensation of uncomfortable breathing and consists of qualitatively distinct sensations of various intensities.

It mainly arises from four primary categories: respiratory, cardiac, neuromuscular, and psychogenic and systemic illness, or a combination of these **(Table 2)**.

Suck-rest-suck cycle may be a manifestation of dyspnea in a newborn and early infancy.

Mechanism of Dyspnea

- *Stimulation of J receptor (supplied by vagal fibers) by stretching due to edema or congestion → Hering-Breuer reflex got activated,* terminating the inspiratory effect.
- *Tachypnea* is defined as respiratory rate of >60 breaths/min in infants aged 0–2 months, >50 in infants 2–12 months, >40 in children 1–5 years, and >20 in children >5 years of age. Respiratory rate can increase 2.6 breaths/min per degree temperature elevation. Quiet tachypnea is often present in left-to-right shunt lesions or CHF, whereas labored tachypnea is observed in patients with *pulmonary disease. Hyperpnea* may be present in congenital heart lesions that result in decreased *pulmonary blood flow.*
- Wheezing or persistent cough at night may be an early sign of CHF.
- *Edema:* Puffy eyelids and sacral edema are signs of systemic venous congestion. Ankle edema, which is commonly seen in adults, is not found in infants.

TABLE 2: Causes of dyspnea.

Respiratory	*Cardiac*	*Neuromuscular*	*Psychogenic*
Asthma, chronic obstructive pulmonary disease (COPD), airway obstruction, pneumonia, pleural effusion	Congestive heart failure, pulmonary edema, acute coronary syndrome, pericardial tamponade, valvular heart defect, pulmonary hypertension, cardiac arrhythmia, or intracardiac shunting	Chest trauma with fracture or flail chest, massive obesity, kyphoscoliosis, central nervous system (CNS) or spinal cord dysfunction, phrenic nerve paralysis, myopathy, and neuropathy	

WEIGHT GAIN, DEVELOPMENT, AND FEEDING PATTERN

Poor weight gain and general developmental delay are noticed in infants and children with CHF or severe cyanosis. Weight is affected more significantly than height. Poor feeding due to dyspnea and increased energy requirement are the cause of wasting. Genetic dysmorphism to be suspected if weight is severely affected and stunting is associated.

CYANOSIS

Characteristics include onset (e.g., at birth, several days after birth) and severity of cyanosis, permanent or paroxysmal nature, parts of the body that were cyanotic (e.g., fingers, toes, lips), and whether the cyanosis becomes worse after feeding.

Time of its appearance (e.g., in the morning on awakening, after feeding), duration of the spells, and frequency of the spells are also important. Most important is whether infants were breathing *fast* and *deep* during the spell or were holding their breath. This helps differentiate between a true cyanotic spell and a breath-holding spell.

PALPITATION

Palpitation refers to experience of rapid heartbeat. It is usually expressed by older children but in mother may be noticed by increased precordial activity. It may be perceived during sinus tachycardia and paroxysms of tachycardia (e.g., supraventricular tachycardia), or single premature beats commonly cause palpitation **(Table 3)**.

SQUATTING

Squatting is usually noticed in congenital cyanotic heart disease with decreased pulmonary flow (TOF physiology).

TABLE 3: Causes of palpitation.

Cardiac cause	*Noncardiac cause*
• Rhythm disturbance—sinus tachycardia, paroxysms of tachycardia (e.g., supraventricular tachycardia), or single or multiple premature beats, heart block—sudden onset, no relation with activity usually except exercise-induced arrhythmias • Volume overload states—regurgitant lesions, left-to-right shunts—more during activity	Hyperdynamic or high cardiac output states like anemia, thyrotoxicosis, anxiety, etc.

Usually it occurs after >2 years; squatting compresses abdominal aorta, increases systemic vascular resistance (SVR), decreases right-to-left shunting, and increases pulmonary blood flow.

SYMPTOMS SUGGESTIVE OF ASSOCIATED COMPLICATIONS

- Symptoms of *bacterial endocarditis*—prolonged fever, clinical predisposition like recent heart surgery or intervention, placement of cardiac implants, central lines, and prolonged IV antibiotic immunocompromised states.
- Clinically history of rash, joint pain—new onset or aggravated heart failure symptoms, embolic phenomenon, hematuria, etc.
- *Renal symptoms:* Decreased urine output in heart failure due to salt and water retention, low cardiac output states, or stenotic lesions and coarctation of aorta; hematuria may be present in infective endocarditis (IE) or embolic cause.
- *GI symptoms:* Jaundice occurs due to congestion due to heart failure. Cardiac cirrhosis and constrictive pericarditis may present with ascites and jaundice. Vomiting and abdominal pain may occur in low cardiac output states due to decreased splanchnic blood flow.
- *Central nervous system (CNS):* Thromboembolic events—poor cardiac function, IE, cyanotic heart disease specially <2 years
  - Brain abscess in cyanotic heart disease >2 years

Other Congenital Malformations or Abnormal Facies

Growth and nutrition: Poor weight gain in left-to-right shunt or increased pulmonary flow states; decreased pulmonary flow states usually no lag is noticed unless severely cyanosed for prolonged period.

Development: Unless patient is syndromic in cardiac disease IQ and development remains normal, some delayed motor milestone may be noticed in patient with significant heart failure or cyanosis due to nutritional deprivation or physical inability.

Antenatal history: History suggestive of maternal diseases includes *diabetes mellitus, phenyl ketonuria, or maternal infection like mumps, rubella in pregnancy like fever, rash,* etc., and *any history of intake of drugs (like anticonvulsant, antidepressant)/exposure (e.g., radiation), etc.* **(Table 4)**.

TABLE 4: Drugs/exposures causing congenital heart disease.

Drugs/exposure	*Disease*
Valproate	ASD, VSD, TOF
Paroxetine	ASD, VSD, ventricular outflow tract obstruction
Nitrofurantoin	HPLHS
Cephalosporins	ASD
Lithium	Ebstein disease mitral atresia
Ibuprofen	TGA
NSAIDs	Premature closure of PDA
Rubella	PDA, ASD, peripheral PS
Diabetes mellitus	TGA, VSD, PDA, cardiomyopathy, septal hypertrophy
Phenylketonuria	VSD, PDA, TOF
Hydantoin	Pulmonic or aortic stenosis, coarctation of aorta, PDA
Fever	Conotruncal and obstructive disease
Alcohol	VSD, TOF
Clomiphene	TOF

(ASD: atrial septal defect; HPLHS: hypoplastic left heart syndrome; PDA: patent ductus arteriosus; TGA: transposition of the great arteries; TOF: tetralogy of Fallot; VSD: ventricular septal defect)

TABLE 5: Functional class—various classifications consisting of different parameters.

NYHA class	*Symptoms*
I	Presence of cardiac disease; no limitation of physical activity and no symptoms on ordinary physical activity
II	Slight limitation of physical activity; comfortable at rest; ordinary physical activity results in fatigue, palpitation, dyspnea, or chest pain
III	Marked limitation of physical activity; comfortable at rest; symptoms on less than ordinary activity
IV	Unable to carry on any physical activity without discomfort; symptoms of heart failure may be present even at rest

Family history: 2–4% recurrence risk (overall low) if one sibling or parent is affected; higher frequency is noticed in a patient with hypoplastic left heart (19%) or coarctation of aorta (9%).

New York Heart Association (NYHA) classification: Most commonly used; it is used to grade the severity of dyspnea, fatigue, angina (chest pain), and palpitation **(Table 5)**.

Other functional classification:

- *Canadian Cardiovascular Society Classification*—for angina
- *World Health Organization (WHO) Modification of NYHA Classification*—for pulmonary arterial hypertension (PAH)
- *Ross Score*—for pediatrics heart failure

Modified Ross Classification for Heart Failure was issued to assess functional status and severity of heart failure in infants and children.

Modified Ross Heart Failure Classification for Children:

1. Class I—Asymptomatic
2. Class II—Mild tachypnea or diaphoresis with feeding in infants, dyspnea on exertion in older children
3. Class III—Marked tachypnea or diaphoresis with feeding in infants or marked dyspnea on exertion in older children and prolonged feeding times with growth failure
4. Class IV—Symptoms such as tachypnea, retractions, grunting, or diaphoresis at rest along with growth failure

Another recent score developed particularly for pediatric population is New York University Pediatric Heart Failure Index for children and adolescents, which yields a weighted score based on physiological indicators and medical therapy.

Examination of the cardiovascular system is best done only after taking a thorough clinical history. Cardiovascular examination starts with visual survey of the child.

Visual assessment (head to toe examination) relevant to cardiovascular system:

- *Built and nutrition:* Anthropometry to be done and sign of macro- and micronutrient deficiency to be assessed; increased pulmonary flow situations lead to more failure to thrived state.
- Note the state of wakefulness, the child's interest in the surrounding, and decubitus.
- Try to recognize whether the child has any syndromic look. Turner syndrome (left-sided heart disease like bicuspid aortic valve, MVP, coarctation of aorta), Down syndrome [endocardial cushion defects, ventricular septal defect (VSD)], Noonan syndrome (pulmonary valve abnormalities), DiGeorge syndrome (conotruncal abnormalities), and Marfan syndrome (aortic root abnormalities)
- Identify degree of respiratory distress and count the respiratory rate before touching the baby. Note if there is any audible grunting, wheeze, and cough.
- Degree of cyanosis visually and then use your pulse oximeter if available. Children of cyanotic heart disease with significant anemia often look acyanotic.
- *Mouth:* Assess the oral cavity. Examine for dental hygiene. Dental caries are important source of IE; lip cracking in Kawasaki disease.
- *Tongue:* Examine the tongue for central cyanosis (in peripheral cyanosis limb extremities, nose tip may be involved but not the tongue), jaundice, and strawberry tongue (Kawasaki disease).
- *Examination of trunk:* Harrison sulcus, Pigeon chest, erythema marginatum, and rheumatic nodules (rheumatic heart disease)
- *Examination of the hand and fingers:* Palmar crease, pallor, cyanosis, clubbing, and xanthomas (dyslipidemia); in IE—Osler nodes (tender swelling of finger tips) and Janeway lesions (flat, painless, red macules or papules that appear on the palms and soles of the feet)
- *Nails:* Splinter hemorrhage in IE

GENERAL TACTILE EXAMINATION

Pulse:

- *Pulse rate:* Count for 15 seconds and multiply by 4. If a pulse oximeter or electrocardiogram (ECG) electrodes are attached to the child, note the pulse rate and rhythm from it. If irregular pulse observed, count for 1 minute.
- Palpate the pulse for volume, quality, or any delay.
- Clinically relevant pulse in children are:
  - *Radial:* For older children
  - *Brachial:* Palpate for infants and toddlers
  - Carotid (never palpate both carotid simultaneously as this can induce syncope)
  - *Femoral:* Note any discrepancies between upper-limb and lower-limb pulse (like in coarctation)
  - Posterior tibial and dorsalis pedis (when you cannot palpate the femoral pulse like after any catheterization procedures)
- *Comment on:*
  - *Rate:*
    - *Tachycardia:* >100 beats/min above 3 years
    - *Bradycardia:* Pulse rate <60 beats/min in older children and <80 beats/min in neonates
  - *Unequal or absent scar:* Suspect coarctation of aorta, arch anomaly, look for scar mark for BT shunt.

- *Radio-radial and radio-femoral delay:* Finding seen in coarctation of aorta
- *Rhythm:*
    - *Regularly irregular:* Wenckebach (common during sleep, rare during awake state); pulsus bigeminus, coupled extrasystole
    - *Irregularly irregular pulse:* Atrial fibrillation, multiple extrasystoles, etc.
- *Volume:*
    - *Small volume pulse:* Low cardiac volume state; severe AS, coarctation of aorta
    - *High volume pulse:* High cardiac output state like anemia, AR, PDA
    - *Collapsing pulse:* AR, PDA
    - *Slow rising and plateau:* Moderate and severe AS
    - *Pulsus paradoxus:* Pulse is weak or disappears on inspiration, e.g., constrictive pericarditis, tamponade, and status asthmaticus.
    - *Jerky pulse:* Normal volume, rapid rising sustained seen in hypertrophic cardiomyopathy (HCM), supravalvular AS

Blood pressure (BP): Hypertension is defined as BP above 95th percentile for age, sex, and height. High blood pressure (HBP) in childhood can be progressive into adulthood and is the strongest predictor of adulthood HBP. HTN increases the risk of end-organ damage, including coronary artery calcifications, ventricular hypertrophy, and increased carotid intima-media thickness.

Difference between 4th report on HTN (2004) and clinical practice guideline of AAP 2017 (5th report) is given in **Table 6**.

Blood pressure measurement: Mercury sphygmomanometer, aneroid, or an automated device is used for BP measurement. Appropriate cuff size: Should encircle three-fourths of the arm circumference and its width should cover two-thirds of the length of the upper arm **(Table 7)**.

Blood pressure was measured after resting at least 5 minutes in the sitting position. Systolic blood pressure (SBP) was determined by onset of the first "tapping" Korotkoff sound, and diastolic blood pressure (DBP) was determined by the fifth Korotkoff sound. An average of three BP measurements at a single occasion was calculated **(Table 8)**.

Primary HTN is now considered the most prevalent type of HTN in childhood, especially in adolescents. Secondary HTN is more common in younger children <6 years of age and children and adolescents with more severe HTN.

For labeling HTN, high BP should be measured on three different occasion. 24-hour ambulatory BP monitoring (ABPM) may be used for further confirmation of diagnosis of HTN and assess pharmacological control **(Table 9)**.

TABLE 6: Assessment of hypertension by 4th versus 5th report.

5th report	*4th report*
Reference values were established based on normal-weight children	Values were based on the entire population, at all weight levels
The sex-specific, age-specific, and height-specific values for screening are lower	Corresponding values are higher than 5th report
HBP was defined as measured SBP and/or DBP at least 95th percentile of age, sex, and height percentiles for children up to 12 years of age; however, for adolescents aged 13–17 years, HBP was defined as at least 130/80 mm Hg, with no adjustment for age, sex, or height	HBP was defined as measured SBP and/or DBP at least 95th percentile of age, sex, and height percentiles for children up to 17 years of age

(DBP: diastolic blood pressure; HBP: high blood pressure; SBP: systolic blood pressure)

TABLE 7: Ideal BP cuff for different age-group.

Age-group	*Width*	*Length*
Neonate	3–4 cm	5–8 cm
Infant	5–6 cm	8–9 cm
Child	7–9 cm	13–18 cm
Adolescent	10–13 cm	24 cm
Large arm	16–18 cm	34–38 cm
Thigh	20 cm	42 cm

TABLE 8: 2017 the American Academy of Pediatrics (AAP) guideline criteria for pediatric hypertension diagnosis.

BP category	*Age <13 years*	*Age ≥13 years*
Normal BP	<90th percentile for age, sex, and height	<120/<80 mm Hg
Elevated BP	90th to <95th percentile for age, sex, and height	≥120/<80 to 129/<80 mm Hg
Stage 1 hypertension	≥95th percentile to 95th percentile plus 11 mm Hg	130–139/80–89 mm Hg
Stage 2 hypertension	≥95th percentile plus 12 mm Hg	≥140/≥90 mm Hg

TABLE 9: BP phenotypes according to office and ambulatory BP.

Category	*Office BP*	*Ambulatory BP*
White-coat hypertension	Hypertension	Normal
Masked hypertension	Normal	Hypertension
Normotensive	Normal	Normal
Ambulatory hypertension	Hypertension	Hypertensive

Masked HTN to be ruled out in cases of solitary kidney, chronic kidney disease, history of coarctation of aorta, obesity, prematurity, and diabetes mellitus patient.

EXAMINATION OF CARDIOVASCULAR SYSTEM

Precordial Areas

- *Apex (also known as apical area or mitral area):* Corresponds to position of the apex beat and its surrounding areas, represents the location for identifying events of mitral valve and left ventricle; examination of apex (i.e., palpation and auscultation) is usually done with patient in left lateral position, except for location of apex.
- *Left lower sternal border (also known as tricuspid area):* Corresponds to left 4th intercostal space just lateral to sternum, represents the location for identifying events of tricuspid valve and right ventricle; examination is done with patient in supine position.
- *Left upper sternal border (also known as pulmonary area):* Corresponds to left 2nd intercostal space just lateral to sternum; represents the location for identifying events of pulmonary valve and main pulmonary artery
- *Right upper sternal border (also known as aortic area):* Corresponds to right 2nd intercostal space just lateral to sternum, represents the location for identifying events of aortic valve and ascending aorta
  - Examination of base of the heart (pulmonary and aortic area) is done with patient sitting and leaning forward.
- *Other areas:* Neo aortic area (left 3rd intercostal space) represents the location for identifying events of aortic valve (particularly AR) and pulmonary infundibulum.

Precordial Examination

Inspection

Inspection should be done from head end or foot end of the patient with patient lying comfortably in supine position.

- *Precordial bulge:* We have to look for whether the precordium or the left hemithorax (usually; may be right hemithorax in case of dextrocardia) is more elevated than the other side. Precordial bulge signifies dilatation of one or more cardiac chambers for a significant period and also the onset is in early childhood. For example, precordial bulge in a 12-year-old boy with mitral regurgitation (MR) suggests that the MR is either congenital or acquired in early childhood, rather than rheumatic or associated with recent-onset dilated cardiomyopathy (DCM).
- *Pulsation:* Any visible pulsation should be noted over the precordial areas (apex, left lower sternal border, left upper sternal border, right upper sternal border), epigastrium, suprasternal notch, and in neck.
- *Scar mark:* Scar mark from previous cardiac surgery should be noted along with its location and extent, e.g., midline scar (involves sternotomy), posterolateral thoracotomy scar (used in PDA ligation, coarctation of aorta repair, etc.).
- *Venous prominence:* Prominent superficial veins over precordium may suggest superior vena cava (SVC) or inferior vena cava (IVC) obstruction.

Palpation

Precordial palpation is carried out over the areas of precordium discussed earlier.

- *Apex:* Cardiac apex is defined as the downmost and outermost part of the precordium where a definite cardiac impulse is felt. It is palpated with the palm and fingers of the outstretched hand with patient in supine position, and then tried to localize with the fingertips. If it is not well discernible, patient should be asked lie in left lateral position for better localization and feeling. But location should only be marked in supine position for accuracy.
  - *Location:* Normally apex is always located just medial to the left midclavicular line at 5th intercostal space (older children and adults) or 4th intercostal space (infants and young children). Only outward shift suggests RV enlargement, whereas downward ± outward shift suggests enlargement of LV.
  - *Character:* Normally LV is apex-forming and the character is known as "tapping". Different other characters of the apex are as follows:
    - *Hyperkinetic:* Forceful and ill-sustained, type of LV apex, seen in LV volume overload/dilated LV

TABLE 10: Types of cardiac apex.

Apex	*LV apex*	*RV apex*
Location/shift	Down ± outward	Outward
Localized	Yes	No
Character	Hyperkinetic or heaving	Diffuse
Retraction	Medial	Lateral

- *Heaving:* Forceful and well sustained, type of LV apex, seen in LV pressure overload/left ventricular hypertrophy (LVH)
- *Diffuse:* Spread over more than one intercostal space and cannot be localized well, characteristic of RV apex, seen in RV volume overload/dilated RV **(Table 10)**
- *Thrill:* Whether present or not; if present, systolic/diastolic (should be included in the palpation of all the areas)

- *Lower left sternal border:* This area is palpated with ulnar border of the examiner's hand or alternately, palm may also be used. Parasternal heave, if found, is graded as follows:
  - *Grade I:* Parasternal pulsation
  - *Grade II:* Parasternal Lift, found in RV volume overload/dilated RV, analogous to hyperkinetic apex
  - *Grade III:* Parasternal heave, found in right ventricular hypertrophy (RVH), analogous to heaving apex
- *Base of the heart:* It includes both aortic and pulmonary areas and should be palpated simultaneously by keeping the examiner's palm along the 2nd intercostal space on both sides of the sternum.
  - Any palpable sound at this area should be considered as P2 unless proved otherwise. P2 is palpable in case of significant PAH.
- *Epigastrium:* Epigastric pulsation should also be looked for and it denotes RV enlargement.

Percussion

- Percussion is the least important step in cardiovascular examination and can very well be omitted if there is no compelling indication (e.g., suspected moderate-to-large pericardial effusion, where left heart border can be delineated well beyond position of the apex).
- Percussion involves determination of right and left heart border by sequential percussion from lateral to medial, parallel to the corresponding heart border. Appearance of dullness indicates that the heart border is reached.

Auscultation

Precordial auscultation should also be performed sequentially according to the precordial areas discussed. But, for the sake of better representation, the findings should be described in the following scheme:

- *Heart sounds:*
  - First heart sound (S1): S1 is produced due to closure of the AV valves (atrioventricular valves). It has two components, M1 and T1, due to closure of the mitral and tricuspid valves, respectively. Clinically separation of these two sounds is not possible and not warranted also. Intensity of S1 needs to be commented upon, whether it is normal, loud or soft.
    - *Loud S1:* Found in MS (loud M1) and tricuspid stenosis (loud T1)
    - *Soft S1:* Found in MR and pericardial effusion (both S1 and S2 are soft or muffled in PE)
    - *Normal S1:* For rest of the conditions, S1 should be described as of normal intensity.
  - *Second heart sound (S2):* S2 is produced due to closure of the semilunar valves. It has two components, A2 and P2, due to closure of the aortic and pulmonary valves, respectively. Splitting of S2 can be appreciated in normal individuals also, which is known as physiological split.
    - *Physiological split:* Physiologically A2 occurs earlier than P2 by 30–40 msec particularly during inspiration due to inspiratory decrease in the impedance of the pulmonary vascular bed allowing prolongation of RV systole. So, physiological split is heard only during inspiration and not in expiration.
    - *Pathological split:* Pathological split can be of the following types:
      - *Wide and variable split:* Split is wider than normal and is heard in both the phases of respiration, but it is still wider in inspiration than in expiration, e.g., severe MR, moderate-to-large VSD (shortened LV systole), severe PS with intact interventricular septum (IVS), and complete right bundle branch block (RBBB) (prolonged RV systole).

- *Wide and fixed split:* Split is wide and there is no respiratory variation, because of fixed stroke volume of RV and LV in all phases of respiration, e.g., large atrial septal defect (ASD).
- *Paradoxical split:* When P2 occurs earlier than A2 particularly during expiration, split is audible only in expiration and not in inspiration. This is known as paradoxical split, e.g., severe AS and complete left bundle branch block (LBBB).

- *Single S2:* S2 can be single because of the following reasons:
  - *Absent P2:* Pulmonary atresia, critical PS, and truncus arteriosus
  - *Absent A2:* Aortic atresia, and critical AS
  - *Fusion of A2 and P2:* VSD with Eisenmenger, single ventricle physiology
- *Intensity of individual components:*
  - *Loud A2:* Intensity of A2 can be increased due to increased pressure in the aorta (e.g., systemic HTN, coarctation of Aorta) or relative anterior displacement of the aorta [e.g., TOF, TGA (transposition of the great arteries)].
  - *Soft A2:* A2 is found to be soft in significant AS or AR.
  - *Loud P2:* Normally, A2 is louder than P2 in left 2nd ICS and P2 is not heard at the apex. If P2 is audible at the apex or is louder than A2 at left 2nd ICS, it is classified as loud P2. Loud P2 usually indicates PAH.
  - *Soft P2:* Soft P2 is a feature of significant PS or PR due to absent pulmonary valve.

- *Third heart sound (S3):* S3 is produced due to resistance of rapid ventricular filling in early diastole by the corresponding ventricle. So, S3 can be produced by either LV (LVS3) or RV (RVS3).
  - It is a low-pitched sound.
  - It is often better palpable than audible.
  - S3 is heard best with the bell of the stethoscope.
  - It is heard over apex (LVS3) or left lower sternal border (RVS3).
  - It is an early diastolic sound heard immediately after S2.
  - Causes:
    - *LVS3:* Conditions with LV volume overload, such as severe MR, significant AR, moderate-to-large left to right shunts (VSD, PDA), LV dysfunction, etc.
    - *RVS3:* Conditions with RV volume overload, such as severe TR, large ASD, right heart failure, etc.
- *Fourth heart sound (S4):* S4 is produced due to stiff ventricles resisting atrial contraction-induced ventricular filling in late diastole. S4 can also be produced by either LV (LVS4) or RV (RVS4).
  - It is also a low-pitched sound like S3.
  - S4 is often better palpable than audible.
  - It is heard best with the bell of the stethoscope.
  - It is heard over apex (LVS4) or left lower sternal border (RVS4).
  - It is a late diastolic or presystolic sound heard immediately before S1.
  - Causes:
    - *LVS4:* Conditions with LV pressure overload, such as severe AS, HOCM, systemic HTN, coarctation of aorta, etc.
    - *RVS4:* Conditions with RV pressure overload, such as significant PAH, severe PS with intact IVS, etc.
- *Gallop rhythm:* It is an auscultatory phenomenon with tripling or quadrupling of heart sounds, which resembles the canter of a horse. Tachycardia is also a prerequisite to produce gallop rhythm. Most common cause is heart failure. The following types are there:
  - S3 gallop (diastolic gallop)—addition of S3 to S1 and S2
  - S4 gallop (presystolic gallop or atrial gallop)—addition of S4 to S1 and S2
  - Quadruple gallop—all the four heart sounds are audible in succession.

- *Additional sounds:*
  - *Ejection click (ECs):* ECs are sounds produced during opening of the semilunar valves. They can be aortic or pulmonary in origin. These are high-pitched, early systolic sounds heard just after S1 at the end of isovolumetric contraction period. Causes include AS (aortic EC) and PS (pulmonary EC); more likely to occur with mild rather than severe stenosis of the corresponding valve.
  - *Non-EC:* It refers to the click originating in the AV valves. Most common example is midsystolic click of MVP, which occurs due to systolic prolapse of MV leaflet into the LA. It is also a high-pitched sound.

- *Opening snap (OS):* This early diastolic sound is produced by forceful opening of the mobile and pliable AV valves at the end of isovolumetric relaxation period. Causes are MS, tricuspid stenosis, etc. In MS, S2–OS gap is inversely proportional to LA pressure, i.e., more severe the stenosis, more the LA pressure, earlier is the OS after S2.
- *Pericardial knock:* It is also an early to mid-diastolic sound, produced due to sudden cessation of ventricular filling in constrictive pericarditis.

▪ *Murmur:* Cardiac murmur is defined as a series of auditory vibrations that can be heard on auscultation. Murmurs are classified according to the phase of cardiac cycle as follows:
  - *Systolic murmur:* A systolic murmur begins at or after S1 and ends before or at S2. It can be further classified into:
    - *Pansystolic murmur (PSM):* It starts with S1 and continues up to S2 or may end just before S2. Causes are VSD, MR, and TR.
    - *Ejection systolic murmur (ESM):* Also known as midsystolic murmur; it starts at a clear interval after S1 and ends at or before S2. It usually follows a crescendo–decrescendo character. Causes are AS and PS.
    - *Early systolic murmur:* It also begins at S1 like the PSM, but ends early, usually before midsystole. Causes are small muscular VSD (defect closes off during ventricular contraction at systole) and acute severe MR (very high LA pressure causes early equalization of LA and LV pressures).
    - *Late systolic murmur:* It starts at around midsystole and continues up to S2. Causes are MVP-associated MR.
  - *Diastolic murmur:* Diastolic murmur is heard between S2 and S1, i.e., during ventricular diastole. It can also be subclassified into:
    - *Mid-diastolic murmur (MDM):* It starts at a clear interval after S2, but continues till S1 or may end just before S1. Causes are MDMs are classically associated with AV valve stenosis, i.e., MS and TS, or due to increased flow across an unobstructed AV valve, e.g., mitral MDM in VSD or PDA and tricuspid MDM in ASD.
    - *Early diastolic murmur (EDM):* It begins with A2 or P2 depending on the site of origin and continues in a decrescendo manner beyond mid-diastole, sometimes up to S1. Causes are AR and PR.
  - *Continuous murmur:* Murmurs that begin in systole and then continue without interruption through the S2 into all or part of the diastole are known as continuous murmurs. Examples are:
    - Communication between high-pressure and low-pressure zone:
      - Restrictive PDA
      - Surgical aortopulmonary shunt (e.g., BT shunt)
      - AV fistula (e.g., vein of Galen malformation, acquired for hemodialysis, etc.)
      - Rupture of sinus of Valsalva (to RA, RV, or LA)
    - Narrowing of artery:
      - Tight coarctation of the aorta
      - Severe peripheral PS
      - Renal artery stenosis
    - Increased flow velocity in veins:
      - Venous hum
      - Supracardiac TAPVC (total anomalous pulmonary venous connection)
  - *Grading of murmur (Levine's):* Murmurs are graded according to severity in a scale of I to VI as follows:
    - *Grade I:* Very faint, may only be heard by an expert, not heard in all positions, no thrill
    - *Grade II:* Soft, heard in all positions, no thrill
    - *Grade III:* Moderately loud, no thrill
    - *Grade IV:* Loud, associated with thrill
    - *Grade V:* Very loud, with thrill, heard with the stethoscope partly off the chest
    - *Grade VI:* Loudest, with thrill, heard with the stethoscope entirely off the chest (just above the precordium, not touching the skin)
  - *Description of a murmur:* Following points should be mentioned while describing a murmur:
    - *Type:* PSM, ESM, MDM, continuous murmur, etc.
    - *Grade:* I–VI
    - *Pitch:* High (murmur of AR), low (murmur of MS), or medium (most of the other murmurs can be characterized as medium-pitched)
    - *Character:* Rumbling (MS), blowing (AR), machinery (PDA), etc. need to be added as a part of classical description of that murmur.
    - *Location (area of maximum intensity):* In smaller children, many murmurs are audible all over the

precordium. But, we need to find out the area where it is heard best.

- *Radiation/conduction:* Radiation means that the murmur is heard at almost the same intensity at an adjoining or nearby area and it follows the direction of the flowing blood which causes that particular murmur, e.g., MR murmur radiates to left axilla, VSD murmur to right lower parasternal area, AR murmur to apex, and AS murmur to neck. On the other hand, conduction refers to transmission of the sound to adjoining areas through chest wall and it is always associated with diminution of intensity.
- *Position of patient:* Supine, left lateral, or sitting and leaning forward, where the murmur is best audible.
- *Diaphragm/bell of stethoscope:* Low-pitched murmurs are best heard with bell, whereas diaphragm is better for medium and high-pitched murmurs.
- *Phase of respiration:* Usually left-sided events are better heard in expiration and right-sided events in inspiration.

CASE SCENARIOS

Case 1: Ventricular Septal Defect

A 4-month-old infant presents with poor feeding, failure to thrive, and recurrent respiratory infections. On physical examination, the infant has tachycardia and is tachypneic with mild intercostal retractions. You auscultate a loud, harsh systolic murmur at the left upper sternal border. There is no cyanosis. Hepatomegaly is present.

Q. What clinical findings are typical for a ventricular septal defect (VSD)? How would you characterize the murmur on auscultation, and what are the next steps in the physical examination and diagnostic workup? What is the origin of the murmur?

Ans. The scenario represents an acyanotic congenital heart disease, in failure. The most common disorder is a VSD. Given that the VSD is causing congestive cardiac failure (tachycardia, hepatomegaly), hyperkinetic pulmonary HTN (respiratory symptoms), and failure to thrive, it is likely to be large.

Typical findings in such a case would be down and out shifted apex beat signifying cardiomegaly, loud P2 (pulmonary HTN), and a grade II–III ESM at the left upper sternal edge, created due to extra flow through a normal pulmonary valve. An additional mid-diastolic murmur at the apex is due to increased diastolic flow through mitral valve.

Note that the VSD itself, being large, leads to equalization of left and right ventricular pressures during systole, and therefore does not produce a murmur.

Initial workup would consist of a chest X-ray, to look for pulmonary plethora, cardiomegaly, ECG for evidence of volume overload of LV, and an echocardiogram for definitive diagnosis and anatomic details.

Case 2: Atrial Septal Defect

A 7-year-old child presents for a routine school physical examination and is asymptomatic. On auscultation, you hear a wide, fixed split S2 and a systolic ejection murmur at the upper left sternal border. The child has no history of fatigue, shortness of breath, or chest pain.

Q. What findings on clinical examination are suggestive of ASD? How would you describe the characteristics of the heart sounds and the murmur? What are the typical ECG findings of the condition?

Ans. Physical examination findings: A fixed, wide split S2 and a systolic ejection murmur at the upper left sternal border are suggestive of an ASD.

Various theories have been proposed for the reason of wide fixed split of the S2, most widely accepted one being that the split S2 occurs due to prolonged right ventricular systole from increased blood flow to the right side of the heart.

Being located between two chambers with minimal pressure difference, the ASD itself is silent, and murmur takes its origin from increased flow through a normal pulmonary valve.

A transthoracic echocardiogram is used to confirm the diagnosis and assess the size of the defect.

Typical ECG findings are rsR' pattern or "crochetage sign" on ECG.

Case 3: Coarctation of the Aorta

A 3-year-old girl presents with complaints of leg weakness and difficulty walking after a mild upper respiratory infection. On physical examination, you measure a significantly higher BP in the upper limbs compared to the lower limbs. You also note absent femoral pulse, with normal radial pulses.

Q. What clinical signs on physical examination raise suspicion for coarctation of the aorta? How would you assess the differential BP readings, and what are the key X-ray findings that help establish this diagnosis?

Ans. The hallmark examination findings include a "discrepancy in BP" between the upper and lower extremities (higher BP in the arms, lower in the legs), and "weak or absent lower-limb pulses".

Typical X-ray findings include rib notching, the "3 sign" or the "E" sign.

Case 4: Tetralogy of Fallot

A 2-month-old infant presents with episodes of cyanosis, particularly during feeding or crying. On examination, you observe a "tet spell" during crying, with a rapid improvement after the baby is placed in a knee-chest position. A harsh systolic murmur is auscultated at the left sternal border.

Q. What are the key clinical findings on examination that suggest TOF? How would you describe the murmur associated with this condition, and what are the characteristic features of "tet spells" that you would look for during a physical examination? Describe the typical X-ray and ECG findings?

Ans. Key clinical findings include cyanosis, clubbing, clinical features of polycythemia, "RV" type of apex (out but not down), soft P2 (may be absent on severe restriction of pulmonary blood flow), and a grade II–III ESM at the left upper sternal edge. Note that the VSD in TOF is always large, and is clinically silent. Longer the murmur, more is the blood flow across the pulmonary valve, and lesser is the degree of cyanosis. The murmur may become shorter, softer, and even absent during a cyanotic or tet spell.

Chest X-ray shows a "core en sabot" or boot-shaped heart due to an upturned RV apex, reduced pulmonary blood flow and no cardiomegaly. ECG shows RV dominance, an "early transition" of QRS complexes.

Case 5: Heart Failure

A 4-year-old boy presents with abdominal pain, increased work of breathing and fatigue of 1-month duration. On physical examination, you note tachycardia, jugular venous distension, hepatomegaly, and intercostal retractions.. He has a gallop rhythm on auscultation. There is no failure to thrive, and parents give a history of upper respiratory tract infection symptoms 2 weeks prior to the onset of symptoms.

Q. What physical examination findings are concerning for this child? What is the significance of the history of upper respiratory tract infection symptoms?

Ans. Physical examination findings of heart failure (tachycardia, distended jugular veins, and hepatomegaly) signify left ventricular/biventricular dysfunction. It is important to note that pain abdomen is a nonspecific but common mode of presentation. Absence of failure to thrive points toward a relatively short duration of ventricular dysfunction.

Upper respiratory tract infection symptoms prior to the onset give a possible etiologic clue about viral myocarditis, which has now led to ventricular dysfunction.

Case 6: Hypercholesterolemia

A 10-year-old child presents for a routine checkup, and lipid screening reveals elevated total cholesterol (250 mg/dL) and low-density lipoprotein (LDL) cholesterol (160 mg/dL). The child is otherwise asymptomatic, with normal growth and development.

Q. What physical examination findings might be suggestive of hyperlipidemia or lipid-related disorders in children? What are the key features of familial hypercholesterolemia that may be evident on clinical examination, and what other tests would you order?

Ans. Physical examination findings: In children with familial hypercholesterolemia, xanthomas (yellowish plaques around the eyes or on the tendons), and in more severe cases, arcus cornealis (a grayish-white ring around the cornea); other associated features of metabolic syndrome (obesity, neck pigmentation, hump of fat on the nape of neck) may be there.

Next steps: Confirm the diagnosis with a lipid panel and genetic testing if necessary. The child should also be evaluated for other cardiovascular risk factors.

Management: Lifestyle modifications, including dietary changes, are recommended. Statins may be considered for children with significantly elevated LDL levels despite lifestyle changes or those with a family history of early heart disease

Case 7: Infective Endocarditis

A 6-year-old boy with a history of repaired congenital heart disease (VSD closure) presents for a routine dental procedure. The dentist asks whether the child needs antibiotics for endocarditis prophylaxis.

Q. What physical examination findings would suggest that this child has an increased risk of IE? What are the key components of a clinical examination that might prompt you to reconsider or reinforce the need for prophylactic antibiotics in this case?

Ans. As per American Heart Association (AHA) IE prevention guidelines (2021), antibiotic prophylaxis is recommended for patients with the following conditions:

- *CHD:*
  - *Unrepaired cyanotic CHD*, including *palliative shunts* and conduits
  - *Completely repaired CHD* with prosthetic material or device (e.g., prosthetic valve or conduit) during the first 6 months after the procedure
  - *Repaired CHD* with residual defects (e.g., VSD, ASD) at the site or adjacent to the prosthetic patch or device
- *Prosthetic heart valves* or *prosthetic material* used for valve repair.
- *History of IE:*
  - A previous episode of IE increases the risk of recurrence.
- *Cardiac transplantation* with *cardiac valvulopathy* (due to immune suppression or altered cardiac function).

Procedures requiring prophylaxis: Antibiotic prophylaxis is recommended for *high-risk patients* undergoing certain *dental* or *nondental invasive procedures* that could potentially cause bacteremia.

Dental procedures:

- Prophylaxis required for:
  - Procedures that involve manipulation of *gingival tissue*, the *periapical region of teeth*, or the *oral mucosa*
  - *Examples:* Extractions, periodontal procedures, dental implants, and root canal therapy
- Prophylaxis not required for:
  - Routine *dental cleanings* or noninvasive procedures (e.g., fillings, X-rays, local anesthesia administration)

Nondental procedures:

- Prophylaxis required for:
  - *Invasive procedures* on infected skin, skin structures, or musculoskeletal tissue
  - *Examples:* Surgical procedures involving prosthetic cardiac valves, prosthetic joints, or other implants
  - *Procedures that involve the respiratory tract* (e.g., tonsillectomy or adenoidectomy in patients with a high risk of IE)
  - Prophylaxis not required for:
    - GI and genitourinary (GU) procedures unless the patient has an active infection [e.g., urinary tract infection (UTI), abscess].
    - Routine procedures like *bronchoscopy* or *cystoscopy* in low-risk patients.

SUGGESTED READING

1. A Practical Handbook on Pediatric Cardiac Intensive Care Therapy—Editors: Dietrich Klauwer et al.
2. Fundamentals of Pediatric Cardiology (Driscoll).
3. Moller's Essentials of Pediatric Cardiology.
4. Moss & Adams' Heart Disease in infants, Children, and Adolescents: Including the Fetus and Young Adult.
5. Nadas' Pediatric Cardiology by John F. Keane (Editor); Donald C. Fyler; James E. Lock.
6. Park's Pediatric Cardiology for Practitioners.
7. Pediatric Cardiology Handbook by Rajveer Bainiwal & Suryalata Kookna.
8. Practical Pediatric Cardiology: Case-Based Management of Potential Pitfalls — Editors: Alan G. Magee, Jan Till, Anna N. Seale.

Examination of the Respiratory System and Its Disorders

Samik Basu

INTRODUCTION

Examination of the respiratory system involves both the upper respiratory tract and the lower respiratory tract: *Do not miss the upper respiratory tract.*

EXAMINE THE CHEST: INCLUDES THE CHEST WALL ONLY

History Taking

Never miss taking a good history, as it will lead you to the relevant part to be examined. You all have a limited time for the examination of the patient.

Always introduce yourself. Take permission to examine and undress the child, and dress the child after examination. Thank the mother and child.

RELEVANT HISTORY

Upper Respiratory Tract

Rhinorrhea, blocked nose, recurrent sneezing, green or bloody nasal discharge, recurrent ear infections, etc.

Lower Respiratory Tract

- History of fever, cough, breathlessness, and chest pain may indicate lung causes such as consolidation, collapse, and empyema.
- History of cough, wheezing, and breathlessness may lead to asthma.
- History of cough, choking, breathlessness may indicate a foreign body.
- History of persistent cough, delayed passage of meconium, short stature, failure to thrive, recurrent infections may lead to cystic fibrosis or ciliary disorders.
- Diurnal variation of symptoms, use of devices, hospitalizations, and ventilation should not be missed.
- A good family/developmental and nutritional history should not be missed to detect congenital/genetic or acquired respiratory ailments.
- History of measles, pertussis, missed immunization, contact with tuberculosis, overcrowding, polluting environment, pets, and cigarette smoking should not be missed.

Remember, a good history will cover the complaints, duration, progression, variations, aggravating factors, and relieving factors, as well as a complete treatment history and a history of allergies (especially in respiratory cases).

The usual symptoms should to be inquired upon are including special symptoms, and relevant history should be taken once you are close to a provisional diagnosis based upon initial history.

COMMON SYMPTOMS

- Cough
- Fever
- Breathlessness
- Wheezing
- Chest pain
- Hemoptysis
- Heaviness in the chest
- Epistaxis, failure to thrive, short stature, recurrent infections, etc.

Apart from examining the patient from head to toe for a few minutes to get a general impression, we start the systemic examination per se.

UPPER RESPIRATORY TRACT (EXTERNAL NARES TO THE TRACHEA)

- Nose (congestion, discharge, hypertrophied turbinate, bleeding spots, and polyp) and nasal septum (deviation); alae nasi (nasal flare).
- Mouth breathing (e.g., adenoids), halitosis, poor dentition (due to mouth breathing), adenoid facies, and drooling.
- Air sinuses (examine for tenderness over the maxilla; ask the patient to sit and lean forward, whether any heaviness on the forehead is complained of or not).

- Pharynx (throat, gum, teeth, palate, posterior pharyngeal wall, postnasal drip), nasopharynx, tonsils with oral hygiene; halitosis present or not
- Larynx, unfortunately, cannot be inspected without sedating the child. This examination cannot be done in children.

Clinical Methods

History of nasal voice:
- *Obstructed nares:* Maybe diagnosed by placing a wisp of cotton below each nostril and observing movement. You can also look for mist in a glass slide or mirror placed under each nose during expiration.
- *Submucous cleft palate:* Can only be diagnosed by palpating the palate.

Other than this, one should try to:
- Look for nasal discharge, deformity, and deviated nasal septum.
- Examine frontal and maxillary sinus tenderness.
- Look for an impacted foreign body if there is foul-smelling discharge/bloody discharge from one nostril.

Examination of the face:
- *If there is a history of asthma/wheeze, try to look for:*
    - Allergic shiners
    - Allergic salute
    - Dennie Morgan's line

EXAMINATION OF THE ORAL CAVITY

- Size of the oral cavity, large tongue, malformed teeth, or caries.
- Uvula, palate, symmetry, size of tonsils, postwall of pharynx (cobblestone/postnasal drip).

Other than this, always palpate the sinuses for tenderness and NEVER forget to examine the ear with an otoscope (If time permits, *do not miss this*).

EXAMINATION OF THE CHEST

Inspection

Examination of the chest is best done in a standing or sitting position. Examine the patient from the front, back, and also above the shoulder. If the patient is supinated, do look over the chest from the head end, leg end, and also from the sides.

Points to note:
- Symmetry, bulge, flatness, shape of the chest as a whole, visible apex beat, if any
- *Shape of the chest:*
    - *Barrel chest:* Emphysema in adults and in severe bronchial asthma.
    - *Unilateral bulging:* Empyema necessitates and tension pneumothorax.
    - *Flattening:* collapse of the lung, congenitally absent pectoralis major
    - *Broad shield-like chest:* Turner's syndrome
    - *Small thoracic cage:* Ellis Van Crevald Syndrome

Pectus excavatum: Funnel chest is the depression of the lower part of the sternum, usually seen in rickets and Marfan syndrome. Severe forms may shift the apex to the left.

Pectus carinatum: Pigeon chest is a marked protrusion of the sternum, seldom seen in large congenital cardiomegaly (untreated), was previously erroneously associated with rickets erroneously.

Harrison's sulcus: Historically associated with rickets, a depression along the attachment of the diaphragm, due to the traction of the diaphragm on a weak chest wall.

Rickety rosary: These are elevated knob like swellings of the costochondral junctions seen in rickets. Scorbutic Rosary is the protrusion of ribs due to displacement; they are sharper than those one in rickets.

- *Abnormalities:* Absent nipple, accessory nipple, scars, aspiration site, indwelling tubes or catheters, pulse oximeters, etc.
- Trachea, sternocleidomastoids, type of respiration, respiratory rate, and movement of accessory muscles of respiration should be noted (alae nasi, contraction of sternocleidomastoids, indrawing of supraclavicular fossa, head bobbing, etc.)
- *Respiratory rate:* Rate can be measured by counting the number of chest rises (inspiration) in a 1-minute cycle. If the child is smaller, you can also gently keep your warm hand on the chest and feel the rise of chest/min.
    - *Respiratory rates in children:* See chart. The normal ratio of respiration to pulse rate is 1:4 it decreases in cases of pneumonia.
    - *Tachypnea:* Usually, seen in excitement during examination, fever, acidosis, heart disease (in fever, for every degree rise in temperature, the rate increases by 5 breaths/min.
    - *Bradypnea:* Usually seen in narcotic poisoning, raised ICT, metabolic alkalosis, and hypothyroidism.

- *Type and rhythm:*
  - Usually, it is abdominothoracic in children.
  - When there is an abdominal pathology, it becomes predominantly thoracic in nature, e.g., massive ascites, large organomegaly, abdominal injury, or mass.
  - *Very rapid and deep breathing:* KUSSMAUL breathing—diabetic ketoacidosis/aspirin poisoning.
  - *Rapid and shallow breathing*—pneumonia and pulmonary edema.
  - *Prolonged inspiration*—upper airway obstruction.
  - *Prolonged expiration*—lower airway obstruction.
  - Gradual increase in breathing, then decrease in breathing, followed by a period of apnea. Cheyne-Stokes breathing is seen in severe heart failure (Unusual in children).
  - If the trachea is shifted to one side, the sternocleidomastoid becomes prominent on that side-TRAIL sign.
- Venous prominence.
- Supraclavicular and infraclavicular fossae.
- Accessory muscles of respiration and intercostal suction.
- *Back:* Scoliosis, kyphosis, drooping of the shoulder, winging of the scapula, venous prominence, sinus or puncture mark.

Palpation

- Surface temperature.
- Tenderness (rib tenderness in trauma, fracture, or secondary metastasis; intercostal tenderness or punch tenderness in liver abscess or empyema thoracis).
- Corroboration of the findings of inspection—examine the spinal deformity, direction of venous flow, details of any swelling present, parietal edema, etc.
- Position of the trachea and the apex beat (i.e., position of the mediastinum).

  Palpate the trachea using the middle finger on the trachea and using the ring and index fingers, assess the space between the trachea and the sternocleidomastoids on either side. The space is narrowed on the side to which the trachea is shifted.

  Shift of the apex beat is to be recorded if there is a massive shift in the mediastinum. Apex beat is difficult to document in cases of obesity, emphysema, pericardial effusion, or if it falls under a rib.
- Movement of the chest (always measure the expansion of the chest with a tape in full inspiration and in full expiration).

  Place your two hands on either side of your chest and stretch your thumbs to the midline. With movement of the chest, note the movement of the thumbs from the midline; asymmetry shows less movement on one side.

  For apical movements of the lung, place your hands on the supraclavicular fossa on both sides from behind the point, bringing the thumb in the midline at the back.

  Placing the patient in the supine position, placing one hand on the chest and the other on the abdomen, and asking the patient to take deep breaths. Usually, both hands should be lifted during inspiration. Paradoxical respiration is seen in Diaphragmatic palsy.
- Vocal fremitus. It is palpated all over the areas of the chest with the ulnar surface of the palm. Actually, palpable vocal resonance. It is difficult to demonstrate in children who have a smaller chest wall. It is not so significant in an examination if you have performed a good vocal resonance later on.

  Is the palpation of laryngeal vibrations on the chest wall when the patient speaks some words repeatedly in a constant tone and voice (e.g., "one, one" or "99, 99"). Place the palm of the hand (thenar and hypothenar eminences) or the ulnar border of the right hand over the intercostal spaces on the chest, comparing the corresponding areas on both sides. Always use the same hand for examining both sides (use the right hand). Avoid the area of cardiac dullness on the left side and place the hand a bit laterally. Start from above downward in the front, sides, and back of the chest.

Different types of fremitus over the chest: Fremitus is synonymous with "palpable vibrations." The different types are:

- Vocal fremitus.
- Rhonchial fremitus (palpable rhonchi; rhonchi are better felt than crepitations).
- Friction fremitus (palpable pleural rub).
- *Tactile fremitus:*
  - Palpable coarse crepitations.
  - Palpable subcutaneous emphysema.
  - Palpable pericardial rub.

PERCUSSION

It is done to note the resonance or dullness of an organ, and also to know the:

- Content (state of underlying tissue, i.e., whether a solid organ, fluid, or gas is present. Usually, by percussion, we get an idea up to a depth of 2 inches). It also indirectly diagnoses tenderness (empyema or liver abscess). Remember, in adults, a lesion <2 cm does not make any change in the percussion note.
- The things we need to note during percussion are percussion notes, liver and cardiac dullness, coin percussion, shifting dullness, tidal percussion, and Traube's space percussion.

Technique

Usually done in the sitting position. From the front, back, and on the apical regions, as well as directly on the clavicle. One may start percussion from the apparently healthy side, or the right side of the chest.

- The dorsal aspect of the middle phalanx of the middle finger of the left hand (the PLEXIMETER FINGER) is kept tightly over the chest wall (i.e., over intercostal spaces), and is struck suddenly with the tip of the middle finger of the right hand (the *percussing* or *plexor finger*) perpendicularly (with "hammer effect"). The entire movement is delivered from the wrist joint, and not from the elbow. Strike once or twice on the pleximeter finger (avoid repeated heavy striking). The other fingers of the left hand should not touch the chest wall.
- Direct percussion is done over bones, and indirect percussion is done for other areas. First percuss the *clavicle* (direct percussion) and then the anterior chest wall along the midclavicular line (MCL). The first palpable interspace in the anterior chest wall is the second intercostal space (ICS). Keep the hands by the side in a resting position while percussing on the anterior chest wall along the MCL.

During percussion of the *axilla* along MAL, the patient's hands are kept over his head.

While percussing the *back*, cross the patient's hands over the knees or shoulders (this position is wide apart the scapulae), and percuss in a bat's-wing or fish-bone pattern.

Lastly, percuss the *apex* of the lung from the back of the patient, keeping the patient's hands by the side.

Always percuss from *above downward* and compare the note on the identical site on the opposite side of the chest.

While percussing on the left side of the anterior chest wall, always follow the left MCL (do not deviate laterally, because the most outer border of cardiac dullness lies 1/2 inch inside the left MCL).

Areas of percussion over the chest:

- *Anterior chest wall:*
    - Over the clavicle (direct percussion)
    - Infraclavicular area (clavicle to third rib)
    - Mammary area (third to sixth rib)
    - Inframammary area (sixth rib to seventh ICS).
- Lateral chest wall (right and left side).
    - Axillary area (fourth ICS to sixth rib).
    - Infra-axillary area (sixth rib to eighth ICS or lower costal margin).
- *Posterior chest wall (right and left side):*
    - Suprascapular (above the upper border of the scapula).
    - Interscapular (between the medial border of the scapula and spine—>T2 to T7 vertebrae—>in a fish-bone pattern' percussion).
    - Infrascapular (below the inferior angle of the scapula—>T7 to Tn vertebrae).
- *Apical (or supraclavicular area):* Always done from the back.

How do you count the ribs and ICS in clinical practice?

First, place the right index finger in the suprasternal notch and then go downward till the *sternal angle* (angle of Louis), which is a transverse bony ridge (junction of the body of the sternum and manubrium sterni). If the finger is moved sideways, it will touch the second rib. Now count the ribs with ICS from above downward.

Posteriorly, the ribs and ICS are counted from below upward (difficulty faced in a muscular body or in an obese patient). If the arms rest by the side of the body, the inferior angle of the scapula lies at the level of the seventh rib.

Note: Angle of Louis or sternal angle (i.e., the level of second costal cartilage) marks the disc space between T4 and T5 vertebrae posteriorly, and anteriorly it marks the tracheal bifurcation.

Percussion Notes

The lung is resonant on percussion, while the abdomen is tympanitic.

When the air in a cavity of significant capacity size is vibrating, the character of the sound becomes tympanitic, e.g., in the case of percussion over the stomach. On the other side, a resonant note is heard over the lung alveoli, which are small pockets of air separated by numerous septa.

Resonant Note

- Tympanitic (abdomen and pneumothorax) of the lung.
- Hyperresonant (emphysema).
- Resonant (normal lung).
- Impaired resonance (thickened pleura).

Tympanitic Note

- Pneumothorax.
- Superficial, big, and empty cavities.
- Over a large emphysematous bulla.

Dull note

- Woody dullness (consolidation
- Stony dullness (pleural effusion)
- Over Traube's space.

Note: Remember, a tympanitic note is elicited on percussion over any hollow viscus.

Hyper-resonant Note

- Emphysema.
- Occasionally, over a lung cyst.

Impaired Note (Slightly Diminished Normal Resonance)

- Thickened pleura.
- Fibrosis of the lungs.
- Collapse of the lung

Dull note:

- Consolidation (woody dullness).
- Pleural effusion, empyema thoracis, and over the "hydro" part of hydropneumothorax (stony dullness).

Traube's Semilunar Space

This is a triangular space or semilunar topographic area in the left lower chest anteriorly, which is bounded by:

- *Laterally:* Left midaxillary line.
- *Above:* Left dome of diaphragm and left lung, i.e., the sixth rib. Below, left lower costal margin.

Importance: Normally, the space is tympanitic on percussion as it contains the fundus of the stomach.

It is lost in:

- Left-sided pleural effusion.
- Enlarged left lobe of liver.
- Massively enlarged spleen or ruptured spleen.
- Situs inversus totalis (Traube's space is present on the right side).

Traube's space is shifted upward in fibrosis or collapse of the left lower lobe of the lung and left-sided diaphragmatic palsy.

Tidal Percussion

While percussing during delineating the lower border of the lung, there is a difference in resonance by one space in full inspiration. It happens to be due to the downward movement of the diaphragm.

Method

The patient will sit with hands crossed over the knees or shoulders. First, *percuss the lower* back along the scapular line at the end of forced expiration, and then percuss the same place at the height of full inspiration. Note the increase in resonance by one space after full inspiration.

Clinical Importance

- Paradoxical resonance, i.e., there is a dull note on inspiration and a resonant note on expiration due to the paradoxical movement of the diaphragm in diaphragmatic palsy.
- Dullness that does not change on inspiration or expiration indicates basal pneumonia, basal pleurisy or subdiaphragmatic abscess.

SHIFTING OF THE UPPER BORDER OF LIVER DULLNESS

To delineate the upper border of liver dullness, percuss the anterior chest wall along the right MCL from above downward. Normally, the upper border of liver dullness is present in the right fifth ICS at MCL.

Lowered or obliterated:

- Emphysema.
- Pneumothorax (right-sided).
- Cirrhosis of the liver (liver becomes small).
- Visceroptosis of the liver.

Elevated:
- Amoebic or pyogenic liver abscess.
- Subdiaphragmatic abscess (right).
- Diaphragmatic palsy (right).
- Pleural effusion (right).
- Basal pneumonia (right).

Auscultation: This is the most important aspect of the examination of the respiratory system. Always use a very good quality pediatric stethoscope. Always warm your hands and the diaphragm before examining a child.

Areas:
- *Upper lobes:* Upper anterior chest.
- *Lower lobe sounds:* Posterior lower chest.
- *Middle lobe and lingula:* Sides of the lower third of the sternum.
- *All lobes:* Lateral chest, in the axilla.

BREATH SOUNDS

Vesicular Breath Sounds

Normal breath sounds over the lungs are vesicular. During examinations, one should note whether they are of normal intensity or reduced intensity. Usually, the breath sounds are louder over the right apical region (anatomical position of the right bronchus); similarly, lower intensity of breath sounds is heard over the left precordium (position of the heart).

Increased intensity of vesicular breath sounds: Excitation, exertion, or on the normal side where the other side is affected by pathology (pl effusion/pneumothorax).

Decreased intensity of vesicular breath sounds: Pleural effusion, pneumothorax, pleural thickening, and respiratory paralysis.

Bronchial Breath Sounds

If you want to hear bronchial sounds, place the stethoscope directly on the trachea. Remember and identify the sound. It is harsher, expiration is equal to inspiration, and *there is a definite gap* between inspiration and expiration.

Types of bronchial breathing:
- *Cavernous:* Lower-pitched over a cavity (C for C).
- *Tubular:* High-pitched, usually heard over a consolidation.
- *Amphoric:* Specialized tubular breathing sound. Sounds like blowing into a bottle with a narrow neck. Usually heard over a large cavity or a communicating bronchus with a pneumothorax.

Rhonchi are continuous (>80 milliseconds in duration), uninterrupted musical (dry) sound produced in the narrowed bronchi or bronchioles as a result of muscle spasm, collection of viscid secretion, mucosal edema, or narrowing by an endobronchial growth.

Monophonic rhonchi: May be inspiratory or expiratory or both, and may change in intensity with change of posture. It is produced due to the narrowing of a single bronchus by a tumor or foreign body (i.e., localized obstruction), which produces a single musical note.

Polyphonic rhonchi: Particularly heard in expiration and are characteristically found in diffuse airflow obstruction, e.g., bronchial asthma or chronic bronchitis. They denote dynamic compression of the bronchi. This is the most common type of rhonchi, where the musical sound (rhonchi) contains several notes of different pitches and results from the oscillation of many large bronchi at a time.

CREPITATIONS OR CRACKLES

Crepitations are discontinuous (<20 milliseconds in duration) bubbling or crackling (wet) sound produced by the passage of air through exudate-filled bronchi, bronchioles, alveoli, big cavity, or due to the sudden snapping open of the relatively stiff alveoli at inspiration.

Fine crepitations (end-inspiratory)—soft, high-pitched, and <10 milliseconds in duration, usually heard in left ventricular failure, fibrosis

Velcro crepitations—sound resembles as if two strips of adhered Velcro tape are being separated.

Coarse crepitations (biphasic)—Louder, low-pitched, and >10 milliseconds in duration, and are produced by exudates in the bronchi, bronchioles, alveoli, or large cavities. Most common conditions associated are acute bronchopneumonia, bronchiectasis, lung abscess, and pulmonary edema.

Recent classification of crepitations: The new terminology for crepitations is "crackles." Nowadays, crepitations are described as follows:
- To note their timing in relation to the respiratory cycle.
- If they are affected by coughing or not. Crepitations in the presence of secretions are confirmed by the observation that they either disappear temporarily or reduce in number after coughing.

Crackles without sputum production indicate interstitial lung disease, whereas crackles with sputum production may indicate pneumonia.

Late crackles: Heard at the end of inspiration. Pulmonary edema.

Coarse crackles: Bronchiectasis

Rhonchi: Rhonchi are continuous (>80 milliseconds in duration), uninterrupted musical (dry) sound produced in the narrowed bronchi or bronchioles as a result of muscle spasm, collection of viscid secretion, mucosal edema, or narrowing by an endobronchial growth. Audible rhonchi is called wheeze.

Classification: Old

- High-pitched rhonchi, which are produced in smaller bronchi or bronchioles, and of squeaky quality, are known as "SIBILANT" rhonchi (end-inspiratory or early-expiratory)—found in bronchial asthma.
- Low-pitched rhonchi, which are produced in larger bronchi and of snoring quality, are known as "SONOROUS" rhonchi (biphasic)—found in endobronchial growth affecting a large bronchus.

Classification (New)

- *Monophonic rhonchi:* May be inspiratory or expiratory, or both, and may change in intensity with a change of posture. It is produced due to the narrowing of a single bronchus by a tumor or foreign body (i.e., localized obstruction), which produces a single musical note. Usually found in foreign body obstruction, lymph node obstruction.
- *Polyphonic rhonchi:* Particularly heard in expiration and are characteristically found in diffuse airflow obstruction, e.g., bronchial asthma or chronic bronchitis. They denote dynamic compression of the bronchi. This is the most common type of rhonchi, where the musical sound (rhonchi) contains several notes of different pitches and results from the oscillation of many large bronchi at a time.

Usually, seen in bronchial asthma.

- *Stridor:* It is a musical, monophonic, high-pitched sound heard without a stethoscope caused by narrowed large extrathoracic airways (obstruction in the larynx and proximal trachea).
- *Grunting:* This is a short, hoarse, crying-like expiratory sound that occurs when a partially closed glottis halts the expiratory flow of air.
- *Snoring:* It is produced due to obstructed air movements in the nasopharynx and oropharynx.
- *Rattle:* It is created by excessive secretions during normal airflow in the central and extrathoracic airways in smaller children and infants and is usually innocuous clinically.
- *Snuffles:* Noisy breathing coming from blocked nasal passages.
- *Pleural rub:* It is a leathery/scratching/grating sound on the stethoscope that needs to be heard in a lifetime to recognize it easily in the future.

It is usually heard at the lower part of the axilla, where movement of the pleura is maximum. This sound is due to thickened pleura of any cause and heard repeatedly at the stage of respiration with no change on coughing, unlike crackles.

It is usually localized to a particular area, which may correspond to localized tenderness to touch or deep inspiration. Sometimes it's so coarse that it may be palpable and is called a palpable pleural rub.

Pericardial rub should be differentiated from a pleural rub by asking the child to hold their breath. Pericardial rub will persist, but pleural rub disappears.

SUCCUSSION SPLASH (HIPPOCRATIC SUCCUSSION)

By the method of percussion, the upper border of dullness is detected in the lateral chest wall along the mid axillary line (MAL), in the sitting position of the patient. Now the diaphragm of the stethoscope is placed on the air-fluid level, and the patient is shaken from side to side vigorously. A splashing sound (like the splashing sound of an intact coconut) is audible with every jerk. Sometimes, the sound can be heard without the help of a stethoscope (unaided ear, i.e., ear placed over the chest wall, and the patient is shaken from side to side). The stethoscope may also be placed in the anterior or posterior chest wall at the air-fluid level to demonstrate succussion splash.

Succussion splash in the chest is always pathological and is found in:

- Hydropneumothorax or pyopneumothorax.
- Herniation of the stomach in the thorax.
- Rarely, over a large cavity in the lung partially filled with exudate.

COIN SOUND

The observer stands at the back. A metallic coin (one rupee coin preferably) is placed over the upper part of the front of the affected chest and is percussed with a similar type of coin when the observer listens at the back (just diametrically opposite to the point of percussion) with the diaphragm of a stethoscope. A high-pitched tympanitic bell-like metallic sound (ringing sound) is heard in a patient with tense pneumothorax.

Do compare the sound with the healthy side (which produces a dull thud as the normal lung does not transmit the ringing metallic sound distinctly).

VOCAL RESONANCE

This is the auscultation of laryngeal vibrations transmitted to the chest wall and nothing but the auscultatory homologue of vocal fremitus.

Method

- The patient will repeat 'one, one' or "99, 99." The patient will speak in a constant tone and voice. Both sides of the chest are auscultated area by area, comparing with the corresponding site on the other side. Auscultation starts from above downward in the front, sides, and back of the chest. Always start from the healthy side; do not auscultate over the bony points.
  - *Diminished:* Pleural effusion, pneumothorax, hydropneumothorax, thickened pleura, fibrosis of the lung, collapse with obstructed bronchus, emphysema, etc.
  - *Increased:*
    - *Bronchophony:* Seems to appear from the earpiece of the stethoscope.
    - Whispering pectoriloquy, even when the patient whispers, the sound is heard clearly.

Bronchophony and whispering pectoriloquy are classically heard over consolidation. It is also heard in collapse with patent bronchus, over a superficial empty cavity, sometimes above the level of pleural effusion, and in an open pneumothorax.

Aegophony: This is a qualitative change in vocal resonance with nasal intonation mimicking the bleating of a goat. It is classically found over consolidation and sometimes, above the level of pleural effusion. Though the speech remains intelligible, the removal of low-pitched elements of the sound explains the nasal bleating quality of aegophony.

CYANOSIS IN CHILDREN

Questions

Q1. Define cyanosis.

Q2. Discuss the pathophysiology of cyanosis.

Q3. Discuss the classification of cyanosis.

Q4. Where to look for central cyanosis?

Q5. What are the causes of cyanosis?

Q6. How to differentiate a cyanosis of cardiac cause from a lung cause?

Cyanosis, derived from the Greek word "kyanos" meaning dark blue, refers to a bluish discoloration of the skin and mucous membranes resulting from an increase in deoxygenated hemoglobin in the blood. In children, cyanosis is a significant clinical finding that often indicates underlying respiratory, cardiac, or hematologic conditions. This chapter provides a comprehensive overview of cyanosis in children, including its pathophysiology, classification, diagnostic approach, and management.

Pathophysiology

Cyanosis occurs when the concentration of deoxygenated hemoglobin in the capillary blood exceeds 5 g/dL. It is more evident in regions with thin skin, such as the lips, nail beds, and mucous membranes. The appearance of cyanosis is influenced by factors such as skin pigmentation, ambient light, and underlying vascular conditions.

The primary mechanisms include:

- *Decreased oxygenation of arterial blood:* Caused by respiratory or cardiac abnormalities.
- *Abnormal hemoglobin:* Hemoglobinopathies such as methemoglobinemia or sulfhemoglobinemia.
- *Impaired circulation:* Peripheral vasoconstriction or stasis leading to local cyanosis.

Classification

Cyanosis can be broadly classified into:

- *Central cyanosis:*
  - Results from systemic hypoxemia due to reduced arterial oxygen saturation.
  - Observed in the lips, tongue, and mucous membranes.
  - *Common causes:*
    - Congenital heart diseases (e.g., Tetralogy of Fallot, transposition of great arteries).

        - Respiratory distress syndrome.
        - Neurological depression affecting breathing.
        - Hemoglobinopathies like methemoglobinemia.
- *Peripheral cyanosis:*
    - Caused by increased oxygen extraction in the extremities due to sluggish blood flow.
    - Affects hands, feet, and nail beds but spares central regions like the tongue.
    - *Common causes:*
        - Hypothermia
        - Shock
        - Raynaud's phenomenon
- *Mixed cyanosis:*
        - Features of both central and peripheral cyanosis.
        - Occurs in conditions like septic shock or advanced congenital heart defects with circulatory collapse.

Causes of Cyanosis in Children

- *Respiratory causes:*
    - Bronchiolitis.
    - Asthma exacerbation.
    - Pneumonia.
    - Foreign body aspiration.
    - Severe laryngomalacia or tracheomalacia.
- *Cardiac causes:*
    - *Cyanotic congenital heart diseases:*
    - Tetralogy of Fallot.
    - Transposition of the great arteries.
    - Total anomalous pulmonary venous return.
    - Tricuspid atresia.
    - Eisenmenger syndrome in untreated congenital defects.
- *Hematologic and metabolic causes:*
    - Methemoglobinemia (e.g., due to nitrate exposure or medications).
    - Sulfhemoglobinemia.
- *Neurological causes:* Central nervous system depression leading to hypoventilation (e.g., sedative overdose).
- *Environmental and miscellaneous causes:*
    - Hypothermia.
    - High-altitude exposure.

Clinical Presentation

The clinical presentation of cyanosis varies depending on the underlying cause, but commonly includes:

- Bluish discoloration of skin and mucous membranes.
- *Respiratory distress:* Tachypnea, grunting, nasal flaring, and retractions.
- *Cardiac signs:* Murmurs, weak peripheral pulses, or gallop rhythm.
- *Neurological symptoms:* Lethargy or altered consciousness in severe hypoxemia.

In congenital heart diseases, cyanosis may worsen with feeding or crying (termed "cyanotic spells"). Peripheral cyanosis typically resolves with warming of the extremities, unlike central cyanosis.

Diagnostic Approach

A systematic approach is essential to determine the cause of cyanosis:

- *History:*
    - Onset and duration of symptoms.
    - Family history of congenital heart disease or hemoglobinopathies.
    - Prenatal history, including maternal infections or exposure to teratogens.
    - Feeding difficulties or failure to thrive.
- *Physical examination:*
    - Assess the location of cyanosis (central vs. peripheral).
    - Respiratory assessment for distress or abnormal breath sounds.
    - Cardiac evaluation for murmurs, thrills, or gallop rhythm.
    - Peripheral pulses and capillary refill time.
- *Investigations:*
    - *Pulse oximetry:* Noninvasive assessment of oxygen saturation.
    - *Arterial blood gas (ABG) analysis:* Determines PaO_2 and acid-base status.
    - *Chest X-ray:* Evaluates lung fields and cardiac silhouette.
    - *Electrocardiogram (ECG):* Identifies cardiac rhythm abnormalities.
    - *Echocardiography:* Visualizes structural heart defects.
    - *Methemoglobin levels:* Assessed if hemoglobinopathy is suspected.
    - *Complete blood count (CBC):* Detects polycythemia or anemia.
- *Advanced testing:*
    - Cardiac catheterization.
    - Genetic testing for syndromic conditions.

Management

The management of cyanosis in children depends on the underlying etiology:

- *Emergency stabilization:*
  - Ensure a clear airway.
  - Administer supplemental oxygen for hypoxemia.
  - Initiate cardiopulmonary resuscitation (CPR) if necessary.
- *Respiratory support:*
  - Mechanical ventilation for respiratory failure.
  - Treat underlying conditions such as pneumonia and bronchiolitis with antibiotics and bronchodilators.
- *Cardiac interventions:*
  - Prostaglandin E1 infusion to maintain ductal patency in duct-dependent lesions.
  - Surgical correction or palliation for structural defects.
- *Management of hemoglobinopathies:*
  - Methylene blue for methemoglobinemia.
  - Exchange transfusion in severe cases.
- *Peripheral cyanosis:*
  - Rewarm extremities in hypothermia.
  - Treat shock with fluids and vasopressors.

Prognosis

The prognosis of cyanosis in children is closely tied to the underlying cause and the timeliness of intervention. Advances in pediatric cardiology and neonatology have significantly improved outcomes for congenital heart defects. Early recognition and prompt treatment are critical to preventing complications such as organ dysfunction or developmental delays.

Conclusion

Cyanosis in children is a vital clinical sign that warrants immediate attention. A systematic approach to its evaluation and management ensures accurate diagnosis and timely treatment. Multidisciplinary care involving pediatricians, cardiologists, pulmonologists, and intensivists often plays a crucial role in improving outcomes for affected children.

CLUBBING IN CHILDREN

Questions

Q1. Demonstrate the clubbing or the method of examining clubbing.

Q2. Discuss the pathophysiology of clubbing.

Q3. What are the causes of clubbing?

Q4. Discuss the grading/staging of clubbing?

Clubbing, also known as digital clubbing or hypertrophic osteoarthropathy, is a medical condition characterized by changes in the shape and structure of the nails and the tips of the fingers or toes. It is an important clinical sign often associated with various systemic diseases, particularly in children, where its presence warrants a detailed evaluation. Understanding the causes, clinical presentation, diagnostic approaches, and management of clubbing in children is crucial for timely intervention and treatment.

Anatomy and Pathophysiology

Clubbing involves structural changes in the distal phalanges, including:

- *Increased nail curvature:* Both longitudinal and transverse.
- *Loss of the angle:* Between the nail bed and the nail fold (Lovibond angle >180°).
- *Bulbous swelling:* Enlargement of the fingertips.
- *Spongy consistency:* Of the nail bed upon palpation.

The pathophysiology of clubbing is not completely understood, but it is thought to involve vascular endothelial growth factor (VEGF) and platelet-derived growth factor (PDGF), which promote vascular proliferation and connective tissue remodeling. This process is triggered by chronic hypoxia, inflammatory mediators, or circulating megakaryocytes bypassing the pulmonary capillary bed due to underlying diseases.

Causes of Clubbing in Children

Clubbing in children may be associated with a range of systemic disorders. These can be classified as follows:

- *Pulmonary causes:*
  - *Chronic suppurative lung diseases:* Conditions such as cystic fibrosis, bronchiectasis, and lung abscesses.
  - *Interstitial lung diseases:* Such as idiopathic pulmonary fibrosis.
  - *Tuberculosis:* Particularly in endemic regions.
  - *Empyema:* Chronic infection of the pleural cavity.
- *Cardiac causes:*
  - *Congenital cyanotic heart diseases:* Such as Tetralogy of Fallot, transposition of the great arteries, and truncus arteriosus.
  - *Infective Endocarditis:* Particularly when associated with congenital heart defects.

- *Gastrointestinal causes:*
  - *Inflammatory bowel diseases:* Ulcerative colitis and Crohn's disease.
  - *Chronic liver diseases:* Such as biliary atresia and primary sclerosing cholangitis.
  - *Celiac disease:* Occasionally associated with clubbing due to chronic inflammation.
- *Hematological and oncological causes:*
  - *Malignancies:* Such as Hodgkin's lymphoma, neuroblastoma, or osteosarcoma with pulmonary metastases.
  - *Chronic anemia:* Including iron-deficiency anemia and hemoglobinopathies in severe cases.
- *Genetic and syndromic associations:*
  - *Primary hypertrophic osteoarthropathy:* Also known as pachydermoperiostosis.
  - *Familial clubbing:* A rare hereditary condition not associated with systemic disease.
- *Miscellaneous:*
  - *Idiopathic clubbing:* Rare cases without an identifiable cause.
  - *Endocrinopathies:* Such as hyperthyroidism.

Clinical Presentation

Children with clubbing may present with:
- *Visible nail changes:* Rounded, convex nails with loss of the normal Lovibond angle.
- *Swelling:* Of the tips of fingers or toes.
- *Spongy nail beds:* Detected upon palpation.
- *Associated symptoms:* Symptoms depend on the underlying disease, such as breathlessness in lung disorders, cyanosis in congenital heart disease, or diarrhea in gastrointestinal disorders.

Stages of clubbing include:
- *Fluctuation of the nail bed:* Early spongy texture.
- *Loss of the Lovibond angle:* Angle becomes obtuse (>180°).
- *Increased nail curvature:* Pronounced convexity.
- *Drumstick appearance:* Bulbous, clubbed fingers, or toes.
- *Hypertrophic osteoarthropathy:* In advanced cases, periosteal bone growth may cause painful swelling of the joints.

Diagnostic Approach

Clubbing in children requires a systematic evaluation to identify the underlying cause:

- *History taking:*
  - *Onset:* Congenital or acquired.
  - *Progression:* Gradual or rapid.
  - *Associated symptoms:* Such as cyanosis, cough, fever, or gastrointestinal disturbances.
  - *Family history:* To rule out familial clubbing.
  - *Environmental and social factors:* Such as exposure to infections or allergens.
- *Physical examination:*
  - Assess for signs of cyanosis, respiratory distress, murmurs, hepatosplenomegaly, or other systemic involvement.
  - Detailed examination of nails and digits.
- *Investigations:*
  - *Blood tests:* Complete blood count, inflammatory markers [C-reactive protein (CRP) and erythrocyte sedimentation rate (ESR)], liver and renal function tests.
  - *Imaging studies:* Chest X-ray, computed tomography (CT) scan, or echocardiogram based on clinical suspicion.
  - *Special tests:* Pulmonary function tests, sweat chloride test (for cystic fibrosis), or biopsy if malignancy is suspected.
  - *Genetic testing:* For syndromic or familial causes.

Management

- *Treatment of underlying cause:*
  - Antibiotics for infections such as tuberculosis and empyema.
  - Surgical correction for congenital heart defects.
  - Anti-inflammatory or immunosuppressive therapy for inflammatory bowel diseases.
- *Supportive care:*
  - Oxygen therapy for hypoxemia.
  - Nutritional support in chronic diseases such as cystic fibrosis.
  - Pain management for hypertrophic osteoarthropathy.
- *Monitoring and follow-up:*
  - Regular assessment of clubbing progression.
  - Monitoring of systemic disease control and complications.

Prognosis and Outcomes

The prognosis of clubbing in children depends on the underlying condition:

- *Reversible causes:* Clubbing may regress after successful treatment of infections or cyanotic heart disease.
- *Irreversible causes:* In chronic or genetic conditions, clubbing may persist.

Early identification and management of the causative disease significantly improve outcomes, emphasizing the importance of a multidisciplinary approach in pediatric care.

Conclusion

Clubbing in children is a vital clinical sign that necessitates thorough evaluation. Its presence should prompt clinicians to investigate potential underlying systemic diseases. By recognizing the stages of clubbing and its associations with various disorders, healthcare providers can ensure timely diagnosis and effective management, ultimately improving the quality of life for those affected.

APPROACH TO THE CASE OF PNEUMONIA IN CHILDREN

Questions

Q1. Discuss the etiology of pneumonia.

Q2. What are the noninfective causes of pneumonia?

Q3. How do you classify pneumonia?

Q4. Define nonresolving pneumonia?

Q5. What are the causes of delayed resolution or nonresolving pneumonia?

Q6. Define recurrent pneumonia.

Q7. What are the causes of recurrent pneumonia?

Q8. Discuss the IMNCI guidelines on pneumonia.

Q9. What are the oxygen delivery devices?

Q10. Discuss the antituberculosis drug (ATD) regimen for pulmonary tuberculosis and the role of steroids in pulmonary TB.

Pneumonia is a significant cause of morbidity and mortality in children, particularly in low- and middle-income countries. A structured approach to diagnosing and managing pediatric pneumonia is essential for improving outcomes. This chapter provides a detailed framework for the evaluation and management of pneumonia in children.

Introduction

Pneumonia is an infection of the lung parenchyma that can affect the alveoli, bronchioles, and surrounding interstitial tissues. In children, pneumonia can present with a wide range of symptoms, from mild respiratory distress to life-threatening illness. Early recognition, appropriate investigation, and timely management are critical to reducing complications.

Etiology

The causative pathogens of pediatric pneumonia vary by age, geographical location, immunization status, and underlying health conditions:

- *Neonates (0–28 days):*
  - Group B *Streptococcus*
  - *Escherichia coli*
  - *Listeria monocytogenes*
  - Herpes Simplex Virus (rare)
- *Infants and young children (1–5 years):*
  - *Viral:* Respiratory syncytial virus (RSV), influenza, parainfluenza, adenovirus, human metapneumovirus
  - *Bacterial: Streptococcus pneumoniae, Haemophilus influenzae type B (HiB),* and *Staphylococcus aureus.*
  - *Atypical: Mycoplasma pneumoniae, Chlamydia trachomatis* (in neonates from maternal infection).
- *Older children (>5 years):*
  - Atypical pathogens such as *Mycoplasma pneumoniae* and *Chlamydia pneumoniae.*
  - Viral infections are still common but decrease in prevalence with age.

Risk factors include malnutrition, incomplete immunization, environmental exposure to smoke, and underlying conditions, such as asthma, cystic fibrosis, and immunodeficiency.

Not all pneumonia is caused by infectious agents.

Children who have severe gastroesophageal reflux (GERD) may develop chemical pneumonitis secondary to recurrent aspiration.

Inhalation of certain chemicals or smoke may cause pulmonary inflammation. Additionally, aspiration pneumonia is more common among children with neurologic impairment, swallowing abnormalities, gastrointestinal motility, or a gastrostomy tube. Oral anaerobic flora, with or without aerobes, is the most common etiologic agent.

Immunocompromised Children

Some children who are immunocompromised, whether secondary to human immunodeficiency virus (HIV) infection/acquired immunodeficiency syndrome (AIDS), an immune disorder, or chemotherapy for a malignancy, are at risk for pneumonias caused by opportunistic agents. Carefully obtained samples for appropriate microbiologic testing are paramount in such patients so that therapy can be optimized.

Children with cystic fibrosis are especially prone to develop infections with *S. aureus*, *Pseudomonas aeruginosa*, *Burkholderia cepacia*, and other multidrug-resistant organisms.

Pneumocystis jirovecii pneumonia (PCP) is common in the most severely compromised children. Adenovirus infections can be severe in these children as well, leading to bronchiolitis obliterans or hyperlucent lung syndrome. In addition, cytomegalovirus (CMV) poses a great risk to immunocompromised patients.

Fungal pneumonia, caused by *Aspergillus*, *Zygomycetes*, or other related fungi, occurs in immunocompromised patients who undergo prolonged hospitalization, have prolonged neutropenia, and/or have received broad-spectrum antibiotics.

Patients with sickle cell disease have problems with their complement system as well as functional asplenia; this predisposes them to infection with encapsulated organisms such as *S. pneumoniae* and *H. influenzae* type B. *M. pneumoniae* is also a common agent of pneumonia in this group of patients.

Classification of Pneumonia

Pneumonia (synonym: pneumonitis) is defined as acute inflammation of the lung parenchyma.

- *Main classification:*
  - "Primary" pneumonia [Streptococcus pneumoniae (most common), *S. aureus*, *H. influenzae*, Klebsiella pneumoniae, etc.]—usually, community-acquired (in normal healthy individuals).
  - *"Secondary" pneumonia (occurs when the host is weakened):*
    - Acute bronchopneumonia, acute lobular, or hypostatic pneumonia.
    - Benign aspiration pneumonia.
    - Suppurative or necrotizing pneumonia (lung abscess)—commonly by *S. aureus* and Klebsiella pneumoniae.
    - Hospital-acquired pneumonia (nosocomial).
    - In an immunocompromised host (*P. jiroveci* infection in AIDS).

Note: Lung abscess may be a part of "primary" pneumonia.

- *Empiricist's classification (most commonly used):*
  - Community-acquired pneumonia (*S. pneumoniae* and *H. influenzae*).
  - *Hospital-acquired pneumonia (nosocomial):* Mainly by aerobic gram-negative bacilli, anaerobes.
  - Pneumonia in immunocompromised host—*P. aeruginosa*, *P. jiroveci*.
- *Anatomical classification:*
  - Lobar.
  - Lobular (bronchopneumonia, if bilateral).
  - Segmental (benign aspiration pneumonia).
- *Etiological classification:*
  - Infective—bacterial, viral, rickettsial, yeast and fungi, and protozoa (*P. jiroveci*).
  - Chemical agents—irritant gases, aspiration of vomitus, kerosene oil, etc., (kerosene oil produces "lipoid pneumonia").
  - Physical agents—irradiation.
  - Hypersensitivity reaction—systemic lupus erythematosus (SLE), Stevens-Johnson syndrome, and Loeffler's syndrome.
- *Radiological classification:*
  - Alveolar or air space pneumonia (pneumococcal mainly)—air bronchogram in chest X-ray.
  - Bronchopneumonia (*H. influenzae*, etc.)—atelectasis is seen in chest X-ray.
  - Interstitial (virus, mycoplasma, etc.)—reticular or reticulonodular pattern in chest X-ray.
- *Behaviorist's classification:* (1) Easy and (2) Difficult: Nonresolving.

Atypical Pneumonia

There is a group of pneumonias that do not behave like lobar pneumococcal pneumonia. This type of "atypical" pneumonia is not severe and is caused by *Chlamydia psittaci (psittacosis)*, *Coxiella burnetii* (Q fever), *Legionella pneumophila*, and *Mycoplasma pneumonias*.

Predominant features are dry cough, constitutional symptoms, abnormality in chest X-ray despite of lack of physical signs in the chest.

Causes of 'Delayed Resolution' of Pneumonia

Delayed resolution means when the physical signs persist for >2 weeks and the radiological features which persist for >4 weeks after proper antimicrobial treatment.

The possibilities are:

- Inappropriate chemotherapy, such as incomplete treatment, suboptimal dose, wrong choice of antibiotics, drug resistance, and irregular intake of drugs.
- Complicated by pleural effusion, suppurative pneumonia, or empyema thoracis.
- Decreased host resistance, such as diabetes mellitus, chronic alcoholism, agranulocytosis, lymphoma, leukemia, multiple myeloma, corticosteroid therapy, hypogammaglobulinemia, AIDS, etc., elderly and debilitated patients.
- Tuberculous pneumonia (needs specific antituberculosis chemotherapy).
- Partial obstruction of the bronchus by a foreign body
- Fungal or atypical pneumonia.
- Pneumonia resulting from connective tissue diseases, pulmonary infarction, etc.
- Recurrent aspiration in gastroesophageal reflux disease (GERD), neurological conditions.

Note: Common causes of "nonresolution" of pneumonia are inappropriate chemotherapy, pneumonia caused by a virulent organism (e.g., staphylococcal pneumonia).

Recurrent Pneumonia in Children

Recurrent pneumonia is defined as two or more episodes of pneumonia in a year or three episodes ever separated by an asymptomatic period of a month or clear chest X-rays. Recurrent pneumonia in children typically has underlying causes.

Underlying causes of recurrent pneumonia in children:

- *Aspiration syndrome* was the most common underlying cause in children with recurrent pneumonia.
- Pulmonary anomalies and structural abnormalities.
- Immune disorders and immunological abnormalities.
- Congenital heart defects.
- GERD
- Sickle cell anemia.
- Asthma
- *Hypersecretory asthma:* Excess production of bronchial secretions.
- *Bronchiectasis:* Causes of bronchiectasis include cystic fibrosis, primary ciliary dyskinesia, immunodeficiency, retained foreign body, and recurrent aspiration

Clinical Features

The clinical presentation varies with the age of the child and the causative organism. Key symptoms include:

- *Neonates:*
  - Nonspecific signs, such as poor feeding, lethargy, irritability, and fever.
  - *Respiratory distress:* Tachypnea, nasal flaring, grunting, and cyanosis.
- *Infants and young children:*
  - Fever, cough, and tachypnoea are hallmark signs.
  - *Respiratory distress:* Chest indrawing, nasal flaring, use of accessory muscles.
  - *Auscultation:* Crackles, decreased breath sounds, or bronchial breath sounds.
- *Older children:*
  - Gradual onset with low-grade fever, persistent cough, and wheezing (more common with atypical pathogens).
  - Pleuritic chest pain or abdominal pain due to diaphragmatic irritation.

Clinical Examinations

- *General survey:*
  - Patient looks toxic and ill, but conscious and cooperative at present.
  - Decubitus—propped-up at 45°.
  - Cyanosis—absent at present.
  - Respiration—42 breaths/min, regular and predominantly abdominothoracic in type.
  - Pulse—86 beats/min, regular (describe other pulse points).
  - *Pulse:* Respiration—2: 1
- *Inspection:*
  - Upper respiratory tract reveals no abnormality.
  - Absence of intercostal suction, but accessory muscles of respiration are working.
  - Absence of fullness or flattening of the chest wall anywhere.
  - Apical impulse—seen below the left nipple, approximately 3" lateral to midline.
  - Diminished movement on the left side of the chest, mainly the lower part of the back and the lateral aspect of the chest.
- *Palpation:*
  - Restricted movement on the left side of the chest.
  - Trachea and apex beat are normal in position (i.e., no mediastinal shift).
  - Vocal fremitus—Increased on the affected side (lower part of the lateral aspect and back mainly).
  - Friction fremitus—Present in the affected part of the back, on the affected side of the chest.

- *Percussion:* Woody dullness on the affected side of the chest (lower part), mainly at the back and lateral aspect.
- *Auscultation:*

  All the positive findings are present mainly in the affected area
  - Tubular breath sound (high-pitched bronchial).
  - Increased vocal resonance—Bronchophony and whispering pectoriloquy.
  - Aegophony.
  - Pleural rub
  - Absence of rhonchi and crepitations (as the lung is solidified and liquefaction has not started
  - yet).

Diagnostic Approach

Clinical Assessment

The cornerstone of diagnosis is a thorough clinical evaluation:

- *Measure respiratory rate and assess for tachypnoea [World Health Organization (WHO) criteria]:*
  - ≥60 breaths/min in children <2 months
  - ≥50 breaths/min in 2–12 months
  - ≥40 breaths/min in 1–5 years
- Look for signs of respiratory distress, such as chest indrawing and grunting.
- *Identify danger signs:* Cyanosis, altered mental status, inability to drink or breastfeed, or severe respiratory distress.

Laboratory Investigations

Investigations should be tailored to the clinical context.

- *CBC:* Leukocytosis with neutrophilia suggests bacterial infection; lymphocytosis favors viral etiology.
- *Blood cultures:* To identify pathogens in severe cases.
- *CRP and Procalcitonin:* May help differentiate bacterial from viral pneumonia.
- *Sputum culture or nasopharyngeal aspirate:* For microbiological identification in older children or severe cases. Bronchoalveolar lavage (BAL) aspirates in difficult cases
- Viral assays [reverse transcription polymerase chain reaction (RT-PCR)], cartridge-based nucleic acid amplification test (CBNAAT) (tuberculosis)
- *Chest X-ray:*
  - Lobar consolidation suggests bacterial pneumonia.
  - Interstitial infiltrates are more common in viral or atypical pneumonia.
  - Pleural effusion or empyema may be evident in complicated cases.
- *Ultrasonography (USG):* This is the best first-line modality to diagnose pneumonia in children's bedside. It also diagnoses pleural effusions, pneumothorax. It is the most important tool nowadays in the hands of a trained technician or doctor. It also helps in draining fluids, diagnosing aspirates, and monitoring the progression of the disease. The BLUE protocol is commonly used.
- Computed tomography (CT) scan of the thorax, if an obstructing tumor is suspected.
  - BAL or transtracheal aspirations.
- Bronchoscopy—may be done whenever there is evidence of a foreign body.
- Lung biopsy—rarely needed. Sometimes, an open lung biopsy is done in patients who are immunocompromised.

Pulse Oximetry

Assess oxygen saturation to detect hypoxemia. Levels <92% on room air indicate the need for supplemental oxygen.

Management:

General principles:

- *Hospitalization criteria:*
  - Severe respiratory distress.
  - Hypoxemia ;[peripheral capillary oxygen saturation (SpO_2) <92%).
  - Infants <2 months.
  - Presence of comorbidities or complications (e.g., empyema).
- *Supportive care:*
  - *Adequate hydration:* Oral or intravenous (IV) fluids as needed.
  - *Nutrition:* Early enteral feeding, if possible.
  - Oxygen therapy for hypoxemic children.

*Antibiotic therapy **(Tables 1 and 2)**:*
Antibiotics should be guided by the likely pathogen, age, and severity:

- *Outpatient treatment:*
  - *First-line:* Amoxicillin (oral).
  - *Alternative:* Macrolides (e.g., azithromycin) for atypical pathogens.

TABLE 1: Integrated Management of Newborn and Child Illnesses (IMNCI) treatment guidelines for children.

Signs	*Classify as*	*Treatment*
Any general danger sign, or chest indrawing, or stridor in a calm child	Severe pneumonia or very severe disease	• Give first dose of IM Chloramphenicol 40 mg/kg/dose (If not possible, give oral amoxicillin 50 mg/kg/dose in 3 divided doses) • Refer *urgently* to the hospital
Fast breathing	Pneumonia	• Give oral cotrimoxazole (8 mg/kg/day of trimethoprim in two divided doses) for 5 days • Soothe the throat and relieve the cough with a safe remedy if the child is 6 months or older • Advise mother to return immediately if child has any of the following signs: not able to drink or breastfeed, becomes sicker, develops fever, has fast breathing, or has difficulty breathing • Follow-up in 2 days
No signs of pneumonia or very severe disease	No Pneumonia: cough or cold	• If coughing for >30 days, refer for assessment • Soothe the throat and relieve the cough with a safe home remedy if the child is 6 months or older • Advise mother to return immediately if child has any of the following signs: not able to drink or breastfeed, becomes sicker, develops a fever, has fast breathing, or difficulty breathing • Follow-up in 5 days if not improving

TABLE 2: Classification and treatment of cough and difficult breathing.

Signs	*Classify as*	*Treatment*
Any general danger sign, or chest indrawing, or stridor in a calm child	Severe pneumonia or very severe disease	• Give first dose of intramuscular (IM) chloramphenicol 40 mg/kg/dose (If not possible, give oral amoxicillin 50 mg/kg/day in three divided doses) • Refer *urgently* to the hospital
Fast breathing	Pneumonia	• Give oral cotrimoxazole (8 mg/kg/day of trimethoprim in 2 divided doses) for 5 days • Soothe the throat and relieve the cough with a safe remedy if the child is 6 months or older • Advise mother to return immediately if child has any of the following signs: Not able to drink or breastfeed, becomes sicker, develops fever, has fast breathing, or difficulty breathing • Follow-up in 2 days
No signs of pneumonia or very severe disease	No pneumonia: cough or cold	• If coughing for >30 days, refer for assessment • Soothe the throat and relieve the cough with a safe home remedy if the child is 6 months or older • Advise mother to return immediately if child has any of the following signs: not able to drink or breastfeed, becomes sicker, develops fever, has fast breathing, or difficulty breathing. • Follow up in 5 days if not improving

- *Inpatient treatment:*
  - *Neonates:* Ampicillin and gentamicin.
- *Infants and children:* IV ceftriaxone or cefotaxime. Add vancomycin if methicillin-resistant *Staphylococcus aureus* (MRSA) is suspected.
- *Duration:* Typically, 7–10 days for uncomplicated cases; longer for severe or complicated pneumonia.
  - *Antiviral therapy:* Consider oseltamivir in children with influenza pneumonia during epidemics.
  - *Tubercular pneumonia* **(Table 3)***:*

Management of Complications

- *Pleural effusion/empyema:* Chest tube drainage and appropriate antibiotics.

TABLE 3: Types of TB cases and their treatment regimen

Type of TB Case	*Treatment regimen in IP*	*Treatment regimen CP*
New	(2) HRZE	(4) HRE
Previously Treated	(2) HRZES + (1) HRZE	(5) HRE

(H: Isoniazid; R: Rifampicin; Z: Pyrazinamide; E: Ethambutol)
Note: Previously treated means that 1 month of therapy was taken earlier.

- *Sepsis or shock:* Aggressive fluid resuscitation and inotropes as needed.

OXYGEN DELIVERY METHODS IN CHILDREN

The administration of oxygen to pediatric patients requires the selection of an oxygen delivery system that suits the patient's age, size, needs, clinical condition, and therapeutic goals.

Oxygen delivery systems are categorized as low-flow systems or high-flow (fixed performance) systems.

With low-flow systems, 100% oxygen mixes with room air during inspiration.

High-flow devices provide such a high flow of premixed gas that the patient is not required to inhale room air.

Supplemental oxygen therapy is often recommended for pediatric patients when peripheral oxygen saturation is consistently below 94%:

- A *nasal cannula* is a low-flow oxygen device. For infants and toddlers who may poorly tolerate a mask, nasal prongs may be a good alternative. The nasal cannula allows breathing through the mouth or nose. A nasal cannula can deliver 24–45% oxygen with appropriate oxygen flow rates of 0.5–2 L/min.
- A *simple face mask* is a low-flow oxygen device. A simple face mask can deliver 35–50% oxygen with an appropriate flow rate of 6–10 L/min. A minimum of 6 L/min of oxygen flow is needed to prevent rebreathing of exhaled carbon dioxide (CO_2).
- A *partial rebreathing mask with a reservoir bag* is a face mask that delivers moderate to high concentrations of oxygen. Side port openings on the mask vent exhaled air on expiration and allow room air to enter on inspiration. The delivered oxygen can be as high as 60%, but the percentage varies, depending on the rate and depth of the patient's breathing.
- A *nonrebreathing mask with a reservoir* is a high-flow oxygen delivery device used for pediatric patients requiring a higher concentration of oxygen. A nonrebreathing mask can deliver a concentration of up to 90% oxygen with an oxygen flow rate of 10–15 L/min.
- A *Venturi mask* is a cone-shaped device with entrainment ports of various sizes at its base. The entrainment ports adjust to deliver various oxygen concentrations. The mask is useful because it delivers a more precise concentration of oxygen.
- A *face tent* is a shield-like device that fits under the patient's chin and encircles the face. It is used primarily for humidification and for oxygen only when the patient cannot or will not tolerate a tight-fitting mask. Because the tent is so close to the patient's face, the concentration of oxygen delivered to the patient cannot be estimated.
- *Oxygen tents and hoods* can provide high concentrations of humidified oxygen, which is useful in a patient with airway inflammation, epiglottitis (croup), or other respiratory tract infections.

Prevention

Immunization

- Routine vaccination against *Streptococcus pneumoniae*, HiB, and influenza.
- Ensure measles and pertussis vaccination

Nutrition: Promote breastfeeding and address malnutrition.

Environmental control: Reduce exposure to tobacco smoke and indoor air pollution.

Prognosis

Most children recover completely with appropriate treatment. Complications such as empyema, abscess formation, and chronic lung disease are rare with timely intervention.

Conclusion

A systematic approach to pediatric pneumonia emphasizes clinical evaluation, targeted investigations, and evidence-based management. Prevention strategies such as immunization and nutritional support play a vital role in reducing the burden of pneumonia in children.

APPROACH TO A CASE OF PLEURAL EFFUSION IN CHILDREN

Questions

Q1. Discuss the etiology of pleural effusion.

Q2. What are the causes of bilateral pleural effusion?

Q3. How will you diagnose pleural effusion?

Q4. How to confirm the type of pleural effusion—any criteria?

Q5. Discuss the management of pleural effusion—indications of thoracentesis.

Q6. Where to put the drain-safety triangle?

Q7. When to remove the drain?

Q8. What are the complications of a chest drain?

Q9. How to manage surgical emphysema with or without pneumopericardium?

Q10. What are the indications of vats and decortications?

Introduction

Pleural effusion in children refers to the accumulation of fluid in the pleural space, the area between the lung and chest wall. It can result from a wide variety of causes, ranging from infections to systemic diseases. The presentation can vary widely, necessitating a systematic approach for accurate diagnosis and management. This chapter outlines the step-by-step approach to evaluating and managing pleural effusion in pediatric patients.

Understanding Pleural Effusion in Children

Pleural effusion can be classified based on:

- *Pathophysiology:* Transudative versus Exudative
- *Composition:* Serous, purulent (empyema), chylous, or hemorrhagic.
- *Etiology:* Infectious, noninfectious, malignant, or idiopathic.

Common pediatric causes include:

- *Infectious:* Bacterial pneumonia (parapneumonic effusion) and tuberculosis.
- *Cardiac:* Congenital or acquired heart disease causing transudates
- *Malignant:* Lymphoma and leukemia.
- *Systemic diseases:* Nephrotic syndrome, connective tissue diseases.

Hemorrhagic pleural effusion (hemothorax):

- Neoplasm—primary or secondary, pleural mesothelioma.
- Chest trauma (during paracentesis or placement of a central line).
- Tuberculous effusion.
- Bleeding diathesis.
- Lymphoma and leukemias.
- Anticoagulant therapy.
- Pleural effusion
- Pulmonary infarction.
- Acute hemorrhagic pancreatitis.

Chylous (milky) pleural effusion: Rare in children

- Tuberculosis.
- Malignancy
- Lymphoma
- Filariasis
- Myxedema (gold paint effusion).
- Trauma to the chest wall.
- Congenital absence of the thoracic duct.

Bilateral pleural effusion:

- Rheumatoid arthritis.
- Bilateral tuberculous effusion (rare).
- SLE
- Pulmonary infarction.
- Lymphoma and leukemias
- Pleural metastases.

Note: Remember, hydrothorax is usually bilateral

Clinical Features

History

A detailed history is vital:

- *Onset and duration:* Acute onset suggests infection; chronic effusion may indicate malignancy or tuberculosis.
- *Associated symptoms:*
  - Fever, cough, and respiratory distress (common in infections).
  - Weight loss and night sweats (suggestive of tuberculosis or malignancy).
- *History of trauma or surgery:*
  - *Family and social history:* Tuberculosis exposure, family history of autoimmune diseases.
  - *Preexisting conditions:* Congenital heart disease, nephrotic syndrome.

Physical Examination

Key findings include:
- *Inspection:* Asymmetric chest expansion, intercostal retractions.
- *Palpation:* Reduced tactile fremitus over the effusion.
- *Percussion:* Dullness over the fluid.
- *Auscultation:* Diminished breath sounds and reduced vocal resonance.

Signs of systemic illness or underlying conditions, such as lymphadenopathy or edema, should also be sought.

Complications of pleural effusion:
- Thickened pleura.
- Empyema thoracis.
- Collapse (compression) of the lung followed by fibrosis later on.
- Spread of infection (tuberculosis) to the pericardium or peritoneum.
- Cardio-respiratory embarrassment as a result of massive pleural effusion.
- Acute pulmonary edema (rare)—as a complication of rapid pleural aspiration.
- Hydropneumothorax—may develop after pleural aspiration.

Investigations

- Blood—CBC, CRP, blood culture goes in favor of tuberculous etiology.
- *Chest X-ray (PA view):*
  - Triangular homogeneous opacity with a curved upper border which is concave medially and upward, and extends up to the axilla.
  - Obliteration of the costophrenic angle (the earliest site of fluid collection).
  - Massive effusion produces unilateral homogeneous opacity.
  - Displacement of mediastinum to the opposite side.
  - A lateral view is done to differentiate it from lobar consolidation.

  Encysted pleural effusion may not obliterate the costophrenic angle.

  A lateral decubitus film may be taken in a suspected patient of subpulmonic effusion.

  Repetition of chest X-ray should be done in all cases after therapeutic paracentesis thoracis.
- *Aspiration of pleural fluid:* For diagnostic purposes, at least 50 mL of fluid should be aspirated. It helps by:
  - Confirmation of diagnosis of pleural effusion.

    Examination of the nature of fluid—Transudate or exudate [physical character (clear in hydrothorax, red in hemorrhagic effusion, milky white in chylous, and purulent in empyema thoracis), biochemical and cytological [red blood cells (RBC), white blood cells (WBC), malignant cells] examination.

    Smear examination—Gram's stain, Ziehl-Neelsen stain, Leishman's stain for microfilaria, or special stains for the detection of malignant cells.
  - Culture of the aspirated fluid (bacteriological, including culture of *Mycobacterium tuberculosis* in Lowenstein-Jensen media. CBNAAT/GENEXPERT is more specific.

    Ultrasonography is done to differentiate an encysted pleural effusion from a pleural tumor and to localize the effusion before aspiration or pleural biopsy. *This should be done as the first step if you diagnose pleural effusion in children (recent advance)*

    Special tests—RT-PCR ASSAYS (polymerase chain reaction to detect organisms, including tubercle bacilli).
- *Sputum examination:* It is done for 3 consecutive days. CBNAAT method.
  - For demonstration of acid-fast bacilli (AFB) (the surest test for tuberculosis)—rarely positive.
  - To diagnose the etiology of pneumonia (if effusion develops from pneumonia).
  - For malignant cells.
- *Mantoux test (not very informative):*
  - Positive in cases of tuberculosis.
  - May be negative in lymphoma.
- Fine needle aspiration cytology (FNAC) or excision biopsy of lymph nodes (axillary, cervical, or scalene node).
- May give a clue to the etiology.
- Imaging—USG, CT scan, or magnetic resonance imaging (MRI) scan detects fluid as small as 50 mL, and may be done as per the latest guidelines.

Minimal collection of pleural fluid for clinical detection: At least 500 mL of fluid is necessary for clinical detection (minimally 300 mL of fluid is required for radiological detection).

Imaging Studies

- *Chest X-ray:*
  - Blunting of costophrenic angles

- Homogenous opacity with meniscus sign
- Mediastinal shift (if large effusion)
- *Ultrasound:*
  - Guides thoracocentesis
  - Differentiates fluid from solid masses
  - Evaluates loculated effusions
- *CT scan:*
  - Detects underlying lung pathology, e.g., masses, abscesses.
  - Evaluates complex or loculated effusions.
- *MRI:* Rarely required but useful for distinguishing pleural from chest wall lesions.

Advanced tests (if indicated):

- Tuberculin skin test or interferon-gamma release assays (IGRAs) for TB
- *Echocardiography:* To rule out pericardial effusion and cardiac causes.
- *Genetic studies:* In suspected familial diseases (e.g., familial chylothorax).

Differential Diagnosis

- *Transudative effusion:*
  - Congestive heart failure
  - Nephrotic syndrome
  - Liver disease (cirrhosis)
- *Exudative Effusion:*
  - Parapneumonic effusion/empyema
  - Tuberculosis
  - Malignancy (lymphoma and leukemia)
- *Other specific types:*
  - Chylothorax (trauma and congenital lymphatic abnormalities)
  - Hemothorax (trauma and malignancy)
  - Rheumatological diseases (e.g., juvenile idiopathic arthritis)

Management

Supportive care:

- *Oxygen therapy:* For respiratory distress
- *Analgesia:* Chest pain management
- *Nutritional support:* Especially in chronic effusions

Intercostal Drainage

If pleural fluid pH <7.2

- Underwater seal drainage. No difference in small bore or large bore. A pigtail catheter is the best option.
- USG-guided implantable cardioverter-defibrillator (ICD) placement is best. Midaxillary line 5/6th intercostal space on the affected side. Negative suction is no longer required.
- Daily monitoring of ICD fluid is mandatory.
- If fluid <1–2/kg/day or <10–20 mL/day for 2–3 days, the ICD can be withdrawn if there is adequate clinical and radiological improvement.

Fibrinolysis (urokinase/streptokinase):

- Loculations and septations within 7–10 days of diagnosis
- Usually instilled through ICD.
- *Contraindication:* Bronchopleural fistula and bleeding diathesis.
- *Side effects:* Fever, intrapleural bleeding, anaphylaxis.

Complications of the insertion of ICD:

- Pneumothorax
- Hydropneumothorax
- Surgical emphysema
- Bronchopleural fistula

Specific Treatment Based on Etiology

- *Infectious causes:*
  - *Antibiotics:* Empiric broad-spectrum antibiotics targeting common pathogens (e.g., *S. pneumoniae* and *S. aureus*).
  - *Drainage:* Chest tube placement for empyema or large parapneumonic effusions.
- *Tuberculosis:* Antituberculous therapy (ATT) based on national guidelines.
- *Chylothorax:*
  - Dietary modification (low-fat diet or medium-chain triglycerides).
  - Octreotide in refractory cases.
- *Cardiac-related effusion:* Diuretics for congestive heart failure.
- *Malignant effusions:* Chemotherapy or targeted therapy based on tumor type.

Surgical Intervention

- *Indications:*
  - When sepsis is not effectively controlled by antibiotics and ICD
  - Respiratory compromise due to pleural thickening
  - ICD drainage output decreases, but clinical and radiological deterioration persists

Flowchart 1: Managing surgical emphysema.

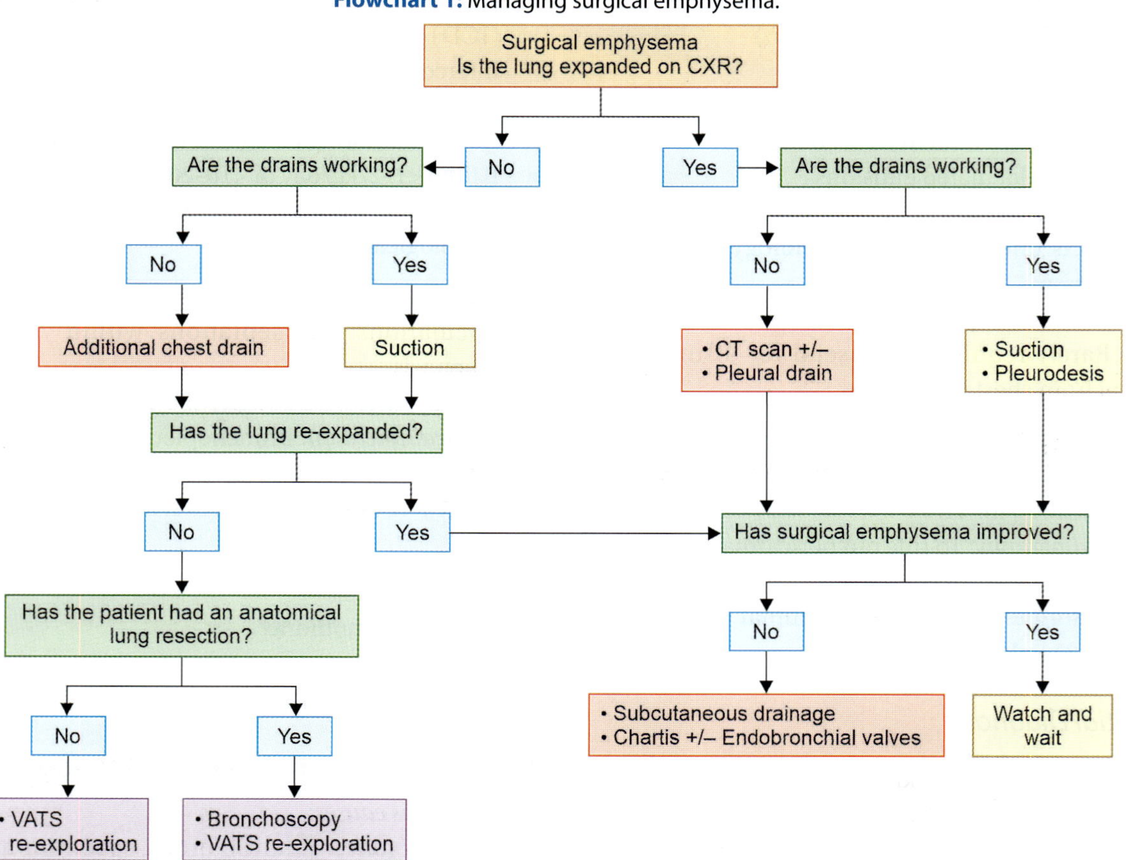

- *Procedures:* Video-assisted thoracoscopic surgery (VATS) and minithoracotomy or open decortication:
  - *Indications:*
    - Thick pleural peel encasing the lung
    - Pleural debris
      - >20% volume
      - <20% volume, but symptoms (fever/tachypnea) are persistent
    - Multiloculated empyema
    - Cavitary lung necrosis
    - Persistent broncho-pleural fistula with collapse of lung.

  Pleurodesis: In recurrent effusions, especially in malignancy.

Postoperative Surgical Emphysema) (Flowchart 1)

- *Monitoring and follow-up:*
  - Regular clinical and radiological assessments to ensure resolution.
  - Evaluate for complications such as fibrothorax, chronic lung disease, or recurrence.
  - Address underlying systemic conditions comprehensively.

Conclusion

Pleural effusion in children demands a multidisciplinary approach that integrates careful history-taking, thorough physical examination, and targeted investigations. Timely and appropriate management tailored to the underlying etiology improves outcomes and minimizes complications.

ARTERIAL BLOOD GAS ANALYSIS

Introduction

Arterial blood gas analysis is a cornerstone of clinical practice that allows healthcare professionals to assess a patient's respiratory and metabolic status quickly and efficiently. The results of an ABG analysis provide critical information that can guide diagnosis, treatment, and monitoring of various medical conditions, particularly those affecting the lungs and the body's acid-base balance. This chapter aims to simplify the complexities of ABG interpretation by breaking down its components, explaining the significance of each parameter, and providing a structured approach to analysis.

What is ABG?

Arterial blood gases are measurements taken from arterial blood to evaluate the levels of oxygen (O_2) and CO_2, as well as the acid-base status of the blood. These measurements are crucial in various clinical settings, including emergency departments, intensive care units, and outpatient clinics. ABG analysis helps clinicians make informed decisions regarding ventilation support, fluid management, and other therapeutic interventions.

How to Draw ABG?

Arterial blood is usually drawn via the brachial or radial artery.

- Inform the client about the procedure and that there is no food or fluid restriction imposed.
- Note if the client is taking anticoagulant therapy or aspirin, as this may affect results.
- Note if the client is receiving oxygen therapy (flow rate, type of administration device), and the client's current temperature.
- Using a heparinized needle and syringe, collect 1-5 mL of arterial blood. Common sites for drawing arterial blood are the radial and brachial arteries.
- Put the syringe with arterial blood in an ice-water bag to minimize the metabolic activity of the sample.
- Deliver the blood sample immediately to the laboratory.
- Apply pressure to the puncture site for 5 minutes or longer.

Components of Arterial Blood Gas

An ABG report typically includes the following key parameters:

- *pH:* Indicates the acidity or alkalinity of the blood. A normal pH range is critical for enzymatic and metabolic processes.
- *Partial pressure of oxygen (PaO_2):* Measures the amount of oxygen dissolved in arterial blood. It reflects the efficiency of oxygen transfer from the lungs to the bloodstream.
- *Partial pressure of CO_2 ($PaCO_2$):* Reflects the amount of CO_2 dissolved in the blood and indicates the respiratory function and effectiveness of ventilation.
- *Bicarbonate (HCO_3^-):* Represents the metabolic component of acid-base balance. It is a buffer that helps maintain the pH within the normal range.
- *Base excess (BE):* Assesses the metabolic component and indicates the amount of excess or insufficient base in the blood. It provides additional information on metabolic disorders.

Importance of Arterial Blood Gas Analysis

Arterial blood gas analysis is vital for diagnosing and managing several conditions, including:

- *Respiratory diseases:* Such as asthma, chronic obstructive pulmonary disease (COPD), and pneumonia.
- *Metabolic disorders:* Including diabetic ketoacidosis and acute kidney injury.
- *Critical care scenarios:* Such as sepsis, trauma, and postoperative complications.

Understanding ABG results can significantly impact patient management and outcomes, making it an essential skill for healthcare practitioners.

Understanding the Normal Ranges

Before interpreting ABG results, it is essential to know the normal ranges for these parameters:

- *pH:* 7.35–7.45
- *PaO_2:* 75–100 mm Hg
- *$PaCO_2$:* 35–45 mm Hg
- *HCO_3^-:* 22–26 mEq/L
- *BE:* –2 to +2 mEq/L

These normal ranges serve as a reference point for evaluating individual patient results.

Interpreting Arterial Blood Gas Results

Step 1: Assess the pH

The first step in ABG interpretation is to determine whether the blood is acidic or alkaline:

- *Acidemia:* pH <7.35 indicates an acidic environment, which can lead to cellular dysfunction.
- *Alkalemia:* pH >7.45 indicates an alkaline environment, which can also disrupt normal physiological processes.

Step 2: Analyze the $PaCO_2$

$PaCO_2$ provides insight into the respiratory component of acid-base balance:

- *Respiratory acidosis:* $PaCO_2$ >45 mm Hg, often due to hypoventilation (e.g., from COPD, respiratory muscle weakness, or central nervous system depression).
- *Respiratory alkalosis:* $PaCO_2$ <35 mm Hg, usually resulting from hyperventilation (e.g., anxiety, pain, or pulmonary embolism).

Step 3: Evaluate the HCO_3^-

HCO_3^- indicates the metabolic component of acid-base status:

- *Metabolic acidosis:* HCO_3^- <22 mEq/L, which can result from conditions such as diabetic ketoacidosis, renal failure, or lactic acidosis.
- *Metabolic alkalosis:* HCO_3^- >26 mEq/L, often caused by prolonged vomiting, diuretic use, or excessive bicarbonate administration.

Step 4: Determine the primary disorder

By correlating the pH with $PaCO_2$ and HCO_3^-, you can identify the primary disorder:

- *Respiratory acidosis:* Low pH, high $PaCO_2$
- *Respiratory alkalosis:* High pH, low $PaCO_2$
- *Metabolic acidosis:* Low pH, low HCO_3^-
- *Metabolic alkalosis:* High pH, high HCO_3^-

Step 5: Assess compensation

The body attempts to compensate for primary disturbances.

Primary acid-base disturbances:

They are:

- *Uncompensated Respiratory Acidosis:* This occurs when there is an increase in the $PaCO_2$ level without a resultant alteration (increase) of the HCO_3^- value. Thus, there will be an acidosis due to respiratory failure (inability to remove excess CO_2 from the blood and the lungs).
- *Partially compensated respiratory acidosis:* This occurs when there is an increase in the $PaCO_2$ level with a resultant alteration (increase) of the HCO_3 value, but the pH is still not within the normal range. Thus, there will still be acidosis due to respiratory failure (inability to remove excess CO_2 from the blood and the lungs).
- *Fully compensated Respiratory Acidosis:* This occurs when there is an increase in the $PaCO_2$ level with a resultant alteration (increase) of the HCO_3 value; thereby, balancing the pH within the normal range. Thus, there will be compensation for the acidosis due to respiratory failure (inability to remove excess CO_2 from the blood and the lungs) with metabolic alkalosis.
- *Uncompensated respiratory alkalosis:* This occurs when there is a decrease in the $PaCO_2$ level without a resultant alteration (decrease) of the HCO_3 value. Thus, there will be an alkalosis due to respiratory failure (excess CO_2 exhalation from the lungs and reduced CO_2 tension in the blood).
- *Partially compensated respiratory alkalosis:* This occurs when there is a decrease in the $PaCO_2$ level with a resultant alteration (decrease) of the HCO_3 value, but the pH is still not within the normal range. Thus, there will be an alkalosis due to respiratory failure (excess CO_2 exhalation from the lungs and reduced CO_2 tension in the blood).
- *Fully compensated respiratory alkalosis:* This occurs when there is a decrease in the $PaCO_2$ level with a resultant alteration (decrease) of the HCO_3 value; thereby, balancing the pH within the normal range. Thus, there will be compensation for the alkalosis due to respiratory failure (excess CO_2 exhalation from the lungs and reduced CO_2 tension in the blood) with metabolic acidosis.
- *Uncompensated metabolic acidosis:* This occurs when there is a decrease in the HCO_3 level without a resultant alteration (decrease) of the $PaCO_2$ value. Thus, there will be an acidosis due to metabolic failure (inability of the kidney to retain adequate bicarbonate).
- *Partially compensated metabolic acidosis:* This occurs when there is a decrease in the HCO_3 level with a resultant alteration (decrease) of the $PaCO_2$ value; but, the pH is still not within the normal range. Thus, there will still be acidosis due to metabolic failure (inability of the kidney to retain adequate bicarbonate).
- *Fully compensated metabolic acidosis:* This occurs when there is a decrease in the HCO3 level with a resultant alteration (decrease) of the $PaCO_2$ value; thereby, balancing the pH within the normal range. Thus, there will be compensation for the acidosis due to metabolic failure (inability of the kidney to retain adequate bicarbonate) with respiratory alkalosis.
- *Uncompensated metabolic alkalosis:* This occurs when there is an increase in the HCO3 level without a resultant alteration (increase) of the $PaCO_2$ value. Thus, there will be an alkalosis due to metabolic failure (inability of the kidney to excrete excess bicarbonate).

- *Partially compensated metabolic alkalosis:* This occurs when there is an increase in the HCO3 level with a resultant alteration (increase) of the $PaCO_2$ value, but the pH is still not within the normal range. Thus, there will be an alkalosis due to metabolic failure (inability of the kidney to excrete excess bicarbonate).
- *Fully compensated metabolic alkalosis:* This occurs when there is an increase in the HCO_3 level with a resultant alteration (increase) of the $PaCO_2$ value; thereby, balancing the pH within the normal range. Thus, there will be compensation for the alkalosis due to metabolic failure (inability of the kidney to excrete excess bicarbonate) with respiratory acidosis.
- *Mixed acid-base disturbances:* This occurs when there is either both metabolic and respiratory acidosis present or metabolic and respiratory alkalosis present at the same time of analyzing ABGs.

SUGGESTED READING

1. APA: Kundu AK. (2023/2024). Bedside Clinics in Medicine: With Colour Photos and Clinical Integration (9th Edition). CBS Publishers.
2. Examination Paediatrics, Edition 5 by Wayne Harris, MBBS, MRCP(UK), FRACP, ISBN: 9780729542517.
3. Light MJ, etal. Pediatric pulmonology, AAP: jaypee brothers: indian reprint: 2013.
4. Pediatric Clinical Examination edited by A. Santhosh Kumar, J Chandra Published 18 April 2009.
5. Pediatric Respirology A Ready Reckoner. Gautam ghosh, pallav chatterjee, subhashis roy, ISBN: 978-81-943206-8-5, 1st edition, noble publication, 2024.

CHAPTER 6

Examination of Gastrointestinal System and its Disorder

Subhamoy Das, Sneha Dasgupta

INTRODUCTION

The gastrointestinal (GI) system stretches nearly 8 m in length—starting at the mouth and ending with the anus. It is a complex system of organs which arise from the endoderm and is unique as it has its own nervous system. The part from the mouth to the ligament of Treitz arises from the foregut, which also gives rise to the liver and pancreas. Midgut gives rise to the third part of duodenum to proximal two-thirds of the transverse colon and the rest of the GI tract is derived from the hind gut. However, when it comes to the examination of the GI system, the kidneys and genitalia are also included. Although, most of the GI complaints are vague, sometimes there are very specific symptoms pertaining to a specific organ.

HISTORY TAKING

Gastrointestinal disease can present with a wide variety of symptoms affecting oral intake, the abdomen, bowel motions, and the patient's constitution. By taking a thorough history, it is possible to narrow down the differential diagnosis and guide clinical examination.

There are few normal GI sensations, e.g., hunger perceived as epigastric discomfort; vigorous peristaltic movements for propelling the gas, food bolus, and liquids is called borborygmi and a sensation of colonic fullness is felt prior to defecation.

The common GI symptoms/complaints are discussed in this chapter.

Dysphagia and Odynophagia

Dysphagia refers to the awareness of something being stuck in the throat while swallowing and gives an unpleasant sensation during the act of swallowing. It is often associated with a significant cause and warrants further evaluation. Most common causes in children constitute esophageal strictures (congenital or acquired, as a sequela of acid/alkali ingestion), rings, webs, vascular impressions, and eosinophilic esophagitis. In such cases, dysphagia is more to solids as compared to liquids, whereas, neuromuscular causes of dysphagia, such as, achalasia, present with dysphagia more to liquids. Often, there is history of maneuvering during swallowing and patient takes a long time to finish meals.

Odynophagia indicates painful swallowing. Esophageal infections such as esophageal candidiasis, human immunodeficiency virus (HIV), and acute stage of acid/alkali burns may have this manifestation.

Heartburn and Dyspepsia

Heartburn or epigastric pain as a result of acid reflux into the lower end of esophagus is relatively rare in children. It may be a symptom of reflux esophagitis or hiatus hernia. There is retrosternal pain and may also cause chest pain. The reflux is often associated with bitter/disagreeable sensation in the mouth.

Dyspepsia is a subjective symptom where there is feeling of fullness, discomfort, and nausea occurring after meals. Frequently, there is no demonstratable cause, but, maybe associated with acid peptic disorders or *Helicobacter pylori* infections which is becoming increasingly common in children.

Anorexia, Early Satiety, and Sitophobia

Loss of appetite is known as anorexia and may be due to many GI diseases including inflammatory bowel disease (IBD), abdominal tuberculosis, and other systemic diseases. There is overall low intake of food and calories thus contributing to weight loss.

Early satiety is felt when appetite is preserved; however, after taking two to three mouthfuls, patient feels full. This may occur as a result of exogenous compression of the stomach such as splenomegaly or a large pancreatic collection pressing on the stomach.

Sitophobia is the fear of developing pain after eating, as a result of which the patient voluntarily consumes less food even though appetite is good. Maybe a sequela of chronic pancreatitis or cholecystitis where pain is triggered by intake of food.

Constipation

Infrequent bowel movement is termed as constipation. Rome IV defines constipation as less than three bowel movements per week. In children, the most common cause for constipation is functional constipation **(Box 1)**. However, one must carefully exclude all the red flags as well **(Box 2)**.

Functional constipation is often associated with history of large diameter stools, retentive posturing, where the child arches their body or crosses their legs or holds onto nearby object. The parents often perceive this as an attempt to pass stools, when in reality it is just a retentive maneuvering. There may also be a history of withholding behaviour where the child hides during potty time.

BOX 1: Rome IV criteria for functional constipation in children.

1. Must include two or more of the following:**
   a. Straining during more than one-fourth (25%) of defecations
   b. Lumpy or hard stools (Bristol Stool Form Scale 1-2) more than one-fourth (25%) of defecations
   c. Sensation of incomplete evacuation more than one-fourth (25%) of defecations
   d. Sensation of anorectal obstruction/blockage more than one-fourth (25%) of defecations
   e. Manual maneuvers to facilitate more than one-fourth (25%) of defecations (e.g., digital evacuation and support of the pelvic floor)
   f. Fewer than three spontaneous bowel movements (SBMs) per week
2. Loose stools are rarely present without the use of laxatives
3. Insufficient criteria for irritable bowel syndrome

**Rome IV Criteria- Ref- Rome Foundation J Neurogastroenterol Moti, Vol. 23, No. 2, April, 2017.

BOX 2: Red flags of constipation.

- Abdominal distension
- Passage of ribbon-like or pellet-like stools
- Passage of meconium >48 hours after birth
- Enterocolitis
- History of blood transfusion
- Failure to thrive
- Developmental delay
- Feeling too hot or too cold
- Inability to move lower limbs
- Loss of bladder control

Diarrhea

Any change in the consistency and frequency of stools is known as diarrhea. Roughly, passage of >300 g/day is labeled as diarrhea. Diarrhea maybe a clinical manifestation of various GI diseases.

Any diarrhea which is acute in onset, but lasts >14 days is known as persistent diarrhea. If insidious in onset, it is termed as chronic diarrhea. The causes include infections like giardiasis, secondary lactose intolerance for persistent diarrhea. The causes of chronic diarrhea are celiac disease, IBD, abdominal tuberculosis, primary or secondary protein losing enteropathy, etc., **(Table 1)**.

Abdominal Pain

This one of the most common GI complaints among the pediatric outpatient department (OPD) visits. As for any other type of pain, it is important to characterize the site, duration, nature and intensity, and radiation of pain along with enquiry regarding the associated features such as vomiting, weight loss, altered bowel habit, pallor, and abdominal distension. Aggravating and relieving factors also need to be asked into **(Table 2)**.

The most common cause of pain in pediatric visits is functional pain which is characterized by being non-specific, poorly localized, and absence of red flags **(Box 3)**.

Vomiting

Vomiting is the forceful expulsion of gastric or intestinal contents through the mouth and is often associated with nausea. Vomiting maybe nonbilious or greenish, i.e., bilious when originating from beyond second part of duodenum.

Effortless expulsion of food from the stomach into the esophagus or mouth is known as regurgitation.

TABLE 1: Small bowel versus large bowel diarrhea.

Small bowel diarrhea	*Large bowel diarrhea*
Large volume watery stools	Small volume diarrhea, often with blood or mucus
Frequency not very high	Frequency >10/day
Not associated with urgency or tenesmus	Associated with urgency and tenesmus
Child often presents with dehydration, micronutrient deficiency, edema, etc.	No such features are seen
Maybe associated with vomiting, weight loss, and flatulence	Uncommon

TABLE 2: Abdominal organs and site, nature, and radiation of pain

Stomach	• Epigastric pain with or without dyspepsia • Maybe aggravated by food intake
Biliary	• Right upper quadrant, severe pain • Lasting >1 hour, often colicky • Radiates to tip of right shoulder
Pancreas	• Epigastric or left upper quadrant • Radiates to the back • Dull severe pain • Associated with vomiting • Increased with intake of food • Often patient feels relief on bending forward
Small bowel	• Periumbilical • Colicky pain • Often associated with vomiting and abdominal distension/constipation

BOX 3: Red flags of abdominal pain.

- Pain >1 hour
- Localized pain (other than around the umbilicus)
- Nocturnal awakening
- Associated with significant weight loss
- Affecting daily activities
- Associated with change in bowel habits or bloody diarrhea

Common causes include gastroesophageal reflux (GER), rumination, etc.

Sometimes, vomiting may be a manifestation of raised intracranial tension and in such cases vomiting is usually not preceded with nausea and is projectile. Other non-GI causes of vomiting may be metabolic acidosis, uremia, etc.

Gastrointestinal Bleed

Hematemesis and Melena

These are a result of upper GI bleed (above the second part of duodenum). Hematemesis maybe painless—variceal bleed or maybe painful—gastric ulcers. Melena is black tarry stools and is produced as a result of colonic bacterial conversion of ferric iron of hemoglobin to ferrous form. For melena to occur minimum 60 mL of blood loss should have occurred and blood should remain in the gastrointestinal tract (GIT) for >6 hours.

Hematochezia

It is the passage of fresh blood per rectum. It indicates source in anal canal, rectum, or sigmoid colon.

Jaundice

Jaundice is the yellowish discoloration of skin and sclera along with mucous membrane. If jaundice is associated with high colored urine or diaper staining, it is likely conjugated jaundice. Unconjugated jaundice may be because of excessive hemolysis [chronic hemolytic anemias, blood group mismatch, and glucose-6-phosphate dehydrogenase (G6PD) deficiency] or maybe physiological in neonates due to immaturity of liver enzymes.

EXAMINATION

General Survey

- *Anthropometry:* Children with chronic liver disease (CLD) may have growth failure and loss of subcutaneous fat. Also, children with chronic diarrhea and malabsorption may have failure to thrive. Recently, metabolic fatty liver disease is on the rise and so children may also present with obesity and an increased waist circumference.
- *Pallor:* May be associated with portal hypertension, chronic diarrhea, or chronic GI blood loss.
- Cyanosis
- *Jaundice:* Is a manifestation of any liver disease and cirrhosis. It is best appreciated in the sclera and mucous membranes.
- *Clubbing:* Noted mainly as a consequence of hepatopulmonary syndrome.
- *Edema:* Is the swelling of the body due to accumulation of fluid in the subcutaneous space. It is palpated above the medial malleolus by pressing the skin for 10–20 seconds. This is known as pitting edema. It may be a finding in CLD and also in chronic diarrheas and protein losing enteropathies.
- *Head to toe examination*:
  - Hair
  - Eyes—to look for cataracts, Bitot's spots, and visible Kayser-Fleischer (KF) rings
  - Skin—spider nevi and xanthomas
  - Rickets

GI SYSTEM SYSTEMIC EXAMINATION—EXAMINATION OF THE ABDOMEN

Inspection

- *Position:* Patient should be lying supine with hands by the side.
- *Exposure:* Ideally, the exposure should be from mid-chest to mid-thigh; however in this era, and considering

the comfort of the patient it is always advisable to modestly expose the patient. In case of examination of a girl child, a female attender as well as the child's mother should be present. Before any examination or exposure, the patient and the guardian should be explained in detail about the examination and verbal consent for the same should be obtained.

- *Points to inspect:* During inspection one is supposed to see the abdomen for:
  - Shape: Whether the abdomen is full/scaphoid. To assess fullness, one must also look at the flanks. A distended abdomen maybe caused by organomegaly, accumulation of ascites, abdominal fat, or gaseous distension. In adolescent girls, pregnancy should also considered as a cause for abdominal distension. A scaphoid abdomen is noted in severe malnutrition and cachexia.
  - Umbilicus: The shape of the umbilicus maybe inverted, which is the normal shape. It may also be flushed or everted, i.e., elevated from the surface. The position of the umbilicus is usually midway between the tip of the xiphisternum and the symphysis pubis and is equidistant from the two anterior superior iliac spines. Any change in the position of the umbilicus is to be noted, usually and intra-abdominal mass such as a large ovarian cyst or omental cyst gives rise to such a finding.
  - Movements of the abdominal wall: The normal breathing pattern in children is abdominothoracic. In case of peritonitis, the movements with respiration are diminished.

    Visible pulsations maybe seen in aortic aneurysm.

    Visible peristalsis maybe seen in intestinal or gastric outlet obstruction. The intestinal movement is seen usually as a step ladder fashion and movement due to gastric outlet appears as a large wave of peristalsis from left to right.
  - Skin surface: In marked abdominal distension, skin appears shiny and stretched.

    Striae atrophicae are whitish wrinkled linear marks produced by stretching of the skin causing rupture of the elastic fibers. It indicated a recent change in the size of the abdomen such as rapid-onset massive ascites, Cushing's syndrome, and sudden onset obesity.

    Scars of previous trauma or surgery need to be looked for and described.

    Venous prominence is to be looked for, particularly, in cases of cirrhosis. If prominent or distended veins are present, the direction of filling of these veins gives an idea as to the etiology. If the veins fill toward the umbilics it signifies portal hypertension (due to portocaval anastomosis).

    Pigmentation of the abdominal skin should also be noted.

    Any visible swelling or lump should be reported. If lump is noted then it is important to note its site, approximate size (which is to be confirmed on palpation), movement with respiration, shape, and surface. Whether the mass is arising from the abdominal wall or intraperitoneal is to be confirmed by straight leg rising test where in case of intraperitoneal mass, it disappears and an abdominal wall mass becomes more prominent. In case the doubt is between an intraperitoneal and retroperitoneal mass, child is kept in knee chest position and with this, the intraperitoneal mass falls forward.
  - Hernial sites and orifices: All hernial sites and orifices including the genitalia should be carefully examined.

Palpation

The abdomen is divided into four quadrants and nine regions. Two lines, one extending from xiphisternum to symphysis pubis, and another line perpendicular to it across the umbilicus divides the abdomen into right upper and lower, and left upper and lower quadrants. The nine regions are right and left hypochondrium, epigastrium, right and left lumbar, periumbilicus, hypogastrium, and right and left iliac fossae.

One should start with superficial palpation for local temperature and any superficial tenderness in any of the quadrants. During this time, any visible mass should also be palpated. Filling of distended veins are to be assessed.

Then the deep structures are palpated. While doing so, the wrist and the forearm should be in the same horizontal plane, even if it requires bending down or kneeling by the patient's bedside. Move flexibly with gentle but firm pressure. The fingers should be straight and one must avoid inadvertent poking.

- Note any deep tenderness:
  - McBurney's point—for appendix and caecum. It is the point between medial two-thirds and lateral one-third of the right spinoumbilical line.

  - Renal angle—T12 vertebra.
  - Murphey's sign—for gallbladder tenderness. This point lies at the tip of the 9th costal cartilage.
- *Palpation of deep structures:*
  - Liver—palpation is to be started gently from the right iliac fossa just lateral to the rectus. The radial border of the hand should be parallel to the ribs. Gradually move up toward the ribs till resistance is felt. When the lower border is palpable, one should trace the whole lower margin and move toward the left to see if left lobe is palpable. Size of the liver should be noted in centimeters from the right costal margin and it should be measured along the right midclavicular line. Once liver is palpated, the margin, surface, and consistency should be noted. Sometimes, in case of acute viral hepatitis or liver abscess, liver may be tender.
  - Spleen—for spleen to be palpable, it must be enlarged to at least double its size. Initial enlargement of the spleen occurs in the superior and posterior direction before it becomes palpable subcostally, after that, it enlarges downward. In children, spleen grows toward the left iliac fossa. If spleen is not palpable in the supine position, patient is to be turned to right lateral position with left had placed over the back and fingers of the right hand to be hooked along the left subcostal margin, known as the hooking method. Once spleen is palpable, it should be differentiated from the left kidney. Spleen characteristically has notches on its surface **(Table 3)**.
  - Kidneys—the kidneys on both sides are palpated bimanually. For the right kidney, right hand is to be placed horizontally in the right lumbar region with the left hand placed posteriorly in the loin. Similarly, during palpation of the left kidney, the hands to be changed. If kidneys are enlarged, then it becomes ballotable.

TABLE 3: Differentiation of spleen versus left kidney.

Left kidney	*Spleen*
Upper pole palpated	Not possible to get to upper end
Smooth surface	Notches palpable
Resonant on percussion	Dull on percussion
Moves very little with inspiration	Moves well with inspiration

  - Abdominal mass—to note the site, size and shape; surface, edge, and consistency; and mobility and attachments.
  - Other structures to be palpated:
    - Urinary bladder if palpable/full
    - Aorta and para-aortic glands are felt by rolling
    - Both groins
    - External genitalia and hernial orifices

Percussion

Defining Boundaries of Solid Organs

- *Liver:* To find the upper border of liver dullness, start palpating from the 2nd intercostal space along the midclavicular line. The total liver span is measured from the upper border of liver dullness to the lower margin.
  - Liver span according to age—roughly
  - Preterm infants 4–5 cm
  - Term infants 5–6.5 cm
  - 1–5 years 6–7cm
  - 5–10 years 7–9 cm
  - 10–16 years 8–10 cm
- *Spleen:* Shifting dullness and fluid thrill

Auscultation

One must auscultate for:

- Intestinal peristaltic sounds (IPSs)
- Venous hum
- Arterial bruit

APPROACH TO CHRONIC LIVER DISEASE IN CHILDREN

Chronic liver disease in children encompasses a wide spectrum of disorders, which include infections, metabolic, genetic, drug induced, idiopathic and structural causes, and can progress to cirrhosis and end-stage liver disease. CLD with neonatal or infantile onset can be due to structural disorder of hepatobiliary system [e.g., biliary atresia (BA) and choledochal cyst], congenital hepatic fibrosis, metabolic disorders (e.g., galactosemia, tyrosinemia, and cystic fibrosis) or intrauterine infections which present as cholestasis of infancy requiring stepwise approach and precise investigations for accurate diagnosis and exact management. Among a wide range of etiologic possibilities, common causes for CLD in children beyond infancy are autoimmune hepatitis (AIH), metabolic disorders like Wilson's disease, and viral infections such as hepatitis B, hepatitis C, and less commonly alpha-1 antitrypsin deficiency.

Clinicians often do not recognize the presence of underlying liver disease, and precise documentation of the disorder can be delayed, leading to a subsequent delay in the initiation of specific therapy. Particularly in case of neonates and infants, early recognition is important because a delay in diagnosis may have a negative effect on the prognosis. Absence of jaundice is not enough to rule out CLD. However a child of CLD with jaundice, hepatomegaly and hepatic encephalopathy requires aggressive management. Sometimes, the condition should be considered in a child with no current or past evidence of liver disease when liver function tests are abnormal on routine medical examination or for complaints unrelated to the liver.

Epidemiology

Chronic liver disease accounts for about 1–5% of different pediatric admissions and accounts for 20% of mortality in our country. The estimated incidence of neonatal liver disease is as high as 1 in 1,000 to 2,500 live births. Availability of definitive etiological and histological assessment and institution of specific and supportive therapy has made prolonged survival with positive impact on quality of life. Affordability and accessible facility for liver transplant in many centers in the country has changed the outcome scenario in the recent decade but this is still in infancy in comparison to the developed world.

Definition of Chronic Liver Disease

A possibility of CLD should be considered in occurrence of intrahepatic and extrahepatic diseases affecting hepatocytes, vascular structure, and biliary structure with clinical, biochemical, and pathological counterparts lasting for >3 months. CLD in case of hepatitis B and C infection is defined as persistence of infection for >6 months. CLD occurs when there is progressive destruction of the liver parenchyma over a certain period leading to fibrosis and cirrhosis. However, any child presenting with features of severe liver disease or physical stigmata of CLD at any point of time may also be considered as CLD. The common causes of CLD in different age groups and the comprehensive list of liver diseases leading to chronicity in children is shown in **Tables 4 and 5**, respectively.

TABLE 4: Age wise distribution of common causes of CLD in children.

Infancy	*1–5 years*	*5–10 years*	*>10 years*
Galactosemia	Tyrosinemia	Wilson's disease	Wilson's disease
Tyrosinemia	HFI	AIH	AIH
HFI	AIH	HVOTO	Chronic hepatitis B/C
PFIC1 and PFIC2	HVOTO	PFIC3	PFIC
Biliary atresia	PFIC1/PFIC2		NAFLD
	ICC		Celiac disease
			PSC

(AIH: autoimmune hepatitis; CLD: Chronic liver disease; HFI: hereditary fructose intolerance; HVOTO: hepatic venous outflow tract obstruction; NAFLD: nonalcoholic fatty liver disease; PFIC: progressive familial intrahepatic cholestasis; PSC: primary sclerosing cholangitis)

The etiological profile of CLD at different centers in India with pediatric gastroenterology and hepatology units is given in **Table 6**.

The clinical spectrum of CLD is quite variable and depends upon the underlying etiology and prognosis of liver disease. The clinical syndromes in CLD has been categorized in **Table 7**.

APPROACH TO CHRONIC LIVER DISEASE

Clinical Presentation

A child with chronic liver may present with or without history of jaundice, however careful elicitation of history is important for any signs of portal hypertensive bleed or ascites or other signs of decompensation in past history which may be suggestive. CLD should also be suspected in a patient who has a previous history of cholestasis in infantile age, history of CLD in a family member, genetic disease or autoimmunity, a relapse of an apparent acute hepatitis, persistence of clinical features of acute hepatitis for >3 months, or a previous history of hepatitis B, C or non-A, non-E hepatitis.

Glycogen storage disorders (GSDs) may present with moderate to massive hepatomegaly without history of jaundice in the past and biochemical parameters suggestive of isolated transaminasemia. Patients with the autosomal recessive liver-specific type may develop cirrhosis after a considerable period. Salient features of CLD are given in **Table 8**.

TABLE 5: Etiology of chronic liver disease.

Chronic hepatitis (hepatocellular causes)	• Viral hepatitis B and C • Autoimmune hepatitis • Sclerosing cholangitis • Drug-induced hepatitis
Cholestasis-related liver disease	• Extrahepatic biliary atresia • Choledochal cyst • Neonatal sclerosing cholangitis • Progressive familial intrahepatic cholestasis (PFIC) • Partial internal biliary drainage (PIBD)
Genetic or metabolic	• Wilson disease • Indian childhood cirrhosis • Hemochromatosis • Glycogen storage disorder • Galactosemia • Tyrosinemia • Mucopolysaccharidosis • Gaucher's disease • Niemen Pick's disease • Wolman disease • Alpha-1 antitrypsin disease • Mucopolysaccharidosis
Congestive disorder	• Budd–Chiari syndrome (BCS) • Veno-occlusive disease • Congestive cardiac failure • Chronic constrictive pericarditis
Portal hypertension-related chronic liver disease	• BCS • Focal nodular hyperplasia • Extrahepatic portal vein obstruction (EHPVO) • Congenital hepatic fibrosis • Non cirrhotic portal fibrosis
Miscellaneous	• Nonalcoholic steatohepatitis (NASH) • Histiocytosis

TABLE 6: Indian scenario of chronic liver disease.

Etiology	*Chennai*	*Pune*	*Chandigarh*	*Lucknow*	*MAMC, New Delhi*	*AIIMS, New Delhi*
Study period	1988–1997	1996–1997	1991–1994	1992–1998	1997–1998	1992–1997
Total patients	236	117	113	144	38	161
Viral	75 (32%)	2 (2%)	9 (8%)	15 (10%)	17 (45%)	29 (18%)
Autoimmune	0 (0%)	7 (6%)	21 (19%)	4 (3%)	1 (3%)	16 (10%)
Metabolic	18 (8%)	50 (43%)	24 (21%)	40 (28%)	4 (11%)	34 (21%)
Others	6 (3%)	14 (12%)	25 (23%)	3 (2%)	2 (5%)	33 (20%)
Unknown	137 (58%)	44 (38%)	34 (31%)	82 (57%)	14 (36%)	49 (30%)

(AIIMS: All India Institute of Medical Sciences; MAMC: Maulana Azad Medical College)

Examination

A thorough clinical examination will be helpful to suggest the presence of chronicity, other than firm hepatomegaly (with or without splenomegaly), a shrunken liver (indicating cirrhosis), an enlarged left lobe of liver or a hard nodular liver is a positive pointer in most cases.

TABLE 7: Clinical syndromes of chronic liver disease (CLD) at presentation.

1. Chronic hepatitis without decompensation	• Patient presenting with features of chronicity in form of firm hepatomegaly and deranged liver function tests • Example, chronic hepatitis B and C
2. Asymptomatic presentation with organomegaly and/or elevated transaminases	• Incidentally detected with firm hepatomegaly with or without splenomegaly • Example, congestive heart failure (CHF) or glycogen storage disorder (GSD)
3. Acute hepatitis in underlying chronic liver disease	• Patient with chronic liver disease may present with jaundice and biochemical parameters suggestive of acute hepatitis with underlying CLD • Example, acute viral hepatitis (A or E) in a patient with undetected CLD like autoimmune hepatitis (AIH) or Wilson's disease
4. Acute on chronic liver failure (ACLF)	ACLF is defined by the Asian Pacific Association for the Study of Liver (APASL) as an acute hepatic insult manifesting as jaundice and coagulopathy, complicated within 4 weeks by ascites, and/or encephalopathy in a patient with previously diagnosed or undiagnosed chronic liver disease
5. Jaundice with cholestasis	• Liver disease associated with cholestasis (biochemically defined as conjugated bilirubin fraction being >20% of total bilirubin or with clinical features of cholestasis) • Example, infantile or neonatal cholestasis syndrome due to various etiology

Other findings include firm splenomegaly; ascites; edema; cutaneous portosystemic shunts; bleeding from portal hypertension; growth failure; muscle wasting; and cutaneous stigmata of CLD. Clinical signs of CLD are given in **Table 9**.

The cutaneous stigmata of CLD includes spider angioma, palmar erythema, diffuse pruritus, caput medusae, etc., are described in **Table 10**.

Extrahepatic autoimmune manifestations such as presence of KF rings in eyes are to be evaluated in etiological workup.

Cirrhosis is the final pathway of a number of CLDs. It is a pathological entity and described as diffuse hepatic fibrosis leading to replacement of normal liver architecture by nodules. However the duration of progression of CLD to cirrhosis is variable from weeks (in complete biliary obstruction) to decades (in chronic hepatitis C). Cirrhosis is one of the leading causes of death from CLD and is debilitating for a child in the most productive period of his life.

Etiological Workup for CLD

Every case with CLD merits a meticulous clinical assessment and complete biochemical and serological sampling including liver biopsy for histopathological assessment in order to reach a conclusive diagnosis.

The laboratory findings of liver injury can be divided broadly into two patterns:

1. Cholestatic or obstructive bile duct injury
2. Injury to hepatocytes or hepatocellular damage

TABLE 8: Salient features in history suggestive of chronic liver disease (CLD) in child.

Prolonged or recurrent episodes jaundice	Hepatotoxic drugs
History of cholestasis	Past history of botulinum toxin (BT)/injection use/tattooing/ surgical Procedures/previous hospitalization
Decompensation (ascites, encephalopathy)	Family history of liver disorder
Upper gastrointestinal (GI) bleed	

TABLE 9: Salient features on examination in chronic liver disease (CLD).

Firm liver on palpation with or without splenomegaly	Cutaneous signs of liver disease
Growth retardation	Prominent abdominal veins
Muscle wasting	Evidence of free fluid (ascites)

However, both types of injury can have considerable overlap in a patient who has liver disease.

The products of hepatocellular system (bile pigments, enzymes, and bile salts), present normally within or eliminated via bile will increase in cholestatic conditions. Hence, alkaline phosphatase (ALP), gamma glutamyl transpeptidase (GGT), and conjugated bilirubin require a clear biliary tree for elimination and will be elevated in cholestatic liver disease. A serum ALP elevation out

TABLE 10: Skin manifestations in chronic liver disease (CLD).

Cutaneous manifestation	*Physiological mechanism and description*
Spider angioma	Central arteriole from which radiating small branches are seen and compression leading to blanching. Exact pathogenesis is not known. More than 2–3 is abnormal.
Jaundice or icterus	Yellowish discoloration of skin and eyes due to deposition of bilirubin in collagen layer
Pruritus	• Itching of palm and sole and diffuse pruritus with excoriation can occur • Deposition of bile acids considered as probable cause
Palmar erythema	Not specific for CLD and appear as mottling of palm and blanching of erythematous palm
Dilated abdominal veins	Due to development of portosystemic collateral channels
Caput medusae	Abdominal wall collateral veins radiating as tortuous vessels from umbilicus
Terry' nail	Proximal or diffuse nail bed pallor
Clubbing	Deformed fingernail bed due to arteriovenous shunt in the lungs

of proportion to level of aminotransferase suggests a cholestatic disorder.

The demarcation between the category of liver injury is not always clear-cut. For example, cholestasis will always lead to a certain degree of hepatocellular damage because of the toxic accumulation of bile within the hepatocytes and the biliary tree. In hepatocellular disease, the reduced bile flow (causing sludge) that results from necrosis of the hepatocytes may cause some rise in serum markers of hepatobiliary obstruction alkaline phosphatase (AP and GGT). Other enzymes that are not routinely tested to detect cholestasis are 5-nucleotidase and leucine aminopeptidase. The baseline investigations done in CLD and further workup done for confirmation of etiology is given here.

Laboratory Parameters

Hematological Investigations

Complete blood count (CBC): Thrombocytopenia in CBC can be found in cirrhosis. Low hemoglobin, total leukocyte count (TLC), and low platelets go in favor of hypersplenism, manifested due to splenomegaly secondary to portal hypertension.

TABLE 11: Biochemical parameters in chronic liver disease (CLD).

Serum bilirubin levels	Bleeding time and clotting time
Liver enzymes	Prothrombin time (PT) and prothrombin index (PI)
Serum protein (total protein and ser albumin)	Blood ammonia
Alkaline phosphatase and gamma glutamyl transpeptidase (GGT)	Renal function Tests

Biochemical Investigations

Biochemical parameters done for workup of CLD are given in **Table 11**.

Liver function tests: Impaired intrahepatic excretion/regurgitation of unconjugated or conjugated bilirubin from hepatocytes of bile ducts results in conjugated hyperbilirubinemia. Bilirubin may be of prognostic value in conditions like fulminant hepatic failure where deep jaundice is associated with increased mortality. Alanine aminotransferase (ALT) or alanine amino transferase is specific for hepatocytes while aspartate aminotransferase (AST) is also secreted by other tissues such as skeletal, cardiac, muscle, kidney, and brain. AST/ALT ratio of >2 indicates CLD. The ratio of AST/ALT < 1 indicates acute hepatic injury. Hepatocytic injury or necrosis following an insult to the liver (e.g., acetaminophen overdose or viral hepatitis) will initially lead to raised enzymes found within the hepatocyte, such as ALT and AST. In toxic hepatitis, viral hepatitis, chronic active hepatitis, and cholestasis hepatitis, ALT can exceed AST. In alcoholic liver disease and Wilson's disease, the ratio of mitochondrial AST: total AST is elevated.

In hepatocellular disease, the serum levels of GGT and AP do not rise to the same degree as the aminotransferases however up to a fourfold elevation of serum ALP can be seen in 75% of patients with cholestasis, of both extrahepatic and intrahepatic pathology. Further evaluation of elevated ALP is to be done by imaging of biliary tract and presence of dilated ducts lead to an elevation of extrahepatic causes of cholestasis while in absence of same, intrahepatic causes are to be considered. The ratio of AP and total bilirubin is low in fulminant Wilson's disease but regardless of cause of acute hepatic failure, a low AP:bilirubin ratio is indication of poor prognosis. Decreased synthetic capacity of liver due to chronic hepatocytic injury is validated by low albumin levels and deranged coagulogram. Normal serum value of albumin ranges from 3.5 to 5 g/dL and a value below 3 g/dL in hepatitis should raise the suspicion of underlying CLD or cirrhosis causing decreased synthesis. However, extrahepatic causes of hypoalbuminemia and coagulopathy should be excluded.

Blood ammonia: Most ammonia in the body is formed by breakdown of protein by bacteria in the gut lumen. The liver converts ammonia into urea, which is then eliminated in urine. Ammonia levels in the blood is elevated when the liver is unable to convert ammonia to urea. This may be caused by CLD going into cirrhosis or severe hepatitis and metabolic liver disease. Hyperammonemia and encephalopathy are findings of liver failure and there is some correlation between the degree of encephalopathy and serum ammonia levels. However, specimen is needed to be drawn in fasting state and quick transport to the laboratory on ice packs is required to avoid falsely high levels.

Radiological Investigation

Ultrasonography (USG) abdomen: B-mode ultrasound supplemented by portal system Doppler and contrast-enhanced ultrasound are the principal techniques in the assessment of liver parenchyma and portal venous hypertension and in surveillance of hepatocellular malignancy. In cirrhosis liver is shrunken, irregular with nodular surface, and dilated splenoportal axis. At conventional B-mode ultrasound, diffuse fatty infiltration or fibrosis results in altered echogenicity of the liver when compared to other organs such as the renal cortex with increased echogenicity of the liver parenchyma, poor or nonvisualization of the diaphragm, intrahepatic vessels, and posterior part of the right hepatic lobe. Qualitative grading can be done as mild, moderate, or severe, or grade 0–3 with 0 being normal.

Ultrasound Doppler study: The major role of Doppler ultrasound is the assessment of portal venous hypertension as a complication of cirrhotic liver or other noncirrhotic condition. Doppler ultrasound of the ligamentum teres showing hepatofugal venous signal (i.e., a patent paraumbilical vein) and hepatofugal flow in the portal vein are considered specific signs with a high positive predictive value for documenting portal hypertension. Assessment of portal venous flow pattern also has role in the diagnosis of portal hypertension. Normal venous blood flow is continuous with hepatopetal direction on Doppler ultrasound with least variations due to cardiac cycle and respiration. Reversed (hepatofugal) portal venous blood flow is expected when intrahepatic resistance is greater than the resistance of portosystemic collaterals. Color Doppler studies in Budd–Chiari syndrome (BCS) may depict no flow or flat flow in the hepatic veins; flow in the reversed direction in hepatic veins, inferior vena cava (IVC), or both and intrahepatic collateral pathways. It is also found that visualization of a caudate vein >3 mm in diameter on grayscale sonography strongly suggests BCS in appropriate clinical setting.

FibroScan: Transient elastography (FibroScan) is a new method of evaluation of fibrosis in CLD which is noninvasive, rapid, and reproducible by liver stiffness assessment. In cirrhotic liver, stiffness quantified ranges from 12.5 to 75.5 kPa. Though the clinical relevance of these values is unknown but availability of appropriate size probe has made this investigation useful for assessing the progression to cirrhosis in case of CLD.

Magnetic resonance imaging: In BCS, MR images obtained with T2-weighted sequences usually show heterogeneously increased signal intensity in the peripheral portion of the liver. Acquisition of T2-weighted gradient-recalled echo sequences shows absence of flow in the hepatic veins and IVC in BCS.

Magnetic resonance cholangiopancreatography (MRCP) can be done to see for obstructive pathology in the hepatobiliary tract [primary sclerosing cholangitis (PSC)] and MRI brain is done in case of Wilson's disease when associated neurological complications is present.

Angiography: Inferior venacavography or hepatic venacavography showing a spiderweb pattern of collateral vessels is pathognomonic of BCS. Angiographic studies can demonstrate the presence of thrombus within the hepatic veins or IVC. Another typical feature of BCS is long segmental compression of the IVC contributed by caudate lobe hypertrophy. The hepatic arteries are seen to be dilated and associated with arterioportal shunts.

Upper Gastrointestinal Endoscopy

Evaluation for portal hypertension is important for prediction or detection of gastroesophageal varices, variceal hemorrhage, ascites, renal dysfunction, portosystemic encephalopathy, hypersplenism, and hepatopulmonary syndrome. Upper GI endoscopy is done

TABLE 12: Endoscopic grade of varices.

Grade I	On inspiration only
Grade II	Both on inspiration and expiration
Grade III	Projecting in lumen <50%
Grade IV	Projecting in >50% of lumen

for detection of varices, portal hypertensive gastropathy (PHG), and ectopic varices. Endoscopic grading of varices can be done in CLD with portal hypertension given in **Table 12**.

Gastric varices are categorized into four types based on their location and relationship with esophageal varices in the stomach:

1. *Gastroesophageal varix (GOV) type 1*: Extension of esophageal varices along lesser curvature
2. *GOV type 2*: Extension of esophageal varices along great curve
3. *Isolated gastric varix (IGV) type 1*: Varices in stomach
4. *IGV type 2*: Varices in duodenum

Ascitic Fluid Analysis

All patients of CLD with ascites should be subjected to diagnostic paracentesis at first presentation and at the beginning of each admission to hospital. Ascitic fluid is evaluated for cell count with differential counts, albumin level, total protein, and culture. Serum-ascites albumin gradient (SAAG) is the best single test for categorizing into portal hypertensive (SAAG > 1.1 g/dL) and nonportal hypertensive (SAAG < 1.1 g/dL) ascites during evaluation.

A neutrophil count of >250 cells/mm^3 is highly suggestive of bacterial peritonitis. Intravenous cefotaxime is the empiric antibiotic of choice. Long-term administration of oral norfloxacin 5–7.5 mg/kg once a day in cirrhotic patients with ascitic fluid protein content of <1 g/dL or prior episode of spontaneous bacterial peritonitis (SBP) is recommended for prevention of SBP.

Serology for Viral Markers

Hepatitis B surface antigen (HBsAg), immunoglobulin M (IgM) hepatitis A virus (HAV), IgM hepatitis E virus (HEV), and anti-hepatitis C virus (HCV) antibody are done for cause of acute insult etiology of CLD or underlying CLD due to some other known or unknown pathology.

Wilson's Workup

The investigations done for establishing a diagnosis of Wilson's disease given in **Box 4**.

BOX 4: Investigations for establishing Wilson's disease.

- Serum ceruloplasmin levels
- 24-hour urinary copper value including baseline and post penicillamine (500 mg BD over 24 hours) levels
- Slit-lamp examination of eyes for Kayser–Fleischer (KF) ring
- MRI brain for copper deposition in basal ganglia
- Liver biopsy and dry weight of copper in liver tissue using atomic absorption spectrometry

Autoimmune Hepatitis Workup

The workup for AIH includes:

- *Serum autoimmune markers*:
    - Antinuclear antibody (ANA)
    - Anti-smooth muscle antibody (ASMA)
    - Anti-liver kidney microsomal (LKM) antibody
    - Anti-soluble liver antigen (SLA) antibody
- Viral markers to rule out hepatitis B or C
- Protein electrophoresis for gamma globulin levels (IgG)
- Liver biopsy

Liver Biopsy

Liver biopsy histopathology by an expert and its correlation with laboratory investigations plays an important role in the diagnosis of CLD. The procedure can be done by percutaneous route only in patients having normal prothrombin time (PT) and or normal platelet count and normal bleeding time (BT), and clotting time (CT). It is preferably to be done under USG guidance with all aseptic precautions by an expert pediatrician or trained radiologist. An expert pathologist should be identified for the study of these biopsy sample. Treatment on patients can be initiated depending on the clinical diagnosis and histopathology. Most histological staging systems for fibrosis and cirrhosis provide five stages, e.g., the METAVIR [4]: Stage 0 (F0) = normal connective tissue; stage 1 (F1) = fibrous portal expansion; stage 2 (F2) = periportal or scanty porto-portal septa; stage 3 (F3) = fibrous septa with architectural distortion; and stage 4 (F4) = cirrhosis. Stages 2 and 3 are considered significant and severe fibrosis respectively.

Workup for Other Disorders

- Protein electrophoresis for α1-antitrypsin deficiency
- α-fetoprotein level to screen for hereditary tyrosinemia and hepatocellular carcinoma (HCC)
- Galactose-1-phosphate uridyltransferase (GALT) assay to rule out galactosemia

- Urine succinyl acetone levels for tyrosinemia
- Serum aldolase B levels for hereditary fructose intolerance (HFI)
- Enzyme study for storage disorders such as GSD and lysosomal storage disorder

Establishing the Diagnosis of Certain Curable Causes of Chronic Liver Disease in Children

Neonatal Cholestasis

Neonatal cholestasis is a serious condition that requires urgent investigation. BA and galactosemia are two common conditions that can be prevented from progression to CLD by early diagnosis and prompt intervention.

Biliary atresia: The most common cause of neonatal cholestasis is extrahepatic biliary atresia (EHBA). In this condition, a timely surgical management relates to outcome of the Kasai procedure. Intrahepatic cholangiogram is the gold standard test for EHBA but liver biopsy can yield up to 90% diagnostic accuracy for BA in experienced hands. Typical features of BA include ductular reaction, bile plugs within bile ductules, and portal tract edema. Liver transplantation may be avoided in only 20% cases even after a successful portoenterostomy (Kasai) procedure.

Galactosemia: The diagnosis of galactosemia is established by erythrocyte GAL-1-PUT activity assay, erythrocyte galactose-1-phosphate (GAL-1-P) concentration, and GAL-1-PUT molecular genetic testing. In classic galactosemia, GAL-1-PUT enzyme activity is <5% of control and erythrocyte GAL-1-P is >10 mg/dL whereas in Duarte variant (D/G) galactosemia, GAL-1-PUT enzyme activity is usually >5% and about 25% of control values. Prenatal testing by using molecular genetic testing is available to initiate treatment at the newborn period. Molecular genetic testing and GAL-1-PUT enzyme activity can be advised for newborn screening.

Glycogen Storage Disorders

Glycogen storage disorders, namely types I, III, IV, and VI, are autosomal recessive metabolic disorders primarily affecting the liver. GSD type I (von Gierke's disease) is caused by deficient glucose-6-phosphatase activity (type Ia) or mutation in the gene encoding the microsomal glucose-6-phosphate transporter (type Ib). The diagnosis of GSD I is established by clinical presentation, abnormal metabolic parameters, molecular genetic testing, and liver biopsy for enzyme activity. The inadequate conversion of glucose-6-phosphate to glucose through normal glycogenolysis and gluconeogenesis, results in the following metabolic abnormalities **(Table 13)**.

TABLE 13: Abnormal metabolic parameters in in glycogen storage disorder (GSD) type 1.

Hypoglycemia	Fasting blood glucose concentration <60 mg/dL (reference range 70–120 mg/dL)
Hyperuricemia	Blood uric acid >5.0 mg/dL (reference range 2.0–5.0 mg/dL)
Lactic acidosis	Blood lactate >2.5 mmol/L (reference range 0.5–2.2 mmol/L)
Hyperlipidemia	• Triglycerides >250 mg/dL (reference range 150–200 mg/dL) • Cholesterol >200 mg/dL (reference range 100–200 mg/dL)

The concept of administering measured amount of uncooked corn starch (UCCS) in GSD in regular interval as treatment is to maintain euglycemia and prevent the stimulus for glycogenolysis.

Progressive Familial Intrahepatic Cholestasis

The diagnosis of progressive familial intrahepatic cholestasis (PFIC) is made on jaundice, elevated serum levels of primary bile acids with low/normal serum GGT activity [familial intrahepatic cholestasis (FIC1) deficiency or bile salt export pump (BSEP) deficiency] or with high serum GGT activity [multidrug resistance protein 3 (MDR3) deficiency], absence of dysmorphism, and pruritus seen after 4–5 months of life when coordinated behaviour appears in an infant. The distinction between three forms of PFIC is based on histological and biochemical differences if full mutational analysis is unavailable. Most medical therapies are of limited value in PFIC 1 and 2. Ursodeoxycholic acid (UDCA) therapy may ameliorate symptoms and normalize biochemical parameters with varying results.

Hereditary Fructose Intolerance

Hereditary fructose intolerance is caused by deficiency of aldolase B enzyme in the liver, kidney, and small intestine with normal activity of aldolase A and C. Initially symptoms appear with the introduction of fruits, juices, vegetables, or sucrose to the infant's diet and even infrequent exposure may produce symptoms (nausea, vomiting, tremors, dizziness, lethargy, and coma). All symptoms on continuous exposure result directly from accumulation of fructose-1-phosphate in liver, small intestine, and kidney. Hypophosphatemia, hypoglycemia, lactic acidosis, and hyperuricemia result from accumulated high levels of fructose-1-phosphate. Tissue toxicity results in hepatomegaly, hepatic failure, and renal compromise.

Hereditary Tyrosinemia Type I

Hereditary tyrosinemia type I (HT-I) is the most common of the three known diseases due to defective tyrosine metabolism with hepatic involvement and renal tubular dysfunction. Elevated urine succinylcholine can establish the diagnosis in an infant or child presenting with features of cholestasis and renal dysfunction. Nitisinone (NTBC) offers an improved means of treatment for patients with HT by preventing acute hepatic and neurological crisis but the impact of NTBC on need for orthotopic liver transplantation (OLT) depends on stage of disease.

Autoimmune Hepatitis

Features of hepatitis with absence of viral marker for hepatitis, elevated IgG levels, positive autoantibodies [ANA, anti-SMA ±, and antineutrophil cytoplasmic antibody (ANCA) in type 1 AIH and anti-LKM type 1 in type 2 AIH] are part of diagnostic criteria for autoimmune hepatitis. Liver biopsy showing interface hepatitis, multilobular collapse, and emperipolesis are also included in scoring system for diagnosis. If liver histopathology is suggestive but antibodies are negative, anti-SLA antibodies can indicate severe disease if found positive. In both types, about 20% of patients can have other autoimmune disorders. Algorithm for approach to undetermined CLD is given in **Flowchart 1** and simplified diagnostic criteria for AIH is given in **Table 14**, respectively.

Isolated partial deficiency of the human leukocyte antigen (HLA) class III complement component C4 can be found in pediatric patients with AIH irrespective of anti-LKM1 or ANA/SMA positive and this phenomenon is genetically determined.

Wilson's Disease

The classic presentation comprises the trio of liver disease plus neurological and ophthalmological involvement. Low ceruloplasmin level is the laboratory test that most often seen (88%) followed by elevated 24-hour urine copper level (71%). In pediatric case series, ceruloplasmin has a sensitivity of 82–88%, while 24-hour urine copper has a sensitivity of 81–100%. So for increasing the sensitivity of diagnostic workup should include ceruloplasmin, serum free copper and urinary copper, and KF ring by slit-lamp examination. Liver biopsy as such is not essential for diagnosis, with the exception of quantitative estimation of copper in tissue, which is significant when elevated to

Flowchart 1: Algorithmic approach to undetermined liver disease.

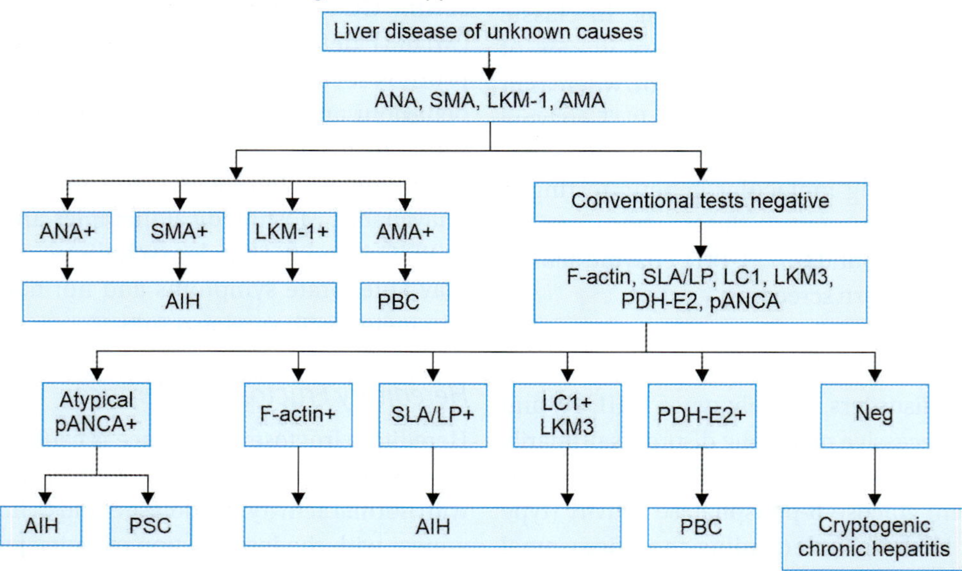

(AIH: autoimmune hepatitis; AMA: antimitochondrial antibody; ANA: antinuclear antibody; LKM: liver kidney microsomal type 1; LP: liver pancreas; pANCA: perinuclear antineutrophil cytoplasmic antibody; PBC: primary biliary cholangitis; PSC: primary sclerosing cholangitis; SLA: soluble liver antigen; SMA: smooth muscle antibody)

>50 μg/g and value >250 μg/g confirms diagnosis in proper clinical setting. The diagnostic algorithm for Wilson's disease is given in **Flowchart 2**.

TABLE 14: Simplified diagnostic criteria for diagnosis of autoimmune hepatitis.

Features/parameter	*Discriminator*	*Score*
ANA or SMA+	1:40	+1*
ANA or SMA+	1:80	+2*
or LKM+	1:40	+2*
or SLA/LP+	Any titer	+2*
IgG or gamma-globulin level	>upper limit of normal >1.1 × upper limit	+1 +2
Liver histology (evidence of hepatitis is a necessary condition)	Compatible with AIH Typical AIH Atypical	+1 +2 0
Absence of viral hepatitis	No Yes	0 +2

AIH: autoimmune hepatitis; ANA: antinuclear antibody; IgG: immunoglobulin G; LKM: liver kidney microsomal; LP: liver pancreas; SMA: smooth muscle antibody; SLA: soluble liver antigen

*Score >6 probable AIH and score >7 definite AIH

Chronic Hepatitis B

Chronic hepatitis B infection have been identified with three phases of host immune response, namely immune-tolerant phase, the immune-active phase, and the inactive hepatitis B virus (HBV) phase. Children with chronic HBV infection may develop active liver inflammation at any age, accompanied by a variable degree of ALT elevation, increasing the risk of severe complications like end-stage liver disease in later life. Current antiviral regimens cannot eradicate HBV but can prevent the progression of liver damage. Chronic HBV infection in an immune-tolerant state with a high viral load and normal levels of aminotransferases are found in majority of children and response to conventional antiviral therapy is poor in them.

Hepatitis C Infection

The natural history of HCV infection in children is not yet well defined, and most children with a normal immune status remain asymptomatic for decades. Most infected individuals (60–80%), irrespective of age at infection, become chronically infected with HCV. Spontaneous resolution in children appears to be infrequent and diagnosis is made by testing for the HCV antibody by

Flowchart 2: Algorithm for diagnosis of Wilson's disease.

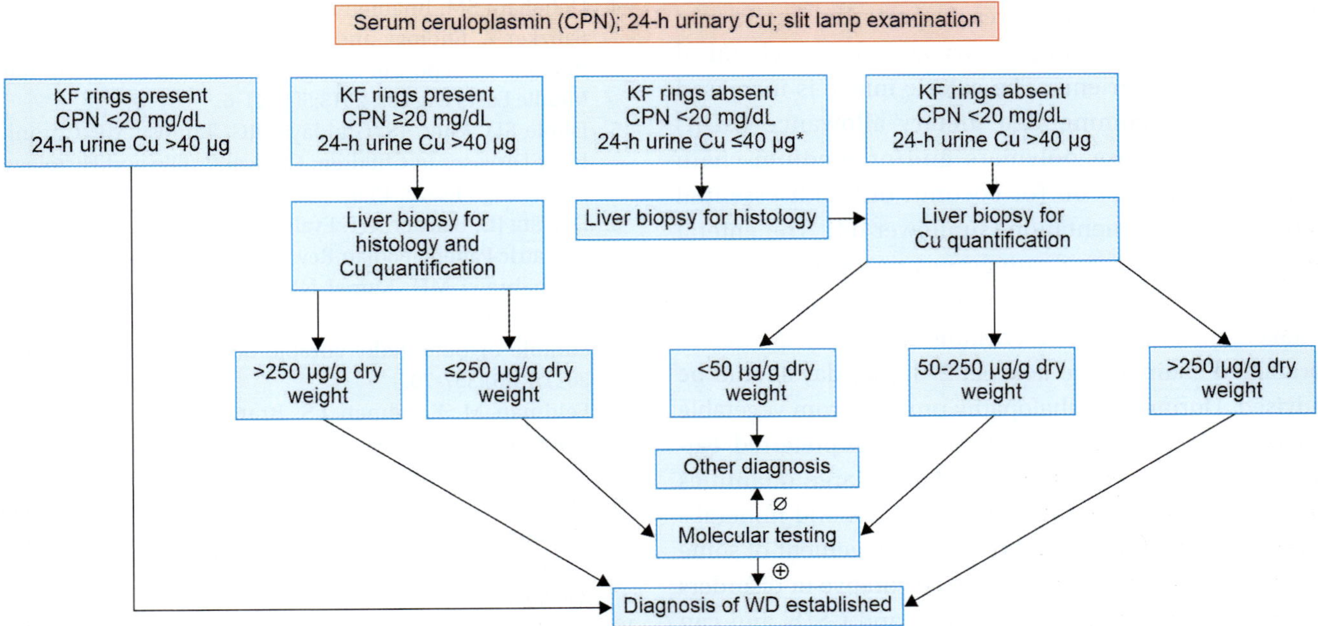

(CPN: ceruloplasmin; KF: Kayser–Fleischer; WD: Wilson's disease)

*2022 Practice Guidance on Wilson disease from the American Association for the Study of Liver Diseases.

enzyme immunoassay, and for HCV RNA by polymerase chain reaction (PCR) method. Only interferon (IFN)-α 2b or pegylated IFN and ribavirin were approved for use in children >3 years of age with chronic HCV hepatitis till very recently when the FDA has approved the use of direct-acting antivirals (DAAs), sofosbuvir and ledipasvir/sofosbuvir for treatment in age group 12–17 years group.

Nonalcoholic Steatohepatitis

Nonalcoholic fatty liver disease (NAFLD) is a condition that includes a form of chronic liver damage from simple fatty infiltration of hepatocytes (steatosis) to the triad of fatty infiltration, inflammation, and fibrosis [nonalcoholic steatohepatitis (NASH)]. NAFLD was mainly associated in older adults (especially females) with central obesity, insulin resistance, and type II diabetes mellitus (DM). The true prevalence in children is unknown as confirmation of diagnosis requires liver biopsy. Serum transaminasemia is not a sensitive or specific markers for NAFLD and current imaging modalities cannot distinguish simple steatosis from NASH. Theoretically, only patients with NASH need to be treated as only NASH may evolve into cirrhosis. Lifestyle modification and gradual weight loss is the initial approach against NAFLD and bariatric surgery is recommended in morbidly obese NASH.

Nutritional Management

A child with CLD requires a periodic nutritional assessment with anthropometry and also biochemical estimation of nutrients. The caloric intake is increased to 130% of recommended dietary allowance (RDA) by adding glucose polymers and/or medium-chain triglyceride (MCT) oil (or coconut oil) with essential fatty acid supplementation (sunflower oil). The enteral route is preferred and sometimes nasogastric and/or nocturnal feeding are required to ensure an adequate intake. In a compensated cirrhotic child proteins rich in branched chain amino acids at 2–3 g/kg/day should be advised. During encephalopathy proteins from vegetable source and restricted intake (1 g/kg/day) is preferred. Fat-soluble vitamins are supplemented in large quantities for cholestasis along with other vitamins and minerals. Dietary therapy is the mainstay of management of some metabolic liver diseases and may be curative in disorders such as galactosemia, fructosemia, and GSDs and can ameliorate symptoms in tyrosinemia.

CONCLUSION

The signs and symptoms of CLD in children ranges from asymptomatic hepatosplenomegaly and growth retardation to acute decompensation in case of end-stage liver disease and cirrhosis. The spectrum of CLD in children is more wider and different from adults and require more meticulous investigation and age wise prioritization for proceeding toward specific etiological workup. The proportion of undefined etiology of CLD in this subcontinent is higher than the data from developed world due to unavailability of laboratory facilities for suspected metabolic and mitochondrial liver diseases in infancy and early childhood. However in the recent years, facility of tertiary care for pediatric liver diseases is expected to suffice for this and early detection of CLD and reaching into specific etiology will determine the utility of medical management or liver transplantation in future.

SUGGESTED READING

1. Bavdekar A, Bhave S, Pandit A. Nutrition Management in Chronic Liver Disease. Indian J Pediatr. 2002;69:427-31.
2. Brancatelli G, Vilgrain V, Federle M, Hakime A, Lagalla R, Iannaccone R, et al. Budd-Chiari Syndrome: Spectrum of Imaging Findings. AJR Am J Roentgenol. 2007;188:168-76.
3. de Andrade Sócio S, Ferreira AR, Fagundes EDT, Roquete MLV, Pimenta JR, de Faria Campos L, et al. Wilson's disease in children and adolescents: diagnosis and treatment. Rev Paul Pediatr. 2010;28(2):134-40.
4. Dehghani SM, Imanieh MH, Haghighat M, Malekpour A, Falizkar Z. Etiology and complications of liver cirrhosis in children: report of a single center from Southern Iran. Middle East J Dig Dis. 2013;5(1):41-6.
5. Dhole SD, Kher AS, Ghildayal RG, Tambse MP. Chronic Liver Diseases in Children: Clinical Profile and Histology. J Clin Diagn Res. 2015;9(7):SC04-7.
6. D'Agata ID, Balisteri WF. Evaluation of Liver Disease in the Pediatric Patient. Pediatr Rev. 1999;20(11):376-89.
7. El-Shabrawi MH, Kamal NM. Medical Management of Chronic Liver Diseases in Children (Part I): focus on curable or potentially curable diseases. Pediatr Drugs. 2011;13(6):357-70.
8. Feldman M, Friedman LS, Brandt LJ. Sleisenger and Fordtran's Gastrointestinal and Liver Disease, 10th edition. Philadelphia: Saunders; 2015.
9. Foucher J, Chanteloup E, Verginol J, Castéra L, Le Bail B, Adhoute X, et al. Diagnosis of cirrhosis by transient elastography (FibroScan): a prospective study. Gut. 2006;55:403-8.
10. Gerstenmaier JF, Gibson RN. Ultrasound in chronic liver disease. Insights Imaging. 2014;5:441-55.

11. Thapa BR, Walia A. Liver Function Tests and their Interpretation. Indian J Pediatr. 2007;74:663-71.
12. Kamath B. Stigmata of chronic liver disease. Hosp Physician. 2003;8:14-6.
13. Lal J, Thapa BR, Rawal P, Ratho RK, Singh K. Predictors of outcome in acute-on-chronic liver failure in children. Hepatol Int. 2011;5:693-7.
14. Medscape. (2017). FDA Clears Two HCV Drugs for Children. [online] Available from https://www.medscape.com/viewarticle/878332. [Last accessed December, 2025].
15. Ovchinski N, Moreira RK, Lefkowitch JH, Lavine JE. Liver biopsy in modern clinical practice: a pediatric point-of-view. Adv Anat Pathol. 2012;19(4):250-62.
16. Roberts EA, Schlisky M L. Diagnosis and Treatment of Wilson Disease: An Update. 2008;47(6):2089-111.
17. Shrivastav A, Chaturvedi A, Gupta RK, Malik R, Mathias A, Jagannathan NR, et al. Minimal hepatic encephalopathy in children with chronic liver disease: prevalence, pathogenesis and magnetic resonance-based diagnosis. J Hepatol. 2016;66:528-36.
18. Sumathi B. Chronic Liver Disease. In: Sumathi B (Ed). Textbook of Pediatric Gastroenterology, Hepatology, and Nutrition, 1st edition. New Delhi: Jaypee Brothers Medical Publishers (P) Ltd.; 2015.
19. Tahir A, Malik F, Ahmad I, Akhtar P. Aetiological factors of chronic liver disease in children. J Ayub Med Coll Abbottabad. 2011;23(2):12-4.
20. Thapa BR, Mehta S. Investigative approach and medical management of portal hypertension. Indian Pediatr. 1992;29:945-54.
21. Vergani GM, Vergani D. Approach to a child with chronic liver disease. J Gastroenterol Hepatol. 2004;14:377-8.
22. Vergani GM, Vergani D. Autoimmune hepatitis in children: what is different from adult AIH? Semin Liver Dis. 2009; 29(3):297-306.
23. Yacha SK, Khanna V. Ascites in childhood liver disease. Indian J Pediatr. 2006;73(9):819-24.
24. Zachou K, Muratori P, Koukoulis GK, Granito A, Gatselis N, Fabbri A, et al. Review article: autoimmune hepatitis—current management and challenges. Aliment Pharmacol Ther. 2013;38:887-993.

CHAPTER 7

Examination of the Central and Peripheral Nervous System

Pradip Prava Paria

PART A: CENTRAL NERVOUS SYSTEM EXAMINATIONS: CLINICAL APPROACH

INTRODUCTION

Infants and young children are not simply smaller versions of adults, and as such, traditional neurological examination methods are often not suitable for children under five years of age. Evaluating neurological function in this age group requires creativity, flexibility, and a playful, unstructured approach to gain the child's cooperation and obtain meaningful results. Like other organ systems, the central nervous system (CNS) in children is constantly growing and maturing. At birth, the brain weighs approximately 70% of its adult size, while the body constitutes only about 5% of adult body weight. Most brain growth takes place during infancy and the early preschool years. Certain neurological disorders, such as developmental delays caused by hypoxia, congenital malformations, and metabolic disorders, are primarily seen in pediatric populations. Additionally, in children, neurological symptoms are more frequently linked to systemic illnesses rather than primary diseases of the CNS.

Just as in adults, the ***neurological evaluation** in infants and young children* requires a comprehensive history, a relevant physical examination, and well-chosen diagnostic tests. The primary aim is to establish the anatomical diagnosis by pinpointing the lesion's location and the pathological diagnosis by identifying the cause of dysfunction.

WHERE IS THE LESION?

While history provides key etiological insights, the neurological assessment and imaging pinpoint the precise anatomical location of the symptoms. The brain and spinal cord, together with the cerebellum, peripheral nerves, and muscles, form a bilaterally symmetrical system aligned along the vertical axis of the CNS. Examination components include mental status assessment for the cortex, cranial nerve testing for the brainstem, coordination evaluation for the cerebellum, and sensory/motor assessment for the spinal cord, muscles, and peripheral nerves **(Fig. 1)**.

WHAT IS THE LESION?

A comprehensive history encompassing present illness, past medical events, family background, and social context enables the clinician to map the progression of the child's condition. Neurological disorders typically exhibit characteristic temporal patterns: acute (within seconds to hours), subacute (over hours to days), chronic (evolving over weeks to months), or paroxysmal (episodic with recovery between episodes) **(Table 1)**.

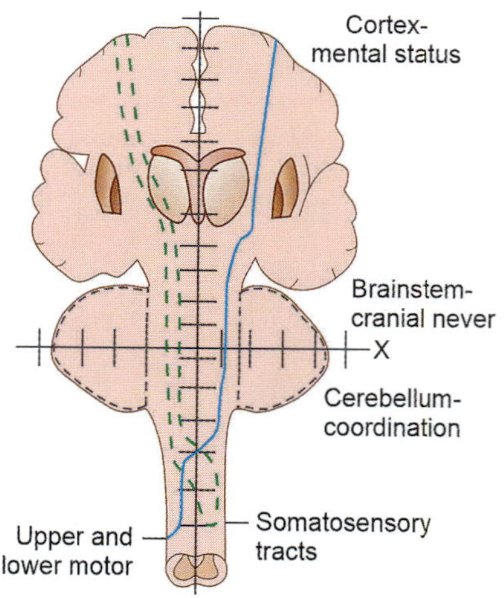

Fig. 1: Neuraxis of neurological localization.

TABLE 1: Temporal profile.

Acute	*Subacute*	*Chronic*	*Paroxysmal*
• Infarct • Hypoxia • Trauma	• Infections • Immune/ inflammation • Toxic/ metabolic	• Congenital • Degenerative • Neoplastic	• Seizure • Syncope • Pain/ headache

AGE-APPROPRIATE NEUROLOGICAL ASSESSMENT IN CHILDREN

The foundation of pediatric neurological assessment lies in adult examination techniques, many of which can be applied to verbal children. However, rigidly enforcing these methods on infants and toddlers can lead to frustration. A flexible approach, considering the child's temperament and developmental level, allows for a more effective assessment, often through observing spontaneous behaviors.

Observe the Child for—

Any obvious dysmorphisms, facial asymmetry, the child's social interaction, presence of hyperactivity. Assess head control, posture, early hand preference, and presence of motor abnormalities. What sounds or words does he or she make?

Once the initial spontaneous observations are complete, the next phase of the examination begins. This is best performed with the infant in the parent's lap. To reduce anxiety and encourage cooperation in children, imaginative strategies, such as turning a reflex hammer into a toy animal, can be highly effective. Adding sound effects to it may make it a nonthreatening game when eliciting muscle stretch reflexes. Finger puppets or brightly colored toys may be offered to the child for playing, which maximizes the information for the clinician. The final stage of the assessment consists of tasks that might cause discomfort or anxiety in the child, such as removing clothing, examining the eyes and ears, evaluating the gag reflex, and checking head size.

RELEVANT HISTORY

A thorough history is essential for neurological assessment. Parents typically serve as the primary informants, but children older than 4 years can often share details about their condition and should be included in the discussion. The history must begin with the caregiver's main concern and be evaluated against developmental expectations for age **(Box 1)**.

Next, the history of the present illness: A thorough and precise neurological history is essential, with symptoms reviewed in chronological order. Assessing the timeline and frequency of symptoms, along with their progression—whether advancing (neurodegenerative diseases), static, or recovering [cerebral palsy (CP)]—is crucial for diagnosis. It is also important to determine whether the condition is acute, subacute, or chronic. Factors that alleviate or worsen symptoms, including medication effects, should be explored. Additionally, assessing how neurological symptoms interact with other organ systems can provide clues about the underlying condition, such as fever and vomiting in meningitis or urinary retention in spinal cord disorders.

Reviewing the *past medical history* is crucial as it may influence the current diagnosis. This includes a record of similar past illnesses, major health issues, surgical interventions, trauma, transfusions, and allergies, and prescribed medications (noting dosage and indication) with response to them.

This is followed by a complete *birth history*, with a review of the pregnancy, including the mother's age, immunization status, any complications during pregnancy [e.g., pregnancy-induced hypertension (PIH), autoimmune hepatitis (AIH), hydramnios, gestational diabetes, and febrile illnesses with rash], use of illicit drugs, cigarettes, or alcohol. Ask about whether the mother had regular antenatal check-ups, ultrasound examination,

BOX 1: Symptoms commonly associated with neurological disorders in children.

- Delayed development—single domain or multidomain, e.g., neurologic—cerebral palsy, non-neurologic—congenital hypothyroidism, and Down syndrome
- Regression of milestones, e.g., neurodegenerative disorder, muscular dystrophy, Rett's syndrome, and epileptic encephalopathy
- Weakness—hemiparesis, paraparesis, or quadriparesis
- Symptoms of raised intracranial tension—headache, vomiting, visual blurring, etc.
- Altered sensorium, e.g., encephalopathy
- Convulsion—motor, sensory, autonomic, provoked, or unprovoked
- Cranial nerve involvement—in the form of vision (II) or hearing impairment (VIII), diplopia, convergent/divergent squint (III, IV, and VI cranial nerves), deviation of the angle of the mouth (VII), dysphagia, drooling of saliva (IX), nasal intonation/ nasal regurgitation of food (XI), etc
- Symptoms of sensory disturbances—pain, paraesthesia, and complete loss of sensation in GBS and TM
- Autonomic disturbances—retention of urine/retention with overflow or fecal incontinence—in spinal disorders
- Loss of postural balance—in cerebellar disorders
- Involuntary movements, such as chorea, athetosis, dystonia, and tremors
- Headache
- Neuromuscular weaknesses

and iron and folic acid intake before or throughout conception. Inquiring about fetal movement, as decreased fetal activity can be associated with hypotonia due to CNS or neuromuscular disorders. The mother's labor history should address, as that was a term or preterm delivery, the place (home or institutional) and mode (normal vaginal vs assisted) of delivery. Birth weight and any complication, e.g., birth asphyxia (Apgar score), should be noted. The baby's consciousness level and history of neonatal issues like seizures or jaundice must be noted. For jaundice, clarify how soon after birth it began and what treatment was employed, typically phototherapy or exchange transfusion. A reliable account of the postnatal period is usually obtainable from the parents, complemented by a review of hospital documentation for any complications. Key areas of inquiry include the infant's general health, feeding and sleeping habits, level of activity, and the nature of the cry.

Evaluating *developmental milestones* **(Table 2)** is a fundamental aspect of neurological history-taking. It involves assessing multiple areas—social, cognitive, linguistic, and motor skills—to identify delays that are isolated or widespread. Any sign of skill regression warrants investigation for possible neurodegenerative or neurometabolic disease.

If parents have difficulty remembering milestone achievements, especially for second or third children, comparing them with the developmental timelines of siblings can be informative. In school-aged children, academic progress often reflects cognitive development, and abrupt changes in performance may signal a neurological problem.

Immunization history is vital as it protects against vaccine-preventable diseases in children. If parents could or cannot remember the vaccine given to the child, it is better to check the immunization card whether there are any missing doses.

Nutritional history plays a significant role in pediatric evaluation, especially in developing countries. Important factors include the mode of feeding (breastfeeding or formula), the introduction of solid foods, and weaning practices. T's better to go for calorie calculation in preillness and during the sickness period. Any form of picky eating (nutritional deficiency) and history of pica (lead poisoning) should be asked for.

Next, the *family history* must be reviewed. A comprehensive family history must include the age at which any neurologic disorders, like developmental delays, seizures, migraines, strokes, or genetic conditions, were diagnosed in close family members. Three generation pedigree charts should be drawn. History should include regarding consanguinity (the chance of metabolic and degenerative diseases is higher in consanguineous marriage) and ethnic background. It is necessary to obtain clear information about miscarriages. or medical termination of pregnancy with specific indication, and also document the sex and gestational age of the relevant embryo or fetus.

A comprehensive *social history* should be obtained, particularly in resource-limited settings. This includes details about living arrangements, crowding, parental occupation and education, and contact with domestic or farm animals. Travel history is especially relevant in urban populations to assess the risk of zoonotic and parasitic

TABLE 2: Key developmental milestones.

Age (mo)	*Gross motor*	*Fine motor and vision*	*Social*	*Language*
3 months	Neck holding	Opens hand spontaneously	Recognizes mother	Coos
6 months	Sits with support	Transfer objects	Stranger anxiety	Monosyllables
9 months	Stands with support	An immature prince grasps	Waves bye-bye	Bisyllables
12 months	Stands without support	Releasing grasp in response to command	Responds to name being called	One to two meaningful words
15 months	Walks alone	A tower of 2 blocks	Jargon	
18 months	Runs	Feeds self from a spoon	Copies parents in the task	8–10-word vocabulary
24 months	Walks up and downstairs	Build a six-block tower	Engages in playing with peers	Two-to-three-word simple sentences

diseases. Additionally, recent stressors, such as family disruptions, sibling birth, and loss of a loved one, should be explored, as they may impact a child's emotional well-being. School and daycare records should also be reviewed to identify any significant changes in academic or social behavior.

GENERAL PHYSICAL EXAMINATION

General appearance, nature of disability, facies, decubitus, build, and nutrition (anthropometry) should be ascertained first, followed by vital signs. Record temperature, pulse, respiration, and blood pressure. Increased temperature and tachycardia may suggest possible infection, including meningitis or encephalitis. Bradycardia, increased blood pressure, and abnormal respiratory pattern may be features of increased intracranial pressure (Cushing response). Tachycardia, along with hypotension, is suggestive of septic shock, as in cases of meningococcemia. Conversely, hypertension may be the cause of encephalopathy or a response to elevated intracranial pressure. An abnormal respiratory pattern may point toward different types of brain herniation.

Look for pallor (leukemia, lymphoma with CNS involvement, and intracranial bleed), cyanosis/clubbing (cyanotic heart disease with cerebral thrombosis or abscess), jaundice (hepatic encephalopathy), and edema.

Skin rash and petechiae in a child with altered sensorium may indicate infection with meningococcus, rickettsia, dengue, etc. Enlarged neck glands may indicate tuberculosis or malignancy with CNS involvement.

HEAD-TO-TOE EXAMINATIONS IN RELATION TO CENTRAL NERVOUS SYSTEM

- *Face:* Dysmorphic features—in Down syndrome or some chromosomal and metabolic disorders (mucopolysaccharidosis, GM1 gangliosidosis, and mucolipidosis).
- *Eyes:* Strabismus, hyper- or hypotelorism, cataract (galactosemia), gaze abnormality, Kayser-Fleischer ring (Wilson's disease), telangiectasia (ataxia telangiectasia)
- *Ears:* Position of the ears (low-set ear in many syndromic children) and any ear tags or skin lesions.
- *Mouth:* Any deviation of the angle of the mouth, drooling, gum hypertrophy, or atrophy of the tongue.
- *Neck:* Check for the presence of neck tilt, webbed neck, implanted shunt, or any scars.
- *Back:* Signs suggestive of occult spinal dysraphism, like midline sacral dimples or localized hair tufts, kyphosis, and gibbus.
- *Skin/neurocutaneous lesions* **(Table 3)**: Hair (kinky-Menkes disease).

Observe for abnormal postures such as hemiplegic limb positioning **(Fig. 2)**, scissoring suggestive of cerebral palsy, and the frog-like posture typical of hypotonia. Identify contractures if present. For ambulant children, gait assessment is essential—look for signs like spastic gait, hemiparetic stride, steppage pattern from sensory deficits, or waddling due to myopathy. Check for hand dominance. Although most children establish handedness by 2 years, a strong preference before this age may be an early sign of asymmetrical motor function or limb weakness.

TABLE 3: Neurocutaneous marker.

Ash-leaf hypopigmented spots, facial angiofibroma, and shagreen patches	Tuberous sclerosis.
Café-au-lait macules along with axillary and groin freckling	Neurofibromatosis type I
Port-wine stain/Nevus flammeus	Sturge–Weber syndrome
Raised verrucous skin lesions in ovoid or linear plaques	Epidermal nevus syndrome

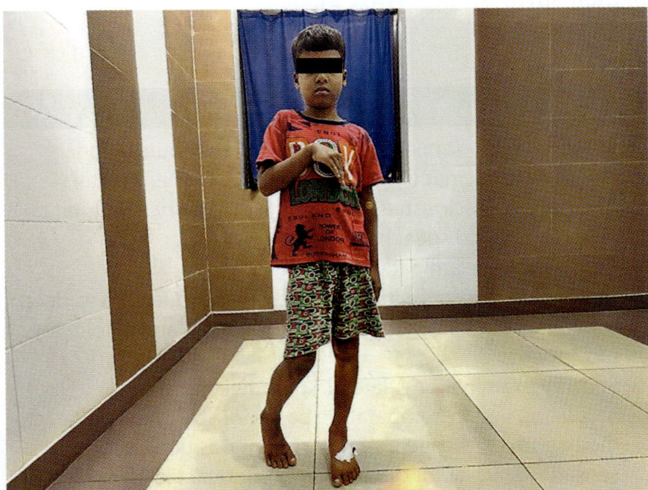

Fig. 2: Hemiplegic posture—arm-adducted and internally rotated at the shoulder; elbow is flexed; forearm semi-pronated, and the wrist and fingers are flexed. Lower limb- slightly flexed at the hip, extended at the knee with plantar-flexed and inverted foot.

OTHER SYSTEM EXAMINATIONS

Abdominal examination should include assessment for hepatosplenomegaly, which can be linked to neurometabolic conditions. A distended bladder, evidence of constipation, or undescended testes may point toward underlying neural tube anomalies. Respiratory functions are mostly compromised in chronic progressive neuromuscular disorders.

NEUROLOGICAL EXAMINATIONS

The neurological examination begins as soon as the interview starts. Observing the child's appearance and movements can provide important clues to underlying conditions. For instance, dysmorphic facial features, abnormal posture, or motor impairments such as hemiparesis and gait disturbances may be noticeable. The exam should take place in a relaxed, child-friendly environment, allowing the child to sit where they feel most at ease—whether on a parent's lap or the floor. The physician should approach gently, saving any invasive. More invasive assessments, such as measuring head circumference or testing the gag reflex, should be saved for the end of the examination. Observing the child's behavior during play and interactions with parents can also provide valuable insights. Typically, a child will play independently at the beginning of the visit but gradually engage in the interview. In contrast, a child with attention-deficit/hyperactivity disorder (ADHD) may display impulsiveness, while a child with autism may seem completely unaware of their surroundings **(Box 2)**.

BOX 2: Key points in neurological examination.

- Mental status—(appearance, behavior, communication, delusion, hallucination, and illusion) and Higher mental function—consciousness, orientation, memory, attention, intelligence, and speech
- Cranial nerve examinations
- Motor system examination—muscle mass, tone, power, deep tendon reflexes and superficial reflexes, gait, and involuntary movements
- Sensory examination—lateral, spinothalamic tract mediating—pain, temperature posterior spinothalamic tract mediating—fine touch, vibration, joint position, cortical sensation (two-point discrimination, and tactile localization)
- Cerebellar functions
- Meningeal irritation signs—neck rigidity, Kerning sign, and Brudzinski sign
- Skull and spinal column

ESSENTIAL TOOLS

Instruments necessary for pediatric neurologic evaluation include colorful cubes, a reflex hammer, a bell, a rubber-adapted penlight, fiberglass tape, items for stereognosis assessment, tuning forks (128 Hz for sensation, 256 Hz for auditory testing), a two-point discrimination device, developmental kits, and an ophthalmoscope.

CONSCIOUSNESS AND HIGHER MENTAL FUNCTION

Scheme of examinations:

- Level of consciousness
- Higher mental functions

Appearance and Behavior

- Delusion/hallucination/illusion
- Intelligence
  - Attention/working memory
  - Language/reading/writing /visuospatial
    - Mood and affect
    - Orientation to place, person, and time
    - Speech
    - Sleep

The examination of selective elements will be discussed here.

The level of consciousness (LOC) refers to a person's awareness of themselves, their environment, and their ability to respond to stimuli. It is classified into two distinct stages-arousal and awareness. Arousal is a function of the reticular activating system (described as whether the sleep-wake cycle is preserved or not). And, awareness is a function of cortical or subcortical structures (expressed in interest in their toys, consolability, eye contact, etc.). Deranged consciousness is thus an impairment in arousal and awareness. Infants under 28 weeks of gestation often do not display predictable alert periods, whereas gentle physical contact can rouse older infants from sleep. In older children, it is particularly important in neurological, medical, and psychiatric evaluations. The levels range from full awareness to a complete lack of responsiveness and are typically described as follows:

- Fully conscious, a person is awake, alert, and oriented to time, place, and person. Normal responses to verbal and environmental stimuli.
- *Clouding of consciousness:* Mildly reduced awareness of the environment. The individual may be confused, distracted, or slow to respond.

- *Drowsiness/lethargy:* There is impaired attention and reduced consciousness; the child responds to verbal or tactile stimulation but drifts back to sleep once the stimulation stops.
- *Obtundation:* More severe reduction in alertness. It is a stage between drowsiness and stupor. The person requires loud verbal or physical stimuli other than pain to respond and may appear confused. Responses are slower and less purposeful.
- *Stupor:* The child responds only to persistent and strong painful stimulation. It is a cerebral response. The child can localize pain and tries to remove the noxious stimuli. Soon after the removal of stimuli, the child slips to the previous condition.
- *Coma:* No response is elicited from the child even with strong and repeated painful stimuli.
- *Delirium:* The child is confused and disoriented, unable to form coherent thoughts, and may be irritable, fearful, agitated, or experiencing hallucinations.

Grading of Consciousness

Glasgow Coma Scale (Table 4)

A numerical scoring system is often used to quantify the LOC in clinical settings.

- *Components:* Eye opening (E)—spontaneous to none (1–4).
- *Verbal response (V):* Oriented to no verbal response (1–5).
- *Motor response (M):* Obeys commands to no motor response (1–6).

TABLE 4: Glasgow Coma Scale.

Score	*Eye-opening (E)*	*Verbal response (V)*	*Motor response (M)*
1	None	No response	No response
2	To pain	Incomprehensible sound	Abnormal extension
3	To speech	Inappropriate words	Abnormal flexion
4	Spontaneous	Confused	Withdrawal from pain
5		Oriented	Localizes to pain
6			Obeys commands

Total score: 3 (deep coma) to 15 (fully alert).

An easy and efficient tool for assessing consciousness is the AVPU scale, often used in initial evaluations where: A stand for alertness, V for response to voice, P for response to pain and U for unresponsive to any stimulus.

Vegetative State and Minimally Conscious State

- *Vegetative state:* Awake but not aware. Retains sleep-wake cycles but lacks purposeful responses to stimuli. For example, a persistent vegetative state (PVS) following severe brain injury.
- *Minimally conscious state:* Severely altered consciousness but with occasional purposeful responses (e.g., following simple commands). For example, the recovery phase from a coma.

HIGHER MENTAL FUNCTION

Higher mental functions refer to the advanced cognitive abilities that distinguish humans from other species. The mental status examination evaluates the function of the cerebral cortex, the highest level of the neuroaxis responsible for integrating perception, cognition, and emotion, ultimately shaping thoughts, feelings, and behavior. In children, the cortex undergoes significant age-dependent development. At the time of birth, most of an infant's actions are controlled by reflexive responses. Mental status assessment should be adapted based on the child's developmental stage.

Appearance and Behavior

As you talk with the parents, casually observe the child for indicators such as cleanliness, responsiveness to the environment, facial affect, sustained eye contact, and overall activity.

Delusions and Hallucinations, Illusion

- *Delusion* is a firmly held mistaken belief that persists even when faced with clear evidence against it.
- *Hallucination* is a false sensory perception that occurs without an external stimulus, originating from the organ of special senses, and is commonly associated with psychiatric, neurological, and substance-related disorders.
- *Illusion* is the mistaken interpretation of what one sees, as if one mistakes a rope for a snake.

Orientation

For older children, orientation can be evaluated by asking them to state the current time, identify their location, and recognize familiar individuals.

Attention

Children with inattention often find it hard to concentrate on tasks requiring focus. Attention can be evaluated by asking the child to recall a sequence of numbers, beginning with two and gradually increasing in length, or to repeat a short list of items until mistakes occur. If a child struggles to repeat six or more numbers correctly, it may indicate attention difficulties. Another method is to ask the child to spell a word in reverse, though this may be influenced by memory problems or learning challenges.

Speech and Language Function

Assess the child's natural speech for clarity of articulation, speech flow, tempo, tone, and volume, while noting any atypical language patterns like made-up words.

Dysphasia refers to an impairment in language abilities, affecting either speech production, comprehension, or both. It usually occurs due to a lesion in the dominant cerebral hemisphere (mostly on the left side). Normally, sounds are recognized as language in the sensory (Wernicke's) area, which is connected to the motor (Broca's) area by the arcuate fasciculus **(Fig. 3)**. The following patterns of aphasia can be recognized **(Table 5)**.

Dysphasia Needs to be Distinguished From

Impairment of voice—dysphonia—may result from vagus nerve palsy or lesions affecting the larynx, altering voice pitch, tone, or volume. Dysarthria, however, is due to poor articulation control, often related to muscle disorders or cranial nerve damage (VII, X, and XII). Evaluating articulation can be done using the "ka, pa, ta" test: 'Ka' comes from the throat, 'pa' from the lips, and 'ta' from the tongue-palate region.

Disorders of Speech

- Stammering/fluency disorder or infantile speech results from psychological factors rather than neurological causes.
- Scanning or staccato speech, characterized by slow, slurred syllables resembling intoxication, is associated with cerebellar disorders.
- Spastic dysarthria, marked by strained or slow speech, is seen in many cases of cerebral palsy.
- Bulbar dysarthria due to bulbar palsy is marked by slurred speech, difficulty swallowing with nasal regurgitation, and pooling of secretions in the throat.
- Nasal speech is typically associated with palatal weakness or congenital anomalies like cleft palate.

Memory

From a clinical perspective, memory is categorized into immediate, recent, and remote types. It can be assessed in children over the age of 5 years. Informal evaluation includes observing how a patient recalls personal details, while formal testing involves asking them to register and recall three objects or perform a digit span test. Additionally, assessing cognitive functions can involve activities such as storytelling, drawing, or solving puzzles.

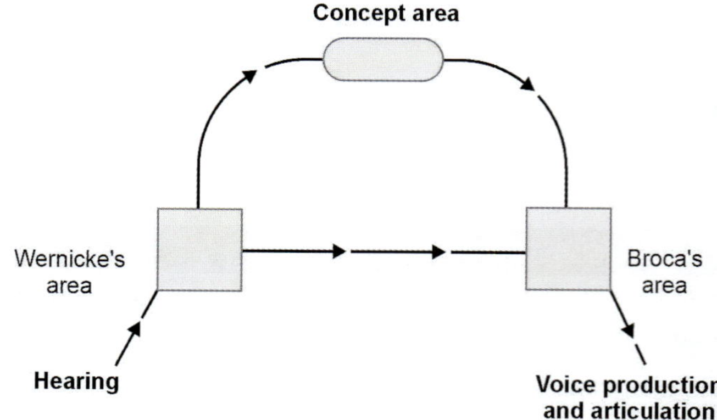

Fig. 3: Speech understanding and output.

TABLE 5: Pattern of aphasia.

Aphasia	*Lesion*	*Characteristics*
Wernicke's aphasia	Superior temporal gyrus	Fluent but nonsensical speech, poor comprehension, unaware of deficits
Broca's aphasia	Inferior frontal gyrus	Effortful speech, difficulty with grammar, and good comprehension
Conduction aphasia	Arcuate fasciculus	Fluent speech, preserved comprehension, and impaired repetition
Transcortical sensory	Temporoparietal junction outside Wernicke's area	As in Wernick's aphasia, with preserved repetition
Transcortical moto	Frontal lobe outside Broca's area	As in Broca's aphasia, with preserved repetition

Immediate memory refers to the ability to recall information after just a few seconds. For example, a child can be asked to repeat a series of digits shortly after hearing them.

Recent memory involves recalling events from the same day, such as answering the question, *"What did you eat for breakfast today?"* It requires retrieving information after a few hours to days.

Remote memory pertains to the recollection of facts or events from months or years ago. This can be assessed by asking questions like, *"What is your teacher's name?"* or *"Which school do you attend?"*

- *Intelligence:* Best assessed by an IQ test. The history of schooling of the child, if age-appropriate, indicates evidence of optimum intelligence. At bedside, interpretation or comprehension of power, problem-solving power can be tested, depending on the child's age.
- *Language:* Age-appropriate language skills—identifying objects, understanding word meanings, and following instructions.
- Reading and writing.
- *Visuospatial:* Copying shapes, illustrating a human figure, and creating a clock drawing.

CRANIAL NERVES

There are 12 pairs of cranial nerves. Of all cranial nerves, I, II, and VIII are pure sensory, III, IV, VI, XI, and XII are purely motor, and the rest of the nerves are mixed in character. The lower part of the face, XI, XII, has cortical control from the opposite hemisphere only. All the other cranial nerves have bilateral cortical control. All the cranial nerves should be examined. However, in infants and children up to 3 years it may not be possible to test all of them.

Olfactory Nerve (Cranial Nerve I)

The olfactory nerves control the sense of smell and are usually tested only when indicated. Ask the child if they can detect odors normally or if they have noticed any changes. Ensure nasal passages are clear. To assess smell, have the child close their eyes and block one nostril at a time while identifying common household scents like chocolate, peppermint, or orange peel **(Fig. 4)**. Avoid strong substances such as ammonia, which can trigger the trigeminal nerve. Smelling perception develops as early as the 32nd week of gestation in newborns.

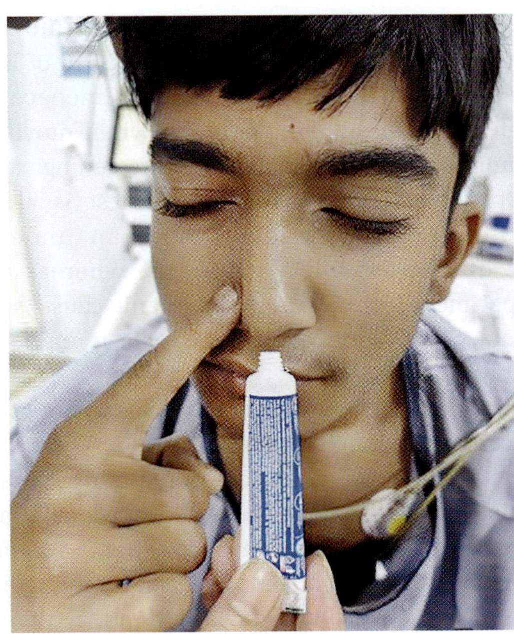

Fig. 4: Cranial nerve I.

Abnormalities: Anosmia, or loss of smell, are often due to nasal congestion, head trauma, meningitis, frontal lobe tumors, or congenital conditions, such as Kallmann syndrome. Distorted smell perception, or parosmia, occurs when pleasant odors are perceived as unpleasant.

Optic Nerve (Cranial Nerve II)

These are the nerves of sight.

Assessment—acuity of vision, field of vision, color vision, and fundus.

- Acuity of vision—at birth—3/60 and by 2 years 6/6.
- *Below 3 years:* There is no standardized protocol for assessing visual acuity in children under 3 years of age. For younger verbal children, the examiner may ask them to identify small objects. In preverbal infants, visual fixation and tracking can be observed using a colored object. Various tools, such as Cardiff acuity cards (7 months to 3 years), tumbling E (3–5 years), or an animal picture Snellen chart, can aid in assessment.
- *Beyond 3 years:* Snellen's chart (placed 6 meters away) is used for distance vision testing, while Jaeger's chart (held 30 cm from the patient) evaluates near vision. Each eye should be tested separately by covering the other. The child's visual acuity is recorded based on the smallest line they can read (e.g., 6/6). If vision is severely impaired, finger counting at 36 cm (14 inches)

is attempted, followed by checking for movement of the fingers, perception, and projection of light, if needed. For an uncooperative child, menace reflex (defensive eye blinking reaction when moving the examiner's fingers suddenly and threateningly toward the patient's eye) may be an option to test visual acuity.

Blindness occurring without an underlying eye disease is called amaurosis, whereas vision impairment resulting from an organic cause, such as cataract, strabismus, or anisometropia, is referred to as amblyopia.

- **Visual fields:** The normal visual pathway is given in **Figure 5,** with the field defect.

To evaluate visual fields, confrontation perimetry is used. Ideally, each eye should be tested individually, but for basic screening, testing both eyes together is acceptable. Position yourself about one meter from the child, making sure your eyes are aligned with theirs. Explain the procedure clearly. Ask the child to cover one eye and focus on your opposite eye. Close your eye corresponding to the child's covered eye. Slowly bring an object from outside their field of vision and have them indicate when they see it. Repeat the process for the other eye. To check for sensory neglect, test both eyes simultaneously **(Fig. 6)**.

To check visual fields in younger children, maintain a toy at the center of vision and slowly move a second, more engaging toy from behind into their peripheral sight. Observe if and when the child shifts their gaze toward the second toy.

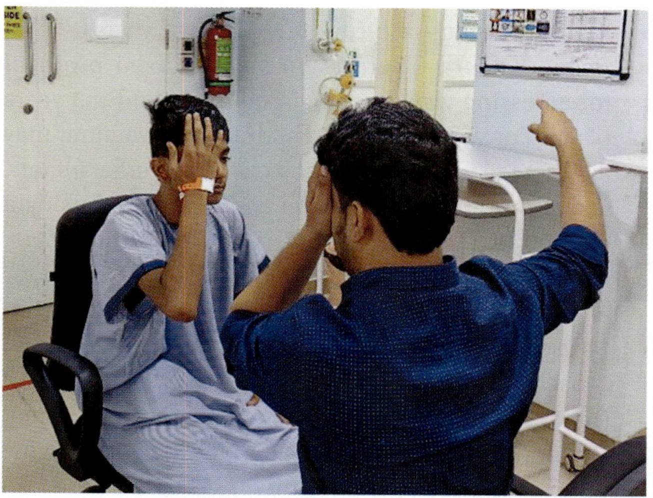

Fig. 5: Examination of the visual field.

Localization of Field Defects

A visual field defect is called homonymous when the identical portion of the visual field is lost in both eyes. For instance, right homonymous hemianopia involves vision loss in the right eye's temporal field and the left eye's nasal field. Conversely, bitemporal hemianopia is a heteronymous defect, affecting the outer (temporal) visual fields of both eyes. When the visual field loss in both eyes matches exactly, the defect is described as congruous **(Table 6)**.

- **Color vision:** Ishihara's chart is used for formal testing. For clinical situations, one may give colored objects and ask the child to name the colors. A 3–4-year-old child will be able to say three colors. Red-green deficiency is the *most common* congenital color blindness. Color testing should be performed in children with acute or chronic vision loss, including optic nerve injury.

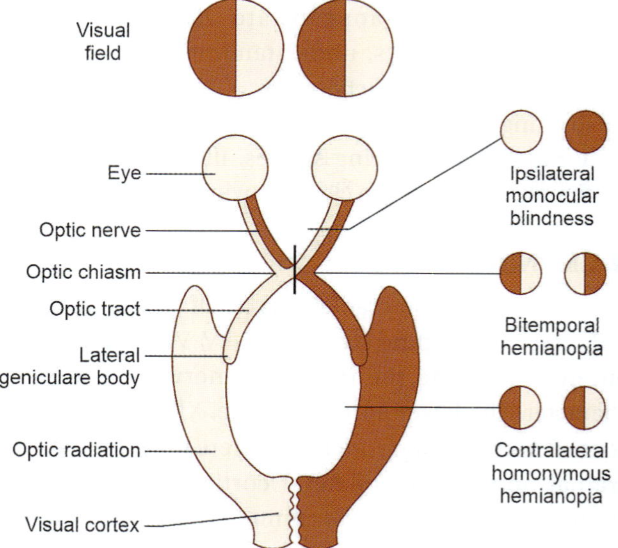

Fig. 6: Lesion in the visual pathway and corresponding visual field defects.

TABLE 6: Field defects with their localization.

Field defect	*Localization*
Monocular	Anterior to optic chiasma
Bitemporal	Lesion in the optic chiasma
Homonymous field defect	Lesion behind the optic chiasm
Incongruous homonymous	Lesion in the optic tract
Congruous homonymous	Lesion behind the lateral geniculate body

- **Fundus:** If necessary (such as when the red reflex is absent), perform a fundoscopic exam at the end of the evaluation. To ease retinal inspection in infants, using a pacifier or gently turning the child's head to one side can be helpful. In children, the optic disc usually has a salmon-pink hue.

Fundoscopy

Dim the room lights by pulling the curtains. Explain to the child that you will be examining their eyes.

Ask the child to fix their gaze on a distant object. Hold the ophthalmoscope in your right hand and approach the child's right eye from the right side, using your right eye to examine. Start the exam about 20 cm away, focusing on the red reflex. An absent or white reflex could suggest serious issues such as cataract, retinoblastoma, and retinal detachment.

Approach the child's head and adjust the ophthalmoscope lens to bring the retina into clear focus. Once the optic disc is visible, evaluate the sharpness of its edges, color, arterial flow, venous pulsations, macula, and surrounding retina. Check for signs of abnormalities such as optic atrophy, papilledema, chorioretinitis, or a cherry-red spot. Then, examine the left eye by holding the ophthalmoscope in your left hand and using your left eye. Although mydriatic drops are usually not needed in older children, they may be necessary for infants.

Abnormalities: Swelling of the optic disc is known as disc edema, and when caused by increased intracranial pressure, it is called papilledema **(Figs. 7A and B)**. Signs to look for are loss of venous pulsation, absence of the physiological cup, engorgement of veins, redness of the disc, and flame hemorrhages. An atrophic disc appears pale yellow to white.

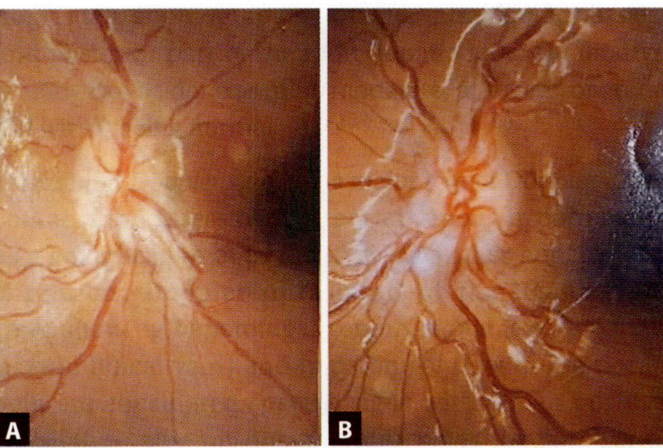

Figs. 7A and B: Papilledema.

Examining the surrounding retina can help identify various childhood conditions, including congenital infections such as cytomegalovirus and toxoplasmosis, acquired infections such as miliary tuberculosis, and retinal hemorrhages. Retinal hemorrhages are observed in 30–40% of full-term newborns and typically resolve within 1–2 weeks. However, their persistence beyond the neonatal period should raise suspicion for nonaccidental trauma. Other conditions that may be detected include retinal dystrophies (e.g., rod/cone dystrophies) and neurocutaneous syndromes, such as tuberous sclerosis.

Evaluation of Vision In Newborns

- At 28 weeks of gestational age, the infant blinks to a bright light.
- At 32 weeks, the infant maintains eye closure until the light source is removed.
- At 29–32 weeks, the pupil reacts to bright light.
- At 37 weeks, the infant turns the head toward a soft light.
- At term—able to fix on and follow a target.

Oculomotor Nerve (Cranial Nerve III), Trochlear Nerve (Cranial Nerve IV), and Abducens Nerve (Cranial Nerve VI)

Nerves - to test for ptosis, nystagmus, strabismus, movement of the eyeball, and light reflexes.

These cranial nerves coordinate eye movements and are evaluated together. The oculomotor nerve (CN III) controls eye adduction (medial rectus), elevation (superior rectus and inferior oblique), depression (inferior rectus), and eyelid elevation (levator palpebrae superioris). It also carries parasympathetic fibers for pupil constriction. The abducens nerve (CN VI) innervates the lateral rectus muscle, allowing for eye abduction, while the trochlear nerve (CN IV) controls the superior oblique muscle, which facilitates downward and inward movement toward the midline **(Fig. 8)**. The initial step in examining these cranial nerves involves watching the child's eyes when looking forward. Both eyes should be aligned, the corneal light reflexes should be symmetrical, pupils equal in size, and the eyelid openings (palpebral fissures) should be the same width.

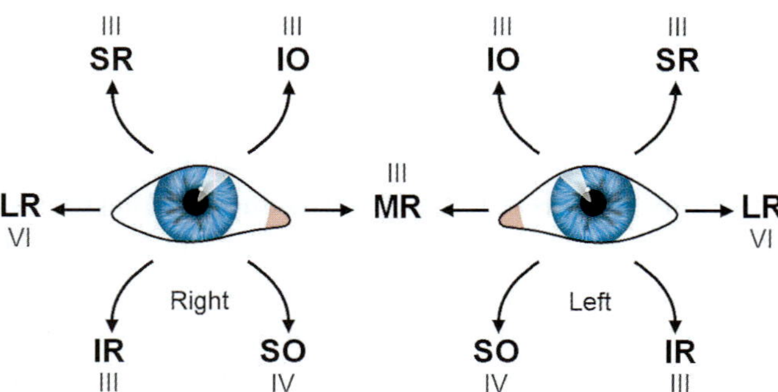

Fig. 8: Function of the extraocular muscles. (MR: medial rectus; LR: lateral rectus; SR: superior rectus; IR: inferior rectus; SO: superior oblique; IO: inferior oblique)

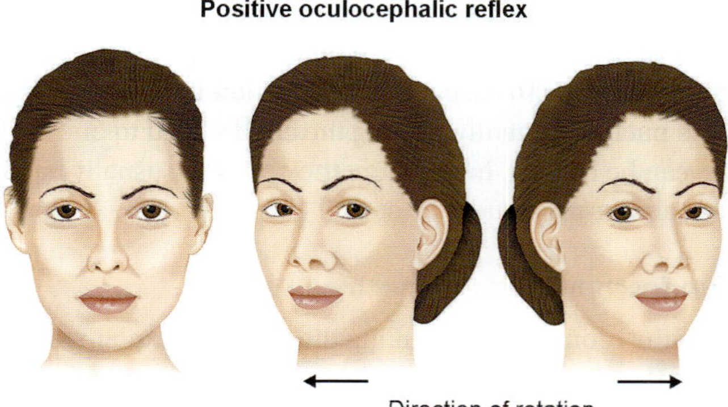

Fig. 10: Oculocephalic reflex.

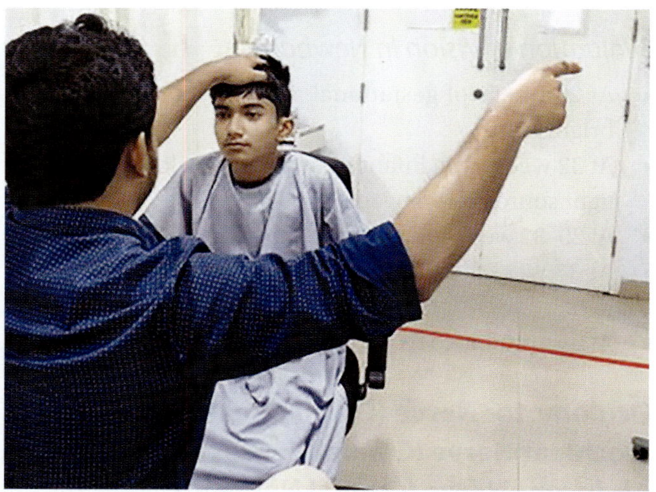

Fig. 9: Examination of movements of the eyeball.

MOVEMENT OF THE EYEBALL

The six extraocular muscles, controlled by cranial nerves III, IV, and VI, coordinate eye movements. To assess these movements in the four cardinal directions, follow these steps: Move your finger or an engaging object across the child's visual field.

Ask the child to track the movement using only their eyes, ensuring they do not move their head (you may need to stabilize it). Avoid extreme lateral gaze, as normal children may exhibit nystagmus. Observe whether eye movements are conjugated. Ask the child if they perceive double vision at any point. When the eye is abducted, the superior and inferior recti function purely as elevators and depressors, while the oblique muscles perform these functions in an adducted position **(Fig. 9)**.

In premature infants beyond 25 weeks of gestation and in comatose patients, eye movement can be assessed using the oculocephalic (doll's eye) reflex. This is tested by rapidly rotating the patient's head horizontally or vertically, observing for reflexive eye movement. Normally, the baby's eyes lag behind, deviating in the opposite direction of the head movement, similar to a doll's eyes. In an awake, alert person, this reflex is absent as voluntary eye movements suppress it. A missing doll's eye response in a comatose child suggests brainstem dysfunction **(Fig. 10)**.

Effects of Paralysis

In oculomotor nerve (CN3) palsy, the affected eye is positioned downward and outward, with restricted movement in adduction, elevation, and depression. Compression of CN3 leads to ipsilateral ptosis and pupil dilation, whereas ischemic CN3 palsy often spares the pupil and causes mild ptosis.

A trochlear nerve (CN4) palsy results in an upward and sometimes outward deviation of the affected eye. Diplopia is most pronounced when looking downward and toward the midline. To compensate, the child tilts their head to the opposite shoulder.

With an abducens nerve (CN6) palsy, the affected eye has a medial deviation and cannot fully abduct. To reduce double vision, the child turns their head toward the affected side.

Diplopia often results from lesions affecting cranial nerves III, IV, or VI. Misalignment of the eyes causes the image to strike different retinal areas, which the brain interprets as separate images.

Supranuclear palsy—lesions of the cortex or midbrain. Cause gaze palsy (paralysis of movement of both eyes in one direction or the other), without paralysis of individual ocular muscles. There is no diplopia. Thus, the presence of diplopia localizes the lesion to the nucleus or infranuclear location [lower motor neuron (LMN) lesion].

Conjugate deviation—means both eyes gaze toward one direction, to the right or left, down or up. A cortical irritative foci (in epilepsy) causes conjugate deviation of the eye to the opposite side, and a cortical destructive lesion (in stroke) causes conjugate deviation of the eyes to the same side. The exact reverse occurs in a pontine lesion.

Internuclear ophthalmoplegia (INO) results from a lesion in the medial longitudinal fasciculus (MLF) of the brainstem, which plays a crucial role in coordinating conjugated eye movements by linking CN VI on one side to CN III on the other. INO is characterized by impaired adduction of the affected eye (medial rectus weakness) and nystagmus in the abducting eye. Ocular motility testing helps distinguish INO from extraocular ophthalmoplegia. Extraocular ophthalmoplegia presents with paralysis of all extraocular muscles, ptosis, and normal pupillary function, whereas INO specifically involves impaired adduction with nystagmus in the contralateral abducting eye **(Fig. 11)**.

Strabismus

Strabismus is a misalignment of the visual axes. If the corneal light reflex is asymmetrical, strabismus should be suspected. It can be classified as paralytic or nonparalytic. Paralytic strabismus results from cranial nerve palsies or brainstem lesions affecting the medial longitudinal fasciculus, whereas nonparalytic strabismus occurs due to eye misalignment with normal extraocular muscle function, often linked to genetic factors, hyperopia, or intraocular abnormalities. In infants younger than two months, a slight resting eye misalignment is normal. When diplopia is present, two key principles help determine the underlying pathology: (1) Diplopia is most pronounced when looking in the direction of the affected muscle's pull, and (2) the displaced peripheral image comes from the affected eye.

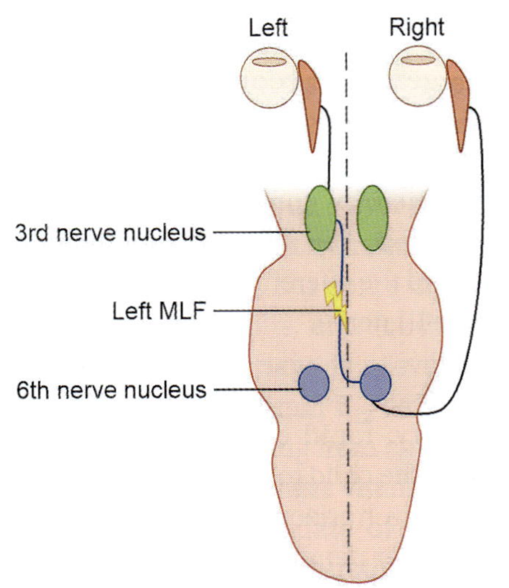

Fig. 11: Internuclear ophthalmoplegia.

To differentiate between paralytic and nonparalytic strabismus, both versions (testing eye movements in six cardinal directions with both eyes open) and ductions (testing each eye separately with the other covered) should be assessed. In paralytic strabismus, such as cranial nerve palsies, abnormal eye movement is evident in both versions and ductions. In nonparalytic strabismus, such as congenital strabismus and misalignment is observed in versions, but a full range of motion is preserved in ductions.

If ductions are restricted, a mechanical cause, such as thyroid eye disease, trauma, and congenital fibrosis, should be considered. Nonparalytic strabismus in children is rarely due to neurological conditions but can lead to amblyopia, which, if untreated, may cause long-term vision impairment.

The cover-uncover test can help diagnose latent strabismus. Instruct the child to focus on your right eye. Cover the left eye, then uncover it while covering the right eye. If the uncovered eye readjusts to refixate, latent strabismus is present, which can be classified as convergent (inward deviation) or divergent (outward deviation) **(Fig. 12)**.

Convergent squint, often due to lateral rectus paralysis (CN VI palsy), is normal in infants during the first few months of life. Divergent squint is usually associated with third nerve palsy (CN III).

When eye movement abnormalities are subtle, the red glass test can assist in identifying the affected muscle. A red glass is placed over one eye, and the patient is asked to follow a white light in various directions of gaze. In areas where eye movement is normal, the patient perceives a single red-white light. However, in the direction of the affected muscle's action, the images separate, with the greatest displacement occurring along the plane of the weakened muscle.

Ptosis

If an eyelid is lower than normal, this is referred to as ptosis. It can be partial or complete. It may be congenital, traumatic, myogenic (myasthenia gravis and myopathy), or neurogenic (III nerve palsy and Horner's syndrome).

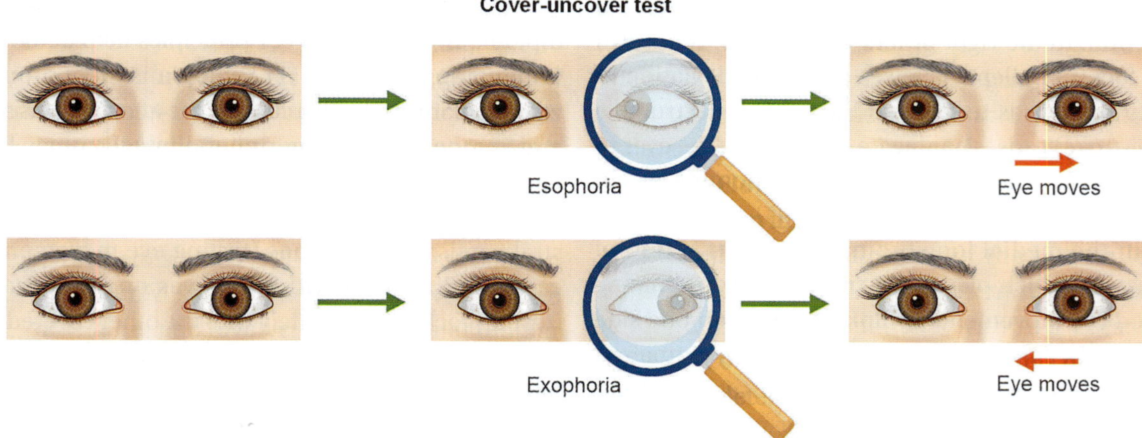

Fig. 12: Cover—uncover test.

Pupillary reflex

Look at the pupils and see if they are equal in size. Pupillary size is controlled by the sphincter pupillae, supplied by the III nerve, and the dilator pupillae, which is supplied by the cervical sympathetics. A constricted pupil is seen in morphine poisoning, organophosphorus exposure, pontine hemorrhage, Horner's syndrome, etc. On the other hand, dilated pupils are seen in optic nerve paralysis, third nerve paralysis, diphtheria, etc., but the most common cause is mydriatic eye drops.

To delineate the pupillary reflex, using a torch, shine the light into one eye to look for constriction (direct reflex). Afferents pass via the second nerve to the lateral geniculate body, and efferents pass from the Edinger-Westphal nucleus through the third nerve to the ciliary ganglion and subsequently to the pupil. Then shine the light in the same eye but look for constriction in the contralateral pupil (consensual reflex) **(Fig. 13)**.

A difference in pupil size combined with an absent direct pupillary response suggests a lesion of the oculomotor nerve. Conversely, if the pupils are equal in size but one pupil shows reduced constriction to light, this indicates possible optic nerve dysfunction, causing diminished light perception. This condition, known as an afferent pupillary defect, is most reliably detected using the swinging flashlight test. During this test, a light moves slowly between the eyes. A pupil with an afferent defect will paradoxically dilate when the light is directed at the affected eye, indicating impaired optic nerve function **(Fig. 14)**.

A fixed and dilated pupil is often seen in optic atrophy, while normal pupillary reactions are preserved in cases of cortical blindness.

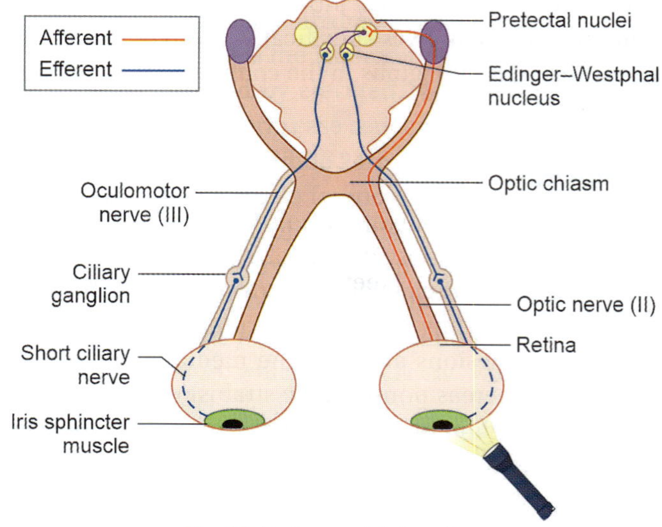

Fig. 13: Pathway of light reflex.

The convergence (accommodation reflex) is performed by asking the child to focus on an object in the midline, which is gradually brought closer to the eyes. This is accompanied by convergence of the eyes and pupillary constriction. The afferent component arises in the frontal lobe, and the efferent from the parasympathetic component of the III nerve.

Nystagmus

It is an involuntary, rapid eye movement that can be assessed by asking the child to follow the examiner's finger as it moves slowly in horizontal and vertical directions. It is classified as either pendular or jerky. Jerky nystagmus is further characterized based on the direction of its fast phase, which may be horizontal, vertical, rotatory, or mixed. A few beats of nystagmus at extreme lateral gaze (end-gaze nystagmus) are common and usually not concerning. However, while horizontal nystagmus can be congenital or drug-related and often involves peripheral vestibular issues, vertical nystagmus is typically a red flag for structural disturbances in central areas like the brainstem or cerebellum. Blind children may exhibit coarse, slow, searching, pendular nystagmoid movements. In cerebellar nystagmus, the fast phase moves toward the side of the lesion.

- *Opsoclonus:* It is a rapid, chaotic, multidirectional eye movement seen classically in neuroblastoma. When these rapid jerky movements are only in the horizontal plane, the term ocular flutter is used.

Trigeminal Nerve (Cranial Nerve V)

These cranial nerves are among the largest and serve both sensory and motor functions. They provide primary sensory innervation to the face, head, oral and nasal cavities, and teeth, while their motor fibers control the muscles of mastication **(Fig. 15)**.

Motor Function

Instruct the child to open their mouth against resistance and then clench their teeth. While they do so, palpate the masseter and temporalis muscles to assess strength. If there is unilateral weakness, the jaw will deviate toward the affected side due to the unopposed action of the healthy pterygoid muscle, and lateral jaw movement will be impaired.

Sensory Function

With the child's eyes closed, assess sensation by gently touching areas corresponding to the ophthalmic, maxillary, and mandibular branches of the trigeminal nerve. Test for light touch, pain, and temperature perception.

Corneal Reflex

The corneal reflex is mediated by the trigeminal nerve (afferent limb) and the facial nerve (efferent limb). It is not routinely tested in children. If necessary, instruct the child to look upward and gently touch the cornea's lateral edge with a fine wisp of cotton, observing for a blink response.

Both the afferent and efferent limbs of the jaw jerk reflex are controlled by the trigeminal nerve. The test is performed by having the child relax with their mouth slightly open while the examiner places an index finger on the chin and taps gently with a reflex hammer. An exaggerated response indicates upper motor neuron (UMN) involvement above the pons.

Facial Nerve (Cranial Nerve VII)

Motor: As a primarily motor nerve, the facial nerve controls the muscles involved in facial expression. Examine the child's resting facial features, noting any unevenness in the palpebral fissures, eyelid closure, nasolabial creases, and the positioning of the lips.

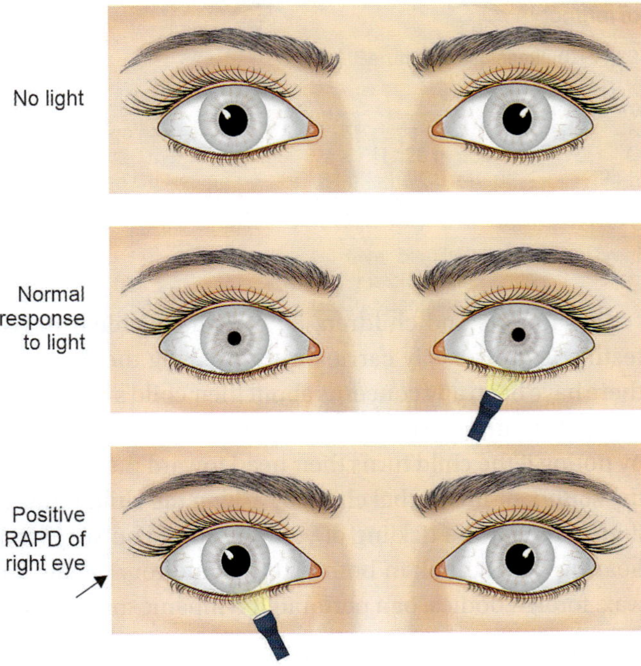

Fig. 14: Normal light reflex and relative afferent pupillary defect (RAPD).

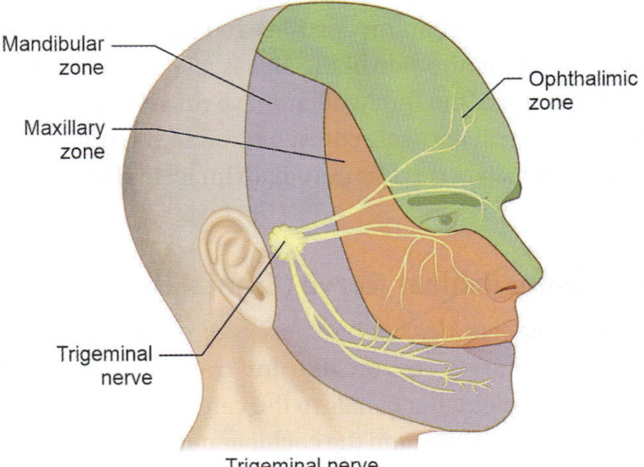

Fig. 15: Trigeminal nerve distribution.

To test, ask the child to raise their eyebrows and observe the forehead. Asymmetrical wrinkling or flattening on one side is a sign of upper facial muscle weakness.

Then ask the child to shut both eyes firmly. Failure to close one eye completely and an increased palpebral gap on that side are indicative of orbicularis oculi weakness. Bell's phenomenon—upward deviation of the eyeball—can also be observed.

Ask the child to show his teeth and to smile (orbicularis oris and levator anguli oris). A normal side can smile; the weak side usually has flattening of the nasolabial fold with drooping of that side of the mouth.

Air leaks on attempted blowing or tapping with lips closed and mouth full of air (buccinator).

When the nerve to the stapedius is compromised within the facial canal, it can result in heightened auditory sensitivity.

Sensory: The Facial nerve conveys taste from the front two-thirds of the tongue via the chorda tympani; if necessary, assess taste using natural flavors such as sweet, salty, or sour agents.

A parasympathetic component supplies the lacrimal gland.

Facial nerve dysfunction can be due to congenital factors, spontaneous idiopathic onset (Bell's palsy), trauma, immune-mediated demyelination (e.g., Guillain-Barré), infectious agents like HSV and HIV, infiltrative or granulomatous diseases, or neoplastic processes. A key differential diagnosis is congenital absence of the depressor anguli oris. Bilateral facial nerve palsy can be challenging to identify, often presenting as a mask-like, expressionless face. It is associated with conditions such as Guillain-Barré syndrome, Moebius syndrome, infantile botulism, and certain myopathies. In cases of LMN facial paralysis, the entire side of the face is affected, whereas in UMN paralysis, the forehead and eye muscles are spared due to bilateral cortical representation of the upper face. Emotional facial expressions remain intact in UMN lesions **(Fig. 16)**.

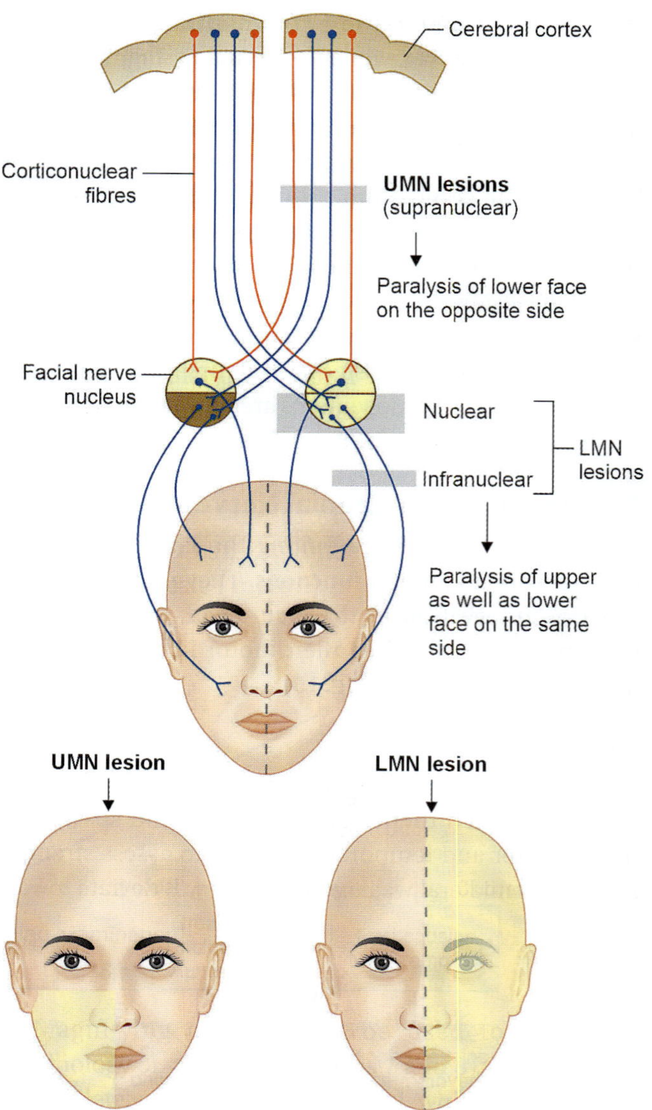

Fig. 16: Facial nerve lesion.

Vestibulocochlear Nerve (Cranial Nerve VIII)

The vestibulocochlear nerve consists of two branches: the vestibular nerve, responsible for transmitting signals from the semicircular canals to the cerebellum to regulate balance and posture, and the cochlear nerve, which carries auditory information from the cochlea to the auditory cortex in the temporal lobe for sound perception.

For infants and children, by bedside cochlear nerve testing is most easily carried out by asking the parent if there have been any concerns about their child's hearing. A soft bell or rattle can be used to check for auditory response by noting if the child turns their head toward the source of the sound, or in a verbal child, by asking the child himself if he can hear the tickling of your watch. If you suspect a hearing deficit, look in both external auditory canals for wax, foreign bodies, or a perforated tympanic membrane.

Cochlear nerve: If hearing impairment is present, assess whether it is due to conductive or sensorineural causes using the Weber and Rinne tests **(Fig. 17)**.

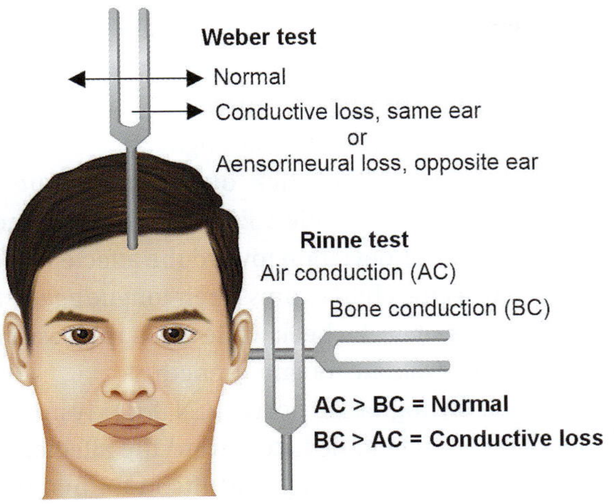

Fig. 17: Weber and Rinne test.

Rinne Test

To conduct the Rinne test, a tuning fork is applied to the mastoid bone until vibrations are no longer felt, then positioned near the ear to determine if air conduction surpasses bone conduction. Since air conduction is more efficient than bone conduction, the child should still perceive the sound produced by the vibrating tuning fork. A positive Rinne test indicates normal hearing, where air conduction exceeds bone conduction. In conductive hearing loss, bone conduction is perceived as louder (negative Rinne), whereas in sensorineural loss, air conduction is still greater than or equal to bone conduction.

Weber Test

In older children, the Weber test is performed by placing a vibrating tuning fork (256 or 512 Hz) on the center of the forehead or incisors and asking if the sound is louder in one ear. Normally, the sound is heard equally in both ears. In sensorineural hearing loss, it localizes to the unaffected ear, whereas in conductive hearing loss, it is louder in the affected ear. The Weber test is ineffective for diagnosing symmetrical hearing loss.

Vestibular

In vestibular dysfunction, the child may experience vertigo or dizziness. Examination often reveals nystagmus, which can be assessed using ice water caloric testing. The test should only be done if the ear canal is clear of wax and the tympanic membrane is intact. The child's head is positioned at a 30° semireclined angle using pillows. Then, 10 mL of cold water (30°C) is gently introduced into the ear canal while nystagmus is recorded via electromyography. During formal testing, the slow phase of nystagmus moves toward the irrigated ear, indicating brainstem activity, whereas the fast corrective phase moves away, reflecting cerebral hemisphere involvement. Ice water caloric testing is commonly used to evaluate brainstem function in a comatose child. If the brainstem is intact, the eyes will turn toward the ear being irrigated, although the corrective nystagmus away from that ear will be absent. The fast, or corrective, phase of nystagmus is observed only in conscious individuals with preserved vestibular function. Absence of response during ice water caloric testing is among the key indicators for confirming brain death.

On Romberg and tandem gait testing, they tend to fall toward the abnormal ear.

Glossopharyngeal Nerve (Cranial Nerve IX) and Vagus Nerve (Cranial Nerve X)

The glossopharyngeal nerve (cranial nerve IX) provides motor innervation to the stylopharyngeus muscle and transmits sensory information from the posterior third of the tongue, pharynx, and tonsillar region. It is an essential component of both the swallowing mechanism and the gag reflex.

The vagus nerve has the widest distribution among cranial nerves, supplying all muscles of the soft palate (except the tensor veli palatini), as well as the pharynx and larynx. It provides both sensory and motor innervation to the respiratory tract, heart, and most abdominal organs through parasympathetic ganglia. These two nerves are closely linked, and it is uncommon for one to be affected without the other.

Assess the child's speech for any hoarseness, nasal resonance, or speech impairment. A combined IX and X nerve lesion can result in an absent swallowing reflex, leading to drooling and choking episodes.

Examine the uvula's movement by asking the child to say "Ahh." If there is asymmetry, the uvula will be pulled toward the stronger side. Also, you can assess the gag reflex by applying light pressure to the lateral oropharynx or soft palate with a tongue blade and noting symmetric palatal movement.

When the UMNs are affected, as in pseudobulbar palsy, the gag reflex becomes exaggerated, often observed in cases of diffuse brain injury or neurodevelopmental disorders. On the other hand, in bulbar paralysis, the cranial nerves IX through XII or their brainstem nuclei in the medulla oblongata are involved. The loss of jaw jerk and gag reflex, along with speech and swallowing difficulties, are key clinical signs of bulbar paralysis, commonly seen in neurological conditions such as Guillain-Barré syndrome and poliomyelitis.

Unilateral vagus nerve dysfunction affects laryngeal function, causing voice hoarseness, while bilateral involvement can severely impact speech and airway control.

Accessory Nerve (Cranial Nerve XI)

The accessory nerve supplies the sternocleidomastoid (SCM) and trapezius muscles. The SCM muscle on one side turns the head to the opposite side, while both SCMs together flex the neck. The trapezius muscle functions to elevate the shoulder and assist in head and neck movement.

Observe the child for any signs of SCM muscle wasting or hypertrophy and palpate to evaluate muscle bulk. Stand behind the child and inspect the trapezius muscles for asymmetry, atrophy, or hypertrophy.

Assess SCM strength by asking the child to turn their head to each side while applying resistance with your hand **(Fig. 18)**. Test the power of the trapezius by instructing the child to shrug their shoulders against resistance.

Muscle atrophy and weakness in these regions are commonly seen in skull base fractures or lesions, motor neuron disease, myotonic dystrophy, and myasthenia gravis; congenital torticollis, however, is associated with SCM enlargement.

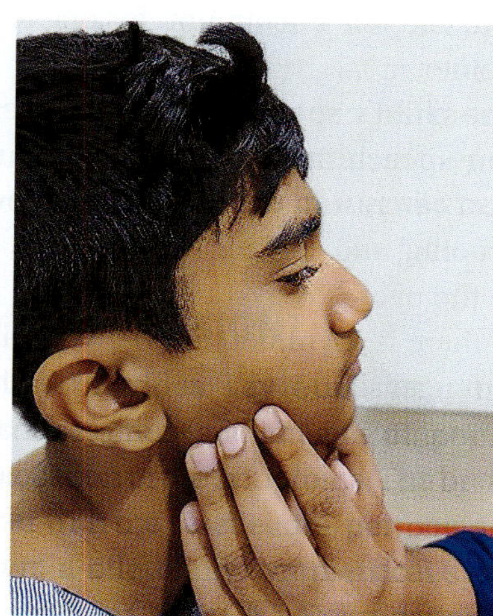

Fig. 18: Examination of sternocleidomastoid.

Hypoglossal Nerve (Cranial Nerve XII)

- The hypoglossal nerve is responsible for tongue function.
- The tongue should be inspected for atrophy, fasciculations and tested for strength.
- Instruct the child to stick out their tongue and sweep it across both sides. Evaluate for asymmetry, fasciculations, or deviation toward the affected side.
- Next, instruct the child to press their tongue against the inner surface of each cheek while you apply resistance externally to evaluate tongue strength.
- Unilateral hypoglossal nerve (CN XII) dysfunction causes the tongue to deviate toward the affected side, while bilateral involvement results in an inability to protrude the tongue, often accompanied by dysphagia. In nuclear or infranuclear lesions, the tongue appears to be wasted and may exhibit fasciculations, with spinal muscular atrophy type 1 being a common cause in children. Proper assessment requires inspecting the tongue while it rests on the floor of the mouth, as the quivering movements seen in a crying infant may sometimes be mistaken for fasciculations.

CRANIAL NERVE EXAMINATION IN INFANT

Cranial Testing Nerve

- *CN2:* Assess visual awareness by noting blink response to bright light. Check for the presence and symmetry of red reflex using an ophthalmoscope.
- *CN 2 and 3:* Evaluate pupillary light reflex for both direct and consensual response.
- *CN3, 4, and 6:* Inspect ocular alignment and conjugate gaze at rest. Perform the oculocephalic reflex ("Doll's eye" maneuver) by gently rotating the infant's head side to side and up and down, observing for compensatory eye movement in the opposite direction.
- *CN5:* Observe rooting and sucking reflexes during feeding. Assess corneal sensitivity using a soft stimulus near the eye and monitor for blinking or grimacing.
- *CN7:* Watch facial movements during spontaneous activity, such as crying and smiling, to assess symmetry.
- *CN8:* Evaluate auditory function by observing startle or turning response to sudden loud sounds.
- *CN9 and 10:* Assess swallowing and coordination during feeding. Listen to the cry quality for hoarseness or nasal tone. Test gag reflex using gentle posterior pharyngeal stimulation.

- *CN11:* Note head turning and shoulder elevation symmetry, especially during spontaneous movement.
- *CN12:* Inspect tongue movements during sucking or when crying; look for deviation, fasciculations, or weakness.

Motor Examination

Assessment of muscle bulk, tone, strength, and involuntary movements.

- **Bulk:** assess three S—(1) the size, (2) shape, and (3) symmetry of a muscle.
  - By inspection—Muscle atrophy, or decreased muscle bulk, can result from disuse or LMN palsy, with neurogenic atrophy typically being more severe than myogenic atrophy. It is important to determine whether the atrophy primarily affects proximal or distal muscle groups and whether it is symmetrical or asymmetrical. Limb circumference should be measured at consistent anatomical landmarks, such as the anterior superior iliac spine or olecranon, to ensure accurate assessment.
  - Muscle hypertrophy is typically a normal physiological adaptation, but in some cases, it can be misleading. Pseudohypertrophy occurs when muscle tissue is replaced by fat and connective tissue, leading to an apparent increase in size but a paradoxical loss of strength, as seen in Duchenne and Becker muscular dystrophies. When muscle weakness is present, palpation is crucial to assess texture and firmness. Muscle tenderness may indicate an inflammatory myopathy, such as dermatomyositis or postinfectious myositis.
- **Tone:** Resistance to passive movement of a joint. From a clinical perspective, muscle tone can be categorized into postural tone and phasic tone.

  Muscle tone fluctuates significantly depending on the child's age and level of alertness.

  In newborns:
  - At 28 weeks of gestation, all four extremities are extended **(Fig. 19)**.
  - *32 weeks:* Flexor tone in the lower extremities
  - *36 weeks:* Flexor tone in both upper and lower extremities
  - A normal term infant's posture is characterized by flexion of all four extremities.

In infants, the range of motion can be quantified using angles (adductor angle, popliteal angle, dorsiflexion angle of foot, and scarf sign), as described in the Amiel-Tison method.

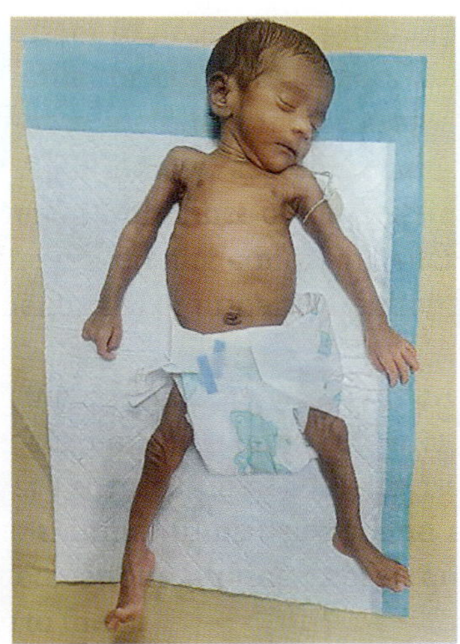

Fig. 19: A preterm baby with universal extension posture.

Amieltison ***(Figs. 20A to E):***

- Adductor angle—in the supine position, the hips are abducted by holding on to the extended knee. The adductor angle is the angle between the thighs. It is <75° below 3 months of age.
- Popliteal angle—measured by flexing the hip to 90° while extending the knee as much as possible. The angle between the thigh and lower leg was recorded.
- Ankle dorsiflexion—angle between the dorsum of the foot and the anterior aspect of the leg when the foot is dorsiflexed.
- Scarf sign—in the supine position, the upper limb is pulled across the chest, holding the flexed elbow. The elbow does not cross the midline below 3 months of age.
- Heel to ear maneuver—lift both the legs of the supine infant without lifting the pelvis from the table and try to bring it to the ear.

Tests for assessing postural tone in infants: Traction response, vertical suspension, and horizontal suspension.

- *Traction response:* Gently holding the infant's hands and pulling them into a sitting position typically reveals a slight head lag, which is expected at this stage. As the infant reaches the upright position, the Head momentarily lags behind before falling forward. This response is considered normal in early infancy, reflecting developing neck and trunk control **(Fig. 21)**.

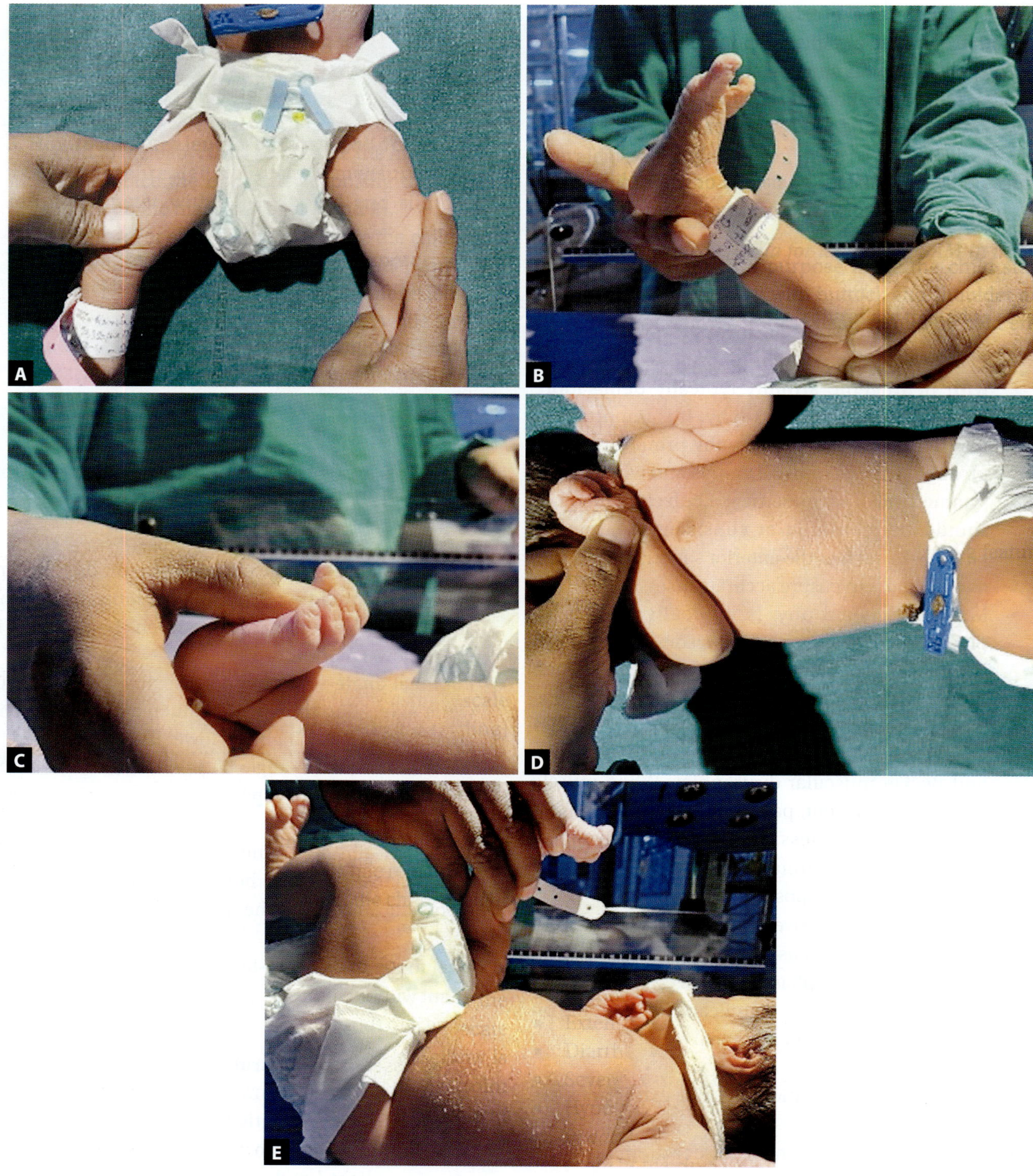

Figs. 20A to E: (A) Adductor angle; (B) Popliteal angle; (C) Ankle dorsiflexion; (D) Scarf sign; and (E) Heel to ear maneuver.

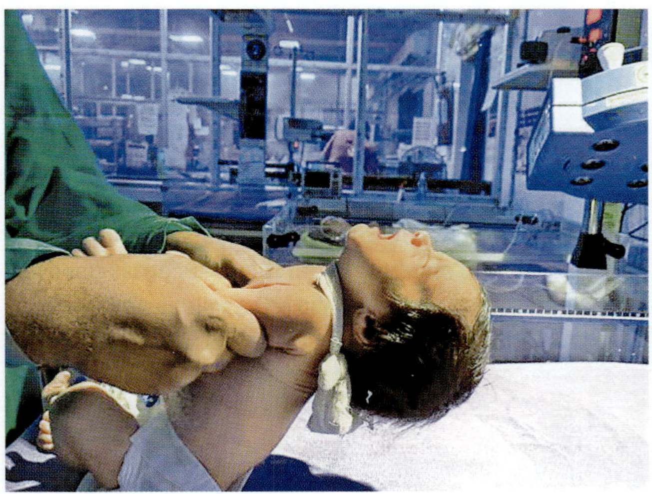

Fig. 21: Traction response.

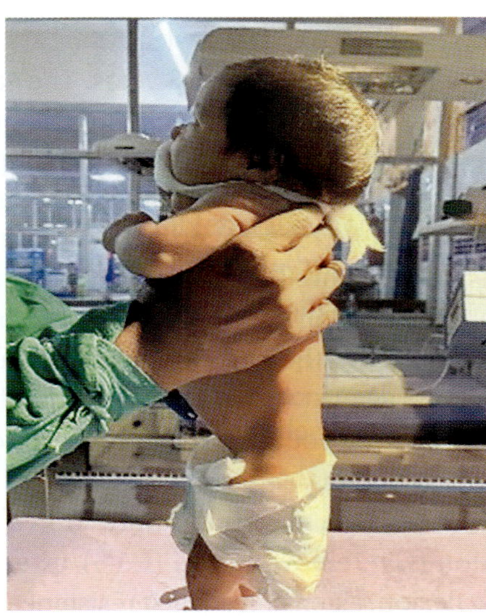

Fig. 22: Vertical suspension.

- *Vertical suspension:* Lifting the infant by the axillae without applying pressure to the thorax should allow the infant to remain suspended, with the lower limbs maintaining a flexed position. In cases of hypotonia, the infant may struggle to maintain this posture and could slip through the examiner's hands due to insufficient muscle tone **(Fig. 22)**.
- *Horizontal suspension:* Supporting the infant in a prone position with a hand placed under the abdomen should prompt the infant to lift the head and flex the limbs. However, in a hypotonic infant, poor muscle tone causes the body to drape over the examiner's hand in a U-shaped posture, indicating weakness **(Fig. 23)**.

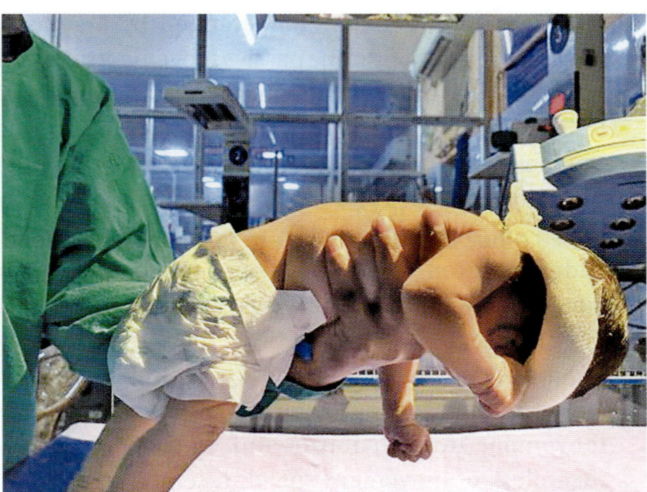

Fig. 23: Horizontal suspension.

TONE ASSESSMENT IN ELDER CHILDREN

- *Posture:* Observe the spontaneous posture of the child when lying down in bed. A floppy hypotonic child lies in a frog-like position (abduction at the hip and flexion at the knee). A hypertonic child will have extended lower limbs and may have scissoring.
- *Feel the muscles:* Normal muscles feel firm. Hypotonic muscles feel flabby and soft. Hypertonic muscles feel stiff.
- Resistance to passive stretching and flap ability—for the upper limb—hold the child's hand and extend and flex the elbow several times. Clasp-knife spasticity will usually be easy to feel (initial stiffness followed by giving way). Then, still grasping the hand, alternate between pronation and supination and flexion and extension of the wrist for lower limb-tested in three ways. (1) Can roll legs from side to side (a good indicator of rigidity); (2) by placing your hand under each knee, abruptly lifting it upward. The heel should remain on the bed. If the heel raises, this indicates increased tone; (3) place one hand on the knee and the other hand around the feet, and unpredictably flex and extend the knee.

Muscle tone must be assessed bilaterally with the head in a neutral position to ensure symmetry. It may be normal, elevated (as in hypertonia—spasticity or rigidity), or diminished (hypotonia).

Abnormalities of Tone

- *Hypertonia:* Elevated muscle tone is often linked to UMN involvement or disorders affecting the basal ganglia.

- *Spasticity:* Spasticity is characterized by a sudden release of resistance during passive movement, referred to as the clasp-knife phenomenon. It results from UMN lesions and typically involves increased tone in flexor muscles of the arms and extensor muscles of the legs. In infants, spasticity in the lower limbs may lead to leg scissoring when the child is suspended vertically. Older children often show persistent commando crawling or walking on their toes due to this increased muscle tone.
- *Rigidity:* Associated with basal ganglia lesions, this condition presents as uniform resistance to passive movement in both flexor and extensor muscles, regardless of movement speed, resembling a "lead-pipe" rigidity.
  Individuals with spasticity or rigidity may develop opisthotonos, a condition characterized by pronounced spinal hyperextension due to excessive paraspinal muscle tone.
- Hypotonia, or reduced muscle tone, is the most frequently observed tone abnormality in neonates with neurological impairment. A hypotonic infant appears floppy and often rests in a frog-leg position. The underlying cause may involve the CNS (cerebral hemispheres, cerebellum, spinal cord) or the peripheral nervous system (anterior horn cells, peripheral nerves, neuromuscular junction, or muscle). In cases of central hypotonia associated with UMN disorders, deep tendon reflexes (DTRs) remain present and are usually exaggerated. Conversely, in neuromuscular disorders, hypotonia is accompanied by absent or diminished DTRs.

Power: Power is the force that can be voluntarily generated.

Formal motor power testing is generally feasible in cooperative older children.

Evaluating a child's posture and performing simple tests can aid in assessing muscle strength. In older children, muscle power can be observed through their movements around the examination room. For upper limb assessment, the child is instructed to extend both arms fully at shoulder height with palms facing upward and maintain the position **(Fig. 24)**.

In cases of a contralateral pyramidal tract lesion, the affected forearm gradually pronates and drifts downward, a sign known as pronator drift. This finding suggests spasticity, and closing the eyes can enhance the effect by further revealing difficulty in maintaining the position.

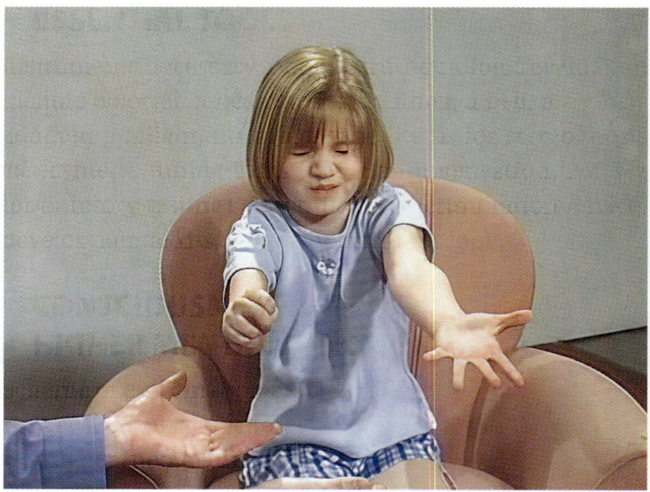

Fig. 24: Pronator drift.

Formal muscle strength testing can typically be performed in children older than 3 years. The easiest way to do this is to put the child's arms into the position of the muscle strength you are testing. For example, if you are testing for shoulder abduction, in the sitting position, stabilize the shoulder, and ask the child to lift the arm. Apply resistance in the downward direction to prevent abduction. Likewise, in the case of the lower limb, to examine the power of the knee extensor, ask the child to extend the knee against the resistance in the downward direction applied by you. Know the root values for the different muscle actions.

- *Upper limb:* Test shoulder adduction (C7, C8)/ abduction (C5), elbow flexion (C5.6)/extension (C7, 8), wrist flexion/extension against resistance. To assess handgrips, request the child to grasp and squeeze the examiner's fingers when prompted. In a pyramidal lesion, flexors are stronger than extensors (the reverse from the legs) **(Figs. 25A to F)**.
- *Lower limb:* Assess muscle strength for hip flexion (L1, L2) and extension (L5, S1), hip abduction and adduction, knee flexion (L3, L4) and extension (S1), ankle dorsiflexion (L4), plantar flexion (S1, S2), as well as foot inversion and eversion **(Figs. 26A to H)**.
- *Neck:* Extend and flex the neck against resistance offered at the occiput and the chin, respectively.
- Intercostal muscles and diaphragm—splint the abdomen below the costal margin with the hand. This will restrict the movement of the diaphragm, and hence, if the intercostals are weak, there will be increasing dyspnea. For the diaphragm, splint the

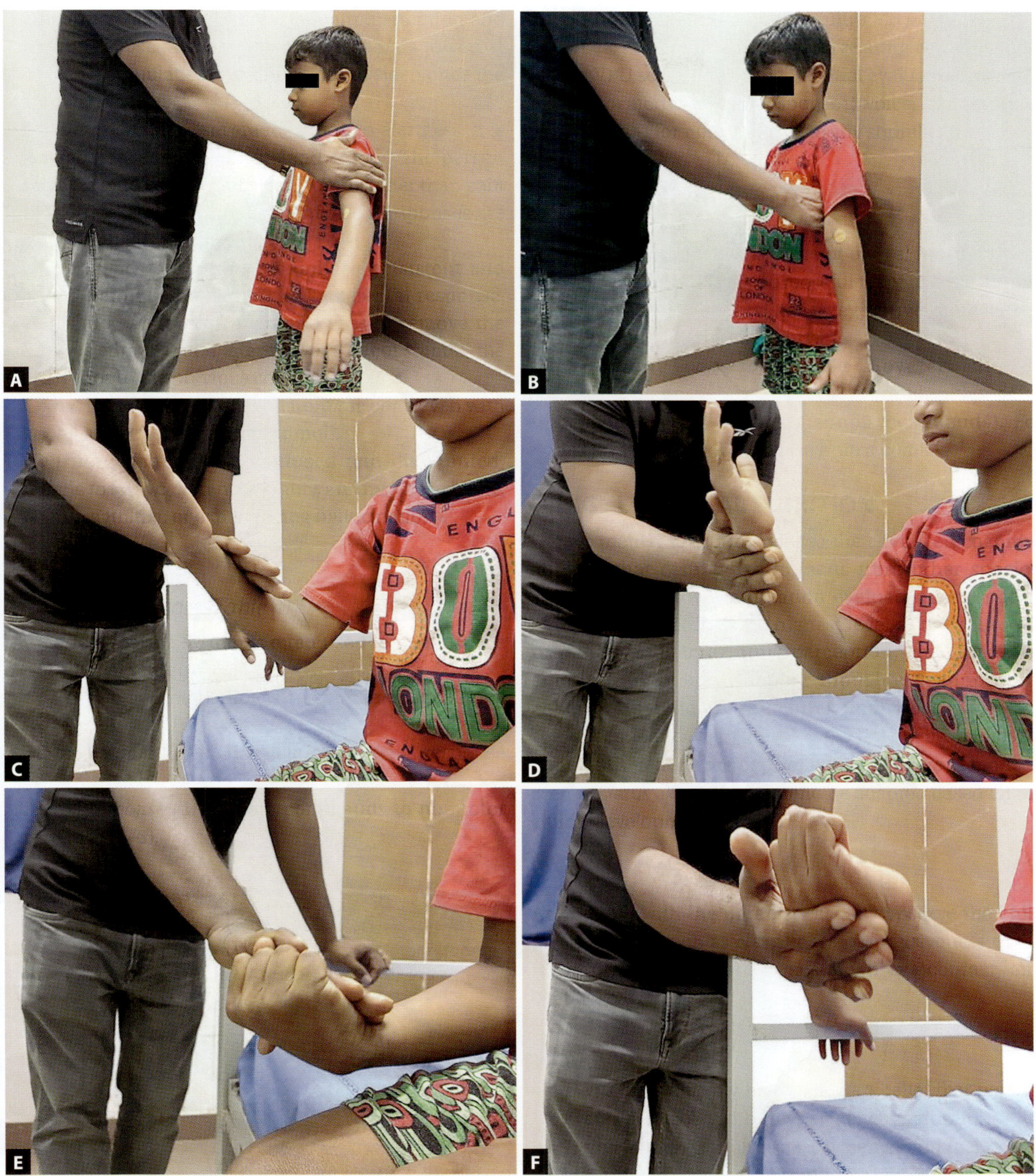

Figs. 25A to F: (A) Shoulder abduction; (B) Shoulder adduction; (C) Elbow flexion; (D) Elbow extension; (E) Wrist flexion; and (F) Wrist extension.

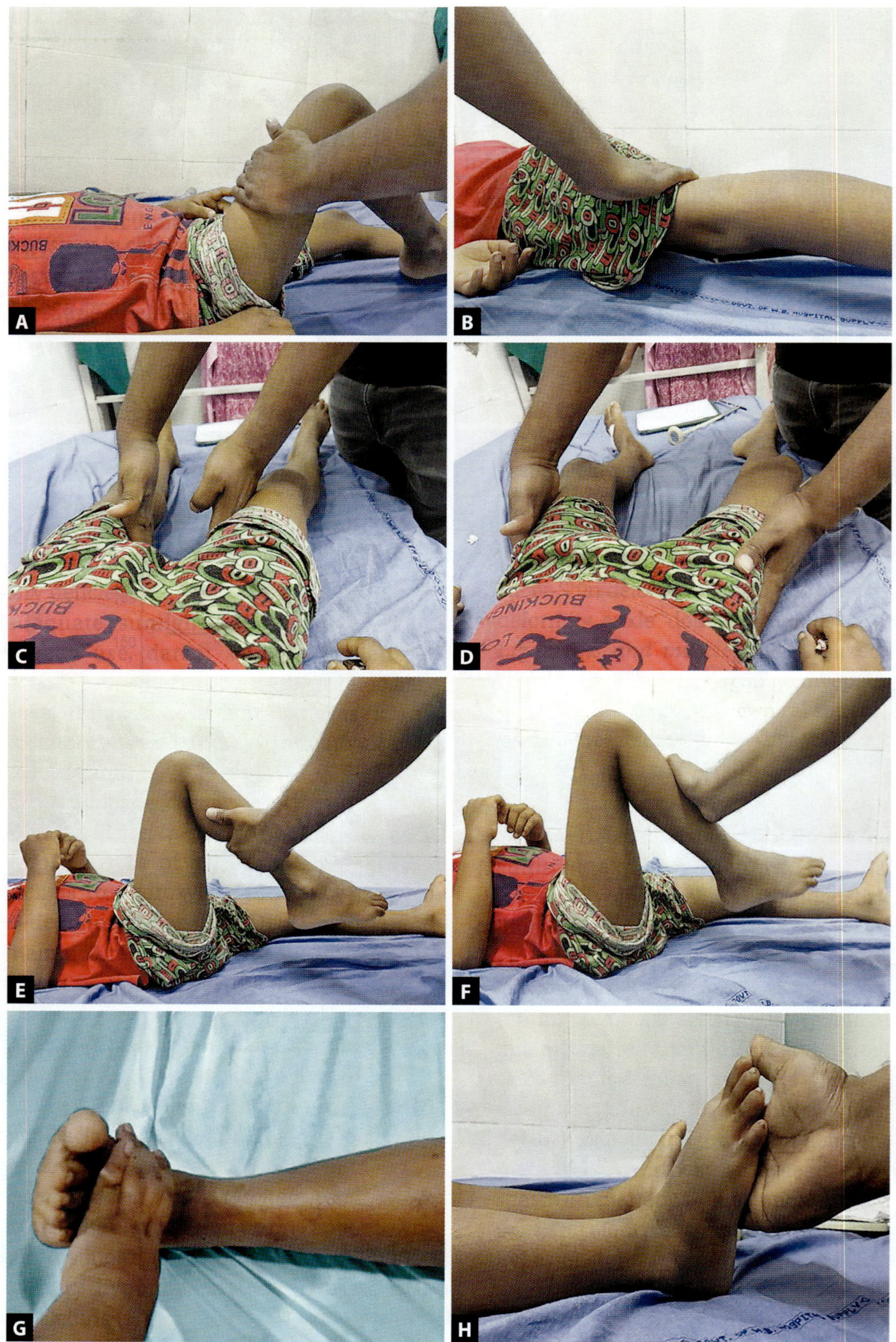

Figs. 26A to H: (A) Hip flexion; (B) Hip extension; (C) Hip adduction; (D) Hip abduction; (E) Knee flexion; (F) Knee extension; (G) Ankle dorsiflexion; (H) Plantar flexion.

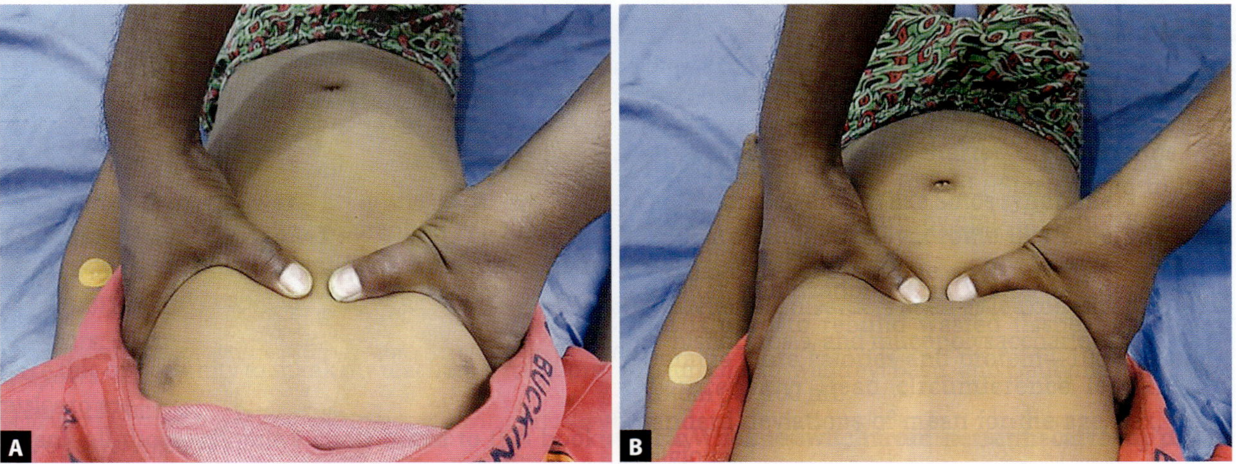

Figs. 27A and B: (A) Intercostal muscle weakness and (B) Diaphragm weakness.

chest by encircling the chest with the examiner's hand. Dyspnea will increase if the diaphragm is paralyzed **(Figs. 27A and B)**.

- *Abdomen:* For the upper abdomen, ask the child to raise the head and chest in the supine position without any support. For the lower abdomen, to raise his extended leg without support. When testing the upper abdomen, if there is upward deviation of the umbilicus (Beevor sign), it indicates bilateral lower abdominal wall paralysis.

Muscle power is graded on a scale of 0–5 as follows (Medical Research Council power scale):

- 0 = No contraction
- 1 = Flicker or trace of contraction
- 2 = Active movement with gravity eliminated
- 3 = Active movement against gravity
- 4 = Active movement against gravity and some resistance
- 5 = Normal power.

Since infants and young children cannot engage in formal strength testing, functional assessments are the most effective approach. Proximal and distal upper limb strength can be evaluated by observing the child reach overhead for a toy and manipulate small objects, providing insight into their motor abilities. Infants with lower extremity weakness often exhibit reduced spontaneous leg movements and struggle to bear weight when held in an upright position. In older children, weakness may present as difficulty with activities such as climbing stairs, jumping, or hopping. When asked to rise from a prone position, they may push against their legs with their hands to assist in standing, a characteristic movement known as Gowers' sign.

For subtle weakness—Ask the child to perform tasks such as hopping on one foot, walking forwards and backwards, toe walking, heel walking, and rising from a squatting or supine position. These activities can reveal subtle weaknesses in the limbs. Additionally, evaluate whether the weakness is predominantly affecting the proximal muscles—as seen in conditions like myopathy, dermatomyositis, or Guillain-Barré syndrome—or the distal muscles, which is more typical of peripheral neuropathies, and note whether the weakness is symmetrical or asymmetrical.

A special mention regarding myotonia, in which the contraction of the muscle persists even after Voluntary efforts have ceased. The child will have difficulty in releasing a handshake. Do not forget to shake hands with parents in those cases—as it may demonstrate myotonia in parents in case of myotonic dystrophy.

Involuntary Movements

Check for unusual movements and determine whether they are present or absent while the child is asleep. All involuntary movements disappear during sleep except hemiballismus and myoclonus.

Most involuntary movements, such as tics, dystonia, chorea, and athetosis, originate from basal ganglia dysfunction. Tremors, however, appear to be an exception, as they are believed to involve the cerebellothalamocortical pathways. Fasciculations, on the other hand, are characteristic of LMN lesions **(Table 7)**.

TABLE 7: Involuntary movements in childhood.

Chorea	Involuntary, quasi-purposive, continuous, writhing, flowing, and irregular movements. These movements primarily affect the proximal joints, becoming more pronounced with excitement and subsiding with purposeful action. Ex- Sydenham Chorea
Ballism	Involuntary, high-amplitude flinging movements, typically generated proximally. Lesion in the subthalamic nuclei.
Athetosis	Slow, writhing, or continuous involuntary movement. It most often affects the distal joints and occurs in association with chorea, hence the name choreoathetosis
Tics	Sudden, involuntary motor or vocal actions that are repetitive and irregular in pattern
Myoclonus	Rapid, shock-like contraction of muscle. Occurs due to lesions in the brainstem or reticular formation
Dystonia	Intermittent and sustained involuntary muscle contractions. Common causes—birth asphyxia, kernicterus, and encephalitis
Tremors	Repetitive, rhythmic shaking of a limb caused by alternating activity in antagonist muscle groups; may occur at rest or with movement
Fasciculations	Brief, involuntary flickers of muscle movement arising from single motor unit activation, typically noted in the lingual muscles of young children

REFLEXES DEEP TENDON REFLEXES AND THE PLANTAR RESPONSE

Involuntary muscle contractions occur when a tendon is tapped with a reflex hammer, causing a brisk stretch of the muscle. Tendon reflexes are heightened in individuals with pyramidal tract lesions, whereas they are diminished or absent in cases of LMN or muscle disorders. Observe for limb movements and visible muscle contractions during the assessment.

Deep tendon reflexes can usually be elicited easily in infants and children. When assessing reflexes in infants, it is crucial to keep the head in a midline position, as turning it to one side may influence reflex tone. Reflex responses are graded on a scale from 0 (absent) to 4+ (markedly hyperactive), with 2+ considered normal. Reflexes graded as 1+ or 3+ may also be normal if they are symmetrical. If a reflex is difficult to elicit, reinforcement techniques such as having the child clench their teeth or interlock their fingers (Jendrassik maneuver) can be used to enhance the response.

Examine for Superficial and Deep Reflexes

Superficial Reflexes

- To evaluate the abdominal wall reflex (T7–T12), gently stroke the abdominal skin from the side toward the midline and watch for contraction of the anterior abdominal muscles. This reflex may be diminished or absent in cases of LMN lesions affecting T7–T12 or UMN dysfunction **(Fig. 28)**.

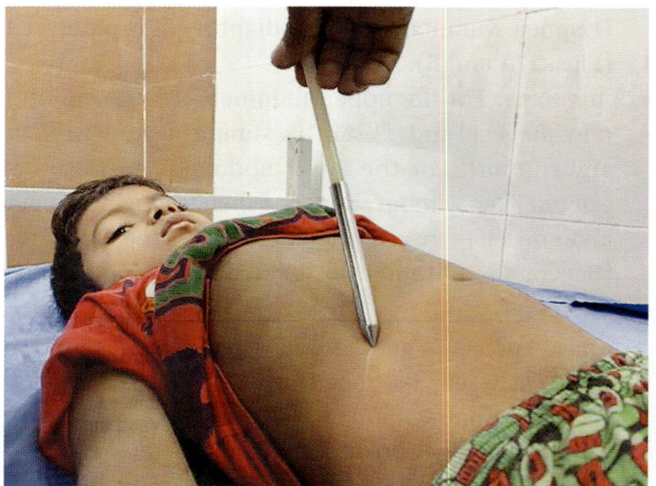

Fig. 28: Abdominal reflex.

- The cremasteric reflex (L1) is tested by stroking the inner thigh while observing for elevation of the ipsilateral testis. A normal response involves the testis rising on the same side as the stimulus. Anal reflex (S3, S4)—elicited by gently stroking the perianal skin. It results in the puckering of the anal orifice.
- The plantar response (S1, S2) is assessed by firmly stroking the lateral sole of the foot with a blunt object or thumbnail. A normal (negative) response consists of plantar flexion of the big toe. Upward movement (dorsiflexion) of the big toe, called a positive Babinski sign, indicates a UMN lesion but is considered normal in infants **(Fig. 29)**.

Deep Tendon Reflexes (Figs. 30A to E)

- With the child in a relaxed state and the head positioned centrally, use a tendon hammer to gently tap each tendon, observing the expected muscle contraction and relaxation. Compare the reflex response on both sides to assess for symmetry and any abnormalities **(Table 8)**.
    - *Upper limb:* Biceps reflex, Triceps reflex, Supinator (brachioradialis) reflex.
    - *Lower limb:* Knee reflex, ankle reflex.

In newborns and infants, the middle finger can be used in place of a reflex hammer to elicit DTRs. Reflex responses tend to be brisk during infancy. When the knee-jerk reflex is tested on one side, a crossed adductor response may be observed, which is considered a normal finding in infants.

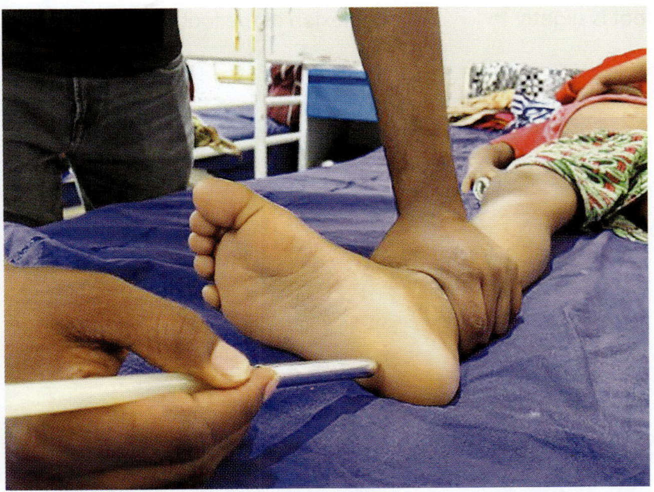

Fig. 29: Plantar response.

CLONUS

The child should be in a relaxed state, with the hips flexed and the knee and ankle in moderate flexion. Support the leg by placing one hand under the knee while grasping the foot from below, then rapidly dorsiflex the foot. In cases of clonus, rhythmic alternating contractions may occur. Sustained clonus is always pathological, but in infants under three months, 5–10 beats may be normal, while in older children, one to two beats can be considered normal if symmetrical.

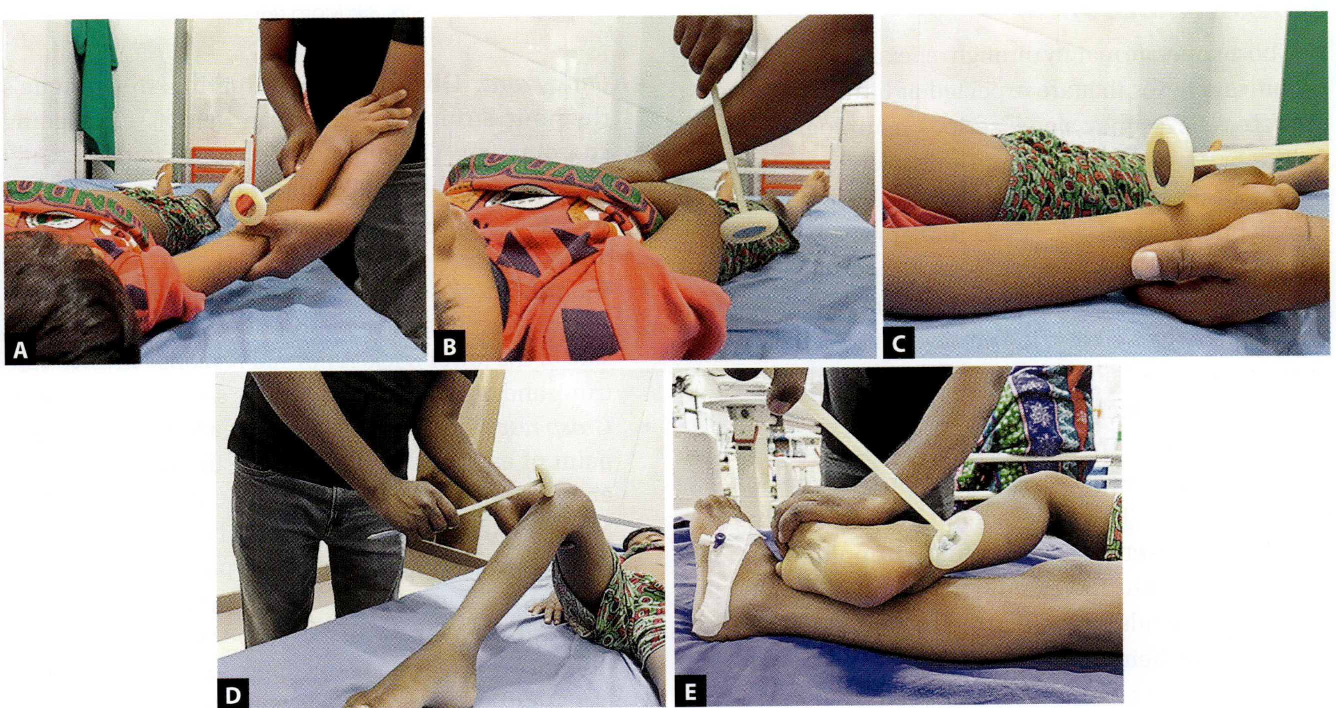

Figs. 30A to E: (A) Biceps reflex; (B) Triceps reflex; (C) Supinator reflex; (D) Knee reflex; and (E) Ankle reflex.

TABLE 8: Deep tendon reflexes and their normal responses.

Reflex	*Spinal level*	*Procedure*	*Normal Response*
Biceps reflex	C5–C6	Tap the biceps tendon in the antecubital fossa	Elbow flexion
Supinator reflex	C5–C6	Tap the brachioradialis tendon near the radial styloid	Forearm flexion or supination
Triceps reflex	C7–C8	Tap the triceps tendon above the olecranon	Elbow extension
Knee reflex	L2–L4	Tap the patellar tendon below the kneecap	Knee extension
Ankle reflex	S1–S2	Tap the Achilles tendon while the foot is slightly dorsiflexed	Plantar flexion of the foot

TABLE 9: Primitive reflexes.

Reflex	*Onset*	*Duration*
Palmer grasp	28 weeks of gestation	2–3 months postnatal
Rooting	32 weeks	1 month postnatal
Moro	28–32 weeks	5–6 months postnatal
Tonic neck	35 weeks	6–7 months postnatal
Parachute	7–8 months postnatal	Remains throughout life

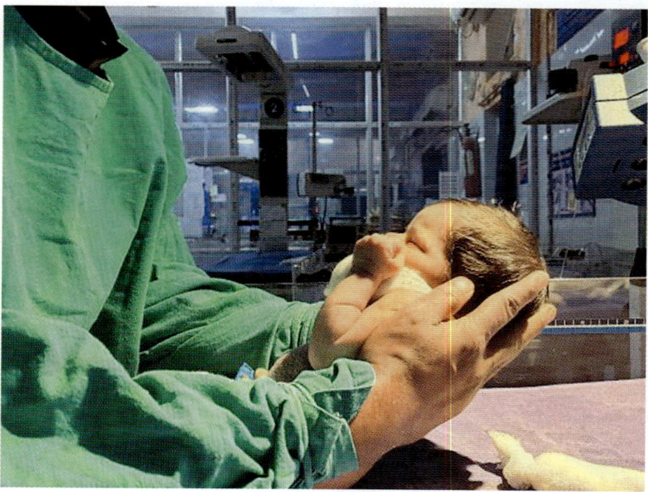

Fig. 31: Moro reflex.

Developmental Reflexes/Primitive Reflexes (TABLE 9)

Newborns operate mainly through reflex actions, exhibiting primitive reflexes that are expected at birth. The absence of these reflexes may signal serious neurological issues. As the brain matures, these primitive reflexes typically diminish, disappearing by around 4–6 months of age. Meanwhile, postural reflexes start to appear, beginning at 3–4 months and completing development by 8 months. These postural reflexes help the infant maintain balance and prepare for walking. If primitive reflexes persist and postural reflexes fail to develop, this may indicate UMN dysfunction in infants.

Persistence or absence outside the normal developmental window suggests neurological impairment.

- *Moro reflex:* The reflex is elicited by holding the infant semi-erect and carefully dropping the head backward onto the examiner's palm. Normally, the infant responds by opening their hands, extending and abducting their arms, then bringing them back in with flexion, often crying. An uneven reaction could signal a clavicle fracture, injury to the brachial plexus, or hemiparesis. Absence of this reflex in a term of infant may indicate generalized CNS suppression **(Fig. 31)**.
- *Suck, root:* Observing or palpating the tongue's rhythmic stripping motion can help assess feeding coordination. The rooting reflex is elicited by gently stroking the infant's cheek near the mouth, causing the baby to open their mouth and turn their head toward the touch.
- *Galant (trunk incurvation):* Support the infant in a ventral suspension position and gently stroke one side of the lower back. A normal response involves the trunk and hips curving toward the side of the stimulus.
- *Grasp response:* Elicited by placing a finger in the open palm of each hand; at 37 weeks, the reflex is strong enough to allow lifting up of the infant from bed. Marked retention of these reflexes beyond 6 months is characteristic of athetoid cerebral palsy **(Fig. 32)**.
- *Asymmetric tonic neck reflex:* This reflex is triggered by turning the infant's head to one side. The expected response is extension of the upper limb on the side the face is turned toward and flexion of the upper limb on the opposite side. A persistent or obligatory tonic neck reflex, where the infant remains fixed in the fencing posture, is always considered abnormal **(Fig. 33)**.

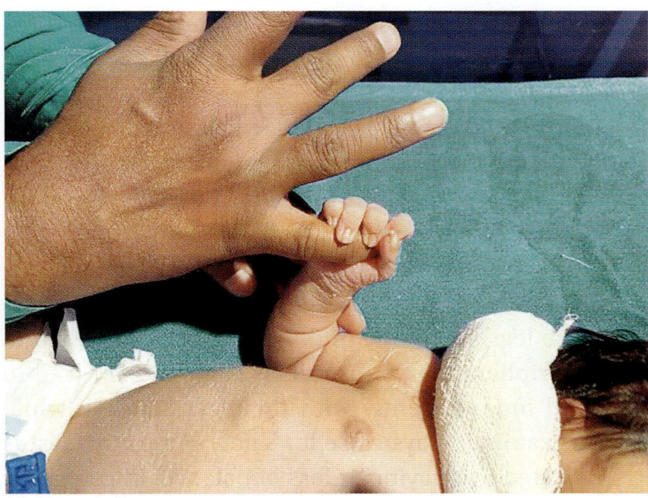

Fig. 32: Grasp response.

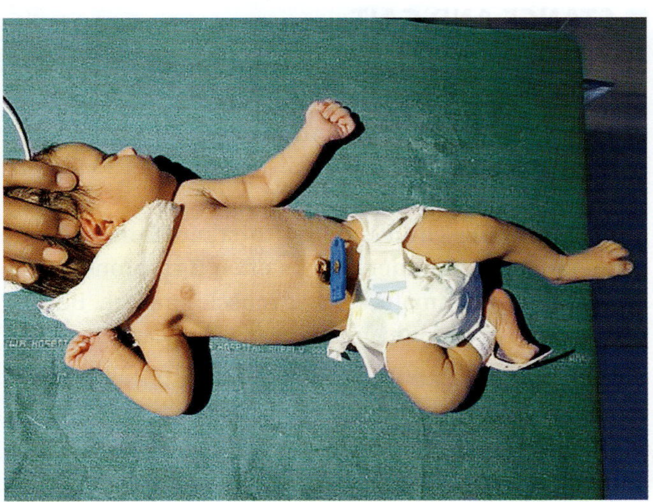

Fig. 33: Asymmetric tonic neck reflex.

Postural Reflexes

- *Landau:* Age of appearance—4–5 months. When held in ventral suspension, the infant demonstrates extension of the head and legs.
- *Parachute reflex:* Hold the child in ventral suspension and suddenly lower him as if he or she were falling. The arms will extend to break the infant's fall. Absent or incomplete response is seen in cerebral palsy.

COORDINATION/CEREBELLAR SIGN

Coordination relies on visual and proprioceptive feedback to execute complex movement patterns and is controlled by the cerebellum. Unlike cortical lesions, cerebellar dysfunction produces ipsilateral rather than contralateral signs. As coordination develops with age, younger children may naturally exhibit some clumsiness. Impairment of the cerebellum disrupts the smooth execution of voluntary movements, leading to ataxia.

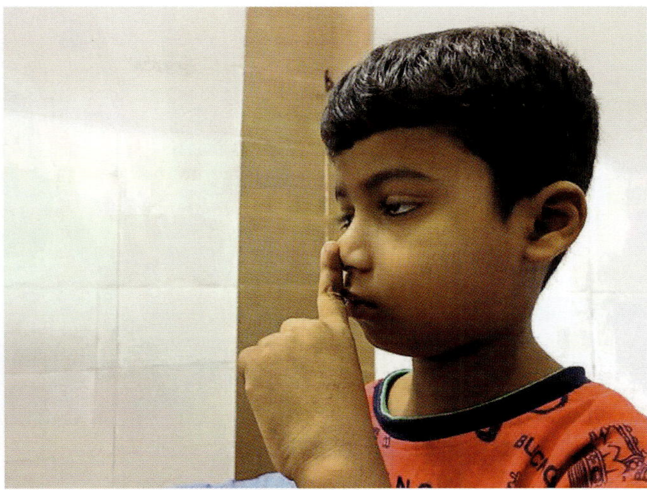

Fig. 34: Finger-nose test.

- *Lesions to the cerebellar vermis:* Result in truncal ataxia, a broad-based gait, or difficulty performing tandem gait assessment.
- *Lesions of the cerebellar hemispheres:* Lead to appendicular ataxia, which becomes evident during tasks such as reaching for objects or performing finger-to-nose and heel-to-shin tests.

Cerebellar disorders often present with hypotonia, preserved muscle strength, and increased fatigability. Speech may be slurred, explosive, and jerky with scanning of syllables. There may be nystagmus and intention tremor.

Of Upper Limbs

Finger–nose test **(Fig. 34)**: This test is done by instructing the child to touch the tip of their nose with their index finger, then reach out to touch the examiner's fingertip. The child should repeat the movement as quickly as possible while the examiner moves their finger to different positions. It is normal for children to do this maneuver repeatedly. But a child with cerebellar affection may have dysmetria or past pointing (errors in judging distance), dyssynergia (irregular, clumsy, uncoordinated motion), and intention tremor (the tremor appears when the child attempts to accurately reach for a target).

Rebound phenomenon: The examiner attempts to extend the patient's elbow while the biceps actively contract against resistance. If the wrist is suddenly released, the

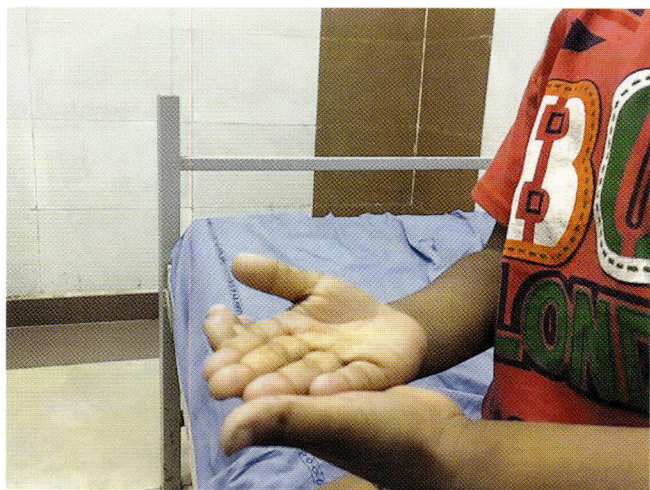

Fig. 35: Dysdiadochokinesia.

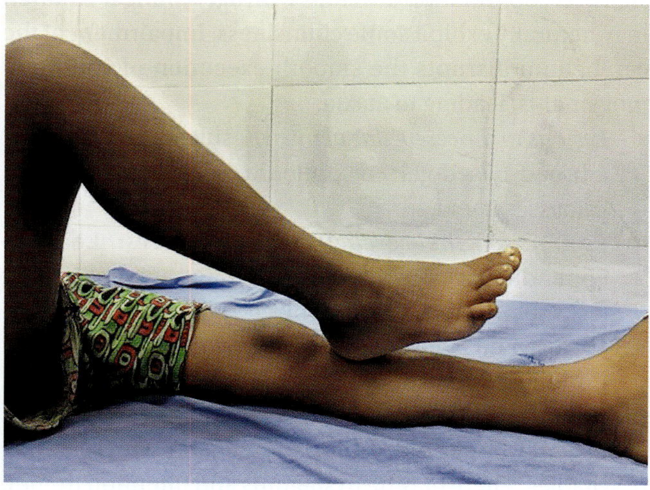

Fig. 36: Heel-shin test.

hand may recoil abruptly and could strike the patient's face.

Dysdiadokokinesia: Instruct the child to rapidly alternate between palm-up and palm-down positions by tapping one hand against the other. Difficulty or inability to perform this movement smoothly is known as dysdiadochokinesia. Swaying or oscillation of the arms held outstretched suggests cerebellar dysfunction **(Fig. 35)**.

For Lower Limbs

Heel–shin test: With the child lying on their back, ask them to slide the heel of one foot down the shin of the other leg repeatedly and rapidly. Observe the accuracy and smoothness of the movement **(Fig. 36)**.

- *Reflexes:* Deep tendon jerks are pendular
- *Gait:* A broad-based, unsteady gait is characteristic of cerebellar ataxia.
  Ask the child to walk heel-to-toe in a straight line, with the toes of the rear foot touching the heel of the front foot at every step. This tandem gait test is useful for identifying subtle balance problems.
- *Romberg's sign:* Although not a cerebellar sign, this test evaluates position sense loss (sensory ataxia) in the legs, often due to dorsal column, spinal cord, or peripheral nerve disorders. The child is asked to stand independently with their eyes closed, while the examiner stays close for safety. A positive test is indicated by swaying or loss of balance. In cerebellar ataxia, instability is present even with the eyes open.

STANCE AND GAIT

Stance refers to how a person stands, while gait describes how they walk. Typically, normal children can stand with their feet close together without swaying. During standing, observe for spinal abnormalities such as kyphosis, scoliosis, or lordosis.

Evaluate the child's ability to stand from a prone position; children under 3 years often turn prone before standing due to immature pelvic muscle strength. Beyond 3 years, if they need this maneuver, it indicates proximal muscle weakness (Gowers sign), wherein the child climbs up his legs to stand due to weakness of the glutei, classically seen in Duchenne's muscular dystrophy.

Evaluate walking and running—by age 5, a normal gait should follow a heel-toe pattern. A toe-heel gait (toe-walking) is often idiopathic but can indicate pyramidal tract dysfunction or pelvic girdle weakness. Subtle gait asymmetries can be detected using Fogs' test, which involves walking on the toes, heels, and the inner and outer edges of the feet.

Gait analysis is most reliable when the child is not self-conscious or aware of being examined. Look for arm swing, pelvic tilt, lurching to one or both sides, length of steps, any asymmetry, and associated movements of the upper limbs. Finally, make him walk in tandem steps and observe.

There are a variety of abnormal gaits **(Table 10)**.

Sensory Examination

The spinal cord contains two main groups of sensory nerve fibers. The posterior column transmits sensory information from the same side of the body, including

TABLE 10: Abnormal gait.

Gait	*Appearance*	*Condition*
Antalgic	The stance phase is briefer than the swing	Musculoskeletal pain
Broad based	Staggering, wide-spread feet	Cerebellar ataxia
Stamping	Wide-based steppage gait	Sensory ataxia
Scissoring	Stiff-legged, drag and cross the midline	Diplegia
Circumduction	Circumduction of the leg, decreased arm swing on the affected side	Hemiplegia
Waddling	Drooping of the hip girdle on the contralateral side	Proximal myopathy
High-stepping	Stepping high to avoid injury to the feet	Lower motor neuron (LMN) foot drop

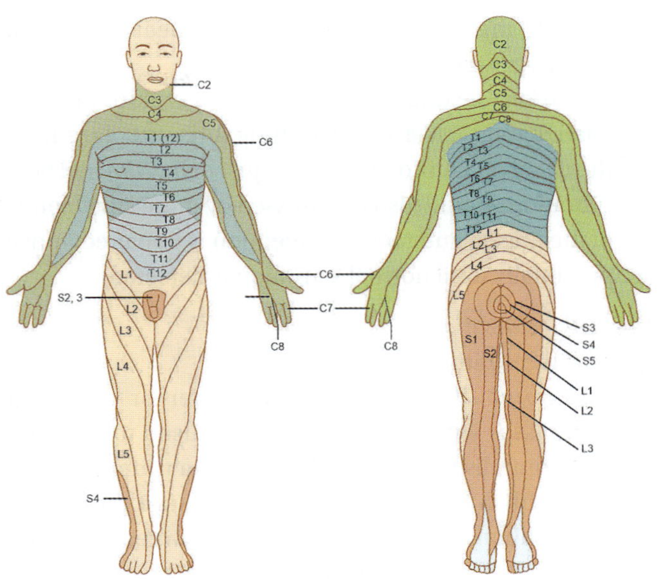

Fig. 37: Sensory dermatome.

stereognosis, proprioception, vibration, and the perception of weight, shape, and size. In contrast, the anterior and lateral columns carry sensory signals for touch, pain, and temperature from the opposite side of the body.

Sensory System Examination

Sensory testing involves assessing touch, pain, temperature, vibration, joint position (proprioception), and cortical sensory processing. These tests require the child to be old enough to cooperate and accurately describe sensations, making sensory examination challenging and often overlooked in young children. Observation can aid in identifying sensory deficits, such as changes in skin color, temperature, or sweating, with the skin appearing cool and dry below the level of injury. A basic assessment can be performed by engaging the child with a toy while gently touching different areas with a cotton swab. Normal infants and children typically respond by crying or withdrawing the affected limb, and isolated sensory disorders are rare in very young children.

- *Sensory level:* Identifying a sensory level is crucial for determining the location of a spinal cord lesion. On examination, the sensory deficit typically appears one to two spinal segments below the actual site of the lesion.
- *For older child:*
    - *Lateral column sensation:*
        - *Touch:* Assess light touch sensation by lightly stroking the skin with a piece of cotton. Ask the child to keep their eyes closed and indicate when they feel the touch. Compare both sides for symmetry.

Remember these important landmarks for dermatomes **(Fig. 37)**:

- C1 gives no supply to the skin.
- C2 The occiput.
- C7 supplies the middle finger.
- T3 in the axilla.
- T10 supplies the umbilicus.
- L3 supplies the knee.
- L5 outer aspect of the tibia
- S1 supplies the little toe.
- S3, 4, 5 around the anus.
    - *Pain:* Assess pain sensation by gently pricking the skin with a fresh pin.
    - *Temperature:* Evaluate the child's response to temperature changes by applying a cooled or heated metal surface. You may also use a cold spray or body warmth as simpler alternatives.

Posterior column sensation:

- *Joint position (proprioception):* Hold the child's big toe by stabilizing the middle segment with one hand and gently gripping the tip from the sides with the other. Move the distal phalanx up and down while explaining the directions to the child. Have the child close their eyes, then repeat the movement several times, pausing at either the up or down position. Ask the child to identify the position of their toe. Repeat the test in various positions.

- *Vibration:* Testing vibration sense in children can be challenging. Use a 128 Hz tuning fork and place it on the distal phalanx of the big toe, just below the nail bed. Vibration should also be assessed over the small joints of the fingers and toes. If perception is impaired, move proximally until normal sensation is detected.

Cortical localization:

Cortical localization includes:

- *Two-point discrimination:* A caliper or a pair of compasses with sharp ends can be used to evaluate two-point discrimination. Begin with a wider distance to establish communication and ensure the child's cooperation. Randomly alternate between touching one or two points, asking the child to distinguish between them. Normal discrimination distances are approximately 2–4 mm on the fingertips, 4–6 mm on the dorsal fingers, 8–12 mm on the palm, and 20–30 mm on the dorsum of the hand.
- *Astereognosis:* (The child is unable to recognize objects of different shapes by touching alone without visual or other sensory input). Use familiar items such as a coin, sharpener, pencil, button, or safety pin. Test each hand separately **(Fig. 38)**.
- *Graphesthesia:* Assess the child's ability to identify letters or numbers drawn on the palm by tactile sensation alone **(Fig. 39)**.

Significant impairments in graphesthesia and stereognosis are commonly associated with contralateral hemispheric lesions, particularly in the parietal lobe.

- *Point localization:* Ability to localize the area touched with eyes closed on the face, arm, hand, leg, and foot. The child is asked to point to the area being touched or tell the area verbally. This is the parietal lobe function.
- *Sensory inattention:* Simultaneous stimulation is performed by pricking two corresponding spots on opposite sides of the body. A patient with a sensory deficit may not perceive the prick on the affected side. In cases of parietal lobe lesions, when both a proximal and distal area (such as the cheek and hand) are touched at the same time, the patient may fail to recognize the distal stimulus due to sensory extinction.

Meningeal Irritation Sign

Meningeal signs are present when the meninges are inflamed from infection or the presence of blood.

Two closely related terms are important in this regard:

- Meningismus is the presence of meningeal signs, found in meningitis, whereas Meningism is the presence of neck stiffness in the absence of meningeal inflammation
- Check for signs of meningeal irritation when appropriate.
- *Neck stiffness:* With the child in a supine position, support the head with one hand and gently attempt to flex the neck. Alternatively, ask a conscious child to bend their neck forward and touch their chin to their chest. Increased resistance or discomfort may indicate meningeal irritation. Neck stiffness is an ominous sign in children suffering from meningitis and meningoencephalitis. However, it may also be

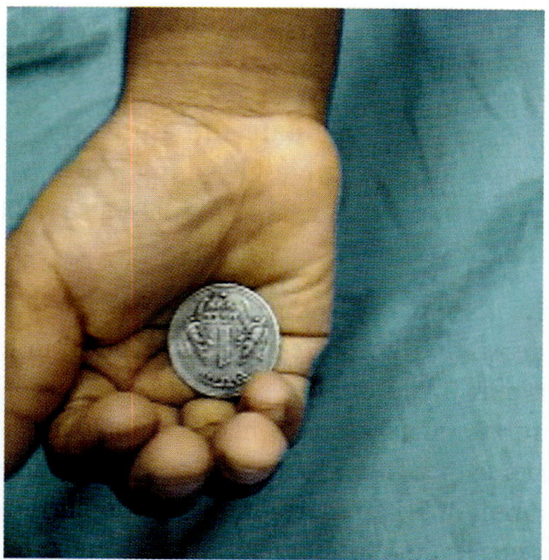

Fig. 38: Stereognosis.

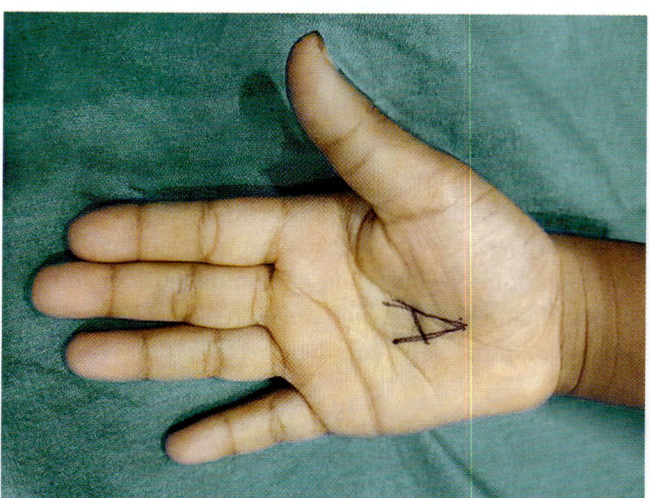

Fig. 39: Graphesthesia.

seen in some children with tonsillitis and cervical lymphadenopathy. It may be absent in the presence of meningitis in young infants and very sick children. To test neck rigidity in a struggling infant, let the head hang off the edge of a table.

Signs Associated with Neck Stiffness

- *Kernig sign:* Position the child supine and flex one hip and knee. While maintaining hip flexion, gently extend the knee. Pain in the posterior thigh and difficulty extending the knee suggests meningeal irritation. Kernig's sign is typically absent if neck stiffness results from local causes rather than meningeal inflammation.
- *Brudzinski sign:* With the child lying supine, support the head with one hand while placing the other hand on the chest to restrict movement. Gently attempt to flex the neck. A positive sign is demonstrated by spontaneous flexion at the hips and knees, pointing toward meningeal inflammation **(Fig. 40)**.

AUTONOMIC FUNCTIONS

The autonomic nervous system regulates involuntary functions by controlling smooth muscles and glands. It consists of central components, including cortical areas, the amygdala, hypothalamic, and brainstem nuclei, as well as peripheral components such as the sympathetic thoracolumbar and parasympathetic craniosacral outflows. These functions operate independently of conscious control.

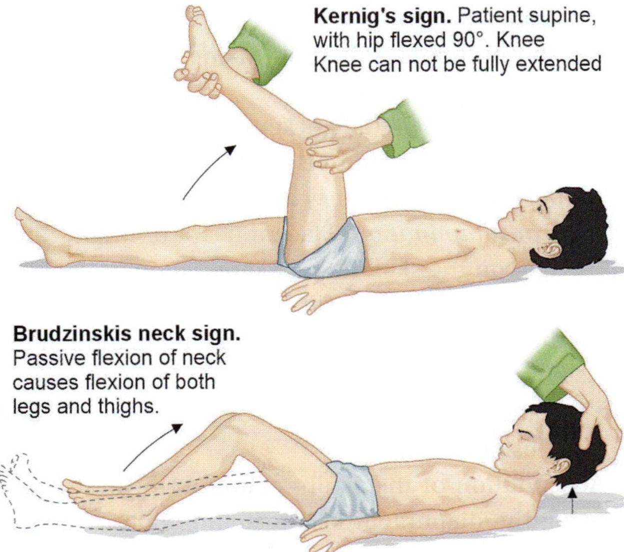

Fig. 40: Kernig and Brudzinski sign.

Symptoms—complain of symptoms related to:

- Orthostatic hypotension—lightheadedness, syncope, and palpitations, which become worse with standing.
- Abnormalities of sweating—excessive or reduced sweating, areas of skin with blanching, etc.
- Dysfunction of the gastrointestinal or genitourinary tracts. Inadequate or absent salivation or lacrimation, alternate diarrhea or constipation, and sphincteric disturbances.

Measure the pulse rate at rest and after six maximal deep breaths. A normal response is a decrease of >15 beats/min, whereas in autonomic dysfunction, the decrease is less than 10 beats per minute. Additionally, in patients with autonomic dysfunction, a drop of >20 mm Hg in systolic blood pressure upon standing from a lying position indicates orthostatic hypotension.

SKULL AND SPINE

The bony framework surrounding the CNS, including the skull and spine, requires close inspection. Look for variations in size, shape, symmetry, swellings, and abnormalities in sutures or fontanelles.

- *Head size:* Head circumference should be measured at every visit for children under 3 years, as it serves as an indicator of brain growth. Then it should be recorded on a suitable growth chart to look for any aberrations. To measure, a plastic nondistensible tape is placed anteriorly over the nasion and supraorbital ridge and posteriorly over the external occipital protuberance surrounding the head **(Fig. 41)**. When a patient presents with an abnormal head circumference, it is

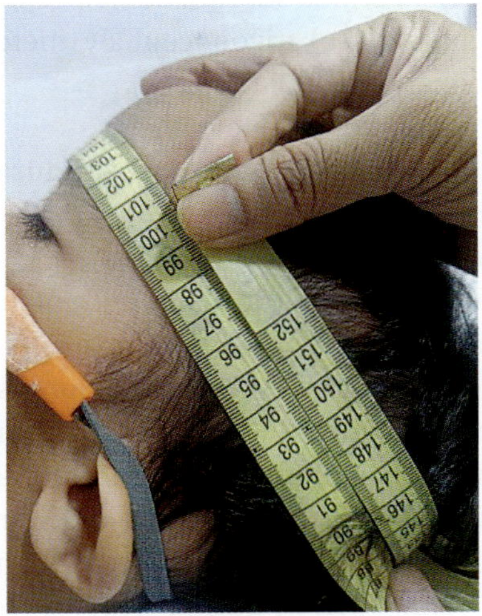

Fig. 41: Occipital frontal circumference (OFC) measurement.

necessary to document the head circumferences of family members, including parents and siblings.

In healthy premature infant's rate of growth of head circumference:

Increases by 0.5 cm per week during the first 2 weeks, 0.75 cm in the third week, and 1.0 cm in the fourth week, continuing at 1 cm weekly until the 40th week

- Head circumference of a term infant: 34–35 cm at birth, thereafter the rate of growth of head circumference:
  - First 3 months @approximately 2 cm/month
  - 3–6 months @1cm/mt
  - 7–12 months @0.5 cm/month
  - 1–3 years @1cm/ 6 months
  - *3–5years @1 cm/year*: The adult head circumference is achieved at around 5–6 years of age.
- *Abnormal size:*
  - *Macrocephaly (large head)*: OFC > 2 SD above the mean for age and sex, most commonly familial or may be a disturbance in growth if there is megalencephaly (enlarged brain, or hydrocephalus
  - *Microcephaly (small head)*: An OFC less than three standard deviations below the mean for age and sex may result from primary reduced brain growth or secondary premature suture closure. It can also be associated with craniosynostosis (premature fusion of cranial sutures).
- *Shape—alteration occurs in:*
  - *Plagiocephaly:* While some skull flattening is normal in infants, it is more pronounced in hypotonic cases.
  - *Craniosynostosis*—cranial sutures fuse prematurely, may be in the form of brachycephaly (premature closure of coronal suture), dolichocephaly (closure of sagittal suture), trigonocephaly (metopic suture), oxycephaly (multiple sutures).
  - *Hydrocephalus*—frontal bulging
  - *Box-shaped heart*—chronic subdural effusion, rickets.
- *Fontanels:*
  - Two fontanelles are normally present in an infant at the time of birth.
    1. *Anterior fontanel:* A soft, diamond-shaped area found where the frontal and parietal bones meet, usually measuring around 2 × 2 cm. It generally closes between 9 and 18 months and is most accurately evaluated when the infant is calm, such as during sleep or feeding in an upright position.

       Normal anterior fontanel: The fontanel is normally slightly depressed and pulsatile. A bulging fontanel may signal increased intracranial pressure (ICP). If the anterior fontanelle is very small or absent at birth, conditions such as craniosynostosis and microcephaly should be considered. Several conditions in infants, including hypothyroidism, rickets, achondroplasia, and Zellweger syndrome, present with large and late-closing fontanels. A depressed fontanel may indicate dehydration, while a full, bulging fontanel is a sign of increased intracranial pressure.
    2. *Posterior fontanel*: Triangular in shape, this fontanel is located at the junction of the parietal and occipital bones and typically closes between 6 and 8 weeks. It is usually small enough to admit the tip of a finger or may already be closed at birth. If it remains open beyond the expected time frame, it may indicate hydrocephalus or congenital hypothyroidism.
- *Shiny skin with prominent, distended veins*—in hydrocephalus, increased intracranial pressure, sinovenous thrombosis.
- *Palpation of a newborn's skull*-may reveal.
  - Overriding sutures (molding)—caused by the pressure applied to the skull as it passes through the pelvis during birth.
  - Premature fusion of cranial sutures leading to restricted skull growth (craniosynostosis)
  - Cranial defects.
  - Thinning and softening of the parietal bones, known as craniotabes.
  - Macewen's sign (a "cracked pot" sound upon skull percussion) should be assessed. It is considered normal in early infancy due to open sutures.
  - *Transillumination:* Place a beam of bright torch light on the skull in a darkened room to look for a halo around the light. if there is hydrocephalus, there will be generalized transillumination in the entire skull.
  - Transillumination may also be positive in subdural effusion.
- Auscultation of the skull—cranial bruit best heard using the diaphragm of the stethoscope. This may appear at the anterior of fontanel, temporal areas, or in the orbital regions.

- Soft, symmetrical bruits can sometimes be heard in healthy children under 4 years old and during fever.
- A loud bruit may indicate severe anemia, raised intracranial pressure, or vein of Galen malformation.
- Spine—to look for any tuft of hair or localized swelling over the spine indicating underlying spina bifida, any sinus, gibbus, kyphosis, or scoliosis. Check for surgical scars on the spine, which may indicate prior to meningomyelocele repair, or on the scalp, which may suggest ventriculoperitoneal shunt placement.

PART B: LOCALIZATION IN NEUROLOGY

INTRODUCTION

"Localization" in neurology relates to the site of lesion in the neuroaxis that possibly explains the presenting clinical features in the child. To understand, we should revise our basic anatomy and physiology knowledge regarding the nervous system.

BASIC ANATOMY (FIG. 42)

The Nervous system can be divided into the central nervous system (brain and spinal cord) and the peripheral nervous system (anterior horn cells, peripheral nerve, neuromuscular junction, and muscle).

The basic structure of the nervous system is the neuron, which comprises of a cell body and an axon that terminates at a synapse. The brain comprises of two cerebral hemispheres—right and left, connected by the corpus callosum, the brainstem, and the cerebellum. Each cerebral hemisphere consists of four lobes—frontal, parietal, temporal, and occipital. The cortical functions of various lobes are listed in **Table 11**.

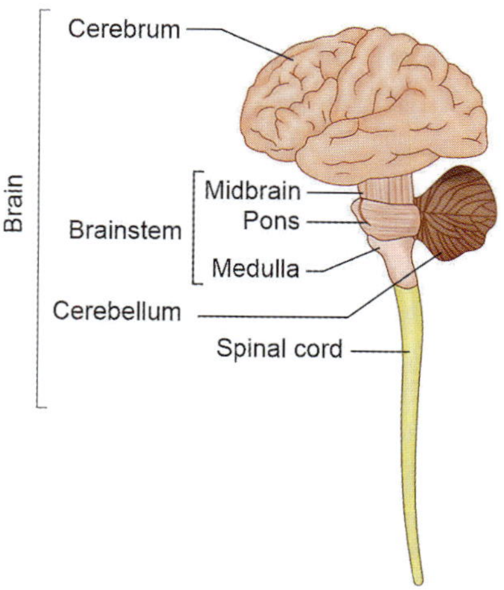

Fig. 42: Basic structures of the central nervous system.

TABLE 11: Functions of lobes of cerebrum.

Lobes	*Functions*
Frontal lobe	Motor functions, personality, emotions, planning, executive functions, and language
Parietal lobe	Sensory input and calculations
Temporal lobe	Auditory reception, memory, and language comprehension
Occipital lobe	Visual reception and interpretation

The left and right hemispheres, though structurally the same, functionally, they are of different attributes. The left hemisphere is the dominant hemisphere in the majority of right and also left-handed persons. It helps in cognition, logic, analytical, language, and communication skills, etc. The right hemisphere is credited with artistic characteristics, like painting, music, dance, creativity, etc.

The brainstem consists of the midbrain, pons, and medulla oblongata. It contains the nuclei of cranial nerves and all the sensory and motor pathways. The cerebellum, often referred to as the small brain, lies below the cerebral hemispheres and posterior to the brainstem. It is responsible for coordination, motor learning, posture, and steady gait.

The brain is wrapped by three membranes: The outermost dura mater, the middle arachnoid, and the innermost pia mater. The subarachnoid space between the arachnoid and pia is filled with cerebrospinal fluid (CSF).

The spinal cord contains afferent and efferent nerve fibers, arranged in functionally separate bundles, and is responsible for motor responses and sensory information for pain, touch, temperature, and proprioception.

Peripheral nerves are made up of large, myelinated axons and smaller, slower unmyelinated axons. The sensory cell bodies of peripheral nerves are situated in the dorsal root ganglia, while the motor cell bodies are located in the anterior horn cells of the spinal cord.

STEPWISE APPROACH FOR LOCALIZATION OF THE LESION

- *Step 1:* Whether the lesion in the upper motor neuron (UMN) or in the lower motor neuron (LMN)?
- *Step 2:* If the lesion is in the UMN, is it in the brain or spinal cord?
  - If the lesion is in the brain, is it in the cerebral cortex, the subcortex, the cerebellum, or in the brainstem.
  - If the lesion is in the spinal cord, find out the spinal level at which this lesion is occurring.
- *Step 3:* If the lesion is in the LMN, where is it exactly located—in anterior horn cells, nerve, neuromuscular junctions, or muscles?

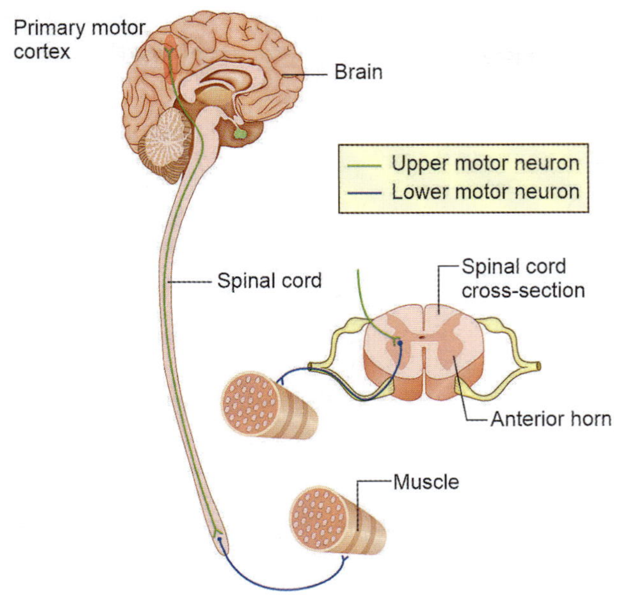

Fig. 43: Upper and lower motor neurons.

Step 1: Whether the Lesion in the Upper Motor Neuron or in the Lower Motor Neuron (Fig. 43)?

We know that there are two basic patterns of weakness—the upper motor and the lower motor type.

Upper motor neuron: A UMN consists of the neural pathways: (1) Above the motor nuclei of the cranial nerves; and (2) above the anterior horn cell in the spinal cord. UMNs travel mainly in the corticospinal tract (pyramidal system); additionally, there are corticobulbar, tectospinal, rubrospinal, vestibulospinal, and reticulospinal tracts, which form the extrapyramidal system, responsible for fine-tuning and modulation of motor activity.

- *UMN weakness lesions* are recognized by spasticity, exaggerated deep tendon reflexes, and extensor plantar response. UMN lesions produce weakness through decreased activation of the LMNs. Distal muscle groups are affected more severely than proximal ones. Axial movements are usually spared unless the lesion is severe and affects bilaterally.
  Spasticity may not be present in some of the UMN lesions in the acute phase (such as spinal shock stage in case of spinal trauma and in acute transverse myelitis). The UMN features appear during the recovery phase from spinal shock.

Lower motor neuron: The LMN constitutes the anterior horn cell of the spinal cord and cranial nerve nuclei in the brainstem. Their axons extend to skeletal muscles via peripheral nerves. They are the final pathway for transmitting signals from the spinal cord and brainstem to muscles.

- *LMN weakness:* LMN lesions are featured by significant weakness, hypotonia, decreased reflexes, and flexor plantar responses. This pattern results from disorders of brainstem motor nuclei and the anterior horn of the spinal cord, or from dysfunction of peripheral nerves, neuromuscular junction, or muscle
  The basic differences are tabulated below **(Table 12)**.

TABLE 12: Differences in upper and lower motor neuron paralysis.

Features	*UMN paralysis*	*LMN paralysis*
Power	Reduced	Markedly reduced
Weakness	Diffuse, symmetric	Patchy, asymmetric
Muscle tone	Spasticity	Hypotonia
Muscle wasting	Minimal or absent	Significant
DTR	Brisk with clonus	Sluggish or absent
Planters	Extensor	Flexor or absent
Convulsion/ involuntary movements	May occur	Fasciculation may occur

(DTR: deep tendon reflexes; LMN: lower motor neuron; UMN: upper motor neuron)

Step 2: Localization in the Upper Motor Neuron Lesion

In a child presenting with features of a UMN lesion, the next step is to decide whether the lesion is in the brain or in the spinal cord.

Features that can help to clinch a UMN lesion above the spinal cord are: Loss of consciousness, derangement in higher mental functions, seizures, hemiparesis, cranial nerve involvement, ataxia, etc., further localization depends on the characteristic clinical features.

Cerebral Cortex ***(Fig. 44)***

Cortical lesions cause contralateral hemiparesis (upper limb > lower limb) with contralateral facial weakness. Both impaired consciousness and seizures are common. There is a loss of cortical sensation. There can be aphasia (if the dominant hemisphere is affected) and/or the presence of a homonymous hemianopia.

It can lead to various neurological deficits, depending on which area of the cortex is affected (frontal, parietal, temporal, occipital).

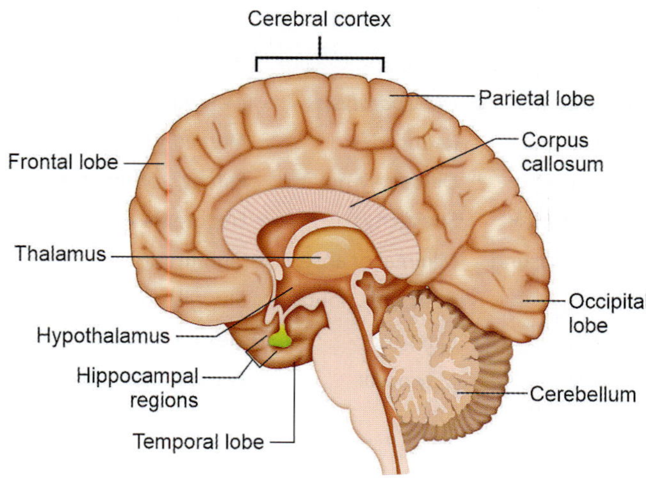

Fig. 44: Structures of the cerebral cortex.

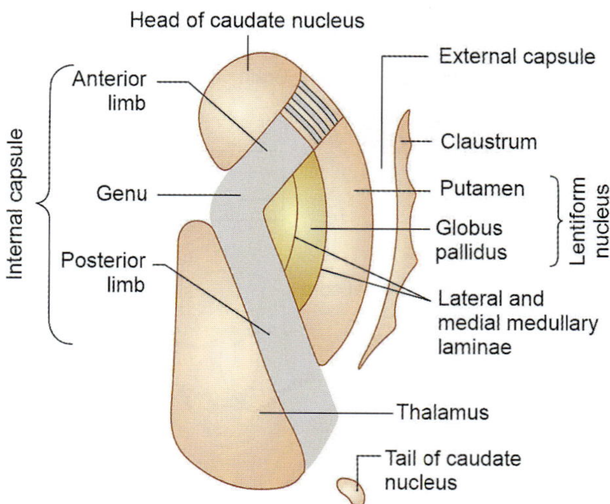

Fig. 45: Subcortical structures- basal ganglia, internal capsule, and thalamus.

- *Frontal lobe lesions:* Affect motor functions, personality, planning, and executive functions. Lesion leads to Weakness or paralysis of the contralateral side (due to motor cortex involvement). There may be cognitive dysfunction in the form of personality changes, poor judgment, and, in some cases, disinhibition.
- *Parietal lobe lesion:* Affects sensory functions (touch, temperature, proprioception) on the contralateral side of the body. There will be Numbness or reduced ability to feel stimuli. The patient may feel difficulties in recognizing objects, drawing, or understanding spatial relationships (agnosia, apraxia).
- *Temporal lobe lesions:* Affect auditory processing and memory. A lesion leads to Hearing loss, hallucinations, and short-term memory loss.
- *Occipital lobe lesions:* Affect vision. There will be a visual field defect—hemianopia (loss of vision in one half of the visual field), or cortical blindness if the occipital cortex is completely damaged.

Subcortical Structures

- *Corona radiata:* contralateral hemiparesis, findings are the same as cortical lesion, except impaired consciousness and seizure are less common.
  Other subcortical structures are the basal ganglia, the internal capsule, and the thalamus **(Fig. 45)**.
- *Basal Ganglia (e.g., putamen, caudate nucleus, and globus pallidus):* Involved in motor control. A basal ganglia lesion leads to extrapyramidal symptoms in the form of rigidity, bradykinesia, and involuntary movement (chorea).
- *Thalamus:* Relay station for sensory information. Lesion leads to contralateral numbness or sensory disturbances, including pain.
- *Internal capsule*: Contralateral dense hemiplegia with contralateral facial weakness. The arm and leg are affected equally. There may be an associated hemisensory deficit.

Cerebellum

Involved in coordination and balance. Cerebellar lesion leads to ataxia, nystagmus, dysmetria, intention tremors, etc.

Brainstem-midbrain, Pons, and Medulla Oblongata

Control vital functions (e.g., breathing, heart rate, swallowing), and house pathways for motor and sensory functions. There are LMN disturbances on the level of the lesion and UMN signs below the lesion.

- *Cranial nerve deficits:* Involvement of the third and fourth cranial nerves suggests midbrain involvement, that of the sixth and seventh cranial nerves suggests lesion in the pons; and involvement of the 9th to 12th cranial nerves is characteristic of involvement of the medulla.
- *Crossed findings:* Ipsilateral cranial nerve findings combined with contralateral body findings (e.g., hemiparesis).
- *Locked-in syndrome:* Damage to the pons may lead to paralysis of all voluntary muscles except for eye movement.

Motor System

- *Pyramidal system (corticospinal tract and corticobulbar tract):* The corticospinal tract mediates the voluntary skilled motor activity. The fibers of the corticospinal pathway arise mainly from the primary motor cortex. After passing through the corona radiata, internal capsule, midbrain, and pons, it decussates at the pyramid of medulla (90% of fibers) and forms the lateral corticospinal tract. The other 10% of the fibers that do not decussate descend in the spinal cord as the anterior (ventral) corticospinal tract **(Fig. 46)**.
    - *Lesions of the pyramidal system* result in spasticity. Spasticity is increased muscle tone that is velocity-dependent. Spasticity generally involves the flexor muscle group of the upper limb and the extensor of the lower limb more.

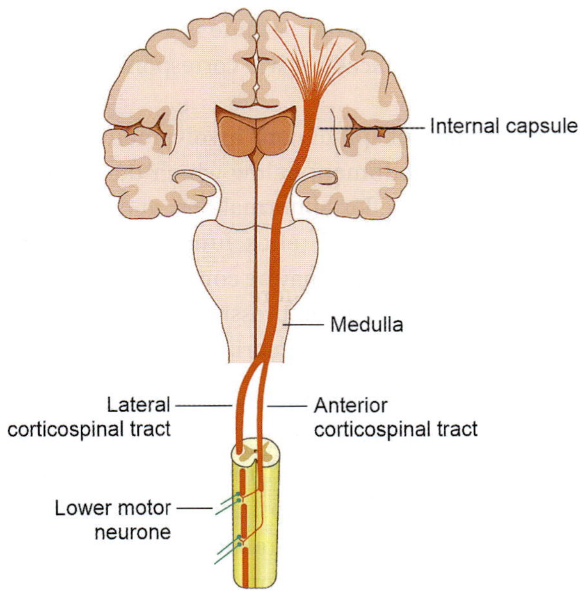

Fig. 46: Corticospinal tract.

Corticobulbar tract—controls voluntary movements of the face, head, and neck by connecting the cerebral cortex to the cranial nerve nuclei in the brainstem. It provides bilateral innervation to most of the cranial nerve motor nuclei except VII (lower face) and XII, which receive contralateral input. So, a unilateral lesion causes mild weakness except for CN VII (contralateral lower face) and CN XII (tongue deviation to the weak side). Bilateral lesion (pseudobulbar palsy) causes severe dysarthria, dysphagia, and emotional lability.

- *Separate portion - pyramidal and extra pyramidal system:* The extrapyramidal system is involved in the control of involuntary and automatic movements. It actually modulates the fine-tuning. It comprises of rubrospinal tract (modifies limb movements), reticulospinal tract (controls posture and locomotion), vestibulospinal tract (maintains balance and head position), tectospinal tract (coordinates head and eye movements), and olivospinal tract (facilitates muscle tone).
- *Lesions of the extrapyramidal tract* result in rigidity. Rigidity involves both agonist and antagonist, and both flexor and extensor muscles. This resistance is felt from the start to the end, and it will not vary with the speed of movement. This is known as lead pipe rigidity. If tremors are superimposed on lead pipe rigidity, that is known as cogwheel rigidity. This often involves neck muscles, trunk muscles, and proximal limb muscles **(Flowchart 1)**.

Flowchart 1: Salient features of the pyramidal and extrapyramidal system.

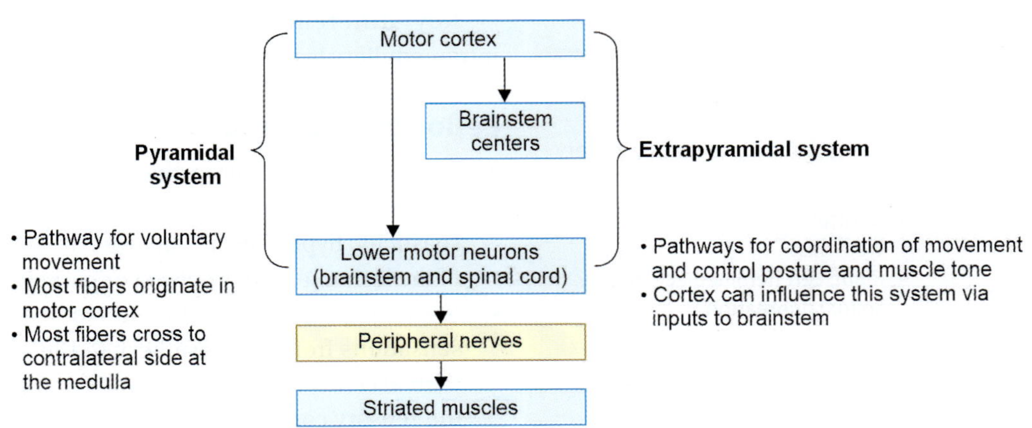

Meninges

- Infections or tumors affecting the meninges (e.g., meningitis and meningioma) can result in:
    - *Headache:* Often due to inflammation or pressure on the meninges.
    - *Nuchal rigidity:* Stiff neck, a classic sign of meningitis.
    - *Cranial nerve palsies:* Due to compression or inflammation affecting cranial nerves.

Vascular Lesions

- *Stroke (Ischemic or Hemorrhagic):* The brain is supplied by branches of the internal carotid—anterior and middle cerebral artery (anterior circulation) and vertebral arteries (posterior circulation) **(Fig. 47)**. Depending on the region of the brain involved, it can cause specific symptoms **(Table 13)**. A stroke can affect areas like the motor cortex (leading to hemiparesis), the thalamus (leading to sensory loss), or the cerebellum (leading to ataxia).

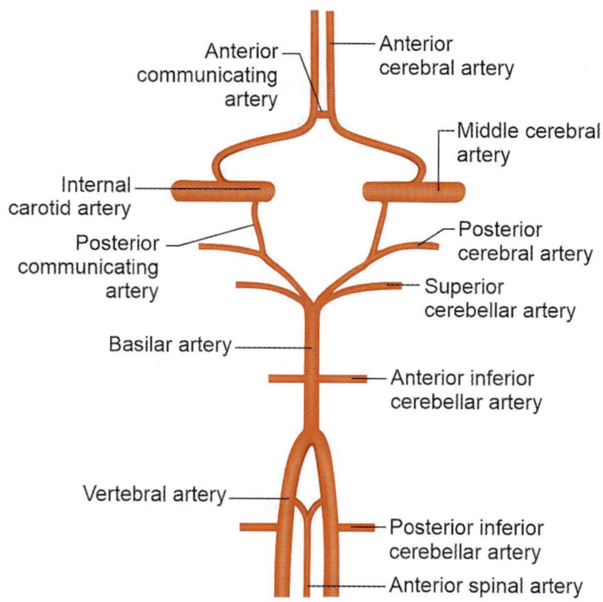

Fig. 47: Circle of Willis—arterial circulation of the brain.

TABLE 13: Features of intracerebral arterial occlusion

Cerebral artery	*Clinical features*
Anterior cerebral artery	Contralateral leg weakness, sensory loss
Middle cerebral artery	• Contralateral face, arm > leg weakness • *Right:* Left hemineglect, apathy, spatial orientation • *Left:* Aphasia
Posterior cerebral artery	Ataxia, vertigo, sensory loss, and cortical blindness

Spinal Cord

The spinal cord has 31 spinal segments: 8 cervical, 12 thoracic, five lumbar, five sacral, and one coccygeal.

The spinal cord ends at the lower border of the first lumbar vertebra. In cases of newborns, it ends at the lower border of L3, but meningeal coverings are carried as far as the second sacral vertebra **(Fig. 48)**. The spinal segments do not correspond numerically with overlying vertebrae, as shown in **Table 14**.

Table 14 highlights the corresponding vertebral and spinal cord levels. Likewise, if there is a lesion at the T10 spinal cord level, clinically, it will correspond to the T7–T8 vertebral level.

The hallmark of spinal cord involvement is a "level" on the chest or abdomen, below which the patient has sensory, motor, or reflex abnormalities; and above which the sensory, motor, and reflex functions are normal. Lesions of the spinal cord may be compressive (secondary to tumor, trauma) or noncompressive (transverse myelitis, etc.). Key differences are summarized in **Table 15**.

Compression of the spinal cord could be extrinsic compression or intrinsic.

- *Extrinsic compression* will result in radicular pain, asymmetric Weakness, ipsilateral hemiplegia with involvement of the ipsilateral dorsal column with loss of joint position and vibration.
- *An intrinsic cord lesion* will result in dissociative pain loss, anterior horn cell involvement, and bladder involvement, considering the proximity of these tracts near the central canal of the spinal cord.

Key differences between extramedullary and intramedullary lesions are given in **Table 16**.

Lesion in Motor and Sensory Pathways

- *Motor pathways:* The corticospinal tract is responsible for voluntary motor control. *Lesions* in the UMN lead to spasticity, hyperreflexia, and weakness below the level of the lesion (e.g., hemiplegia or paraplegia).
- *Sensory pathways:* The sensory system relays sensations from the periphery to the spinal cord and then ascends up to the thalamus and finally relays to the sensory cortex. There are two major sensory tracts:

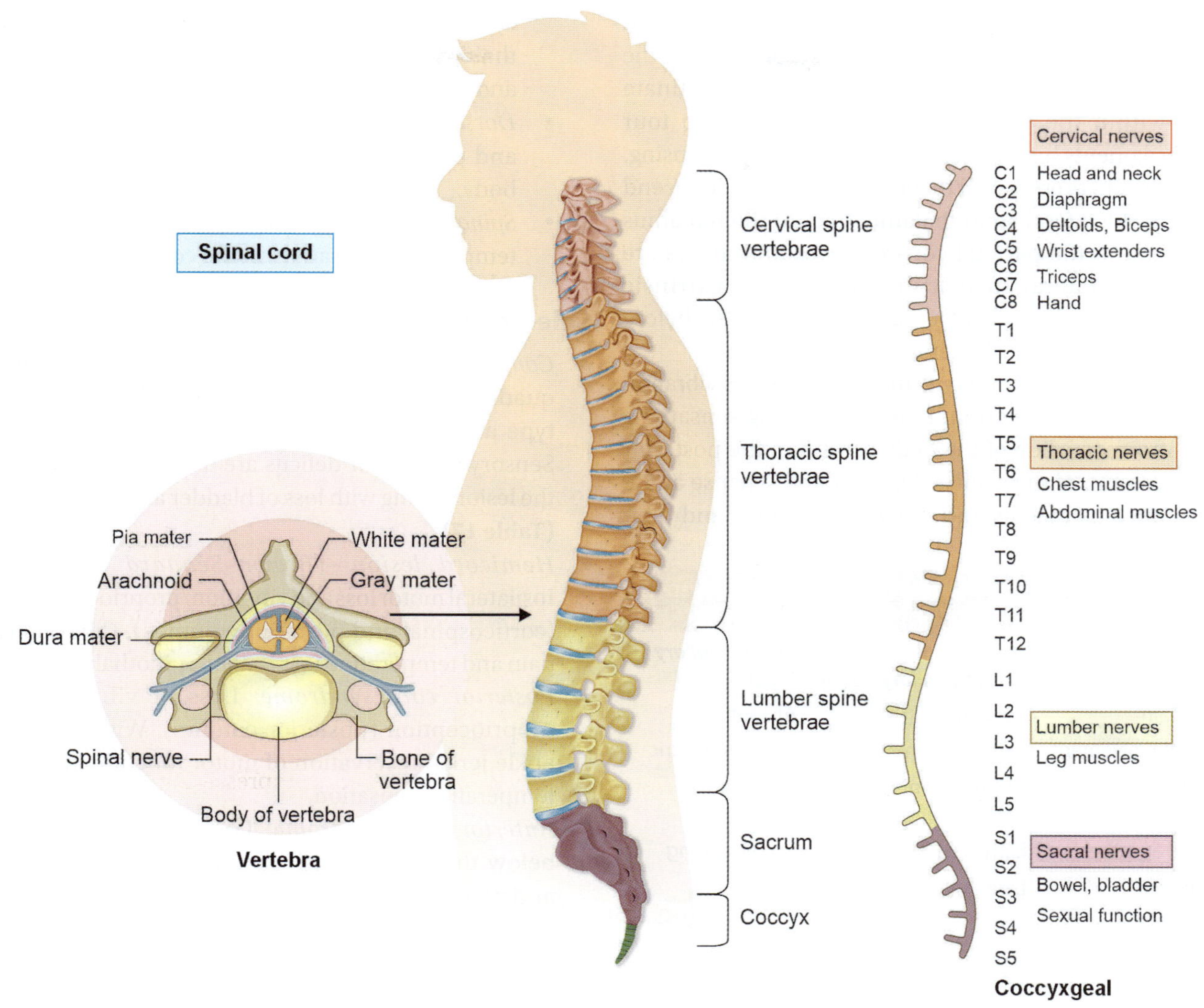

Fig. 48: Basic structures of the spinal cord.

TABLE 14: Relationship of the vertebral body and the corresponding spinal segments.

Vertebral body	*Spinal segment*
Cervical	Add 1
First six dorsal	Add 2
Seventh to ninth dorsal	Add 3
10th dorsal	L1–L2
11th dorsal	L3–L4
12th dorsal	L5 and sacral segments

TABLE 15: Differences between compressive and noncompressive myelopathy.

Feature	*Compressive*	*Noncompressive*
Onset	Gradual	Maybe acute
Symmetry	Asymmetrical	Symmetrical
Bony deformity and tenderness	Present	Absent
Root pain	Present	Absent
Girdle-like sensation	Present	Absent
Bladder and bowel	Early	Late

- *Lateral spinothalamic tract*—that carries pain and temperature; fibers conveying sensation enter the spinal cord via the posterior root and terminate within the posterior horns within two to four segments higher on the same side. After synapsing, the fibers cross over to the opposite side and ascend in the lateral spinothalamic tract to the thalamus and to the parietal cortex. Lower limb fibers are most lateral in distribution. Hence, extrinsic compression will affect sacral sensory fibers before affecting cervical fibers.
- *Posterior spinothalamic tract*—that carries vibration and proprioception. Fibers conveying sensations from one side of the body ascend in the posterior column of the same side, enter and synapse at the nucleus gracilis and nucleus cuneatus, and then cross over to the opposite side and terminate in the thalamus. The lower limb fibers are most medial, and the upper limb fibers are most lateral **(Fig. 49)**.
- *Dorsal column lesion:* Results in loss of vibration and proprioception on the ipsilateral side of the body.
- *Spinothalamic tract lesion:* Leads to loss of pain and temperature sensation on the contralateral side.

TABLE 16: Differences between intra- and extramedullary spinal cord lesions.

Features	*Extramedullary lesion*	*Intramedullary lesion*
Root pain	Present	Absent
Motor involvement	Early, asymmetric	Late, symmetric
Sensation	All are diminished	Dissociative sensory loss
Saddle anesthesia	Early	Sacral sparing
Sphincter involvement	Late	Early
Trophic changes	Absent	Common

Selected Pattern in Spinal Cord Lesion

- *Complete spinal cord lesion:* Can lead to paraplegia or quadriplegia depending on the level of injury (LMN type at the level and UMN type below the lesion). Sensory and motor deficits are usually bilateral below the lesion. along with loss of bladder and bowel control **(Table 17)**.
- *Hemicord lesion—(Brown-Séquard syndrome)*: Ipsilateral motor loss and vibration/proprioception loss (corticospinal and posterior columns). Contralateral pain and temperature loss (lateral spinothalamic tract).
- *Posterior cord syndrome:* Loss of vibration and proprioception (posterior column). With preserved ankle jerk. Preservation of motor function and pain/temperature sensation.
- *Anterior cord syndrome:* Loss of motor function below the lesion (corticospinal tract). Loss of pain and temperature sensation (spinothalamic tract). Preserved vibration and proprioception (posterior column).

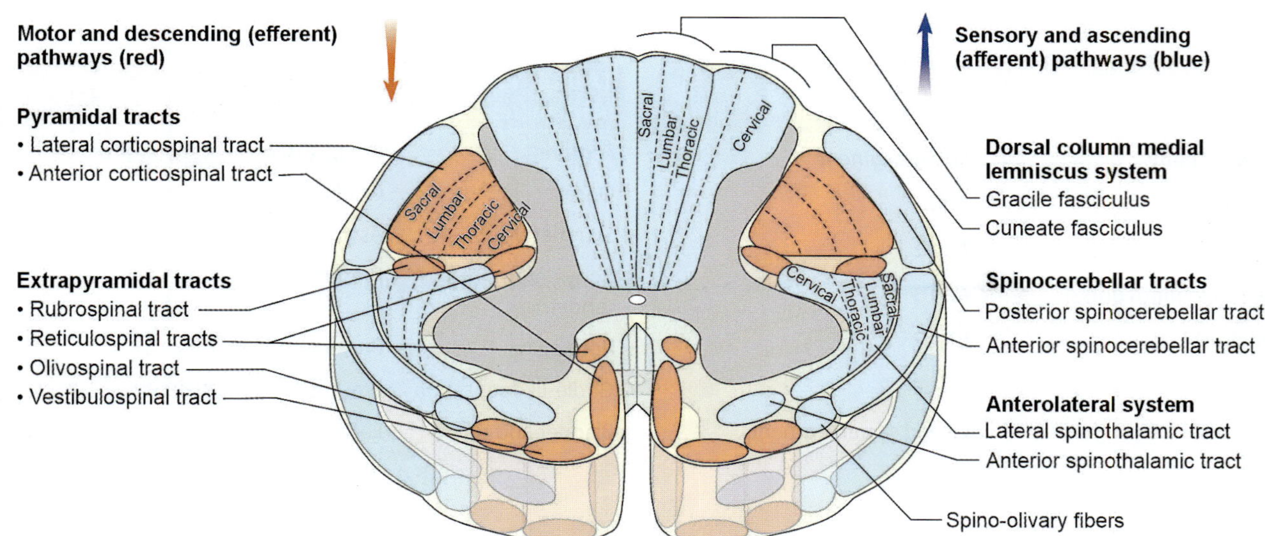

Fig. 49: Representation of motor and sensory pathways in the spinal cord.

TABLE 17: Pattern of injury in complete spinal cord lesion.

Features	*Cervical*	*Thoracic*	*Lumbar*	*Sacral*
Weakness	Quadriplegia	Paraplegia	Weakness in lower limbs, flaccid > spastic	Absent
Sensory loss	Present, below the lesion	Present, below the lesion	Saddle anesthesia	Saddle anesthesia
Reflexes	Hyperreflexia below the lesion	Hyperreflexia and spasticity in the lower limbs	Loss of reflexes (areflexia) in the lower limbs	Present
Bladder/bowel dysfunction	Absent	Present (depending on the level of lesion)	Common	Common
Special features	Respiratory compromise if high cervical levels (C3–C5) involvement	Autonomic symptoms, such as dysregulated sweating and hypotension	Nothing specific	Sexual dysfunction
Common causes	Trauma, tumor, syringomyelia, and multiple sclerosis	Trauma, transverse myelitis, or epidural abscess	Disc herniation, tumors, or vascular lesions	Cauda equina or conus medullaris syndrome

- *Central cord syndrome:* Weakness is greater in the upper limbs than in the lower limbs. Commonly caused by hyperextension injuries or syringomyelia.
- *Cauda equina syndrome:* Peripheral nerve root involvement leads to LMN signs with radicular pain and later onset of bowel/bladder issues.
- *Conus medullaris syndrome:* Central spinal cord involvement leads to mixed UMN and LMN signs with early bowel/bladder dysfunction and symmetric presentation.

Functional Localization Summary of Upper Motor Neuron Lesion

- *Motor deficits:* Suggest a lesion in the motor cortex, basal ganglia, cerebellum, or descending motor pathways (corticospinal tract).
- *Sensory deficits:* Point to damage in the sensory pathways, whether cortical, thalamic, or spinal.
- *Cognitive deficits:* Often indicate frontal or temporal lobe dysfunction.
- *Visual disturbances:* Can indicate occipital lobe, optic nerve, or brainstem involvement.
- *Cranial nerve signs:* Suggest a lesion in the brainstem or localized to the specific cranial nerve pathway.
- *Ataxia:* Localizes to the cerebellum but can also involve proprioceptive pathways.

At a Glance

Clinical features in different levels of injury of the central nervous system **(Table 18)**.

Step 3: Localization in Lower Motor Neuron Lesion

Lower motor neurons extend from the anterior horn cells in the spinal cord (or brainstem nuclei for cranial nerves) to the skeletal muscles they innervate **(Fig. 50)**. LMN lesions are characterized by the following:

- *Muscle weakness:* Flaccid weakness in the affected muscle group.
- *Atrophy:* Wasting of muscles due to denervation.
- *Fasciculations:* Visible twitching of muscle fibers due to spontaneous discharge of motor units.
- *Hypotonia:* Reduced muscle tone.
- *Hyporeflexia or areflexia:* Decreased or absent reflexes in affected regions.

Disease Prototype

- Anterior horn cell involvement (e.g., spinal muscular atrophy) is associated with wasting, fasciculation, and hyporeflexia. There is no sensory loss.
- *Root disease (radiculopathy):* Root pain is the clue; it occurs in the particular dermatome involved and may radiate to the limbs. The pain can be

TABLE 18: Clinical features in different levels of injury of the CNS.

Site	*Motor symptom*	*Characteristics*	*Associated symptom*	*Etiology*
Cortical/subcortical	Hemiplegia, diplegia, quadriplegia	Distal > proximal weakness—deficits rarely complete	Seizures, Cortical sensory loss, aphasia/apraxia, pseudobulbar palsy	• Mono/hemiplegia—stroke, granulomas—demyelination Encephalitis • Quad/diplegia—HIE, PVL, and leukodystrophies
Internal capsule	Hemiplegia	Complete deficits involving the upper and lower limbs	Hemisensory deficits, Hemianopia, Dystonia	Stroke, TBM, Encephalitis
Brainstem	Hemiplegia/Quadriplegia	Complete deficits	Ipsilateral CN deficits, Ipsilateral ataxia	Glioma, Encephalitis, Leigh's disease
Spinal cord	Paraplegia/quadriplegia/hemiplegia	Complete deficits–severe spasticity–LMN signs at the level of the lesion; UMN signs below the lesion	Bladder/Bowel involved (earlier in intramedullary lesion)–sensory level -ipsilateral position/vibration loss, contralateral pain/temperature loss	Myelitis, trauma, meningomyelocele, neoplasm

(CNS: central nervous system; HIE: hypoxic-ischemic encephalopathy; LMN: lower motor neuron; UMN: upper motor neuron; PVL: periventricular leukomalacia; TBM: tuberculous meningitis)

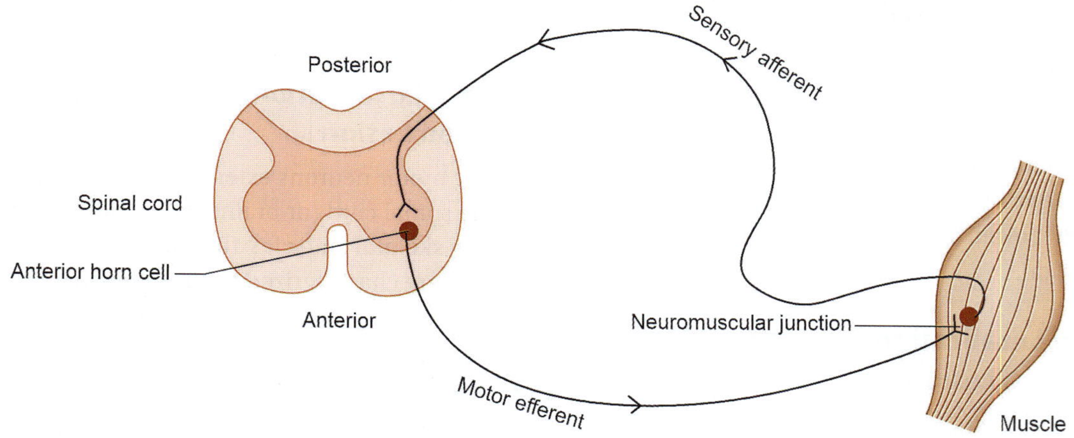

Fig. 50: Structures of the lower motor neuron.

provoked by particular movements or positions (such as a straight leg raise). There are associated sensory symptoms in the form of hyperesthesia, tingling, and numbness. Neurological findings are usually asymmetric and involve muscle atrophy, weakness, loss of deep tendon reflexes, and sensory loss only in the concerned dermatomes and myotomes.

- Peripheral nerve involvement (e.g., hereditary sensory and motor neuropathies) is associated with predominant distal weakness, distal wasting, hyporeflexia, and sensory involvement.
Sensory symptoms are usually the presenting symptoms of neuropathy and include positive (burning, pain, walking on cotton wool, band-like sensation on feet or trunk, stumbling, tingling, pins and needles) and negative symptoms (numbness, loss of sensation) in hands and feet (glove and stalking distribution).
- Neuromuscular junction involvement (e.g., myasthenia gravis) is associated with hallmark fatigable and

TABLE 19: Features of LMN lesions.

Site of lesion	*Anterior horn cell*	*Peripheral nerve*	*NMJ*	*Muscles*
Weakness	generalized	Distal	Facial and extraocular muscles	Proximal
DTR	Absent	Decreased/absent	Normal	Decreased
Fasciculation	Present	Absent	Absent	Absent
Sensory system	Spared	May be affected	Spared	Spared
Fluctuation in weakness	Absent	Absent	Present	Absent

(DTR: deep tendon reflex; LMN: lower motor neuron; NMJ: neuromuscular junction)

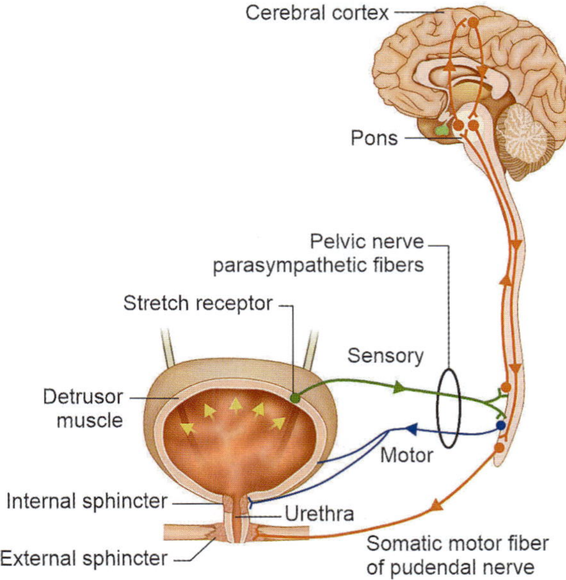

Fig. 51: Neural control of micturition.

fluctuating weakness. The weakness improves after a period of rest. The facial and extraocular group of muscles are often affected by disorders of the neuromuscular junction as in myasthenia gravis.

- Muscle disease (e.g., muscular dystrophies) is associated with proximal and symmetrical weakness and normal to decreased deep tendon reflexes. Atrophy of muscles in myopathy often occurs in late stages. There may be a selective atrophy of one group of muscles with hypertrophy of another group in cases of muscular dystrophy.

Distinguishing features depending upon the site of lesion in LMN lesions **(Table 19)**.

Bladder and Bowel Lesion Localization

Bladder dysfunction can arise from lesions in various parts of the nervous system. Understanding bladder control mechanisms and neural pathways helps in localizing these lesions **(Fig. 51)**.

Neuroanatomy of Bladder Control

- *Parasympathetic nervous system (S2–S4):* Controls bladder contraction (detrusor muscle) for voiding.
- *Sympathetic nervous system (T11–L2):* Controls bladder relaxation and contraction of the internal urethral sphincter for urine storage.
- *Somatic nervous system (S2–S4):* Via the *pudendal nerve,* controls the external urethral sphincter for voluntary continence.
- *Cortical centers:* Frontal micturition center (voluntary control). Lesion leads to urge incontinence
- *Pontine micturition center (PMC):* Coordinates the switch between storage and voiding phases.

Micturition

In infants, accumulation of urine in the bladder activates stretch receptors in the bladder wall, which generate sensory (afferent) impulses that are transmitted to the spinal cord, and ultimately, a spinal reflex is initiated. This stimulates involuntary contraction of the detrusor and relaxation of the internal urethral sphincter and helps to force out urine from the bladder: the whole process is known as micturition. When bladder control is established in older children, the micturition reflex is still stimulated, but sensory impulses also pass upwards to the brain (cortical and pontine micturition center), and there is awareness of the need to pass urine as the bladder fills (around 300–400 mL in adults). By learned and conscious effort, contraction of the external urethral sphincter and muscles of the pelvic floor can inhibit micturition until it is convenient to pass urine. Incontinence is the involuntary loss of urine after bladder control has been established.

Clinical Syndromes

- *Spastic bladder (UMN lesion):*
  - *Cause:* Lesions above the sacral spinal cord (e.g., cervical or thoracic spinal cord injury).
  - *Symptoms:* Small-capacity bladder, involuntary contractions, urge incontinence. In the acute setting of spinal cord injury, the bladder is flaccid and does not contract. This leads to urinary retention and overflow incontinence. Over time, a UMN pattern emerges, whereby the bladder is spastic. It contracts too much, leading to urgency and incontinence.
- *Flaccid bladder (LMN lesion):*
  - *Cause:* Sacral spinal cord, cauda equina, or peripheral nerve lesions.
  - *Symptoms:* Large-capacity bladder, urinary retention, and overflow incontinence.
- *Detrusor-sphincter dyssynergia:*
  - *Cause:* Lesions between the PMC and sacral spinal cord.
  - *Symptoms:* Lack of coordination between detrusor contraction and sphincter relaxation, resulting in urinary retention.

Bowel involvement is usually characterized by constipation and retention of feces, irrespective of the level of lesion. The lesion at the sacral level, however, is usually associated with relaxation of the external rectal sphincter, leading to fecal incontinence.

PART C: CEREBRAL PALSY

- Definition of cerebral palsy
- Classification of cerebral palsy
- Causes of cerebral palsy
- Early markers of cerebral palsy
- Red flags of cerebral palsy
- Associated problems of cerebral palsy
- Treatment of cerebral palsy
- Team for management of cerebral palsy

INTRODUCTION

What is it? Cerebral palsy (CP) is a nonprogressive disorder that affects movement, posture, and muscle coordination, often associated with seizures and abnormalities of speech. Vision and intellect. It results from brain damage that occurs before, during, or shortly after birth. Although damage to the brain is static, clinical manifestations may change over time. Early diagnosis and intervention play a crucial role in improving the quality of life for individuals with CP.

How common? CP is the most common motor disability in childhood, affecting about 2–3.5 per 1,000 live births in high-income countries, with a boy/girl ratio of 1.4:1.

HOW WILL YOU CLASSIFY? (TABLES 20 AND 21) (FIG. 52)

Functional classification is based on the extent of possible activity in a child with CP **(Table 22) (Fig. 53)**. It helps in planning treatment and rehabilitation.

- *Causes behind **(Table 23)**:* 80% of CP is caused by an in utero brain injury, 10% occurs during the time of birth, and 10% occurs in early childhood.
- *Pathology behind*: CP is caused by an insult to the developing brain, any time before, during, or after birth. Any significant ischemic-hypoxemic insult triggers an excito-oxidative cascade leading to secondary energy failure in the mitochondria. Hypoperfusion causes protective redistribution of blood to the brain, heart, and adrenals. During reperfusion, there is a massive influx of free oxygen radicals and calcium ions in the affected areas due to damaged ion channels. This ionic imbalance causes neuronal membrane depolarization and glutamate transporter failure in the presynaptic glia. When the increased synaptic glutamate spills over into the extracellular spaces, excitatory glutamate/N-methyl-D-aspartate (NMDA) receptors get stimulated,

TABLE 20: Classifications according to topography and physiology.

Topographic	*Physiological*
Monoplegia, hemiplegia, diplegia, all four limbs involved (LL > UL), quadriplegia, and triplegia	• Spastic type (70–80% cases), for example, diplegia, paraplegia, quadriplegia, etc. • *Dyskinetic:* (10–15%) dystonic and choreoathetoid • Hypotonic • *Ataxic:* 4% • *Mixed:* 10%

TABLE 21: Classification based on site of lesion. The type of cerebral palsy depends on the site of the brain involved.

Type of cerebral palsy	*Causes*	*Symptoms*	*Radiological findings*
Spastic quadriplegia	Perinatal asphyxia	Microcephaly, seizure, intellectual disability, vision, and hearing impairment	Cystic encephalomalacia
Spastic diplegia	Prematurity	Normal intelligence, toe walking	Periventricular leukomalacia
Spastic hemiplegia	Vascular event	Preserved intellect	Porencephaly
Dyskinetic	Asphyxia, kernicterus	Intellect preserved, rigidity, dystonia, drooling	Basal ganglia involvement
Ataxic	Cerebellar malformation	Cerebellar sign	Cerebellar malformation
Mixed	Asphyxia	Both spastic and dyskinetic types	

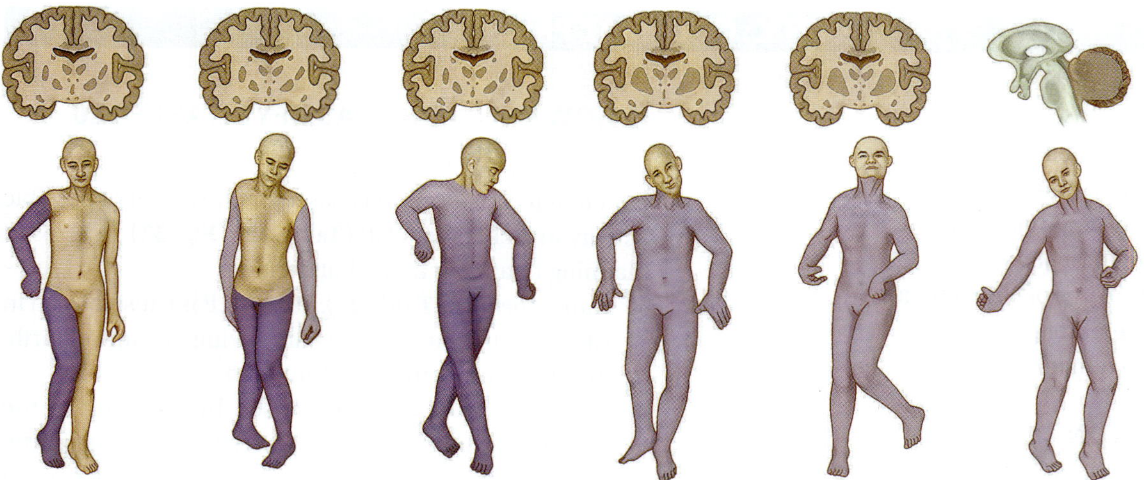

Fig. 52: Types of cerebral palsy and areas of brain involvement.

TABLE 22: Gross motor functional classification system (GMFCS).

Level	*Activity*	*Comments*
I	Walks without limitations	Perform gross motor skills like running and jumping, but with reduced speed, balance, and coordination compared to peers
II	Walks with limitations	May use handrails for stairs or mobility aids for long distances
III	Walks using a Hand–Held mobility device	Walk indoors with assistive devices (e.g., crutches and walkers)
IV	Self-mobility with limitations	Primarily rely on powered mobility or physical assistance for mobility
V	Transported in a manual wheelchair	Severe limitations in head and trunk control. Depends on a caregiver for mobility

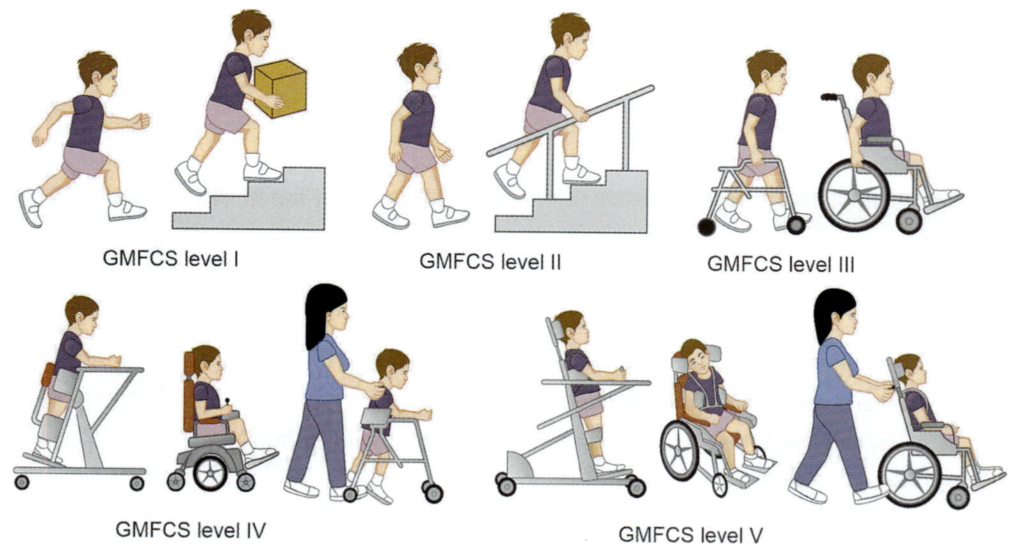

Fig. 53: Gross motor functional classification system (GMFCS).

TABLE 23: Causes of cerebral palsy.

Prenatal	*Natal*	*Postnatal*
• Genetic-chromosomal anomalies, Neuronal migration disorder • Multiple pregnancy, maternal malnutrition, advanced maternal age, iodine deficiency, hypoxia (placental insufficiency, and eclampsia), Drug and teratogenic • Infection chorioamnionitis, TORCH infection • Intrauterine Cerebral infarction/ hemorrhage	• Prolonged labor • Hypoxia • Birth trauma • Low birth weight and prematurity/IUGR • Multiple birth	• Toxins • Trauma • Metabolic: – Hypoglycemia – Hyperbilirubinemia • Meningitis/encephalitis • Hydrocephalus • Neonatal seizure

(IUGR: intrauterine growth restriction; TORCH: toxoplasmosis, rubella, cytomegalovirus, and herpes simplex virus)

which causes the release of more free radicals and worsens the oxidative stress. Enzyme-mediated cellular damage and release of proapoptotic cytochrome C and apoptosis-inducing factors stimulate pathways leading to neuronal apoptosis. Lactic acid accumulation also disrupts the mitochondrial respiratory chain. The cumulative effect is apoptosis and necrosis of brain cells, with glia being more susceptible than neurons. The inflammatory cascade is triggered by maternal infection and makes the brain more sensitive to hypoxemic-ischemic injury.

HOW DO THEY PRESENT?

Clinical Features

Spastic Cerebral Palsy

It is the most common type of CP (70–80%). There is damage to the upper motor neuron (pyramidal or corticospinal tract) pathway, characterized by persistently increased limb tone (spasticity) with brisk deep tendon reflexes and extensor plantar responses. Spasticity tends to present early in the infancy period. Sometimes there may be initial hypotonia, and spasticity develops later on.

There are three main types of spastic CP:

1. *Unilateral involvement (hemiplegia):* There is unilateral involvement of the arm and leg. The arm is usually affected more than the leg, with the face unaffected. Affected children often present before 12 months of age with fisting of the affected hand, cortical thumb adduction, and hand preference. Gait is circumductive when they start to walk. Epilepsy and intellectual disability are relatively common.
2. *Bilateral (quadriplegia):* All four limbs are affected, often severely; the trunk is also involved with poor head control and low central tone. There is a tendency to opisthotonus (extensor) posturing. The most severe form of CP is often associated with seizures, microcephaly, and moderate or severe intellectual impairment.
3. *Bilateral (diplegia):* All four limbs are affected, but the legs are affected more than the arms. Initial indicators are difficulties in diapering and the commando crawl. Intellectual disability and epilepsy are less common. Diplegia is usually associated with preterm birth due to periventricular leukomalacia.

Differentials—hereditary spastic paraplegia, leukodystrophy, metabolic (arginase deficiency, abetalipoproteinemia, sulfite oxidase/molybdenum cofactor deficiency), Aicardi–Goutieres syndrome.

Ataxic Cerebral Palsy

The site of the lesion is the cerebellum and the adjacent brainstem. Most are genetically determined. They usually present with early trunk and limb hypotonia, poor balance, and delayed motor milestones. Incoordination, intention tremor, and an ataxic gait may be noticeable later.

- *Differentials*: Hereditary ataxia, Ataxia telangiectasia, Friedreich's ataxia, Wilson disease, hydrocephalus, posterior cerebellar tumor, glucose transporter type 1 (GLUT1) deficiency, mitochondrial cytopathies, and Angelman disease.

Dyskinetic Cerebral Palsy

Initially, hypotonicity gradually evolves into dystonia, rigidity, and abnormal postures. Intellectual disability and epilepsy are less common. Muscle tone is variable, and primitive motor reflex patterns may be frequent. There may be associated greenish discoloration of teeth, intermittent opisthotonic posture, sensorineuronal hearing loss, and upward gaze palsy.

- *Differentials*: DOPA-responsive dystonia, GLUT1 deficiency, glutaric aciduria 1, Neuronal brain iron accumulation (NBIA), cerebral folate deficiency, and Lesch-Nyhan syndrome.

Hypotonic Cerebral Palsy

It is very rare. There may be a frontal lobe and basal ganglia lesion. The injury occurs in the early gestational period or soon after birth due to asphyxia. Atonic CP can be seen in the evolving stage of dyskinetic and spastic CP.

Differentials: Muscular dystrophy and Werdnig-Hoffman disease.

Mixed Cerebral Palsy

It may present with both pyramidal and extrapyramidal features in the form of spasticity and choreoathetosis, along with ataxic movements.

EARLY POINTERS OF CEREBRAL PALSY

- Delayed milestones—with poor head control, and floppy or stiff extremities cortical thumb, changes in tone and posture, abnormal movements, asymmetry of hand function/hand preference abnormal gait once walking is achieved, e.g., toe-walking.
- Persistence of primitive reflexes, Presence of pathological reflexes.
- Failure to develop protective reflexes (parachute by 9 months)
- Feeding difficulties; sleep disturbance.
- Inconsolable cry/easy irritability.

Red flags in CP: The signs that indicate motor impairment is not CP, and which should prompt further assessment and investigations:

- Absence of risk factors
- Family history of CP or a progressive neurological disorder, dysmorphism
- Loss of cognitive or developmental abilities
- Development of focal neurological signs
- Magnetic resonance imaging (MRI) findings not in keeping with clinical signs or diagnosis of CP.

ASSOCIATED PROBLEMS

- Global developmental delay/intellectual disability, hyperactivity, speech disorder (50%), and microcephaly (5%).
- Epilepsy (20%)
- *Hearing problem:* Sensorineural deafness in dyskinetic type.
- *Ocular defect*—refractory errors, strabismus, amblyopia. Homonymous hemianopia. nystagmus sensory impairment.
- *Gastrointestinal*: Constipation, reflux, esophagitis, feeding problems, and growth failure.
- Skeletal deformities and joint contractures, low-impact fracture, limb length discrepancy, chronic pain.

INVESTIGATIONS

- For determining etiology and timing of insult—neuroimaging.
  - CT scan of brain-detects major congenital anomalies, cerebral atrophy, porencephaly, hydranencephaly
  - MRI—for further delineation, detects neuronal migration disorders such as lissencephaly and schizencephaly, anatomical defects (such as agenesis of corpus callosum), periventricular leucomalacia, and lesions in the basal ganglia and the brain stem, ischemic changes.
- *To rule out other disorders:*
  - GELAAK (glucose, electrolytes, lactate, ammonia, acid-base status, and urine ketone), trimethylsilyl derivatization (TMS)/gas chromatography-mass spectrometry (GCMS), to rule out inborn error of metabolism (in case of consanguinity, recurrent sibling loss, abnormal urinary order, unexplained encephalopathy) thyroid function test
  - TORCH (toxoplasmosis, rubella, cytomegalovirus, and herpes simplex virus), venereal disease research laboratory (VDRL)—to rule out intrauterine infections calcium and phosphate levels, renal and liver function tests, genetic evaluation, if suspicion of CP mimics
- *Assessment of comorbidities*:
  - Cognition—Bayley's scale of infant development screening, Wechsler Intelligence scale
  - Visual—visual acuity, strabismus. Fundus examinations, visual evoked potentials.

- Hearing—otoacoustic emission (OAE) and auditory brain evoked response (ABER).
- An electroencephalogram (EEG) is done to look for epileptic potentials.

Hip radiograph—to look for hip subluxation, maldevelopment of the acetabulum.

TREATMENT

The aim of treatment is not a cure but to mitigate the disability and achieve maximum possible functions for daily living. It is basically a multidisciplinary approach. The pediatrician is the coordinator of the team. Other team members may be a pediatric neurologist, therapist (physiotherapy, speech therapy, and occupational therapy), or psychologist. Ophthalmologist, ear, nose, and throat (ENT) surgeon, neurosurgeon, orthopedic surgeon, teacher, and social worker. Parents are important members of this group. The child is assessed for their capabilities and disabilities. Motor impairment, speech, vision, hearing, and psychological disabilities should be addressed. The following lines of management should be followed:

- *Early stimulation* **(Table 24)**—early stimulation programs are useful in infants under 12 months of age. It helps in dendritic and synaptic proliferation. Lack of stimulation results in neuronal extinction.
- *Treatment of comorbid conditions* ***(Table 25)***.
- Development activation and disability limitation—physiotherapy, occupational, and speech therapy. Together, they ensure holistic development, addressing the child's physical, cognitive, and social needs.
  - *Physiotherapy:* Physiotherapy in CP—it improves gross motor function, prevents secondary complications like contractures and joint deformities, and helps in independent movement and participation in daily activities.
    - *Interventions:*
      - *Stretching and range of motion (ROM): Exercises to* prevent muscle tightness and contractures. It should be done at least three times a day with a joint above and below. During the daytime, passive and active movements of the joint occur through the full range of motion. Splinting at night. For adductor contracture—carry the child on the loin side of the mother. Keep a pillow between the thighs during sleep.
        Hydrotherapy (water) may also be used to reduce spasticity and improve ROM.
      - *Strengthening exercises*: Weight-bearing activities, resistance exercises. It targets weak muscles to improve muscle control. For core strengthening, sitting on a therapy ball.
      - *Assistive devices* and gait training: Enhances walking patterns using assistive devices. Orthoses [e.g., ankle foot orthosis (AFOs), knee, and knee-ankle-foot orthosis] for foot positioning. Wheelchairs, standing frames, walkers/ crutches for mobility.
      - *Functional exercises*: Incorporate daily activities to improve motor function. Example: Playing games, reaching for objects.
  - *Occupational therapy:* Enhance **fine motor skills** for daily activities (e.g., eating and dressing).

TABLE 24: Types of early stimulation.

Type of stimulation	*Stimulus*
Vision	Use high-contrast patterns or brightly colored toys to engage the infant's attention. Show the baby mirrors to explore their reflection
Hearing	Expose the infant to a variety of sounds, including music, speech, and natural sounds. Talk, sing, and play music
Tactile	• Touch the baby • Use different textures (soft cloths, rubber toys) to stimulate tactile exploration
Sensory	Rub the body and scalp gently
Speech	Talk to the child
Motor	• Increase tummy time • Opportunity to kick and move freely
Social and emotional	Face-to-face interaction plays peak a boo, responds to coos or cries

TABLE 25: Comorbidities and treatments.

Conditions	*Treatment*
Spasticity	Baclofen, benzodiazepine, tizanidine, botulinum toxin
Dystonia	Trihexyphenidyl, levo-dopa, gabapentin, baclofen, diazepam, and tetrabenazine. DBS in refractory cases
Convulsion	Anticonvulsant
Behavioral problems	Atypical antipsychotics—risperidone and aripiprazole
Salivation	Oral physiotherapy, glycopyrrolate, and transdermal scopolamine
Hyperkinetic behavior	Clonidine, stimulants—methylphenidate, and atomoxetine
Contracture	• Dynamic—casting, splinting, and botulinum toxin • Fixed contracture- tendon lengthening surgery
Feeding difficulties	Oral physiotherapy, shallow spoon, frequent small feed, antigastroesophageal reflux disease (anti-GERD) measures, percutaneous endoscopic gastrostomy, and feeding jejunostomy
Constipation	High fiber diet, polyethylene glycol
Sleep disturbances	Good sleep hygiene, Melatonin
Bracing and orthosis	Ankle foot orthosis (AFO)

Promote **independence** in self-care, school, and play.

- *Interventions:*
  - *Fine motor skill development:* Activities to improve hand-eye coordination and dexterity. *Example*: Picking up small objects, drawing, or threading beads. In advanced cases, splinting and casting provide support and improve hand function.
  - *Constraint-induced movement therapy (CIMT)*: Movement of the affected side is constrained with casts so that the impaired limb is forced to perform undermotivation repetitive movements in hemiplegia.
- *Sensory integration therapy*: Example: Activities using different textures or sensory tools.
- *Self-care training*: Focuses on dressing, grooming, and feeding using special utensils, adaptive spoons, seating systems, etc., or communication devices.
- *Environmental modifications*: Adaptations at home or school to improve accessibility and safety. Example: Installing grab bars, creating a clutter-free workspace.

- *Speech and language therapy:* Improve speech clarity and communication. Address feeding and swallowing difficulties (dysphagia).
  - *Interventions:*
    - *Speech exercises*: Focus on strengthening oral muscles to improve articulation. Example: Repetition of sounds, words, and phrases. For non-verbal children. Devices like communication boards, tablets, or eye-gaze technology may be used for alternative communication
    - *Breathing and voice control training*: to improve voice strength and quality. Example: Blow bubbles or use whistles.
    - *Language development*: For vocabulary building and sentence formation. Example: Storytelling, answering questions, or naming objects.
    - *Swallowing therapy*: Manages feeding difficulties through positioning and oral motor exercises.

- Behavior modification—for associated autistic features, hyperactivity, and aggression in the child. Parental counselling to cope up with psychosocial stress. Social awareness to make the child as independent as possible.
- *Correction of associated defects*:
  - Refractory errors-correct with proper lens, corrective surgery for squint.
  - Hearing loss-hearing aids.
- *Appropriate school placement*: Children with normal intellect should attend regular schools. Those with borderline intelligence or mild impairment benefit from integrated schooling. Others require special schools and vocational training.
- Appropriate training for self-employment.

TABLE 26: Prognosis according to motor functions.

If a child can sit	Likely, they will be able to walk unaided by age 6 years
Cannot sit but can roll over	May be able to walk unaided by age 6 years
Cannot sit or roll over	Unlikely to be able to walk unaided

PROGNOSIS

It should be emphasized that although not curable, CP is definitely treatable, and with appropriate intervention, the quality of life can be good. An infant with early diagnosis and intervention, good family support, and absence of associated problems is a good prognostic factor. Though hemiplegia or diplegia have relatively better ones, hypotonic quadriplegia CP have worse outcomes.

A child's motor ability at 2 years of age can be used as a rough guide to future ambulation **(Table 26)**.

Hemiplegic CP with no other deficit almost always walks by 2 years of age, while 50% of those with spastic diplegia walk by the age of 3 years, in 50% of cases. In quadriplegia, only 33% eventually walk.

APPROACH TO A CASE OF CEREBRAL PALSY

Salient Points in History and Examinations

Cerebral palsy is a group of permanent disorders affecting movement and posture due to nonprogressive disturbances in the developing brain. The approach involves identifying the type, severity, associated conditions, and management strategies to optimize quality of life.

History

- *Parental concerns (presenting complaints)*:
  - Motor manifestations—developmental delays.
  - Comorbid conditions—seizure, vision/hearing impairment.
  - Bladder and bowel habits.

Prenatal and Perinatal History

- Maternal age, consanguinity, infections (TORCH), drug/alcohol exposure, gestational diabetes, oligo/polyhydramnios, or placental issues. Prelabor rupture of membranes (PROM) and foul-smelling liquor.
- Prematurity, low birth weight, birth asphyxia.
- Seizure or neonatal jaundice, or hypoglycemia.

Developmental History

- *Delayed motor milestones*: Head control, rolling, crawling, sitting, and walking.
- *Quality of movements*: Asymmetry, abnormal muscle tone, or unusual postures.

Family history (three pedigree trees): Family history of genetic or metabolic disorders.

Any similar history in siblings, sibling death, or recurrent abortions.

Associated symptoms: Cognitive delays, vision or hearing problems, seizures, feeding difficulties, or behavior concerns.

Examination

General Examinations

Anthropometry, especially for microcephaly, wasting, and stunting dysmorphology, Neurocutaneous markers, Amiel-Tison angles (by a goniometer), Orthopedic complications (joints and spine).

Objective assessment of development:

- Head to toe.
- Eye—squint, nystagmus, and cataract.
- Chest-rachitic rosary and deformities.
- Abdomen—organomegaly.

Neurological Assessment

- *Tone abnormalities:* Hypertonia (spastic CP) or hypotonia (ataxic CP) or variable (dyskinetic)
- *Reflexes:*
  - Persistence of primitive reflexes (e.g., moro or grasp reflex).
  - Hyperreflexia in spastic CP.

Abnormal gait: Crouched (hip flexion, knee flexion, and ankle dorsiflexion) in diplegic CP and circumductive (hip and knee extension, ankle plantar flexion)—hemiplegic CP. Excessive adductor spasm causes scissoring (diplegic CP).

Characteristic upper limb postures include elbow flexion with pronation of the forearm, flexion of the wrist and fingers, and thumb in palm hemiplegic CP.

Callosity, limb length or size disparity (appreciated by comparing thumbs or big toes side by side), vasomotor changes (hemiplegia), scissoring (diplegia and quadriplegia).

Hip subluxation or contracture—if present, dynamic or fixed.

Movement patterns: Asymmetry, dystonia, or choreoathetosis (dyskinetic CP).

Associated System Examination

- *Vision:* Strabismus or visual field defects.
- *Hearing:* Auditory responses to sound.
- *Speech:* Dysarthria or delay.
- *Growth:* Monitor for failure to thrive or malnutrition.

Final Diagnosis—How to Write in Practical Sheet

A X-year old child, a case of static encephalopathy: Physiological classification (spastic/dyskinetic/ataxic/mixed), topographic classification (hemiplegia/diplegia/quadriplegia) with functional level [gross motor functional classification system (GMFCS)] with or without comorbid conditions (seizure/visual or hearing impairment, etc.) with a developmental age (DQ) with patient evaluation measure (PEM)/lower respiratory tract infection (LRTI)/contracture and the most probable etiology being (antenatal/natal/postnatal) insult secondary to.

PART D: FLOPPY BABY

- Classification of floppy baby/infant.
- Clues to differentiate peripheral versus central.
- Assessment of the tone of the baby/infant.
- Investigations to confirm your etiology.
- Types of spinal muscular atrophy (SMA).
- Symptoms and problems of SMA.
- Investigations and management of SMA.

INTRODUCTION

Hypotonia is decreased muscle tone, involving the axial musculature, appendicular or both. It can result from a wide range of neurological, muscular, and systemic conditions. It is helpful to divide the localization into two broad groups: (1) The supraspinal conditions (including the brain, brainstem, and cervical spinal junction) that can be called central hypotonia, and (2) motor unit hypotonia (including anterior horn cell, peripheral nerve, neuromuscular junction, and muscle). A structured approach helps narrow down the underlying cause.

ETIOLOGICAL CLASSIFICATION: MAY BE CENTRAL, PERIPHERAL, OR MIXED

Central (Central Nervous System) Hypotonia (More Common—80%)

- *Features:* Normal or increased reflexes, no significant weakness, known as floppy or strong
- *Causes:*
  - *Genetic/chromosomal disorders:* Down syndrome, Prader-Willi syndrome, DiGeorge syndrome
  - *Brain malformations:* Lissencephaly, hydrocephalus.
  - *Hypoxic-ischemic encephalopathy (HIE):* Perinatal asphyxia.
  - *Metabolic disorders: Inborn error of metabolism,* aminoaciduria, organic acidemia, Urea cycle defects, mitochondrial diseases. Fatty acid oxidation disorder (FAOD) and mucopolysaccharidosis.

Peripheral Hypotonia

- *Features:* Weakness, reduced/absent reflexes, muscle atrophy. Known as floppy weak.
- *Causes:*
  - *Spinal cord lesions:* Spinal muscular atrophy (SMA).
  - *Neuropathies:* Charcot-Marie-Tooth disease. Congenital hypomyelinating neuropathy.
  - *Neuromuscular junction disorders:* Congenital myasthenic syndromes. Botulism.
  - *Muscle Disorders:* Congenital muscular dystrophies or myopathies.

Mixed-motor Unit Disorders

Mixed-motor unit disorders with superimposed hypoxia, Pompe disease, mitochondrial disorders, and infantile neuronal degeneration.

Systemic Causes

Hypothyroidism. Sepsis, inborn errors of metabolism.

APPROACH

History

A thorough history is crucial:

- *Prenatal/perinatal history:*
  - Maternal infections, drug use, complications, or prematurity. History of reduced fetal movements, polyhydramnios, and breech presentation
  - *Perinatal history*: History of resuscitation, weak cry, respiratory distress, hip dislocation, and arthrogryposis indicates in utero hypotonia in the infant.
- *Developmental history:* Delayed milestones, feeding difficulties, or regression of skills.
- *Family history:* Genetic disorders or similar presentations in relatives. Consanguinity, previous fetal loss.
- *Onset:* Congenital (present from birth) or acquired (after a period of normal development). Acute, chronic, or episodic. Is there any diurnal variation
- *Associated symptoms:* Weaknesses, seizures, cognitive delay, or organ involvement.

Clues from history to differentiate between the central nervous system (CNS) and peripheral nervous system (PNS) involvement **(Table 27)**.

Examination

General Appearance

- Dysmorphic features (e.g., Down syndrome and Prader-Willi syndrome). Usually indicates a CNS origin. Except for myopathic facies, a long, narrow face may be due to PNS involvement.

- Organomegaly (suggests metabolic or storage disorders).
- Physical examination of parents—in transient neonatal myasthenia, myotonic dystrophy.

Neurological Exam

Examine the child's posture, head shape, size, and spontaneous movements, along with assessment of the higher functions and cognition. Floppy infants often lie with their limbs abducted and extended, along with plagiocephaly, due to the head on one side. The tone is readily assessed by passive movements. The techniques to elicit abnormal tone are pulled to the seat. Ventral, vertical suspension, and scarf sign. Deep tendon reflexes (DTR) is exaggerated in central hypotonia and diminished or absent in peripheral hypotonia. Assess for bulbar involvement (e.g., facial weakness and poor suck/swallow).

Clinical features **(Tables 28 and 29)**:

Salient features of PNS involvement:

- Anterior horn cell—signs of denervation may be there in the form of weakness, loss of reflexes, fasciculation, and wasting.
- *Neuropathy:* Motor neuropathy will give weakness, sensory neuropathy will give impaired perception of pain, touch, and temperature, with a loss of reflexes in both
- *Neuromuscular junction*—as end-plate acetylcholine stores become depleted, there is diurnal worsening of symptoms through the day, leading to fatiguability, weakness.

TABLE 27: Differences between central and peripheral nervous system involvement.

Central	*Peripheral*
Motor delay associated with social/cognitive delay	Only motor delay. Relative normality of the social/cognitive domain, except for congenital muscular dystrophy
• Dysmorphism, visual/hearing impairment, and spinal dysraphism • History of (H/O) perinatal asphyxia, birth trauma, hypoglycemia, seizure, and lethargy	Family history of neuromuscular disorder or maternal myotonia

TABLE 28: Features of hypotonia.

Frog-like posture	Poor quality of spontaneous movements with legs fully abducted and arms lying by the side of the body, either flexed or extended
Pull to sit	Excessive head lag and a rounded back
Vertical suspension	Minimal support with a sensation of slipping through the hands
Ventral suspension	Inverted U position/ragged doll posture
Paradoxical breathing	Intercostal muscle paralysis with intact diaphragm

TABLE 29: Difference between central and peripheral hypotonia.

	Central hypotonia	*Peripheral hypotonia*
Level of lesion	Proximal to the anterior horn cell	Motor unit
Dysmorphism/seizure	Present	Absent
Tone	Reduced	Reduced
Deep tendon reflexes (DTR)	Normal or brisk	Depressed or absent
Weakness	+	++
Antigravity movement	Present	Absent
Contracture/ foot deformity	Absent	Usually, present

- *Myopathy:* There is often proximal weakness, wasting, diminished or normal reflexes, and gait disturbance

Developmental Milestones

- Motor, cognitive, and social delays suggest central causes.
- Isolated motor delays may lead to neuromuscular disorders.

Systemic Exam

- Cardiac (e.g., cardiomyopathy in Pompe disease, myotonic dystrophy).
- Respiratory (e.g., diaphragmatic weakness in SMA).
- Skin (e.g., café-au-lait spots in neurofibromatosis)
- Eyes are affected in myotonic dystrophy, congenital muscular dystrophy (CMD).
- Liver—mitochondrial disease, Pompe disease, carnitine deficiency, and lysosomal/glycogen storage disease.

Investigations

When central causes are suspected, depending on the case, the choice of investigation is neuroimaging, for which MRI is distinctly preferred. Karyotype, fluorescence in situ hybridization (FISH), microarray, or specific genetic tests, metabolic screening (Ammonia, lactate, glucose, plasma amino acid, urinary organic acid, blood acyl carnitine profile), and endocrine testing (hypothyroidism) may also be processed. Electroencephalogram (EEG), infection screen [cerebrospinal fluid (CSF) and blood].

If peripheral causes are suspected, the first investigation would be creatine phosphokinase (CPK), followed by electrophysiology such as electromyography (EMG), nerve conduction study (NCS), and repetitive nerve stimulation. EMG studies are used as an important diagnostic tool to differentiate whether the disorder is myopathic, neuropathic, or a denervating process. Muscle and nerve biopsy is the gold standard for structural myopathies and peripheral neuropathies.

Management

- *Supportive care:*
  - Physical and occupational therapy to prevent contractures.
  - Respiratory support if needed (e.g., ventilation).
- *Specific treatments:*
  - Genetic counseling for inherited disorders.
  - Enzyme replacement in metabolic conditions (e.g., Pompe disease).
  - Neuromuscular therapies (e.g., anticholinesterases for myasthenia).
  - Gene therapy for SMA (e.g., nusinersen).
- *Endocrine causes:* Thyroid hormone replacement.

Salient points of SMA and differentials of peripheral neuropathies: Spinal muscular atrophy is a genetic disorder that affects the motor neurons in the spinal cord, leading to muscle weakness and atrophy. It is caused by mutations in the *SMN1* gene (survival motor neuron 1 gene), which is essential for the survival of motor neurons. Without a functional *SMN1* gene, located on chromosome 5q13. These neurons progressively deteriorate, impairing the body's ability to control muscle movements. SMA, a progressive, autosomal recessive condition, has an incidence of one in 6,000–10,000 live births, and the carrier frequency is 1 in 50.

SPINAL MUSCULAR ATROPHY

Types of Spinal Muscular Atrophy

Spinal muscular atrophy is classified into five main types based on the severity and age of onset **(Table 30)**.

Variants of SMA, not due to the *SMN* gene mutation:

1. SMA with congenital arthrogryposis and bone fracture
2. SMA with respiratory distress
3. Fazio-Londe disease
4. Brown-Vialetto-Von-Laere syndrome
5. Kennedy's disease (x-linked recessive bulbospinal neuronopathy)

Symptoms

- Muscle weakness and wasting (proximal muscles are more affected).
- Difficulty with motor tasks, such as sitting, standing, and walking.
- Breathing and swallowing challenges in severe cases.
- Reduced reflexes and muscle tone (hypotonia).
- Intellect is preserved in all types of SMA.

Diagnosis

- *Genetic testing* is confirmatory. The diagnosis of SMA currently relies upon demonstrating a homozygous deletion affecting exon 7 of *SMN1*. *SMN1*, the gene

TABLE 30: Classification of spinal muscular atrophy (SMA).

SMA type	*Age of onset*	*Milestone achieved*	*Life span*
0	Prenatal	None	Zero to <6 months
1 (Werdnig–Hoffmann)	< 6 months	Neck control, proximal > distal weakness, tongue fasciculations	<2 years
2 (Dubowitz)	< 18 months	Sits independently, cannot stand	Two to three decades
3 (Kugelberg-Welander)	>18 months	Stand and walk Polyminimyoclonus	Normal expectancy
4	Adolescent or adult	May complain of muscle pain or fatigue	Normal expectancy

mutated in SMA, has a nearly identical copy, known as *SMN2*, on the same chromosome. The SMA phenotype depends on the interactions of the SMN1 mutation and the number of copies of SMN2. Children with type 1 SMA have one or two copies of SMN2, whereas those with type 2 or 3 tend to have three or more.

- *EMG and NCSs*: NCS may be normal. EMG—shows features of denervation, and motor unit action potential (MUAP) shows large amplitude, long duration, polyphasia with reduced recruitment (neurogenic pattern)
- Muscle biopsy is required in rare cases—evidence of denervation atrophy.

Treatments

Recent advances have significantly improved outcomes for SMA patients. Treatments include:

- *Gene therapy: Zolgensma:* A one-time intravenous therapy that delivers a functional copy of the *SMN1* gene.
- *SMN2-targeted therapies:*
    - *Nusinersen:* An intrathecal medication that increases SMN protein production from the *SMN2* gene.
    - *Risdiplam:* mRNA splicing modifier of SMN2.
- *Supportive care:*
    - *Neurorehabilitation*: Physical therapy and use of orthosis to maintain mobility. Occupational and speech therapy. Prevention of contracture, prevention of osteopenia, and fractures.
    - Respiratory support [e.g., bilevel positive airway pressure (BiPAP) or ventilators]. Cough assist device for impaired cough. Frequent suctioning, chest physiotherapy, and prevention of aspiration. Influenza and pneumococcal vaccination.
    - Nutritional management and feeding tubes/ gastrostomy or jejunostomy if needed.

Prognosis

The prognosis varies significantly depending on the SMA type and access to treatment. With advances in therapies, especially early intervention, many individuals experience improved quality of life and extended life spans.

Other Differentials

- *SMA*—presented with severe proximal weakness, tongue atrophy, fasciculation with absent DTR. Preserved social interaction. EMG/NCV—showed anterior horn cell involvement. Diagnosed by the detection of the *SMN* gene by the polymerase chain reaction (PCR) technique.
- *Peripheral neuropathy*: Weakness predominantly involves the distal musculature with absent deep tendon reflexes and pes cavus.
  Investigations: NCV showing demyelinating or axonal pattern. Diagnosed by molecular deoxyribonucleic acid (DNA) testing for specific conditions. Sural nerve biopsy in rare cases.
- *Congenital myasthenia*: Greater involvement of oculomotor and bulbar muscles. True congenital myasthenia due to receptor defect is rare, presenting with ptosis, episodic weakness, recurrent feeding and respiratory difficulties, and easy fatigability. Transient neonatal myasthenia is due to the transplacental passage of the antibody of a mother suffering from myasthenia. Genetic studies are usually used for congenital myasthenia. They are less responsive to acetyl choline esterase inhibitors.
- *Congenital muscular dystrophy*: It is presented with hypotonia, weakness, and contracture. Associated with brain and eye abnormalities. *Investigations*: Brain MRI for structural and white matter abnormalities. CPK is usually elevated. A muscle biopsy with specific (like merosin) staining and mutation helps in diagnosis.

- *Congenital myotonic dystrophy:* There may be a history of polyhydramnios and decreased fetal movements. Neonate presents with hypotonia, inverted V appearance of the mouth, myopathic facies with temporal wasting. Distal > proximal weakness. Examination of the mother is important with evidence of grip myotonia. The EMG of the mother shows features of myotonia. Diagnosed by triplet-primed polymerase chain reaction (TP-PCR) for cytosine-thymine-guanine (CTG) repeats.
- *Congenital myopathy:* It presents with hypotonia and feeding problems at birth. Weakness is not progressive. Nemaline, central core, myotubular myopathy. CK, EMG—not so helpful for diagnosis. Muscle biopsy is used for definitive diagnosis. Mutation analysis is also available.
- *Pompe disease:* It is presented with unexplained heart failure, enlarged heart, large tongue, and hepatomegaly. In a very floppy infant, typical ECG and ECHO changes. Diagnosed by acid maltase assay in cultured fibroblast or mutation analysis.

PART E: REGRESSION OF MILESTONES IN CHILDREN

- What is neuroregression?
- How will we classify neuroregression?
- How will you approach for diagnosis?

INTRODUCTION

Milestone regression refers to the loss of previously acquired developmental skills in children, signaling a serious underlying condition. A structured approach is essential to identify the etiology and guide management.

The initial step in clinical evaluation is to rule out pseudoregression in all cases. Apparent regression may occur without an underlying neurodegenerative disorder due to factors such as poorly controlled seizures, excessive anticonvulsant medication, intercurrent systemic illness, or secondary neurological complications in a static encephalopathy.

Neuroregression may be due to gray matter degeneration (poliodystrophies) or white matter disorders known as leukodystrophy.

ETIOLOGICAL CLASSIFICATION

Regression in a child below 2 years:

- *Without extracranial involvement:*
  - *Gray matter involvement:* Neuronal ceroid lipofuscinosis (NCL), and biotinidase deficiency, and mitochondrial disorders (Leigh disease)
  - White matter involvement
    - *Macrocephaly:* Alexander, Canavan, megalencephalic leukoencephalopathy with subcortical cyst (MLSC).
    - *With peripheral neuropathy:*
      - *Large head:* Metachromatic leukodystrophy (MLD)
      - *Small head:* Krabbe disease
      - *Prominent nystagmus:* Pelizaeus-Merckbacher disease (PMD)
- *With extracranial involvement:*
  - Hepatomegaly, intolerance to carbohydrate—galactosemia, fructosemia.
  - *Hepatosplenomegaly, skeletal abnormalities*: Mucopolysaccharidosis (MPS), Niemann-Pick disease (NPD), peroxisomal disorder, Gaucher disease, and GM1 gangliosides.
  - Cardiac Pompe, glycogen storage disease
  - *Muscle involvement*: Pompe, mitochondrial disease
  - *Coarse facial features, hypothyroidism*: MPS, GM1 gangliosidosis.
  - Hair-woolly, kinky-Menkes disease. Alopecia—biotinidase deficiency

2.5 years age group:

- *Gray matter*: MPS and mucolipidosis.
- *White matter*: MLD, adrenoleukodystrophy (ALD).
- *Ataxia*: Ataxia telangiectasia, mitochondrial disorders.
- *PME phenotype*: NCL, myoclonic epilepsy with ragged red fibers (MERRF)
- *Extrapyramidal*: Pantothenate kinase-associated neurodegeneration (PKAN), Lesch-Nyhan syndrome, Glutaric aciduria

5–15 years age group:

- *Ataxia*: Friedreich ataxia, spinocerebellar ataxia, and abetalipoproteinemia.
- *PME phenotype*: NCL, MERRF, and subacute sclerosing panencephalitis (SSPE).
- *Extrapyramidal*: Wilson disease, PKAN, and Huntington's disease
- *White matter*: ALD and multiple sclerosis (MS)

How to approach—under this history, examinations etc.

HISTORY

Developmental History

- *Nature of regression*: Isolated (e.g., speech loss) or global (motor, cognitive, and social skills).
- *Timeline*: Acute (e.g., infections and trauma) or gradual (e.g., neurodegenerative conditions).
- *Skills lost*: Motor, language, social, or self-care abilities.

Family History

Genetic disorders, consanguinity, or similar presentations in relatives.

Prenatal and Perinatal History

- Maternal infections, drug use, or complications.
- Birth trauma, asphyxia, or prematurity.

Associated Symptoms

- *Neurological*: Seizures, ataxia, or vision/hearing loss.
- *Systemic*: Vomiting, hepatosplenomegaly, or abnormal growth patterns.

- *Behavioral*: Regression in autism spectrum disorders, epileptic encephalopathy [Lennox-Gastaut syndrome (LGS) and Landau-Kleffner Syndrome (LKS).

EXAMINATION

General Examination

- *Growth parameters*: Microcephaly or macrocephaly.
- *Dysmorphic features*: Syndromic associations (e.g., Rett syndrome and Down syndrome). Mucopolysaccharidosis (MPS).
- *Skin findings*:
  - Hypopigmented macules (tuberous sclerosis), café-au-lait spots (neurofibromatosis, Gaucher, Hunter). Angiokeratoma—Fabry disease, hyperpigmentation-adrenoleukodystrophy, fat pad, focal atrophy—a congenital disorder of glycosylation
  - Hair findings—alopecia—biotinidase deficiency, pigmentary changes—PKU and Menkes disease.

Neurological Examination

- *Tone and reflexes:* Hypertonia (central causes) or hypotonia (metabolic, peripheral causes). Dystonia (metabolic cause, like glutaric aciduria)
- *Gait:* Ataxia or spasticity.
- *Vision and hearing:*
  - Retinitis pigmentosa-gray matter disease (peroxisomal disorder, mitochondrial, NCL, MPS).
  - Optic atrophy—white matter disease
  - Cherry red spot—Tay-Sachs disease, Niemann-Pick disease, GM1 gangliosidosis.
  - Cataract—galactosemia, Zellweger disease, and Wilson disease.
  - Hearing loss—MPS, ALD, mitochondrial disorders, and peroxisomal disorders.
- *Cranial nerves:* Bulbar dysfunction and facial weakness.

Systemic Examination

- *Abdomen:* Hepatosplenomegaly (storage disorders).
- *Cardiac:* Cardiomyopathy (Pompe disease). Lysosomal storage disorder.
- *Respiratory:* Signs of aspiration or respiratory compromise.

INVESTIGATIONS

Basic Investigations

- *Blood tests:*
  - Metabolic panel [glucose, ammonia, lactate, arterial blood gas (ABG), and urine ketone].
  - Liver function tests, renal function tests, and creatine kinase (CK).
  - Vit B_{12}, E
  - Heavy metals, lead, mercury
- *Infection screen:* TORCH panel if perinatal infections are suspected.
- Thyroid function tests.

Advanced Investigations

- *Neuroimaging:*
  - MRI brain with spectroscopy—to assess structural abnormalities or white matter changes.
  - Radiography—for skeletal surveys in storage disorders. Example, dysostosis multiplex in MPS
- *Electrophysiology:* EEG—for epileptic encephalopathies or subclinical seizures. NCV/EMG—to exclude central or peripheral nervous system involvement. Visual evoked potential (VEP), auditory brainstem evoked response (ABER), and somatosensory evoked potentials.
- *Genetic testing:* Chromosomal microarray, targeted genetic panels/whole exome sequencing for syndromic conditions.
- *Metabolic testing:*
  - Urine organic acids, plasma amino acids.
  - Enzyme assays. In cases of inborn error of metabolism, such as lysosomal storage disorders and biotinidase deficiency.
  - *Very long-chain fatty acids (VLCFA) and plasmalogen levels*: Peroxisomal disorder.
  - *Urine copper, serum ceruloplasmin*: Wilson disease.
  - *Urine MPS*: mucopolysaccharidosis.
- *Cerebrospinal fluid (CSF) analysis:*
  - For infections, inflammation, or neurotransmitter abnormalities.
  - Glucose, lactate, pyruvate, and amino acids.

Histopathological and ultrastructural information from selected biopsies:

- *Bone marrow:* Storage cells are seen in Niemann-Pick disease, Gaucher disease. Conjunctival, skin, rectal biopsy: Neuronal ceroid lipofuscinosis:

- *Hair microscopy*: Menkes disease
- *Serology*: Human immunodeficiency virus (HIV), subacute sclerosing panencephalitis (SSPE).

Management

It is never appropriate to declare a disease as "untreatable," as such statements can lead to feelings of distress, isolation, and hopelessness for the parents. There is almost always something that can be done to support the child. Supportive care plays a crucial role in enhancing the quality of life for children with neurodegenerative disorders. Interventions aimed at reducing spasticity, managing seizures and pain, optimizing nutrition, preventing constipation and pressure sores, and improving mobility can significantly benefit the child. These measures not only improve the child's well-being but also positively impact on the lives of their parents and unaffected siblings.

Symptom-specific Management

- *Seizures:* Antiepileptic drugs tailored to the epilepsy syndrome.
- *Spasticity:* Physiotherapy, baclofen, or botulinum toxin.
- *Behavioral changes:* Behavioral therapy and educational support.

Disease-specific Treatment (Table 31)

- *Metabolic disorders:*
  - Dietary modifications (e.g., low-protein diet in phenylketonuria).
  - Enzyme replacement therapy (e.g., Gaucher disease and Pompe disease).
- *Autoimmune disorders:* Immunomodulation with steroids or intravenous immunoglobulin (IVIG).

TABLE 31: Specific management of some neurodegenerative disorders.

Disease	*Therapeutic event*
• Gaucher disease, Fabry disease • Mucopolysaccharidosis type I (MPS I), Pompe disease	Enzyme replacement
Ataxia (Co-Q deficiency)	Coenzyme Q10
Ataxia with vitamin E deficiency	Vitamin E
X-linked adrenoleukodystrophy, MPS 1H-Hurler disease	Bone marrow transplant
Glycogen storage disease	Liver transplant
Glutaric aciduria–II and biotinidase deficiency	Cofactor replacement

- *Neurodegenerative disorders:* Supportive care, as these are often progressive.

Supportive therapies:

- *Multidisciplinary approach:* Neurologist, geneticist, metabolic specialist, and developmental therapist.
- *Family support:*
  - Genetic counseling and psychological support.
  - Always consider and rule out treatable causes of neuroregression, such as hydrocephalus, HIV infection, hypothyroidism, and lead toxicity. It is important to remember that several neurodegenerative disorders have treatment options available.

Prevention

One of the very important aspects of the management of a child with neurodevelopmental disorder (NDD) is to accurately establish the diagnosis. This becomes important not only for proper care and prognostication but also for accurate prenatal diagnosis to prevent further children from being affected by the same disease. The diagnosis may also help identify pauci or presymptomatic siblings or other family members who may benefit from early therapy, e.g., zinc therapy in Wilson's disease. It would be wise to refer the parents for prenatal diagnosis to an equipped center before they plan any future pregnancies.

Prognosis

- Varies based on the underlying cause.
- Early identification and intervention can improve outcomes in reversible or treatable conditions.
- A subset of children experiences recurrent episodes of neurological decline followed by periods of apparent recovery, which is characteristic of conditions such as organic acidurias, mitochondrial disorders, and urea cycle disorders.
- Moreover, HIV encephalopathy should always be considered, and a thorough assessment of risk factors should be conducted systematically.

Final Diagnosis—How to Write in Practical Sheet

X-year-old boy/girl, with insidious loss of previously attained milestones, with/without visual, hearing impairment, spasticity/hypotonia, macrocephaly, with/without seizure/involuntary movements suggestive of gray/white matter involvement, with/without organomegaly. The most probable diagnosis is:

PART F: HEMIPLEGIA

- What is your diagnosis?
- Type and site of lesion.
- Neurological examination of cranial nerves and systemic neurology
- Types of stroke and how to differentiate a hemorrhagic stroke from an ischemic stroke
- Investigations first line and second line
- Management for stroke in children

INTRODUCTION

Hemiplegia is a condition characterized by weakness or paralysis of one side of the body, including the arm, leg, and usually the face. Anatomically it is classified as contra lateral or crossed hemiplegia **(Table 32)**. It is commonly associated with cerebral palsy (CP), but other neurological conditions can also cause it **(Table 33)**. The condition significantly impacts a child's motor function, coordination, and overall development. Early diagnosis and intervention play a crucial role in improving functional outcomes and quality of life.

Though most commonly, CP leads to hemiplegia in children, we will restrict our discussion to acute ischemic stroke and its differentials **(Table 34)**. Hemiplegic CP and its management, discussed in the cerebral palsy chapter.

CHILDHOOD STROKE

Childhood stroke is a medical condition where there is an interruption of blood flow to the brain in children or infants, leading to brain damage. An acute-onset focal neurologic deficit is stroke, unless proved otherwise. Although stroke is more commonly associated with adults, it can occur at any age, including during pregnancy, infancy, and childhood. Early recognition and treatment are crucial to minimizing long-term effects. The reported incidence of strokes in pediatric patients is between 1.3 and 13/100,000/year and up to 25–40/100,000/births in neonates.

Types of Childhood Stroke

Childhood stroke may be broadly classified as ischemic, 55% and hemorrhagic, 45%. Ischemic stroke is due to either thrombosis or embolism. The third type of stroke may be due to cerebral sinovenous thrombosis. They are usually sudden, worst in onset, and gradually improve. Almost 20% of childhood strokes are recurrent.

The most common vessels involved are the middle cerebral and anterior cerebral arteries.

Causes

- Vasculopathy (inflammatory and noninflammatory)—trauma to the carotid vessels or the vertebral artery. *Infection:* Bacterial, fungal infection, mycoplasma, noninfective—SLE, PAN, postvaricella angiopathy, noninflammatory vasculopathy—Marfan, moyamoya disease, other connective tissue disease, focal cerebral arteriopathy. Autoimmune conditions (e.g., vasculitis).

TABLE 32: Anatomical classifications.

Type	*Site of lesion*
Contralateral hemiplegia	Cerebral cortex, corona radiata, internal capsule
Crossed hemiplegia (paralysis of the ipsilateral cranial nerve with contralateral hemiplegia	Brainstem with cranial nerve involvement (Weber syndrome and Benedict syndrome)
Cruciate hemiplegia (paralysis of the arm on one side and leg on the other side)	decussation in medullary corticospinal fibers
Cord hemiplegia	Cervical spinal cord

TABLE 33: Causes of hemiplegia—according to the time of onset.

Sudden (minutes)	Acute (1–2 days)	Subacute (many days)	Chronic	Paroxysmal
Stroke—(mc)-Hemorrhage, embolism	Meningitis, encephalitis, thrombosis	TB meningitis, brain tumor, acute disseminated encephalomyelitis (ADEM)	Brain tumor, abscess, and cerebral palsy	Todd's palsy, migraine

TABLE 34: Differential diagnoses for neuropsychomotor impairments.

Condition	*Clinical features*	*Neurological findings*	*Diagnostic clues*
Intracranial hemorrhage	Sudden onset headache, vomiting	Impaired consciousness, rapid evolution	Imaging may identify the etiology, such as an arteriovenous malformation or, aneurysm. Bleeding diatheses should be ruled out
Arterial ischemic stroke	Abrupt or stuttering onset; Preceding chicken pox, febrile illness, cardiac condition, head or neck trauma	Consciousness is generally preserved. Note neurocutaneous features	Arteriopathy, cardiovascular or hematological causes
Meningitis/ meningoencephalitis	Fever, headache, and systemic symptoms	Fever, neck stiffness, reduced level of consciousness	• It shows multiple areas of involvement, not confined to the vascular territory • CSF—shows pleocytosis, increased protein, and an organism may be isolated
Acute disseminated encephalomyelitis (ADEM)	• Fever, headache • Subacute onset	Fever, neck stiffness, reduced level of consciousness, and focal neurological deficits	White matter involvement in a patchy distribution, variable diffusion restriction
Posterior reversible encephalopathy syndrome (PRES)	Seizures, drug intake, such as cyclosporine and tacrolimus	Reduced consciousness, arterial hypertension	Patchy grey and white matter involvement in the posterior head region
CNS tumor	Chronic/subacute history of neurological symptoms followed by an acute change	Increased intracranial pressure, focal neurodeficit	Contrast-enhanced imaging delineates
Metabolic	Developmental delay/regression, hypotonia, encephalopathy, vomiting	Movement disorder, seizures	Symmetric basal ganglia/brainstem involvement, white matter changes, deranged metabolic panel
RCVS	Thunderclap headache, history of ingestion of vasoactive drugs	Focal neurologic deficit	Angiogram shows diffuse segmental narrowing of intracranial arteries, complete reversal after reimaging in 3 months
Hemiplegic migraine	Headache, history of recurrent episodes with normal imaging, and family history	Hemiparesis generally resolves in 72 hours (rarely longer)	Normal imaging: Genetic testing may be considered
Post ictal	History of (H/O) seizure	Complete reversal usually within 24 hours (Todd's palsy)	Normal imaging and electroencephalography may be helpful
Nonorganic	Fluctuating weakness, disproportionate effect on function	Examination findings do not confirm	Normal investigations

- Congenital/structural heart defects, infective endocarditis, rheumatic heart disease, cardiomyopathy, and cardiac surgery.
- Hematological—polycythemia, hemoglobinopathy, and lymphoreticular malignancy.
- Prothrombotic state—protein C, protein S, anti-thrombin III deficiency, MELAS, Leigh disease, organic acidemia, and hyperhomocysteinemia.
- Blood clotting disorders (e.g., sickle cell disease and thrombophilia).
- Trauma or head injury.
- *Drugs*: Cocaine, amphetamine, triptans, and ergots.
- Arteriovenous malformations (AVMs) or aneurysms.
- Miscellaneous—iron deficiency anemia, and mineralizing angiopathy.
- Age related risk factors are described in **(Table 35)**.

Symptoms

Symptoms vary by age and the stroke's location, but may include **(Table 35)**:

- *In infants*: Seizures, excessive sleepiness, poor feeding, or weakness on one side of the body.
- *In older children*: Sudden weakness or numbness on one side of the body, difficulty speaking or understanding speech, vision problems, headaches, or difficulty walking.
- Many children, especially infants and young children, also manifest nonspecific features like headache, drowsiness, irritability, and behavioral abnormalities. Isolated extrapyramidal symptoms, such as hemidystonia may be a presenting symptom in infants with subcortical strokes involving perforating arteries.
- *Perinatal arterial ischemic stroke (PAIS)*: Seizures (focal and unilateral), cardiorespiratory symptoms, altered consciousness, failure to thrive, and feeding intolerance

Diagnosis

Diagnosis often involves: A step to confirm the vascular nature of the disease, followed by possible etiology and risk factors.

- *Imaging tests*: Magnetic resonance imaging (MRI) [T1, T2, Fluid-Attenuated Inversion Recovery (FLAIR), and diffusion-weighted imaging (DWI) sequences] and magnetic resonance angiography (MRA). DWI—most sensitive in early ischemic infarcts. As early as 4–6 hours. Magnetic resonance venography (MRV) if necessary. CT (in emergencies, and to detect calcification—mineralizing angiopathy, hemorrhage), digital subtraction angiography (DSA) (gold standard to diagnose vasculopathy, dissection) in specific conditions.
- *Transcranial Doppler (TCD)*—to measure blood flow velocity in major cerebral vessels, especially in sickle cell diseases.
- *Blood tests:* To identify underlying conditions, complete blood count with peripheral smear, erythrocyte sedimentation rate (ESR)/C-reactive protein (CRP), serum iron studies, and sickle cell screening.
- *Heart tests*: ECG, echocardiogram to assess heart function.
- *Cerebrospinal fluid tests*: To detect infections or inflammation.
- *Coagulation profile*: Protein C, protein S, antithrombin III, and homocysteine.
- *ANA, anti-ds* DNA, antiphospholipid antibody.
- *Inborn error of metabolism-arterial blood gas (IEM-*ABG), ammonia, lactate, and tandem mass spectrometry (TMS)/gas chromatography–mass spectrometry (GC-MS).

Treatment

Immediate care: If you suspect a stroke in a child, seek medical attention immediately. The acronym *FAST* (Face drooping, Arm weakness, Speech difficulty, Time to call emergency services) is also applicable to children.

- Treatment of seizure, hypo/hypertension, meningitis.
- Thrombolysis (clot-busting drugs) or surgery in selected cases, in adolescents.
- *Preventive measures*: Medications such as anti-coagulants [low-molecular-weight heparin (LMWH)—arterial dissection, structural heart disease, inherited prothrombotic state] for 3–12 months. Or antiplatelet agents—aspirin (3–5 mg/kg), managing underlying conditions, and lifestyle adjustments.
- Revasculization surgery for moyamoya disease/syndrome.
- Emergency craniectomy in malignant infarct with impending herniation.

TABLE 35: Age-related risk factors.

Age group	*Risk factors*
Perinatal	Primipara, oligohydramnios, chorioamnionitis, PROM, asphyxia, hypercoagulable state
1–11 months	CNS infection, cardiac disease, severe dehydration
1–5 years	Moyamoya disease, cardiac disease, and inflammatory vasculopathy
6–11 years	Moyamoya disease, a prothrombotic condition, and metabolic disease
≥12 years	Cardiac disease, prothrombotic condition, and metabolic disease

(CNS: central nervous system; PROM: premature rupture of membranes)

- *Ongoing care*: Physical, occupational, and speech therapy to aid recovery.

Prognosis

The outcome depends on factors such as the stroke's cause, severity, and how quickly treatment begins. Early intervention can significantly improve recovery and reduce long-term complications. Recurrence risk—20%.

The common neuropsychomotor impairments include motor developmental delay, gait disturbances, epilepsy, learning difficulties, feeding and swallowing difficulties, drooling, and scholastic difficulties from various factors.

Salient Points in History and Examinations

History: To elicit etiology.

- *Hematological:* History of stroke in family members, similar complaints in the past.
- Bleeding in the past, rash, joint pain, fever, and bone pain. Cardiac—history of (H/O) rheumatic heart disease, cyanosis/squatting spells, h/o hypertension or previous cardiac surgery
- H/O infection—herpes, chicken pox, TB, h/o connective tissue disease, head injury.
- Features suggestive of raised intracranial pressure (ICP), convulsions, headache, vomiting, bradycardia, and hypertension.

Birth and developmental history, mainly in hemiplegic CP.

Family history—similar complaints in parents/siblings [sickle cell anemia, homocystinuria, and MELAS (mitochondrial encephalomyopathy), h/o epilepsy or migraine.

General examinations: Comment on consciousness, typical posture.

- Pulse characteristics, blood pressure (BP)—hypo/hypertension, four limb BP.
- Pallor—anemia, sickle cell anemia, connective tissue disease, massive IC bleed.
- Cyanosis—in critical congenital heart disease (CCHD) (cerebral thrombosis <2 years, cerebral abscess >2 years).
- *Anthropometry*: Occipitofrontal circumference (OFC), limb length discrepancy, and Marfanoid habitus.
- Head to toe examination—fundus (papilledema, choroid tubercles, bleed), lymphadenopathy, BCG scar, joint bleed, skin—neurocutaneous markers, hemangioma, rash, and petechiae.

Examination of CNS:

- Higher mental functions—level of consciousness, behavior, memory, speech, and handedness.
- *Cranial nerves*:
  - Second nerve—look for homonymous hemianopia (site of lesion-internal capsule or above)
  - Seventh nerve—UMN palsy localizes lesion above pons, most likely on the same side. LMN facial palsy may localize the lesion to the pons.
- *Motor system*:
  - Bulk—measure asymmetry. Limb length discrepancy may differentiate between congenital and acquired hemiplegia.
  - Tone—clasp knife spasticity. Assess and grade power. To test for subtle hemiplegia, walk on heels, walk on the inside of feet (Fog test), or walk outside of feet (reverse Fog test). Ask the child to keep their hands outstretched for 30 seconds; the weak side will drift down. In infants, the cover test—covering the face with a cloth and finding which hand the child uses to remove the cover.

DTR—exaggerated. Look for clonus. Absent abdominal reflex on the side of the lesion with extensor plantar.

Gait—circumduction

Sensory—in older children, cortical sensation (parietal lobe)

Cerebellum—in the posterior circulation stroke

Other system—cardiovascular disease (CVS)—evidence of heart disease, murmur, and carotid bruit.

Abdomen—hepatosplenomegaly, renal bruit.

Final diagnosis—how to write in practical sheet: Cerebrovascular accident, hemiplegia (right/left), with or without cranial nerve/other deficits, localization (cortical/subcortical/internal capsule), pathology (bleed/thrombus/embolism), etiology (risk factors), complications, and functional status.

PART G: PARAPLEGIA

- Enumerate causes of paraplegia.
- Common causes of spinal lesions.
- Management of paraplegia.

INTRODUCTION

Paraplegia refers to weakness of the trunk and lower limbs, whereas quadriplegia refers to weakness of all four limbs. They may occur due to lesions in the cerebrum, spinal cord, peripheral nerve, neuromuscular junction, or muscles. Cerebral lesions are upper motor neuron (UMN) type, spinal lesions may cause UMN or lower motor neuron (LMN) type of lesions, and peripheral nervous system lesions are LMN type—localization described in the previous chapter.

CAUSES

- Cerebral lesion involving the parasagittal or periventricular region causes spastic paraplegia or quadriplegia. Common causes are cerebral palsy, hydrocephalus, degenerative brain disease, anterior cerebral artery stroke, and sagittal sinus thrombosis.

  Features of cortical lesion—seizure, alteration of sensorium, and features of raised intracranial pressure.
- *Spinal:* These may cause acute or slowly progressive symptoms. Cervical cord lesions present as quadriplegia, and lower lesions cause paraplegia. Spinal paraplegia or quadriplegia may be asymmetric in onset. Lower motor neuron signs are present at the level, and upper motor signs are present below the lesion, along with bladder and bowel dysfunction. An acute transverse lesion of the cord may cause loss of all motor, sensory, or reflex activities below the lesion, presenting as a spinal shock for a few weeks, after which UMN signs appear. Chronic spinal lesions are present as a clumsy gait, stunted limbs, foot deformity, and bladder dysfunction.

  Malformations such as meningocele and meningomyelocele have been obvious since birth. Skin overlying the dysraphism may show a tuft of hair, sinus, lipoma, etc. Atlantoaxial dislocation may cause slowly progressive quadriplegia, either as an isolated condition or as a part of a syndrome, such as Down syndrome and mucopolysaccharidosis.
- Common causes of spinal lesions—they may be compressive or noncompressive.
- Noncompressive—transverse myelitis, anterior spinal artery infarction, encephalomyelitis, vitamin B_{12} deficiency, polio, trauma, and familial spastic paraparesis.
- Compressive—extradural and intradural (extramedullary/intramedullary) **(Fig. 54)**.

Extradural-epidural abscess or hemorrhage/hematoma, meningioma, disc prolapse or fracture, caries spine, bony metastasis, cauda equina syndrome (compression by central disc herniation)

Intradural extramedullary—neurofibroma, dermoid cyst, subdural abscess/hemorrhage, meningioma, meningomyelocele):

Intradural intramedullary—ependymoma, astrocytoma, hematoma, and syringomyelia.

Localization and clinical distinguishing features are described in the localization chapter **(Table 36)**.

Features of spinal lesion **(Fig. 55)**

No seizure, no alteration of sensorium, normal higher function, UMN-type of features below the level of lesion, LMN-type of features at the level of lesion, sensory changes below the level of lesion with a definite upper level, nerve root irritation signs at the level of lesion (root pain). Bladder involvement-retention or retention with overflow.

Lower motor neuro lesions

Anterior horn cell disease—with hypotonia and areflexia. Example, spinal muscular atrophy (SMA).

Peripheral nerve disorders—Guillain-Barré syndrome (GBS) and other types of polyneuropathies usually present acutely with symmetric ascending paralysis and areflexia with or without sensory involvement. There may be transient bladder and bowel involvement in the early stages. Hereditary sensorimotor polyneuropathy (Charcot-Marie-Tooth disease) usually presents with a slowly progressive chronic lesion.

Neuromuscular junction disorder—prototype disease is myasthenia gravis. Presents with ptosis and weakness of extraocular muscles, worsening in the evening. They may rarely present with generalized weakness.

Muscle disorder—these causes proximal weakness with preserved deep tendon reflexes. Example, muscular dystrophy, myopathy

Pseudoparalysis—surgery, osteomyelitis, fracture, and myositis.

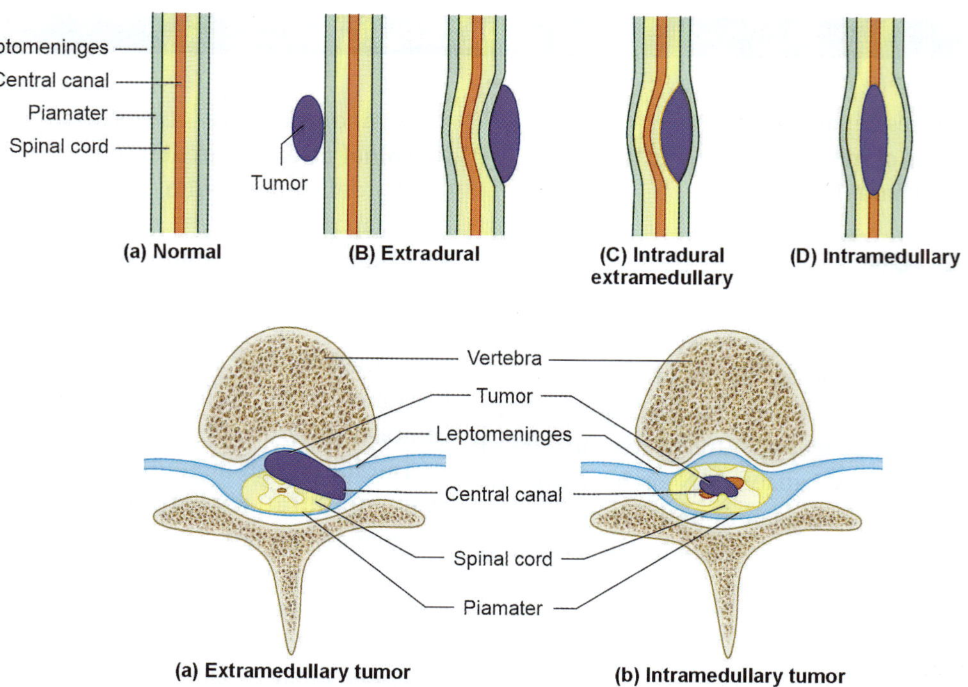

Fig. 54: Types of compressive lesions in the spinal cord.

TABLE 36: Salient features—involvement of the cord.

	Corticospinal (motor)	*Spinothalamic (pain/temperature)*	*Dorsal columns (vibration/proprioception)*
Hemicord (Brown–Sequard)	Affected ipsilateral	Contralateral loss	Ipsilateral loss
Anterior cord	Affected bilateral	Affected bilateral	Unaffected
Central cord	Unaffected	Affected bilateral	Unaffected
Posterolateral	Affected bilateral	Unaffected	Affected bilateral

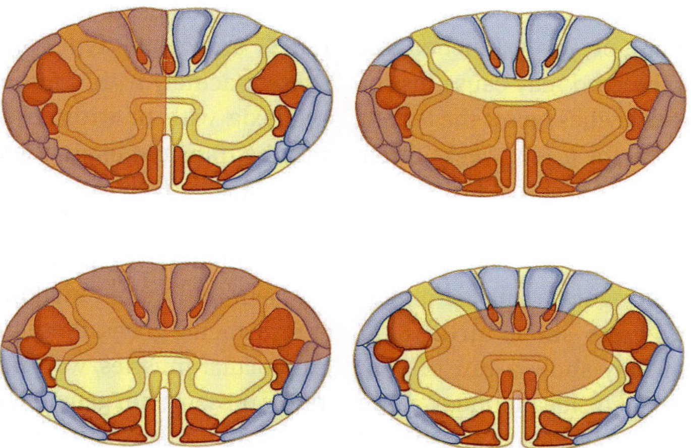

Fig. 55: Clinical features with spinal cord lesions.

APPROACH TO MANAGING PARAPLEGIA IN CHILDREN

A thorough and accurate diagnosis is crucial for determining the cause of paraplegia and planning the treatment.

History and Physical Examination

History Taking

- *Onset and progression:*
  - *Acute:* Trauma, infections, GBS. Transverse myelitis.
  - *Chronic:* CP, SMA, or leukodystrophies.
- *Birth history:* Prematurity, perinatal asphyxia, or neonatal complications.
- *Family history:* Neuromuscular or genetic disorders.
- *Associated symptoms:* Sensory loss, hyperesthesia/ paraesthesia, bowel/bladder dysfunction, feeding difficulties, respiratory symptoms.
- *Recent illness:* Preceding infections or fever (e.g., GBS and transverse myelitis).

Physical Examination

General examination: Evidence of TB and BCG scars.

Skin: Neurocutaneous marker (café-au-lait spots).

- *Neurological exam:* Assess muscle tone (spasticity vs. flaccidity).
  - Reflexes (hyperreflexia in CP vs. hyporeflexia in GBS/SMA).
  - Cranial nerve involvement (e.g., bulbar palsy in SMA or GBS).
- *Motor function:* Strength and range of motion in all four limbs. UMN features in the lower limbs in the spinal lesion. (However, the first few days may have flaccidity due to spinal shock). Flaccid paraplegia in the LMN lesion.
- *Sensory exam:* Determine sensory levels (e.g., spinal cord injury).
- *Posture and deformities:* Contractures, scoliosis, or joint subluxations.
- *Bladder/bowel involvement:* Bowel involvement is unlikely. Regarding the bladder, ascertain whether it is retention, retention with overflow, whether bladder fullness awareness is appreciated whether voluntary initiation of micturition is possible.
- *Spine:* Tuft of hair, sinus, mass, and gibbous.

Investigations

- *Neuroimaging:*
  - *MRI brain and spine:* Detects CP, trauma, tumors, or demyelinating lesions.
  - *CT scan:* For acute trauma or bleeding.
- *Electrophysiological studies:* Nerve conduction studies (NCS) and electromyography (EMG)—differentiate between neuropathies, myopathies, and motor neuron disorders.
- *Laboratory tests:*
  - *Genetic testing:* SMA, Duchenne muscular dystrophy (DMD), or leukodystrophies.
  - *Metabolic workup:* Mitochondrial or metabolic disorders.
  - *Infection markers:* Cerebrospinal fluid (CSF) analysis, serologies (e.g., GBS and encephalitis).
- *Respiratory function tests:* Assess diaphragmatic and intercostal muscle strength in neuromuscular disorders.

Management

Acute Management

- *Spinal precautions:* If trauma is suspected, the child should be immobilized with a collar and backboard to prevent further injury **(Fig. 56)**.
- *Airway management and respiratory support:*
  - Ensure the child has adequate respiratory function, especially if there's involvement of the diaphragm or chest muscles (e.g., cervical spine injury).

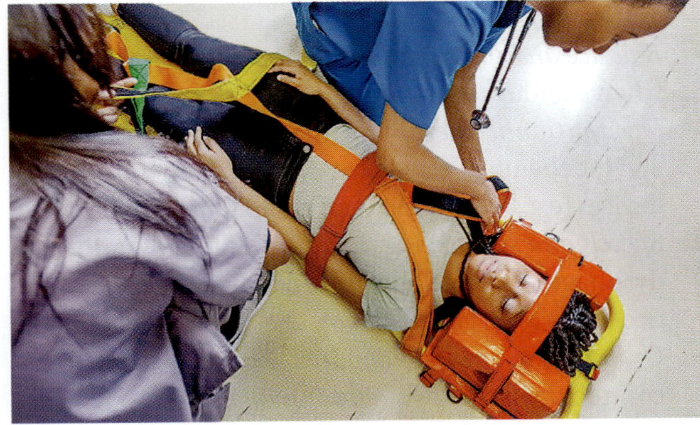

Fig. 56: Immobilization in the case of spinal cord trauma.

Neuroprotective strategies: If the paraplegia is due to acute spinal injury, interventions such as high-dose corticosteroids (methylprednisolone) may be considered to reduce inflammation and secondary injury, although the benefits remain debated.

Pain management: Administer pain relief for acute spinal injuries, fractures, or associated muscle spasms.

Further management, according to etiology:

- *Infections:* Antibiotics or antivirals.
- *GBS:* Intravenous immunoglobulin (IVIG) or plasmapheresis.
- *Trauma:* Immobilization or surgery. Surgical management may be required depending on the cause of paraplegia:
  - *Decompression surgery:* If there is a spinal cord compression due to a herniated disc, tumor, or vertebral fracture.
  - *Spinal stabilization:* If there is vertebral instability, surgery may be necessary to stabilize the spine.
  - *Spinal cord injury repair:* In cases of traumatic spinal cord injury, surgery may be performed to address fractures or dislocations that could further damage the spinal cord.

LONG-TERM MULTIDISCIPLINARY CARE

Physiotherapy

- *Strengthening exercises* for the unaffected parts of the body.
- *Range-of-motion exercises* to maintain joint mobility and prevent contractures.
- *Mobility training:* Use of mobility aids such as wheelchairs and braces, or training for independent ambulation if possible.
- *Balance and coordination training* to improve stability when standing or sitting.
- *Occupational therapy:* Enhance fine motor skills and independence in daily tasks. Recommend adaptive devices (e.g., feeding aids and communication devices).
- *Speech and swallowing therapy:* Address dysarthria or dysphagia. Introduce alternative feeding methods if necessary (e.g., gastrostomy).
- *Orthopedic management:* Prevent and treat contractures, scoliosis, and hip dislocations. *Assistive Devices*: Wheelchairs, orthoses, or splints to improve mobility and comfort.
- *Nutrition and growth monitoring:* Address feeding challenges and ensure adequate caloric intake. Monitor for malnutrition or obesity.
- *Psychological support:* Provide counseling for the child and family to cope with the condition. Engage in social and educational activities to improve the quality of life.
- *Bladder care:* Antibiotic prophylaxis if neuropathic bladder and clean intermittent catheterization

Pharmacological Management

- *Spasticity management:*
  - *Oral medications:* Baclofen, diazepam, or tizanidine.
  - Botulinum toxin injections for focal spasticity.
  - Intrathecal baclofen for severe cases.
- *Pain management:*
  - Analgesics for joint or muscle pain.
  - Prevention of clots-physiotherapy, special inflatable pumps placed over the legs to improve circulation, etc.
  - *Bedsore:* Wound care including debridement, special mattresses (ripple mattresses, waterbed, etc., to prevent bed sores.

Regular Monitoring

- Assess functional status and adjust interventions.
- Monitor for complications, such as infections, osteoporosis, and pressure ulcers.

Prognosis

- Prognosis depends on the underlying cause and severity of impairment.
- Early diagnosis and comprehensive care can improve outcomes and quality of life.

Final Diagnosis—How to Write in Practical Sheet

Paraparesis, anatomical level—vertebral (extradural/intradural/intramedullary), etiology (compressive/vascular/infective/demyelination), complication, and functional status.

PART H: ABNORMAL HEAD SIZE AND SHAPE

- Define macrocephaly
- Causes of macrocephaly
- Define microcephaly
- Causes of microcephaly
- What is craniosynostosis
- Assessment/investigations for deformed head
- Management of deformed head/possibilities for craniosynostosis cure
- Define hydrocephalus
- Pathogenesis of hydrocephalus
- Etiology and types of hydrocephalus
- Management and types of shunt surgery

ABNORMAL HEAD SIZE AND SHAPE

Abnormal head size and shape in infants and children can indicate various conditions, which may be benign or serious neurological disorders. Here is a simplified approach to evaluating and managing these cases.

Abnormal Head Size

Abnormal head size may be divided into two main categories:

- *Macrocephaly (large head)*: An unusually large head, measured as more than two standard deviations above the population mean **(Fig. 57)**.

Causes

Hydrocephalus and megalencephaly under this heading. Neurocutaneous, soots, metabolic condition are different points:

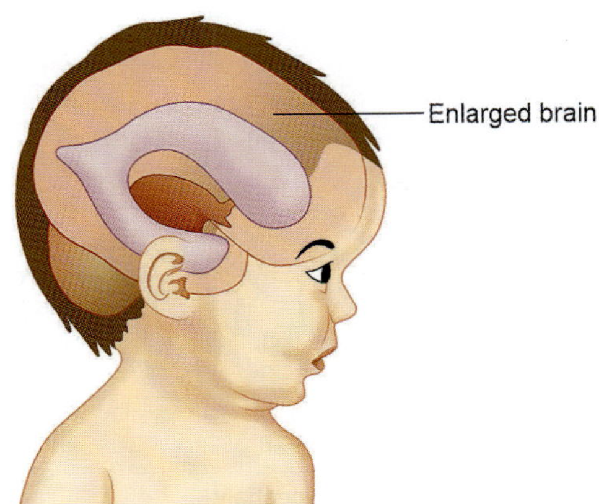

Fig. 57: Macrocephaly.

- Increased brain volume:
  - *Hydrocephalus*: Accumulation of cerebrospinal fluid (CSF) in the ventricles. Symptoms may include a bulging fontanelle, irritability, vomiting, and poor feeding in infants.
  - *Megalencephaly*: An increase in brain size due to underlying neurodevelopmental or metabolic abnormalities, often associated with childhood-onset seizures, delayed motor skills, cognitive delays, or intellectual impairment. It may be present in disorders like:
    - The neurocutaneous spectrum includes conditions, such as neurofibromatosis, tuberous sclerosis, and Sturge-Weber syndrome.
    - Sotos syndrome, also known as cerebral gigantism.
    - Metabolic abnormalities, including leukodystrophy, lipid accumulation disorders, and histiocytosis.
- Increased extracranial volume:
  - Subdural hematoma*: Benign familial macrocephaly*: A hereditary condition where there is a large head with no associated neurological deficits. In this scenario, always measure parents' head circumferences to confirm the condition.
  - Benign enlargement of extradural spaces.
- Metabolic conditions, such as mucopolysaccharidoses, where macrocephaly is associated with other systemic manifestations, such as organomegaly and corneal clouding.
- *Microcephaly (small head)*: A head circumference that is more than three standard deviations below the mean for the child's age and sex **(Fig. 58)**.

Causes of microcephaly include:

- *Primary/genetic microcephaly*: Present from birth, this condition results from a static developmental brain anomaly, characterized by an underdeveloped cerebral cortex and intellectual disability.

  Two variants—autosomal dominant and autosomal recessive and X-linked:

  1. *Autosomal dominant:* It is relatively rare. As a rule, each child of an affected parent has a 50% risk of inheriting the abnormal gene. There is abnormal development of the brain with pachygyria and small cerebellar and cerebral hemispheres. Intellectual

impairment is less severe than autosomal recessive microcephaly, X-linked inheritance of microcephaly carries a 25% chance of affecting male offspring.

2. *Autosomal recessive:* It is the most common type. As a rule, both parents are unaffected carriers of the microcephaly gene. Microcephaly is evident since birth. The brain is small in size, with a small cerebral cortex, and characteristic facial features include a sloping forehead, prominent nose, and protruding ears. Most of them are suffering from seizures and severe intellectual disability.

- *Syndromes*
  - *Genetic causes*:
    - *Chromosomal abnormalities*: Conditions such as Down syndrome, Angelman syndrome, and Cri-du-chat syndrome.
    - *Single gene disorders*: Such as Smith-Lemli-Opitz syndrome and Rett syndrome.

- *Secondary/nongenetic microcephaly*: Caused by an injury to the brain during fetal development or in the early years of life when brain growth is rapid.
- *Prenatal factors*:
  - *Infections*: In utero exposure to Zika virus, rubella, cytomegalovirus, or toxoplasmosis.
  - Maternal substance use: alcohol (Fetal Alcohol Syndrome), certain drugs (phenytoin), or smoking during pregnancy.
  - Radiation exposure
  - Metabolic—hypoglycemia, radiation exposure, maternal phenylketonuria.
  - *Poor intrauterine growth*: Due to placental insufficiency or maternal malnutrition.
  - Hypoxic ischemic encephalopathy

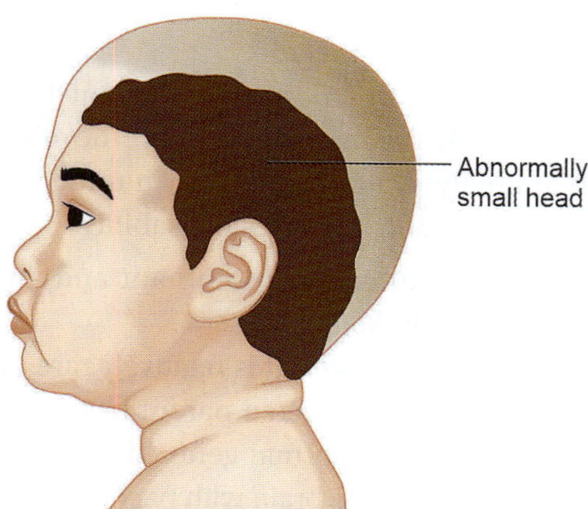

Fig. 58: Microcephaly.

- *Postnatal/environmental factors*:
  - *Nutritional deficiencies*: Severe malnutrition in infancy or childhood.

Abnormal Head Shape

Head shape abnormalities can be categorized into two main groups:

1. *Positional head deformities*: These occur when a child's head shape changes due to external forces (e.g., pressure from lying on one side).
   Common causes:
   - *Positional plagiocephaly*: Flattening on one side of the head, often associated with supine sleeping. This is a cosmetic issue and typically resolves with repositioning.
   - *Brachycephaly*: A broad, flat head shape due to excessive lying on the back.
   - *Scaphocephaly*: A long, narrow head shape, due to lying on one side constantly in infants.
2. *Craniosynostosis*: It refers to early fusion of one or more cranial sutures, resulting in abnormal skull morphology.

There are several types of craniosynostosis **(Fig. 59)**:

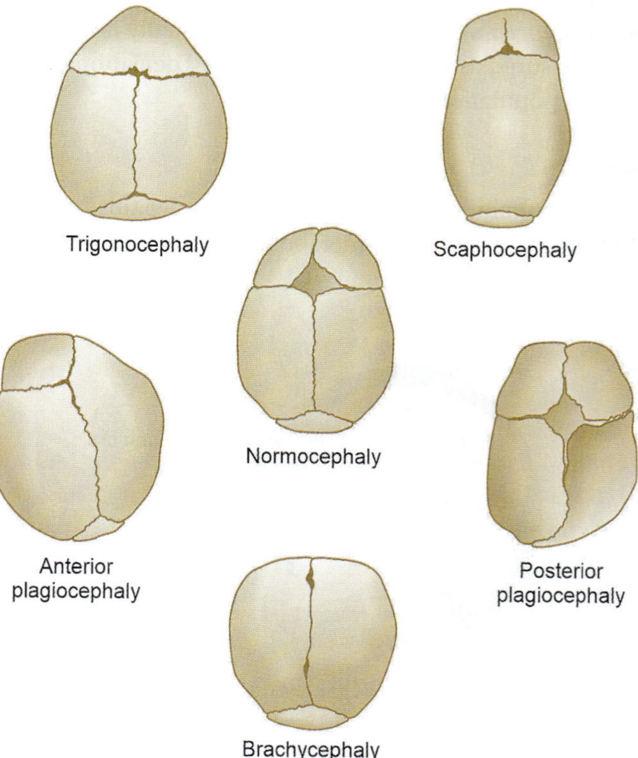

Fig. 59: Craniosynostosis.

- *Scaphocephaly/dolicocephaly*: Premature closure of the sagittal suture, leading to a long, narrow skull.
- *Brachycephaly*: Premature closure of the coronal sutures, resulting in a broad and short head.
- *Trapezoid head*: Premature closure of one coronal suture.
- *Trigonocephaly*: Triangular head (pointed forehead), premature closure of metopic suture
- *Turricephaly*: Tall head, shaped like a tower.
- *Oxycephaly*: Cone-shaped head.
- *Plagiocephaly*: Caused by unilateral closure of the coronal or lambdoid sutures, leading to a flattened side of the head and facial asymmetry.

Craniosynostosis may occur as an isolated condition, involving only the skull, or as part of a syndrome linked to genetic disorders, such as Crouzon, Apert, and Pfeiffer syndromes.

Assessment

Initial Assessment

The first step in evaluating abnormal head size and shape is to take a thorough medical history and perform a physical examination.

Chief complaint: Increased size of head, developmental delay, and features of raised ICT.

History Taking

- *Prenatal and birth history*: Regarding complicated pregnancy or delivery (e.g., prematurity, intrauterine growth restriction, and delivery trauma)
- *Growth and developmental history*: Is the head size and shape changing over time? Is there a history of delayed milestones or developmental delays?
- *Family history*: Regarding similarly affected family members, consanguinity or any genetic conditions in the family (e.g., craniofacial abnormalities, dysmorphism, and inborn error of metabolism).
- *Symptoms associated with head shape change*: Is there any neurodeficit, signs of increased intracranial pressure (ICP) (e.g., vomiting and irritability), or visual disturbances?
- *Feeding and growth patterns*: Is the child growing at a normal rate, and are there any concerns with feeding or weight gain?
- *Central nervous system (CNS) history:* Sensorium, cranial involvement (second and sixth), involuntary movements, ataxia, family history—siblings/family members, tuberculosis (TB) contact, measures parents' head circumference.

Physical Examination

- *General examination*—any dysmorphism (achondroplasia and sotos), neurocutaneous disorders.
- *Vitals*: Hypertension, bradycardia, respiratory problem, increased ICP.
- *Anthropometry*: Protein-energy malnutrition (PEM) is likely in intrauterine infection, inborn errors of metabolism (IEM), occipital frontal circumference (OFC), and measuring parents' head circumference also.

Head to foot:

- Head-shape, microcephaly, macrocephaly, craniosynostosis, plagiocephaly. Frontal bossing- obstructive hydrocephalus. Parietal prominence in subdural collection. Prominent occiput in Dandy-Walker malformation or posterior fossa cyst
- Head circumference measurement: how to measure. The head circumference is plotted on a growth chart to assess trends over time.
- Palpate fontanelles, sutures, and shunts—anterior, posterior, and other fontanelles, sutural separation, dilated scalp veins. Assess AF tension, look for craniotabes, and the McEwan sign.
- If a shunt is palpable, try to trace the shunt and try to find out if the shunt is working by pressing the shunt
- Transillumination
- Auscultate - bruit over the eyeballs, temporal fossa, and retroauricular area.
- Eyes-ptosis, nystagmus, squint, face—dysmorphism. Spine-evidence of dysraphism [neglected tropical diseases (NTD) or scar, scoliosis]. Abdomen—abdominal scar of ventriculoperitoneal (VP) shunt. Organomegaly in storage disorders. Skin-neurocutaneous markers:
- *CNS examinations*:
  - Sensorium and speech.
  - Cranial nerves-optic nerve includes visual acuity and fields, fundus for papilledema/optic atrophy, chorioretinitis, cherry red spot
  - Pupil- and third, fourth, and sixth nerves
  - Hearing-impaired in postmeningitis hydrocephalus, mucopolysaccharidoses (MPS).

- Limbs—spasticity (lower limb > upper limb).
- Gait—may be an ataxic gait.
- Reflexes, lower limb—exaggerated.
- Cerebellar sign—may be there.

Diagnostic Work-up

To confirm the diagnosis, appropriate investigations should be performed:

- *Imaging*:
  - Computed tomography (CT) scan of the head: This can evaluate cranial sutures for early closure (craniosynostosis), hydrocephalus, intracranial calcifications [TORCH (Toxoplasmosis, Rubella, Cytomegalovirus, and Herpes Simplex Virus) infection], or other intracranial structural abnormalities.
  - Magnetic resonance imaging (MRI): May be helpful for assessing brain structures—hydrocephalus, brain malformations, or neuronal migration disorders.
- Screening for TORCH infection.
- *Genetic testing*: A karyotype or targeted genetic testing may be indicated.
- *Metabolic testing*: For suspected metabolic disorders, tandem mass spectrometry/gas chromatography-mass spectrometry (TMS/GC-MS), testing of urine or blood for specific metabolites [urinary glycosaminoglycans (GAG), oligosaccharides in storage disorder], and maternal phenylalanine level in microcephaly evaluation.

Management

Management depends on the underlying causes:

- *Positional head deformities*: Repositioning, increase in tummy time, and occasionally the use of a helmet.
- Craniosynostosis: Surgical correction is often required, typically between 6 and 12 months of age, to prevent increased ICP and to correct the head shape.
- *Hydrocephalus*: placement of a VP shunt or ventriculostomy
- *Microcephaly*: There is no specific treatment for microcephaly, but early intervention with developmental therapies (speech, occupational, and physical therapy) is important.
- *Genetic and metabolic disorders*: Management involves treating the underlying disorder, if possible, and providing supportive therapies and genetic counseling.

Follow-up and Monitoring

To monitor:

- *Head circumference of growth*: Tracking progress on growth charts.
- *Developmental milestones*: Monitoring for delays or abnormal neurological signs.
- *Psychosocial support*: Offering support to the family and providing resources for genetic counseling or social services if needed.

Hydrocephalus

Hydrocephalus in infants and children is marked by abnormal CSF buildup within the ventricular system, which can raise ICP. Timely intervention is vital to reduce the risk of permanent complications.

Circulation of CSF: CSF is primarily produced by the choroid plexus within the lateral ventricles, with additional secretion from the capillary endothelium of the brain parenchyma. The choroid plexus receives innervation from both adrenergic and cholinergic fibers—adrenergic stimulation reduces CSF production, while cholinergic activity enhances it. CSF flows from the lateral ventricles through the foramina of Monro into the third ventricle, then continues via the cerebral aqueduct (aqueduct of Sylvius) into the fourth ventricle. From there, it exits to the cisterna magna through the foramina of Magendie and Luschka. CSF is absorbed in the subarachnoid space by arachnoid villi, which drains into the superior sagittal sinus **(Fig. 60)**.

Pathogenesis

The normal rate of CSF production is approximately 20 mL/day. Hydrocephalus can result from one or more of the following mechanisms, acting individually or together:

- Hypersecretion of CSF, which may occur in the presence of a choroid plexus papilloma.
- Impaired flow of CSF through the ventricular system
- Decreased absorption

Etiology of Hydrocephalus

Congenital

- Intrauterine infection causes an inflammatory reaction of the ependymal lining, resulting in obstruction of the CSP flow. Like in toxoplasma, rubella, CMV
- Congenital malformation—cause:

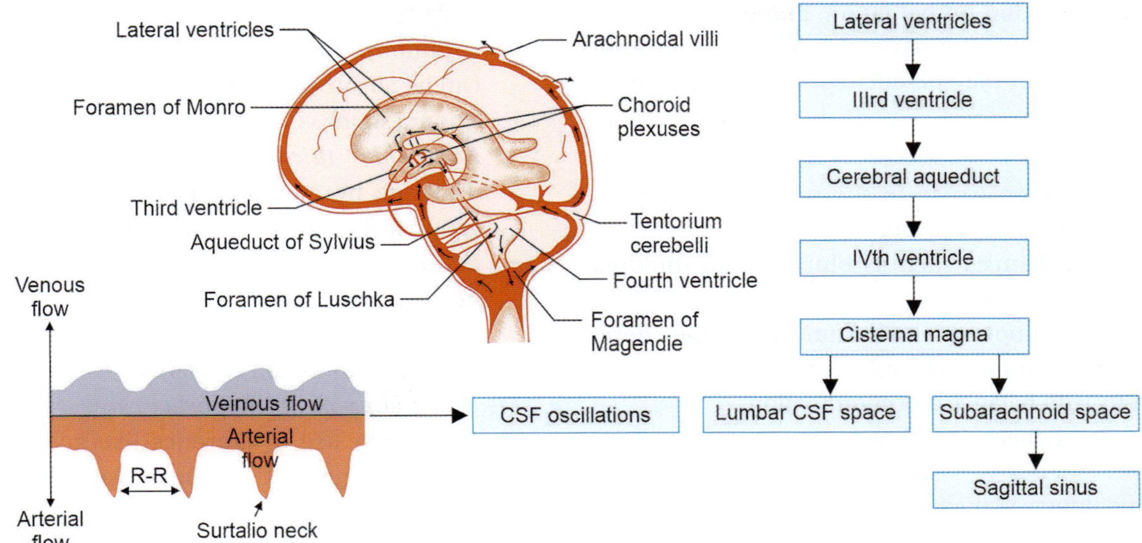

Fig. 60: Cerebrospinal fluid (CSF) circulation.

- In Arnold-Chiari malformation types 1 and 2, part of the cerebellum descends into the foramen magnum, obstructing the normal flow of CSF.
- Arteriovenous malformation, such as the vein of Galen, obstructs the CSF flow.
- Atresia/stenosis or obstruction of the aqueduct of Sylvius.
- Cranial defects—sinovenous pressure is increased in achondroplasia, platybasia, and craniostenosis.
- Dandy-Walker syndrome has a posterior fossa cyst that opens in the fourth ventricle, with a prominent occiput, along with hydrocephalus

- *Acquired causes:* Infections cause hydrocephalus by aqueductal gliosis. Infections may be bacterial meningitis, tuberculosis, viral (Mumps), congenital, TORCH infections, or neurocysticercosis.
  - Inflammatory lesion presenting as a brain abscess.
  - Posthemorrhagic hydrocephalus occurring after traumatic brain injury or subarachnoid bleeding.
  - Choroid plexus epithelial papilloma
  - Posterior fossa tumors such as medulloblastoma, astrocytoma, and ependymoma presenting as mass lesions.
  - Sagittal sinus thrombosis

TYPES OF HYDROCEPHALUS

- Communicating hydrocephalus, also known as nonobstructive hydrocephalus, can be congenital or acquired and results from impaired CSF absorption outside the ventricular system, particularly at the arachnoid villi or basal cisterns. This impairment is typically due to scarring and fibrosis caused by infection, inflammation, or hemorrhage within the subarachnoid space. Common causes include bacterial or tubercular meningitis, sarcoidosis, brain hemorrhage, Arnold-Chiari malformation, and idiopathic conditions, such as normal pressure hydrocephalus.
- *Noncommunicating (obstructive) hydrocephalus*: In this type. There is a block in the circulation within the ventricular system, at various sites like the foramen of Monro, outlet of the fourth ventricle, and aqueduct of Sylvius (most common). It can also be congenital or acquired. It is seen in the following conditions, such as tumors (medulloblastoma, astrocytoma), cysts, abscesses, hematoma, Arnold-Oriari malformation, Klippel-Feil syndrome, etc.

Clinical Features

Symptoms vary based on the child's age and the severity of hydrocephalus:

In infants:

- Rapidly increasing head size.- >1 cm every fortnight.
- Irritability, poor feeding, vomiting, and lethargy.
- Bulging or tense fontanelles.
- *Scalp:* Skin over the scalp became thin and shiny with loss of hair. Veins are easily visible and dilated.
- *Downward gaze ("sunsetting" eyes)*: Failure of upward gaze results from compression of the tectal region through the suprapineal recess, leading to upward gaze palsy.

- Sutural separation on palpation, and on percussion (a sharp tap over the parietal bone), the crackpot (Macewen) sign may be elicited. Transillumination may be positive

In older children:

- Headache (often worse in the morning) becomes better on sitting. Nausea and vomiting.
- Visual disturbances such as blurring and diplopia caused by papilledema.
- Horizontal diplopia due to dysfunction of the lateral rectus muscle unilaterally or bilaterally.
- Difficulty with balance and coordination.
- Behavioral changes or decline in school performance.
- Seizures
- Pyramidal signs in the lower limbs

Differential diagnosis

Subdural effusion, subdural hematoma, megalencephaly, and hydranencephaly (absence of cerebral hemispheres replaced by fluid-filled sacs).

Diagnosis

- *Clinical assessment*:
  - Detailed medical history and physical examination.
  - Measurement of head circumference in infants.
- *Imaging studies*:
  - *Ultrasound*: For infants with open fontanelles.
  - *CT scan or MRI*: Preferred for detailed imaging of the ventricles and detecting blockages, tumors, or malformations.
- *Other tests*:
  - Lumbar puncture (in rare cases) to measure CSF pressure or test for infections.
  - Genetic testing if a hereditary condition is suspected.

Management of Hydrocephalus

The primary goal is to reduce CSF buildup and alleviate symptoms. Treatment is typically surgical:

- *Surgical Interventions:*
  - *Shunt*: A tube is placed to divert excess CSF from the brain to another part of the body, e.g., the abdominal cavity, peritoneum (VP shunt, most common), pleura, or the right atrium, where it can be absorbed. Example, Upadhyaya shunt and Chopra shunt.
  - *Endoscopic third ventriculostomy* enables CSF drainage by creating an opening in the third ventricle floor, bypassing the obstruction.
  - *Endoscopic third ventriculostomy with choroid plexus cauterization (ETV/CPC)*: A combined procedure to reduce CSF production and facilitate drainage (often used in infants).
- *Medical management (supportive care)*:
  - Temporary use of diuretics like acetazolamide (dose—50 mg/kg/day). Or furosemide to reduce CSF production.
  - Treatment of underlying causes (e.g., antibiotics for infections and surgery for tumors).
  - If the hydrocephalus gets arrested, no treatment is needed.

Postoperative Care and Follow-up

- *Monitoring for complications*:
  - Shunt malfunction or infection.
  - Overdrainage or underdrainage of CSF.
  - Neurological deficits or developmental delays.
- *Rehabilitation*:
  - Physical, occupational, and speech therapy to address developmental challenges.
  - Supportive educational interventions.
- Regular Follow-up

Final Diagnosis- How to Write in Practical Sheet

X-year-old child with progressive increase in head size, with or without signs of raised ICP, with/without focal neurological deficit, with/without developmental delay, with/without seizure. Diagnosis is hydrocephalus (communicating/noncommunicating), probable etiology being.

PART I: APPROACH TO THE CASE OF MUSCULAR DYSTROPHY

- Localization of neuromuscular disorders
- Differentials
- Muscular dystrophies with onset in infancy, childhood, and adolescence
- Investigations for muscular dystrophy
- Management of muscular dystrophies

INTRODUCTION

Common clinical manifestations of pediatric neuromuscular (NM) diseases include a floppy infant and difficulty in walking, according to different ages of presentation. In infancy, they present as a Floppy baby, which varies from a subtle delay in the attainment of motor milestones to severe hypotonia with associated respiratory distress, feeding difficulty, etc. On the other hand, older children may present with difficulty in walking, abnormal gait, enlargement of muscles, or pain in muscles. Other clinical presentations of neuromuscular disorders include effort intolerance, easy fatigability, and acute rhabdomyolysis.

For precise diagnosis, accurate localization **(Table 37)** in the neuroaxis is the key approach, as neuromuscular disorders result from a defect in the motor unit comprised of anterior horn cells, axons, nerve, neuromuscular junction, and muscle fiber.

DIFFERENTIALS

- Anterior horn cell-spinal muscular atrophy (SMA).
- *Neuropathy*: Peripheral neuropathy.
- *Neuromuscular junction*—myasthenia gravis.
- Muscle-muscular dystrophy [Duchenne muscular dystrophy (DMD), but there are other types, including Becker muscular dystrophy (BMD), limb-girdle muscular dystrophies, facioscapulohumeral muscular dystrophy (FSHD)], congenital myopathy, metabolic myopathy, congenital muscular dystrophy (CMD), congenital myotonic dystrophy.

In general:
- Proximal weakness is an indicator of myopathy (except congenital myotonic dystrophy), whereas distal weakness goes in favors neuropathy [exception is SMA type III].
- Most of myopathies have symmetrical weakness.
- Wasting of muscle could result from long-standing myopathy or secondary to neuropathy.
- Muscular hypertrophy could result from a wide range of neuromuscular disorders such as DMD, BMD, myotonia congenita, or SMA type III, and cysticercosis.
- The presence of fasciculations is an indicator of involvement of anterior horn cells, classically seen in SMA.
- Disorders of neuromuscular transmission cause fatigable weakness with a predilection for cranial and proximal muscles.
- In children with plexopathy, like brachial plexus injury, both proximal and distal muscles are involved with diminished sensation and DTR.
- Presence of sensory loss, distal atrophy resulting in stork-like legs with absent DTR and foot deformities like hammer toe are hallmarks for hereditary neuropathies like hereditary motor sensory neuropathy.

MUSCULAR DYSTROPHIES WITH ONSET IN INFANCY, CHILDHOOD, OR ADOLESCENCE

- *DMD:* A type of dystrophinopathy with onset in early childhood, causing severe, progressive systemic weakness. It is an X-linked recessive disorder, primarily affecting males. Females are usually carriers

TABLE 37: Key clinical features for localization in neuromuscular disorders.

Clinical features	*Anterior horn cell*	*Nerve*	*Neuromuscular junction*	*Muscles*
Weakness	P = D	P < D	P = D	P > D
Muscle atrophy	Yes	Yes	No	Late stages
Tone	Decreased	Decreased	Decreased	Decreased
DTR	Absent	Absent/diminished	Normal/diminished	Normal/diminished
Plantar response	Mute or flexor	Flexor	flexor	Flexor
Sensory	Normal	Diminished	Diminished	Diminished

but can have mild symptoms on rare occasions (2–8%). DMD affects 1 in every 3,300 live-born males. Early signs appear in childhood, typically between ages 2 and 5. Muscle weakness begins in the hips, thighs, and shoulders with difficulty in walking, running, or climbing stairs. Enlarged calf muscles (pseudohypertrophy) are a typical finding with lumbar lordosis. There may be a history of frequent falls and difficulty in standing up from the floor (Gower's sign). Progressive loss of ambulation often requires a wheelchair by adolescence. Respiratory problems and cardiomyopathy are the causes of death.

- *BMD:* Becker dystrophy is allelic (caused by different mutations in the same gene) with DMD. Compared to DMD, some functional dystrophin is produced in this condition. They usually present in adolescence, with lower limb weakness, calf hypertrophy, pelvic girdle weakness, and cardiomyopathy. Progresses more slowly than DMD and can be associated with a near-normal life span.
- *Myotonic dystrophy:* A dominantly inherited disease, due to trinucleotide repeat expansion of *CTG* in the *DMPK* gene. Neonates present with hypotonia, bulbar dysfunction, typical inverted 'V' shaped upper lip. There may be facial diplegia, grip myotonia, learning disability, and progressive distal weakness in children. It is a multisystem disorder with male pattern baldness, cataracts, intellectual disability, cardiac abnormalities, diabetes mellitus, etc. There can be anticipation through generations.
- *Fascioscapulohumeral dystrophy:* Usually presents in late adolescence, with asymmetric facial and shoulder girdle muscle weakness. Strong family history with autosomal dominant inheritance, due to a deletion on chromosome 4. There may be associated sensorineural hearing loss.
- *Limb girdle dystrophy:* A heterogeneous genetic disorder (AD/AR) with variable onset and progression, causing proximal lower extremity weakness. The proximal upper extremity is also involved with scapular winging. Cardiomyopathy may be associated. Plasma creatine kinase (CK) is usually raised.
- *CMD:* A heterogeneous disorder with variable patterns of inheritance. Most are present at birth or in early infancy with weakness, hypotonia, or contractures. Weaknesses are slowly progressive with a tendency to contracture. Feeding difficulties and breathing difficulties may be associated. Some of the variants may have associated eye and brain disorders with muscle abnormalities (e.g., Fukuyama muscular dystrophy). Muscle biopsy shows dystrophic features.

Initial Assessment and Diagnosis

Age at onset, whether the illness is progressive or static, whether it is confined to the neuromuscular alone, or whether central nervous system (CNS) is also involved.

History taking: The first step in diagnosing muscular dystrophy is to take a detailed history:

- *Birth history*: History of polyhydroamnios, decreased fetal movement, kick count, breech presentation, congenital dislocation of the hip, and contracture.
- *Family history*: Of muscle weakness, difficulty walking, or early childhood deaths. The history of consanguinity and the generation pedigree chart are very informative. Some of the disorders are autosomal dominant (AD) in inheritance [FSHD, limb girdle muscular dystrophy (LGMD), and myotonic dystrophy], some are autosomal recessive (LGMD and metabolic myopathy), and X-linked (DMD and BMD)]. Most mitochondrial myopathies are inherited from the mother.
- *Developmental milestones*: Presence of developmental dissociation with isolated motor delay with preserved cognition and language favors a neuromuscular disorder. Coexistence of cognitive delay, speech delay, vision, hearing impairment, or the presence of seizure is an indicator of CNS involvement. It is not uncommon to have muscular disease along with CNS involvement, as in DMD, alpha dystroglycanopathies [including Fukuyama CMD], myotonic dystrophy, and mitochondrial disease.
- *Presenting complaints:* Broadly, neuromuscular complaints could be divided into negative symptoms (weakness, muscle atrophy, fatigue, exercise intolerance) and positive symptoms (myalgia, cramps, contractures, myotonia, myoglobinuria). History of abnormal gait, frequent falls, difficulty in getting up from the floor, and difficulty in climbing stairs points towards muscular dystrophy. Specific muscle group affection (e.g., hips, shoulders, and legs) can help differentiate types of MD. Pain is uncommon in most pediatric neuromuscular disorders except in dermatomyositis and polyradiculoneuropathy. Muscle cramps and muscle stiffness are nonspecific

TABLE 38: History to identify the type of weakness.

Weakness	*Pattern*
Getting up from a sitting position, walking upstairs or downstairs (upper limb), raising arms over head, or combing (lower limb)	Proximal limb weakness
Difficulties in buttoning/unbuttoning and wearing slippers	Distal limb weakness
Difficulties in blowing, closing eyes completely	Facial muscles
Difficulties in swallowing, choking, nasal regurgitation, and recurrent aspiration	Bulbar weakness
Inability to lift the head off the bed while attempting to get up from the lying-down position	Neck flexor weakness
Turns to one side and takes support to get up from the sitting position	Truncal weakness

complaints, unless when precipitated by exercise and associated with myoglobinuria. In case of metabolic myopathy) **(Table 38)**.

- *Age at onset*: Neuromuscular weakness that manifests at birth and early neonatal period includes SMA, congenital myotonic dystrophy, congenital myopathy, CMD, congenital myasthenic syndrome, glycogen storage disease, and carnitine deficiency. Whereas other muscular dystrophies, inflammatory myopathy, and metabolic myopathy could manifest in early childhood.

Onset:

- Acute/subacute—AIDP. Myositis, drug-induced myopathy.
- Chronic/insidious—muscular dystrophy, metabolic myopathy, congenital myopathy, endocrine myopathy.
- Episodic—myasthenia gravis, metabolic myopathy, mitochondrial myopathy.

Extent and pattern of involvement:

Pattern of weakness:

- Proximal limb weakness—muscular dystrophy, inflammatory myopathy, juvenile SMA, metabolic/ endocrine myopathy.
- Distal weakness—neuropathy, distal myopathy (myotonic dystrophy).
- Scapuloperoneal weakness—scapuloperoneal dystrophy.
- Ptosis—myasthenia gravis, centronuclear, and nemaline myopathy.
- Neck extensor weakness—inflammatory myopathy and FSHD.

Precipitating factors:

- Weakness precipitated by fasting or fever—fatty acid oxidation disorders (FAOD).
- Precipitated by a high-carbohydrate diet—hypokalemic periodic paralysis.
- Pain, weakness, passage of red urine after exercise—metabolic myopathy.

Physical examination:

- Anthropometry—wasting of muscles.
- Dysmorphism, neurocutaneous marker, asymmetric face (FSHD), Gottron papules, heliotrope rash (dermatomyositis).
  - *Muscle strength and tone*: Assess for signs of muscle weakness, including the *Gowers' sign*.
  - *Muscle hypertrophy*: In *DMD*, certain muscles, particularly the calves, may appear enlarged due to pseudo-hypertrophy (the enlargement is due to fat and connective tissue replacing muscle tissue).
  - *Posture and gait*: Children may develop a waddling gait or difficulty with balance due to muscle weakness. Assess their ability to rise from the floor, walk on tiptoe, and perform other tasks that involve muscle strength.
    - *Waddling gait:* DMD
    - *Stamping gait*- peripheral neuropathy
    - Toe walking may be an indicator of muscular dystrophy
    - Lordotic posture and Gowers' sign- proximal hip girdle weakness

Involvement in the upper limb and trunk:

- Neck flexor weakness (DMD), paraspinal contracture (rigid spine syndrome), winged scapula (FSHD), contractures of the elbow (Emery–Dreifuss muscular dystrophy), and hyperextensibility of distal joints as seen in the Ullrich variant of CMD.
- *Lower limb:* Inverted Champagne bottle (peroneal muscular atrophy), hypertrophy of extensor digitorum brevis (EDB) (DMD), pes cavus (Friedreich's ataxia), and talipes equinovarus (DMD).

- Evidence for myotonia in the mother (ask the mother first and then open it suddenly) and features of myasthenia (ptosis and weakness).
- *Other findings*: Atrophy of sternocleidomastoid, trapezius, winging of scapula. Atrophy of the intrinsic muscles of the hands. Anterior compartment of legs, tightness of heel cords, pes cavus, pes planus, and presence of foot drop.

Other systems examinations:

- *Cardiac involvement:* DMD, BMD, EDMD, and Pompe disease.
- *Respiratory involvement:* Congenital myopathy, CMD, SMA, and mitochondrial disorders.
- *Hepatic:* Pompe, debrancher enzyme deficiency.
- *Facial dysmorphism:* Congenital myopathy.
- *Ocular involvement:* CMD and mitochondrial.

Diagnostic Work-up

Three basic investigations for any neuromuscular disorders: (1) CPK, (2) thyroid profile, and (3) EMG.

Serum CK levels: Elevated *CK* levels in the blood are often indicative of muscle damage. Levels are typically very high in *DMD.*

Interpretation:

- CK—elevated—muscular dystrophy.
- CK—normal indicates myopathy (congenital, mitochondrial, and metabolic). SMA and myasthenia gravis.
- CK—variable, with rash, calcinosis—dermatomyositis.
- CK normal, and EMG—showed pure motor disease—SMA.
- CK—normal, but clinically there is a sensory abnormality; EMG/NCV—showed abnormal neuropathy—CMT.
- EMG—myopathic—muscle disease. Go for a muscle biopsy and a specific stain.
- CK normal, fluctuating weakness, Repetitive nerve stimulation test (RNST) (3hz—decrementing)—NMJ disorders (myasthenia gravis).
- *Electromyography (EMG)*: EMG testing may help rule out other causes of muscle weakness, such as neuropathy or myopathy. Brief duration, small amplitude, polyphasic potential with increased recruitment is suggestive of myopathy.
  EMG testing may help rule out other causes of muscle weakness, such as neuropathy or myopathy. Brief duration, small amplitude, polyphasic potential with increased recruitment is suggestive of myopathy.
- Metabolic profile—in suspected metabolic myopathy—serum ammonia, lactate, arterial blood gas (ABG), blood glucose, urine ketone, trimethylsilyl derivatization followed by gas chromatography-mass spectrometry (TMS/GC-MS), as necessary.
- *Genetic testing:* Genetic testing is the cornerstone of diagnosis in muscle disorders. Testing for *DMD* and *BMD* involves identifying mutations in the *Dystrophin gene (DMD) by multiplex ligation-dependent probe amplification (MLPA). For other MD types, whole exome sequencing (WES) is the preferred one (LGMD, FSHD, congenital myopathy, and CMD).* TP-PCR is used for myotonic dystrophy. If a female child has suspected MD, genetic testing can also determine whether she is a carrier of an X-linked form like DMD.
- *Muscle biopsy:* In some cases, especially when genetic testing is inconclusive, a *muscle biopsy with immunohistochemistry* may be performed. Dystrophinopathy, calpainopathy, congenital myopathy, and mitochondrial disorder may be detected with a specific stain. Electron microscopy helps to confirm the diagnosis in cases of congenital myopathy.
- *Other investigations*: MRI with short tau inversion recovery (STIR) frequency—for inflammatory myopathy
- Enzyme analysis—muscle phosphorylase—McArdle disease, Pompe-acid maltase, TMS-carnitine palmitoyl transferase deficiency.
  Antibody testing: AChR, anti-MuSK (Myasthenia gravis), antimyositis antibody-dermatomyositis.
- *Cardiac and pulmonary evaluation*:
  - *Electrocardiogram (ECG) and echocardiogram*: Children with MD, particularly *DMD/BMD*, LGMD, and myotonic dystrophy, are at risk for *dilated cardiomyopathy or arrhythmia.* Routine monitoring with an ECG/echocardiogram is important, especially as the child ages.
  - *Pulmonary function tests*: Many of the muscular disorders, when they progress, respiratory muscle weakness can leading to difficulty breathing. Pulmonary function tests (PFTs) can assess the severity of respiratory impairment and guide the need for respiratory support.

Differential Diagnosis

While *muscular dystrophy* is a common cause of progressive muscle weakness, several other conditions should be considered, including:

- *SMA*: A neurodegenerative disorder that causes muscle weakness and atrophy due to anterior horn cell degeneration. Type 3 or 4, with adolescent or adult, may be present with calf muscle hypertrophy. They are ambulatory with normal life expectancy and normal cognition, but may complain of intermittent muscle pain and fatigue. They have hyporeflexia or areflexia, and tongue fasciculations. Diagnosed by *SMN1* gene analysis.
- *Myopathies*: Inflammatory (e.g., *juvenile dermatomyositis*) or metabolic disorders (e.g., *glycogen storage diseases, mitochondrial myopathies*). Dermatomyositis—presents insidiously with symmetric, proximal weakness affecting arms and legs. Characteristic skin findings that suggest dermatomyositis include periorbital heliotrope, rash, and erythematous, eczematoid rash over the knuckles of the fingers or toes (Gottron papule). Markers of muscle inflammation, including ESR or serum CK, can be normal or elevated; Other measures of muscle involvement (aldolase or serum creatinine) can be elevated in the absence of an elevated CK. Biopsy of affected muscles shows perifascicular muscle cell atrophy and inflammation.
- *Neuromuscular junction disorders*: Conditions such as *myasthenia gravis* can mimic muscle weakness. MG occurs due to interference with acetylcholine transmission at the neuromuscular junction. The juvenile form begins with fluctuating systemic weakness, ptosis, diplopia, dysarthria, and dysphagia. The diagnosis can be suspected by a decremental response to repetitive nerve stimulation (RNST) and confirmed by detection of AChR or anti-muscle-specific kinase (anti-MuSK) antibody.
- *Congenital myopathies*: These may present with muscle weakness at birth or early childhood, with characteristic muscle histopathology. These conditions present with defects primarily affecting skeletal muscle fibers, causing muscle weakness and/or hypotonia. They are static or slowly progressive. Plasma CK is normal or only mildly elevated.

Management and Intervention

Management of muscular dystrophy is multidisciplinary, aimed at improving function, preventing complications, and enhancing quality of life.

Pharmacological Management: Duchenne Muscular Dystrophy

- *Corticosteroids*, such as *prednisone (0.75 mg/kg/day)* or *deflazacort* (0.90 mg/kg/day), can slow the progression of muscle weakness by reducing inflammation and preserving muscle function. They may help extend ambulation and delay the onset of severe disability.
- *Disease-modifying therapies*:
  - *Exon skipping therapies* (e.g., *eteplirsen*): exon 45, 51, 53—antisense oligonucleotide. These aim to bypass specific mutations in the dystrophin gene to allow for the production of a shorter but functional dystrophin protein.
  - *Stop codon read through—ataluren.*
  - *Gene therapy*: Investigational therapies aim to deliver a correct copy of the dystrophin gene or use *gene editing* technologies.
  - *Others:* Utrophin regulator, myostatin inhibitor.

Physical and Occupational Therapy

- *Physical therapy (PT)*: Regular physical therapy helps to maintain muscle strength, joint mobility, and flexibility. Stretching exercises and strength training can delay joint contractures and improve function.
- *Occupational therapy (OT)*: Helps with the use of adaptive devices, assists with daily activities, and provides strategies to maximize independence as the disease progresses.
- *Bracing and assistive devices*: Orthopedic interventions, such as night splints, ankle-foot orthoses (AFOs), or powered wheelchairs, are used to improve mobility and reduce complications, such as joint deformities.

Respiratory Management

- *Noninvasive ventilation*: In later stages of MD, respiratory function may decline. Noninvasive ventilation [e.g., bilevel positive airway pressure (BiPAP)] can help children with *DMD* manage sleep-disordered breathing and daytime hypoventilation.
- *Cough assist devices*: These help clear secretions and improve respiratory function.

- *Pulmonary rehabilitation*: Regular respiratory therapy and monitoring are essential for maintaining lung function and preventing respiratory failure.
- *PFT, every 6 months if nonambulatory and annually if ambulatory child.*

Cardiac Management

- *Cardiology follow-up*: Regular cardiac monitoring is crucial, with ECG/echocardiography, as *Duchenne MD* can lead to *cardiomyopathy* and heart failure. Medications such as angiotensin-converting enzyme (*ACE) inhibitors, beta-blockers*, or *diuretics* may be used to manage heart failure.
- *Serum calcium, phosphate, vitamin D3 (biannually), dual-energy X-ray absorptiometry (DEXA) scan,* annually

Surgery

Orthopedic surgery: In cases of significant contractures or scoliosis, surgery may be required to maintain function or prevent deformities.

Genetic Counseling and Family Support

- *Genetic counseling*: For families affected by MD, counseling can help them understand inheritance patterns, risks for future children, and options like prenatal genetic testing.
- *Psychosocial support*: Affected children and their families may experience emotional and psychological challenges. Support groups, counseling, and therapy are often beneficial for coping with the social and emotional impact of MD.
- *Cognitive function*: Some forms of MD, especially *Duchenne MD*, can have associated intellectual disabilities or learning difficulties, requiring an assessment of cognitive development.

Follow-up and Long-Term Care

Regular follow-up is required to monitor disease progression, adjust treatment plans, and provide appropriate interventions:

PART J: TUBERCULAR MENINGITIS IN CHILDREN

- What is your diagnosis?
- Points in favor of diagnosis
- Pathophysiology of tubercular meningitis
- What are the stages of TBM
- Investigations to confirm your diagnosis

INTRODUCTION

Tubercular meningitis (TBM) is a severe manifestation of *Mycobacterium tuberculosis* infection, involving the meninges surrounding the brain and spinal cord. It is more common in children, especially in areas where tuberculosis (TB) is endemic. About 1% of total TB cases and 5–10% of extrapulmonary TB cases develop central nervous system (CNS) TB. Incidence is higher in young children and human immunodeficiency virus (HIV)-infected patients. The estimated mortality of tuberculous meningitis in India is about 1.5 per 100,000 population. Risk factors for CNS TB include younger age, HIV co-infection, malnutrition, recent measles or pertussis infection, the use of immunosuppressive agents, and high disease prevalence in the community.

PATHOPHYSIOLOGY

- TB bacilli reach the brain via hematogenous spread from a primary focus (lungs, lymph nodes).
- They form small tubercles in the brain or meninges, which may rupture, causing inflammation and exudation.
- This leads to *basilar meningitis*, vascular complications, and hydrocephalus.
- Predisposing factors—young age, household contact, prior measles, and protein-energy malnutrition.

Chief complaint: Fever (high/low grade, evening rise, and long duration).

- Seizure (focal/generalized).
- Altered sensorium/lethargy (sudden/insidious).
- Focal neurological deficits.

CLINICAL FEATURES

Stages of TBM (modified Medical Research Council classification) **(Table 39)**:

- *Stage I (prodromal)*: 1–4 weeks.
  - Nonspecific symptoms such as fever, irritability, malaise, and headache.
  - Anorexia, vomiting, or lethargy may be present.
  - Subtle neurological signs (e.g., personality change).
- *Stage II (meningitic stage)*:
  - *More pronounced symptoms*:
    - Persistent headache, fever, and vomiting.
    - Neck stiffness, photophobia, and Kernig's/Brudzinski's signs.
  - *Neurological signs*:
    - Cranial nerve palsies (commonly III and VI).
    - Increased intracranial pressure (papilledema, seizures).
- *Stage III (advanced)*:
  - *Severe neurological impairment*:
    - Coma, hemiplegia, and quadriplegia.
    - Decerebrate or decorticate posturing.
  - Life-threatening complications such as hydrocephalus or brain herniation.

DIAGNOSIS

Acute/subacute/chronic encephalopathy, meningoencephalitis of infective etiology with/without paresis, with/without cranial nerve palsy, with/without vision, hearing involvement, with/without evidence of increased intracranial pressure, involuntary movements, malnutrition grade, and vaccination status, probably etiology being TBM.

Differentials: Partially treated meningitis, viral encephalitis, typhoid encephalopathy, brain abscess, tumor, chronic subdural hematoma.

INVESTIGATIONS

- *Clinical suspicion*: Based on symptoms, history of TB exposure, or immunosuppression.

TABLE 39: Severity of TBM (modified MRC scale).

Stage I	Alert, oriented without any focal neurological deficit
Stage II	GCS 10–14 with/without focal neurological deficit or GCS 15 with focal neurological deficit
Stage III	GCS < 10 with/without focal neurological deficit

(MRC: Medical Research Council; GCS: Glasgow Coma Scale; TBM: tuberculous meningitis)

- *Cerebrospinal fluid (CSF) analysis (lumbar puncture):*
  - *Appearance*: Clear or straw-colored. Cobweb coagulum
  - Increased protein (100–500 mg/dL).
  - Decreased glucose (<40 mg/dL or <2/3 of blood glucose).
  - *Lymphocytic pleocytosis* (10–500 cells/mm^3).
  - Smear for acid-fast bacilli (AFB): Low sensitivity.
- *Imaging (CT/MRI brain)*:
  - Basal meningeal enhancement.
  - Hydrocephalus.
  - Infarcts (especially in the basal ganglia).
  - Tuberculomas.
- *Microbiological tests*:
  - CSF *GeneXpert MTB/RIF*: Detects TB and rifampin resistance.
  - Culture (gold standard but slow).
  - PCR for TB DNA.
- *Other investigations*:
  - *Chest X-ray*: Look for pulmonary TB.
  - *Mantoux test (PPD)*: Positive in 50% of cases.
  - *ESR and CBC*: Nonspecific markers of inflammation.

MANAGEMENT

Antitubercular Therapy

- *Intensive phase (2 months)*: Isoniazid (INH), rifampin, pyrazinamide, and ethambutol.
- *Continuation phase (10 months)*: Isoniazid and rifampin. Ethambutol.

Treatment duration: *12 months* for TBM.

Corticosteroids

Reduce inflammation and intracranial pressure. Prednisolone or dexamethasone for 4–8 weeks, then taper.

Management of Complications

- *Hydrocephalus*: Ventriculoperitoneal (VP) shunt or external ventricular drain (EVD).
- *Seizures*: Antiepileptic drugs.
- *Raised ICP*: Mannitol or hypertonic saline.
- *Cranial nerve palsies,* including vision and hearing loss.
- *Focal neurological deficits.*
- *Behavioral abnormalities and learning disabilities.*

Supportive Care

- Nutritional support.
- Physical therapy for motor deficits.

PROGNOSIS

- Mortality is high without early treatment. Stage 1: 100% recovery, stage 2–80% recovery, but 50% had neurological sequelae, stage 3—50% survive, and 80% have sequelae.
- Neurological sequelae (e.g., cognitive deficits and motor impairments) are common in advanced stages.
- Early diagnosis and treatment significantly improve outcomes.
- Hydrocephalus, optic neuritis, spinal block, infarction, epilepsy, intellectual disability, blindness, endocrinopathy.

Picture courtesy: Dr Arindam Ghosh, Dr Habib Mostofa, Dr Suman Mondal, some adapted from Internet source.

SUGGESTED READING

1. Amlie-Lewin J, Onesto C. A practical approach to acute hemiparesis in children. Dev Med Child Neurol. 2015; 57(11):1017–24.
2. Ashwal S, Rust RS. Disorders of the nervous system. In: Kliegman RM, St Geme JW III, Blum NJ, Shah SS, Tasker RC, Wilson KM, editors. Nelson textbook of pediatrics. 21st ed. Philadelphia: Elsevier; 2020. p. 3550-60.
3. Aulakh R, Chopra S. Pediatric tubercular meningitis: a review. J Pediatr Neurosci. 2018;13(4):373–82.
4. Campbell WW, Barohn RJ, editors. DeJong's The Neurologic Examination. 8th ed. Philadelphia, PA: Lippincott Williams & Wilkins (Wolters Kluwer); 2019.
5. Davis LE, King MK. Clinical approach to neurological localization. Am Fam Physician. 2015;92(7):528–36.
6. Graham HK, Rosenbaum P, Paneth N, Dan B, Lin JP, Damiano D, et al. Cerebral palsy. Nat Rev Dis Primers. 2016; 2:15082.
7. Hatherley C, Chavada G, Bowrey DJ, et al. Acute paediatric paraplegia: a case series review. Eur J Paediatr Neurol. 2013; 17(6):620-24.
8. Mercuri E, Pane M, Cicala G, Brogna C, Ciafaloni E. Detecting early signs in Duchenne muscular dystrophy: comprehensive review and diagnostic implications. Front Pediatr. 2023;11:1276144.

9. Patel D, Bovid KM, Rausch R, Longmire BE, Goetting M, Merrick J. Cerebral palsy in children: a clinical practice review. Curr Probl Pediatr Adolesc Health Care. 2024; 54:101673.
10. Peredo DE, Hannibal MC. The floppy infant: Evaluation of hypotonia. Pediatr Rev. 2009;30(9):e66. (Older but frequently used clinical context and differential diagnosis framework).
11. Slater GE, Swaiman KF. Muscular dystrophies of childhood. Neurology review article.
12. Swaiman KF, Ashwal S, Ferriero DM, Schor NF, Finkel RS, Gropman AL, Pearl PL, Shevell MI, editors. Swaiman's Pediatric Neurology: Principles and Practice. 6th ed. Edinburgh: Elsevier; 2018.
13. The child with macrocephaly, microcephaly, or head shape abnormality in Symptom-Based Approach to Pediatric Neurology. Kumar I, McNamara N (eds). Springer; 2023:463-85.
14. Walsh P, Jordan E. Fifteen-minute consultation: A practical approach to developmental regression in children. Arch Dis Child Educ Pract Ed. 2018;103(1):43–50.

CHAPTER 8

Examination of Genitourinary System and Its Disorders

Sumantra Kumar Raut

PART A: HISTORY TAKING

Kidney diseases constitute a chunk of general pediatric practice. In India, approximately 8–10% of total outpatient attendance and 12% of pediatric ward admissions have renal issues. Carefully eliciting the history and vigilance during case examination are key to success to reach a provisional diagnosis for majority of cases similar to any other subspecialties in clinical medicine. Congenital anomalies, urinary tract infection (UTI), inherited nephropathies, and glomerulonephritis (GN) are the leading causes encountered on daily basis. Alarmingly, 58% of children with renal failure presented at end stage highlighting the importance of a good history and examination for early diagnosis in such cases.

- As discussed in chapter of "History Taking" by our previous author in pediatrics, usually parents (more reliable) or grandparents (better data on family history) are major informants. In some case of infant with working mother history can be better provided by the primary caregiver.
- Age gives some clue about phenotype such as congenital nephrotic syndrome (cNS), Bartter syndrome (BS), renal tubular acidosis (RTA), nephronophthisis (NPHP) type 2, severe hydronephrosis (HDN) present at infancy. Idiopathic NS, postinfectious glomerulonephritis (PIGN), chronic kidney disease (CKD) due to congenital abnormality of kidney and urinary tract (CAKUT), and complement mediated atypical hemolytic uremic syndrome (aHUS) mostly happen during early or late childhood. Juvenile NPHP, primary hypertension (HTN), and lupus nephritis are more prevalent during teenage.
- Sex recognition is important as some X-linked recessive diseases might spare the girls or may have less severe phenotype. For example, Dents disease (tubulopathy with nephrolithiasis), Fabry disease (inborn error with proteinuria and CKD, heart, vasculature, and the nervous system involvement), Lowe syndrome (mother of those boys may have cataract), and Alport syndrome. In X-linked dominant diseases like some variant of Alport syndrome, affected females generally experience symptoms that are less severe and manifest at a later age compared to males. Antenatally diagnosed bilateral HDN with bad bladder may lead to suspicion of posterior urethral valve (PUV) in case of male child. Urinary tract infection (UTI) in infancy is more common in boys; whereas in older kids, it is more common in girls. Continuous incontinence of urine is more common in duplex ureters in girls than boys. Disorder of sex determination may happen in diseases like *WT* gene-related WAGR syndrome, variants of congenital adrenal hyperplasia.
- *Address*: Hypertension in children is commoner in urban kids. Renal stone is more common in North-Western India in comparison to Southern part due climate and other issues. D+ HUS epidemics may follow some geographical area with high burden of cholera or diarrhea.
- *Religion*: Certain genetic diseases such as tubulopathy, congenital nephrotic, and genetic complement abnormalities are common in religions with higher incidence of consanguineous marriage like Muslims and descendent of Jews.
- *Chief complaints*: Most of the patients with renal disorders pointing toward specific pathology though there are few overlaps between pathology of different parts of kidney involved and as well with other systems involvement. Many of the patients may remain asymptomatic till advance stage of renal disease. Repeated blood transfusion for anemia of CKD can be misdiagnosed as congenital hemolytic anemia unless looked carefully **(Table 1)**.

TABLE 1: Various complaints in patients with kidney disease.

Complaints	*Probable etiology*	*Comments*
Anasarca, puffy face	NS, acute glomerulonephritis (AGN), AKI, CKD	*D/Ds:* Heart failure, liver failure, hypothyroidism, angioedema, malnutrition
Syndromic face	CAKUT, cNS	*Cushingoid face:* Steroid effect
Low urine output	NS, AGN, renal failure, bladder outlet obstruction	Palpable bladder may differentiate postrenal causes
Red urine	UTI, renal stone, AGN, collagenopathy, renal/bladder tumor, renal vessel thrombosis, kidney cyst rupture	Routine urine if have no RBC but blood + then hemoglobinuria; if blood and RBC both nil then likely various dye (foods/drugs)
Lower urinary tract symptoms	Dysuria, poor stream, urgency, incontinence, straining	UTI, bladder dysfunction, PUV in male child
Failure to thrive	CKD, tubulopathy	Long-term drug effect (steroid)
Polyuria, polydipsia	Tubulopathy (RTA, Bartter), ciliopathy (NPHP)	
Abdominal mass, with/without pain abdomen	Wilm tumor, hydronephrosis, ADPKD (polycystic kidney disease)	
Frothy urine	Proteinuria (NS)	
Pallor	CKD, dRTA with hereditary anemia	
Fever	UTI, renal abscess, lupus	
Seizure	HTN, HUS, collagen vascular disease	
Rash, arthritis	PIGN, collagen vascular disease, HSP	PIGN has resolving rash
Constipation	Comorbidity with UTI, bowel bladder dysfunction (BBD), neurogenic bladder	
Abnormal hearing	RTA, Alport syndrome	Ototoxicity by frusemide
Abnormal vision	Night blindness: pRTA; photophobia: cystinosis	

(ADPKD: autosomal dominant polycystic kidney disease; AKI: acute kidney injury; CKD: chronic kidney disease; CAKUT: congenital anomalies of the kidney and urinary tract; D/D: differential diagnosis; HTN: hypertension; HUS: hemolytic uremic syndrome; PIGN: post-infectious glomerulonephritis; RTA: renal tubular acidosis; UTI: urinary tract infection)

- *History of present illness (HOPI)*: Symptoms to be stated as per chronology as discussed in "History Taking" chapter. In case of disease course with multiple relapses like NS or repeated UTI with neurogenic bladder, history starts when first symptom was noticed and not only from current episode. History should be in patient own language so instead of hematuria, it should be red urine. Comorbid history to be asked for other system too as congenital abnormalities may point toward CAKUT, etc., if parents are maintaining uristix and drug diary for NS that has to be checked.
- *History of past illness*: History of similar episode under different spectrum (like prior UTI with no known risk factor) or different episode but having some relevance to be mentioned. Past history of AKI ever in lifetime carries relevance in case of CKD. History of renal biopsy if done for any reason to ask for.
- *Treatment history*: Treatment for current or prior illness [various immunosuppression, e.g., levamisole, cyclophosphamide (usually not to be repeated in lifetime for renal causes if received full course once), mycophenolate, tacrolimus, cyclosporine, monoclonals for long course NS; prior antibiotics therapy or prophylaxis for repeated UTI]. Long-term antihypertensive empty pill count to be done to check compliance.
- *Birth history*: Polyhydramnios (aBS), oligohydramnios (PUV, renal dysplasia), and antenatal USG scan reports if available to ask for antenatal hydronephrosis [PUJO (pelviureteric junction obstruction), VUJO (vesicoureteric junction obstruction), VUR (vesicoureteric reflux), and PUV]. Perinatal history for preterm birth (future HTN, CKD, Barker hypothesis), birth asphyxia (AKI), umbilical vessel cannulation

(HTN, renal vein thrombosis) to enquire. Death or disparity of one of the twin to ask for twin to twin transfusion syndrome (renal tubular dysgenesis).

- *Development history*: Global developmental delay may be a part of chronic disease (CKD, tubulopathy) or associated neurological ailments (nephronophthisis may be associated with Joubert syndrome or Meckel Gruber syndrome). Development quotient up to 5 years and scholastic performance after 5 years to be compared with peers.
- *Immunization history*: Any missed routine vaccine due to ongoing immune-suppressive therapy for long course NS to be asked for. Optional vaccines like varicella, pneumococcal, and flu shots to be checked from card. For CKD patients, double dose hepatitis B vaccine records and also periodic anti-HbS antibody titer to be checked.
- *Family history*: Positive family history for consanguinity, renal stone in early age, CKD, AGN, tubulopathy, renal transplant, and late improvement of bed wetting to be asked for. Deafness with kidney failure in maternal uncle to be asked for X-linked Alport syndrome. Family history of tuberculosis in last 5 years to asked before starting long-term steroid for NS.
- *Nutritional history or diet history*: 24 or 72 hours recall method is ideal to check child's protein and calorie intake of weekdays. CKD patients with FTT should be receiving higher protein (1.2–1.5 g/kg body weight) and calorie (110–140% of current weight). Salt craving to enquire for tubulopathy and polydipsia for tubulopathy and ciliopathy (NPHP). Amount of liquid intake in-between dialysis session for end-stage renal disease (ESRD) patient and gastrostomy feed volume in CKD patients to be asked for.
- *Socioeconomic status*: PIGN and other infectious related GN, snake bite are more common in poor overall hygiene of living. ESRD patients on CAPD (chronic ambulatory peritoneal dialysis) should have a single room without pet while performing peritoneal dialysis. Older child on clean intermittent catheterization (CIC) should have privacy in washroom. Financial status regarding maintenance of long-term medications (e.g., post kidney transplant, cystinosis, hypophosphatemic rickets) has to be checked.
- *Bowel bladder habit*: Proper bowel habit regarding timings, posture, seat arrangements since late infancy to be asked for (risk factor for repeated UTI). If child with neurogenic bladder is on bowel wash proper technique, timing and volume of wash have to be enquired.

SUGGESTED READING

1. Gulati S, Mittal S, Sharma RK, Gupta A. Etiology and outcome of chronic renal failure in Indian children. Pediatr Nephrol. 1999;13:594-6.
2. Harambat J, van Stralen KJ, Kim JJ, Tizard EJ. Epidemiology of chronic kidney disease in children. Pediatr Nephrol. 2012;27:363-73.
3. Jain S. Rationale, requirements and recommendations for best facilities and better future. World J Nephrol. 2023;12(1):10-20.
4. Kanitkar M. Chronic Kidney Disease in Children: An Indian Perspective. Med J Armed Forces India. 2009;65:45-9.

PART B: GENERAL SURVEY

After an excellent elicitation of history, a proper general examination and thorough systemic examination are the key to success for arriving at a good provisional diagnosis and a guidance for choosing investigations to reach final diagnosis after ruling out differentials.

- *Consciousness and well-being:* The consciousness can be semiquantitatively measured by age appropriate Glasgow coma scale. Child with seizure [HTN, uremia, HUS, neurological lupus, cortical sinus venous thrombosis (CSVT) in NS, dialysis disequilibrium syndrome (DDS)], etc. Psychosis in an older child may be due to steroid or CNI adverse effect. It is an art to calm the smaller kids and make them comfortable in mother lap before examining them or measuring blood pressure (BP).
- *Decubitus:* Child with severe anasarca with pleural effusion due to NS, collagenopathy, or child with heart failure due to renal failure might prefer to sit and may be restless.
- *Pallor:* Pallor because of anemia may be due to CKD, HUS, dRTA with hereditary ovalocytosis. For crying child, it may be looked into the palms and overall skin surface. NS can cause pallor without anemia. In NS with hypovolemia, hemoglobin (Hb) may be very high due to hemoconcentration but it usually does not manifest as hyperemia.
- *Icterus:* May be positive in leptospiral infection with AKI, acute hemolysis with cast nephropathy, hepatitis viral induced nephropathy (membranous or membranoproliferative) or secondary kidney injury due to hepatorenal syndrome.
- *Cyanosis*: Congenital cyanotic heart disease may present with cyanotic glomerulopathy with proteinuria and high serum uric acid. Central cyanosis with normal near-normal oxygen saturation in finger pulse oximeter may be possible in methemoglobinemia (happens when hemodialysis unit water treatment is done by activated chlorine agents recently; or patient with UTI with G6PD deficiency receives cotrimoxazole/nitrofurantoin).
- *Clubbing:* CKD may rarely cause pseudo clubbing due to secondary hyperparathyroidism.
- *Edema:* Edema due to renal condition is usually pitting and may start with localized involvement but may subsequently leads to anasarca. NS, AGN, AKI, or CKD may cause anasarca mostly with low urine output, differentiating it with cardiac and hepatic conditions. Edema mostly starts with eyelids, faces (rarely neck, forehead) in kidney diseases **(Figs. 1A to E)**. It may also involve scrotum in and in sacral area for infants **(Figs. 2A and B)**. Scrotal edema (and not penile edema) in NS if present is considered as severe edema and requires diuretics and hospitalization. Edema may coexist with hypovolemia (thready pulse, cold extremities, pain abdomen). NS patients with anasarca treated with diuretics may show pedal edema with sunken eyes simultaneously. NS and AGN patients treated with steroid and in remission may have cheek swelling (cushingoid) which may be confused as edema. Pedal edema in kidney ailment may also be due to side effect of amlodipine.
- *Facies:* Various syndromic patients may have different types of kidney disorders ranging from CAKUT to cystic renal disease, ciliopathy or even nephrotic syndrome. Congenital NS with microcoria (*LAMB2*) may indicate Pierson syndrome. Ear tags, potter facies may be seen in CAKUT. Lupus nephritis may have butterfly rash. Hair loss may be seen in lupus and VDDR type 2.

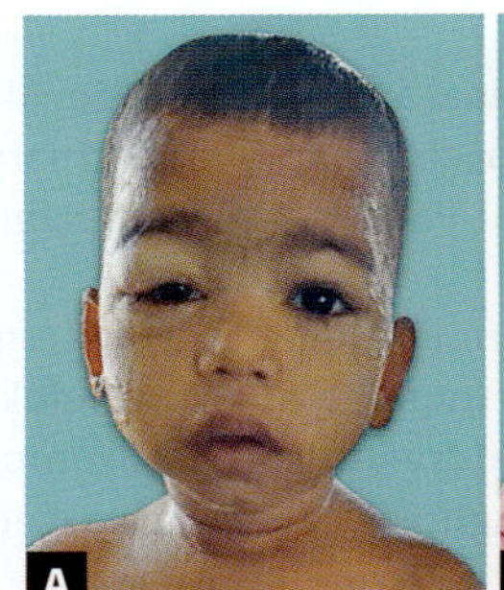

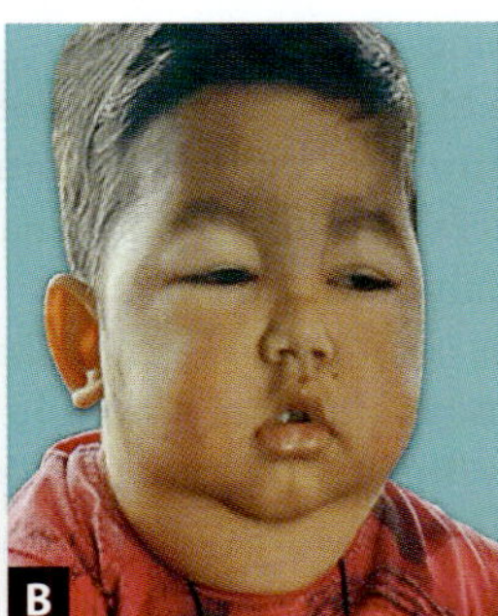

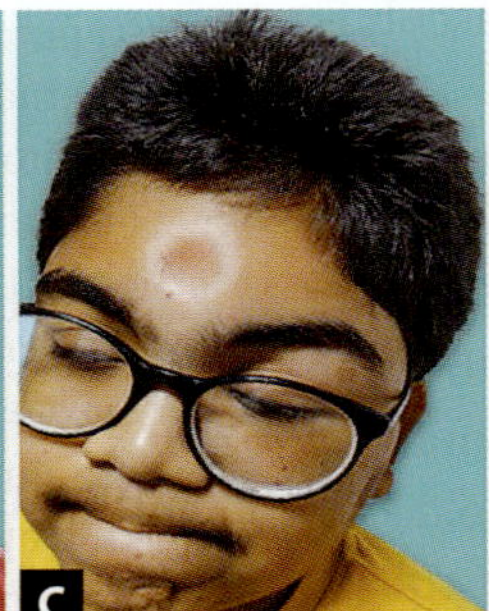

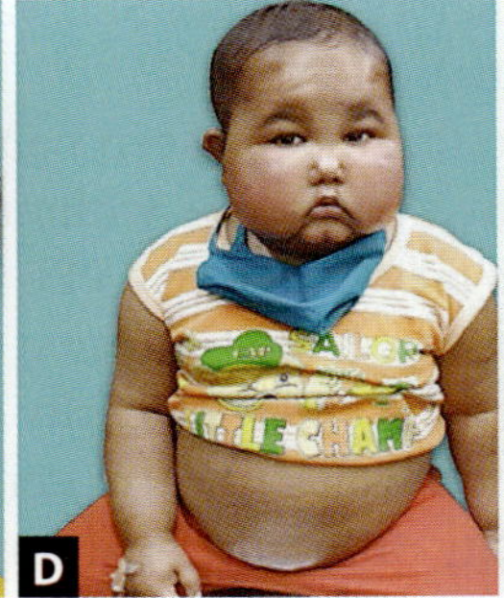

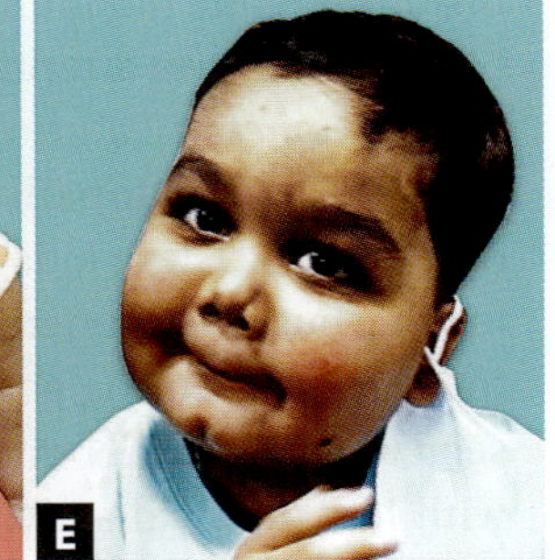

Figs. 1A to E: Edema in nephrotic children at different sites: (A) Eyelids; (B) Front of neck; (C) Forehead; (D) Facial puffiness with ascites plus cushingoid; (E) Cushingoid facies, no puffiness.

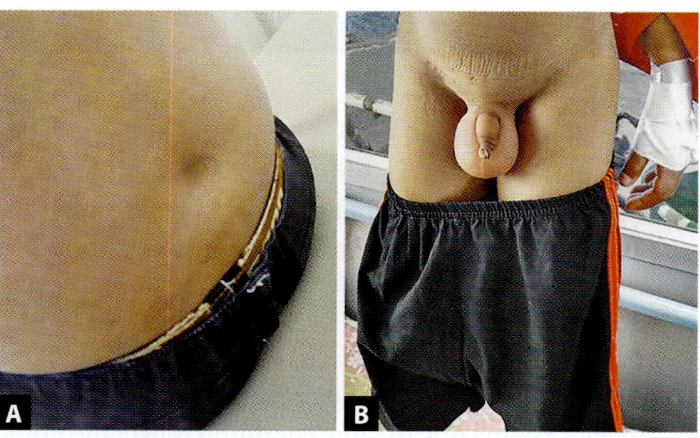

Figs. 2A and B: (A) Sacral edema; (B) Scrotal edema.

Cataract may be visible in Lowe syndrome (pRTA) and prolong steroid therapy in NS, AGN, and post-renal transplant kids. Aniridia (*WT1*) may be seen in WAGR syndrome (Wilm's tumor, aniridia, genital abnormality, and growth retardation).

- *Eyes:* Bitot spot may be seen in proximal RTA due to vitamin A loss in urine. Photophobia may be seen in cystinosis due to corneal cystine crystal deposit.
- *Vitals:* Thready pulse in otherwise nonseptic child with NS may signify hypovolemia. Differential pulse volume in 4 limbs my points toward Takayasu arteritis. Tachypnea in a NS child may be due to gross pleural effusion as a part of nephrotic anasarca or pneumonia owing to its immune-suppression or pulmonary thromboembolism owing to its prothrombotic state. Blood pressure should be checked in all OPD visit for all children with kidney diseases irrespective of age. HTN is common with AGN, NS, reflux nephropathy, renal failure, HUS, renovascular disease, connective tissue disorders, drug-induced (steroid, CNI) repeated UTI (owing to renal scars), monogenic HTN, etc.; and is less commonly found in renal tubule-interstitial disease. Fever besides infection is also a manifestation of autoimmune inflammatory state like SLE, vasculitis (ANCA, Takayasu arteritis).
- *Anthropometry:* Failure to thrive is seen commonly with CKD, tubulopathy, VUR even without renal dysfunction. These kids may also have a PEG tube or feeding buttons inserted over epigastric region that not to be missed during general survey. Obesity may be seen with NS or AGN who are on long-term steroid and with less physical activity or in postrenal transplant state (owing to improve appetite, prolong daily steroid therapy, more home confinement).
- *Bony deformity*: Rickets may be seen with normal renal function with acidosis (RTA) or normal pH (hypophosphatemic rickets, VDDR, and prolong steroid therapy) or in renal failure advance stage. Congenital NS with iliac horn is seen in nail patella syndrome. Broad hands may be seen in Bardet–Biedl syndrome. Thoracic cage deformity may be seen in Jeune syndrome (nephronophthisis associated with asphyxiating thoracic cage).
- *Neck nodes and neck veins*: Neck veins may be prominent and pulsatile in CCF due to renal failure (CKD, AGN) meriting urgent needs for diuretics or RRT. Nonpulsatile neck engorgement may be due to unilateral thrombosis of neck lines for hemodialysis or a proximally made AV fistula. Neck nodes may be generalized with tuberculosis which is more common in CKD patient in comparison to general population or in NS, AGN, or post-transplant patients due to immune-suppression. Kikuchi and Kimura diseases may have NS with enlarged neck nodes.
- *Skin appearance*: Stria in lower abdominal wall or proximal limbs may occur due to rapidly developing edema in NS, AGN, or owing to steroid therapy. There may be spontaneous rupture of skin and leakage of subcutaneous fluid in case of intense parietal edema in NS. Dry dehydrated skin may be seen in DI, RTA, and Bartter syndrome. Hyperpigmentation (café au lait spots in neurofibromatosis) or hypopigmentation (ash leaf patch in tuberous sclerosis) may be associated with renal vessel stenosis or renal cysts. Generalized itch marks in skin may be seen due to uremic pruritus.
- *Nails:* Half and half pigmented nails are signs of under dialysis in ESRD patients though more common in adults.

SUGGESTED READING

1. Arora P. Chronic Kidney Disease (CKD) Clinical Presentation. In: Batuman (Ed). Drugs & Diseases in Nephrology. 2024
2. Geetha M. Evaluation of the Renal Patient. Professional/Genitourinary Disorders/Approach to the Genitourinary Patient/Evaluation of the Renal Patient. Missouri: Saint Louis University; 2022.
3. National Institutes of Health. Chronic Kidney Disease Tests & Diagnosis. [online] Available from https://www.niddk.nih.gov/health-information/kidney-disease/chronic-kidney-disease-ckd/tests-diagnosis. [Last accessed December, 2025]
4. Rault R, Carpenter B. Pseudoclubbing in chronic renal failure. Q J Med. 1989;73(271):1063-9.

PART C: EXAMINATION OF GENITOURINARY SYSTEM

After a proper history elicitation and general examination, a thorough systemic examination is required to narrow down the provisional diagnosis which will guide for further investigations to reach to the final diagnosis. Genitourinary (GU) system examination usually comes under per abdominal examination and classically described under the heading of inspection, palpation, percussion, and auscultation. Here, we will touch upon the key points of GU system related findings.

Inspection

- Any renal mass in lumber area—hydronephrosis, MCDK (multicystic dysplastic kidney), cystic diseases [ADPKD (autosomal dominant polycystic kidney) and ARPKD], renal tumors (Wilm's tumor, nephroblastoma).
- Suprapubic distension may suggest full urinary bladder [bladder outlet obstruction (BOO), PUV (posterior urethral valve)].
- Ascites may be seen as a part of anasarca in case of renal failure either acute or chronic or in case of nephrotic syndrome (NS) or acute glomerulonephritis (AGN) even in absence of much renal failure. Cellulitis of anterior abdominal wall or scrotal wall may be seen due to complication of NS. Genital edema is considered as severe edema in respect to anasarca unless any local cause exists **(Figs. 3A to E)**. Spontaneous clear fluid leak can happen from tight abdominal wall if ascites if huge along with parietal edema in nephrotic state. Purpuric ecchymotic rashes in abdominal wall or buttock may be seen in vasculitis like HSP of lupus or ANCA-mediated vasculitis. It may also be seen due to low platelets in HUS/TTP. Striae can be seen in lower abdomen and inner thighs if there is sudden increase in abdominal girth due to development of huge ascites suddenly in NS in recent past. Again, ascites has to be differentiated from obesity/cushingoid in a NS child on high dose steroid. In ascites, the umbilicus will be a horizontal slit or everted while in cushingoid obesity, it is inverted as in case of normal child.
- Look for urine leaking or nonleaking stoma like ureterostomy [in case of vesicoureteric junction (VUJ) obstruction or vesicoureteric reflux (VUR) management], suprapubic cystostomy (in case of BOO), weeping umbilicus of patent urachus (urine coming through umbilicus), or leak of urine from penis tip or its ventral part (hypospadias) or dorsal part (epispadias), or an open bladder (bladder exstrophy), or any other fistula orifice. Patients with neurogenic bladder may be doing CIC (clean intermittent catheterization) through a Mitrofanoff (appendico-vesicostomy created for easy and often self-assisted bladder catheterization).
- To take note of any catheter, its type, duration of dwelling, and its health status regarding infection (exit point skin color change, any discharge, tunnel swelling, and redness). Catheter may be for per urethral catheterization Foley's/NG tube (for urinary retention), nephrostomy pigtail catheter (pyonephrosis drainage), Mickey button (for cystostomy and CIC through it); peritoneal dialysis catheter (temporary stiff PD catheter or permanent soft Tenckhoff PD catheter), PEG tube/button (for gastrostomy feeding in CKD/tubulopathy child), etc.
- Genital examination may reveal any DSD (disorder of sex determination). Examples are micropenis in boy with Denys–Drash syndrome, enlarged clitoris in female child with congenital adrenal hyperplasia **(Figs. 3A to E)**.

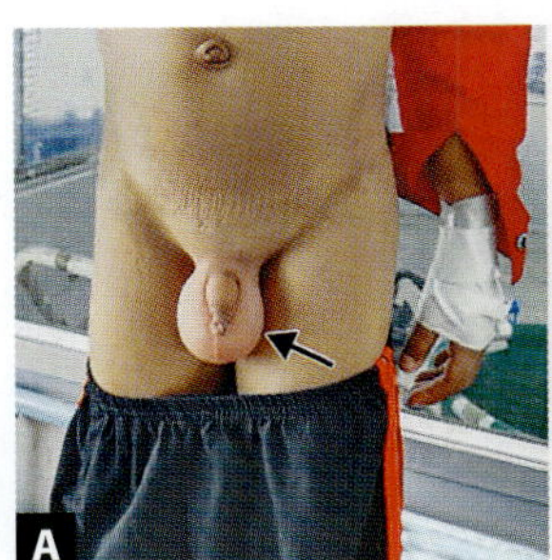

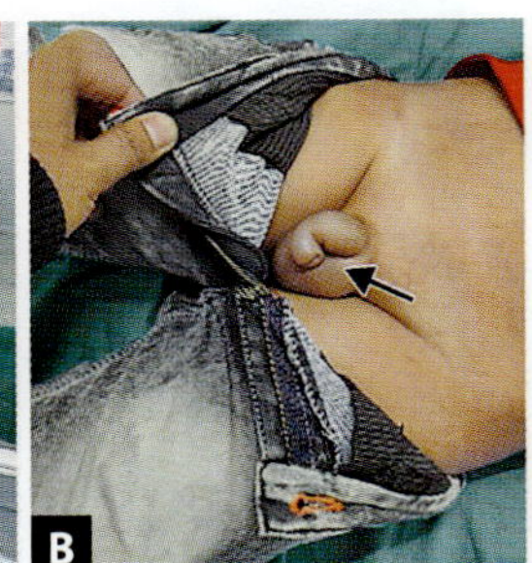

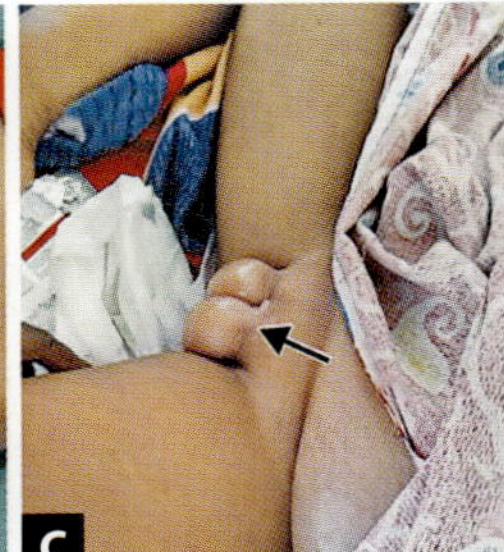

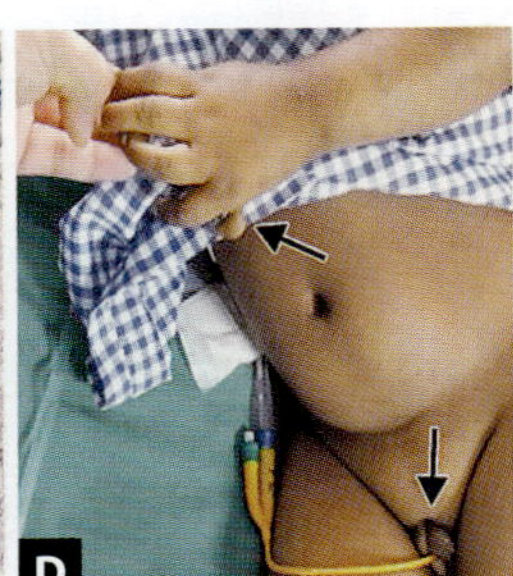

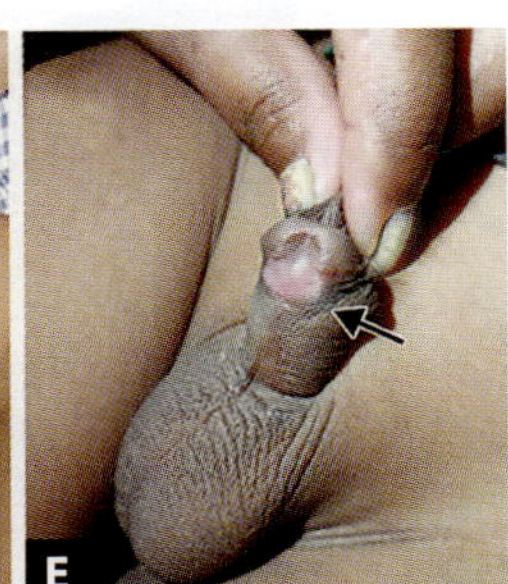

Figs. 3A to E: Examination of genital under genitourinary system: (A) Scrotal edema; (B) Penile edema; (C) Vulvar edema; (D) Micropenis with polydactyly (Bardet Biedl syndrome); (E) Hypospadias.

- Varied degree of hypospadias causes inward urine stream while epispadias may cause outward stream and may be associated with ectopia vesicae. In boys, phimosis may be present since birth and may be a trigger for repeated urinary tract infections (UTIs) while paraphimosis may be acquired later in life, mostly iatrogenic.
- In girls, labial adhesion can cause dysfunctional void, poor stream, and may lead to repeated UTIs. Also vesicovaginal fistula can cause leaking of urine through vagina or continuous urine leak may be seen in females in case of duplex kidney with upper moiety draining beyond sphincter.
- Inguinal hernia may be secondary due to persistently increase abdominal pressure due to constipation or straining during urine or may be a sequel of congenital hydrocele.
- Inspection of spine may reveal lump, pits, fistula opening in midline or paramedian area or may be tuft of hairs suggesting meningomyelocele (overt or occult) **(Fig. 4)**.
- Any prior operative scar (PUJ obstruction, ureteric reimplant, bladder surgery for stone of neck repair), suprapubic catheter scar, or prior peritoneal dialysis catheter scar has to be noted if present **(Fig. 5)**.
- A re-emphasis on privacy during examination of private part in older children and adolescent to be kept in mind. Keeping a female attendant alongside while examining an older girl child by a male doctor is also a prerequisite. Also, consent or assent from patient as appropriate for age is needed. One need to explain the benign nature of the examination process to gain confidence of the older child and also about the painless nature of some inconvenient examination like per rectal examination. Infants are preferably examined in their parent's lap.

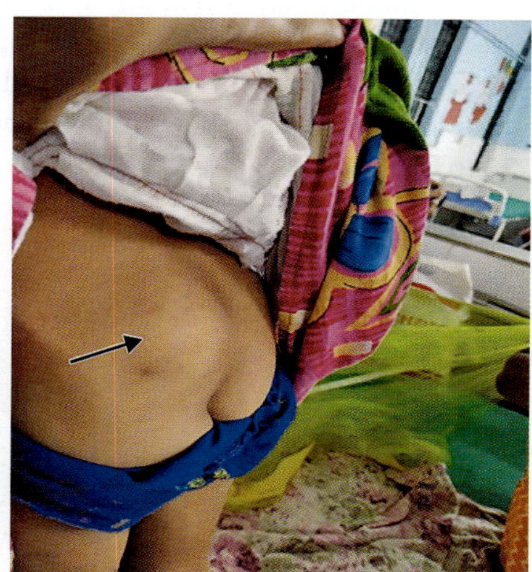

Fig. 4: Examination of back (meningomyelocele).

- To take note of bladder or bowel incontinence if an older child arrives with a diaper giving a hint to voiding or filling dysfunction of bladder or as a part of neurogenic bladder. Consider yourself fortunate if a male (or even female) infant passes urine during examination so as to directly visualize the stream which may be weak in voiding dysfunction or PUV.

Palpation

- *Superficial palpation*: Any tenderness in abdomen usually with ascites may suggest peritonitis or hypovolemia (due to mesenteric ischemia) in a nephrotic child in relapse or a renal failure patients on peritoneal dialysis. Tenderness over redness suggests cellulitis, another complication in NS patients.
- *Renal angle tenderness:* Gently pressing on the back side at the angle between lower ribcage and back muscle (Erector spinae) may produce pain in pyelonephritis, pyonephrosis, perinephric abscess, renal vessel thrombosis, obstructed or infected renal stone. Patient might be in lateral decubitus, upright or prone posture **(Fig. 6)**.
- *Deep palpation*: Ascites may be evaluated in case of anasarca in NS, AGN, AKI, or CKD patients. Milder ascites may be missed with fluid thrill or shifting dullness and puddle sign may help conveniently in older children.
- Fecolith or impacted fecal mass may be palpable in severe constipation that may put the child into risk of repeated UTI.

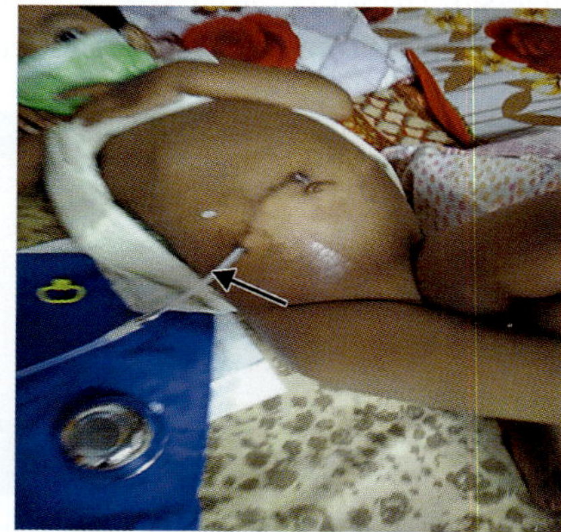

Fig. 5: ESRD child on peritoneal dialysis catheter.

- Phimosis or labial adhesion can be reconfirmed during palpation but gently.
- Renal mass may be felt in lumber area.

Q1. How to differentiate between renal versus nonrenal mass in lumber area?

Ans.

- *Bimanual palpation*: To examine any mass in right lumber area, patient will be in supine position, left hand of examiner in patient's loin while approaching from the right side of patient, right hand in anterior abdominal wall in lumber area. When examiner tries to approximate both the hands gently an enlarged or un-ascended kidney might be felt moving between both the hands through rubbing movement during respiration. Similarly for left sided mass, examiner may perform same maneuver while standing on the right side of patient or more conveniently can move to left side of the patient and can keep the right hand posteriorly and left hand anteriorly, doing the rest of the procedure similarly as on right side **(Fig. 6A to C)**.
- *Ballotable*: To examine ballottement of an intra-abdominal viscus while taking the position similar to bimanual palpation examiner may push the viscus with a gentle stroke by the left hand put at the back, try to feel if the structure is touching in the right hand placed anteriorly and dropping back to touch the left hand. Kidney can be ballotable or bimanually palpable if enlarged [ADPKD, HDN, MCDK, renal tumor, storage disorder (amyloidosis, etc.)] or unascended normal size kidney. Rarely gastric or pancreatic tail masses can also be ballotable. In infant or thin built children, kidneys may be normally palpated particularly the right lower pole during full inspiration.

Q2. How to differentiate between kidney and spleen/liver when enlarged?

Ans.

- Finger can be insinuated between lower ribs and kidney but not between ribs and spleen/liver.
- While percussing from above downward over the palpated organ, an intervening resonant structure (colon) suggests that the viscus might be kidney and not spleen/liver mass.
- Anal tone may be checked in a child with neurogenic bladder to assess for bowel incontinence.

Percussion

- Moderate ascites may be examined by shifting dullness or fluid thrill.
- Colonic resonance over a suspected left lumber mass may suggest renomegaly over splenomegaly.
- Full bladder will produce a dull note on percussion over suprapubic area.

Auscultation

- Renal bruit may be heard as a whooshing sound with a stethoscope approximately 1 inch superolateral to the umbilicus **(Fig. 6A to C)**. It can also be heard from the back near renal angle. It is a sound created by turbulent blood flow, due to renal artery stenosis (Takayasu disease, fibromuscular dysplasia, neurofibromatosis, and tuberous sclerosis). Though it is not specific

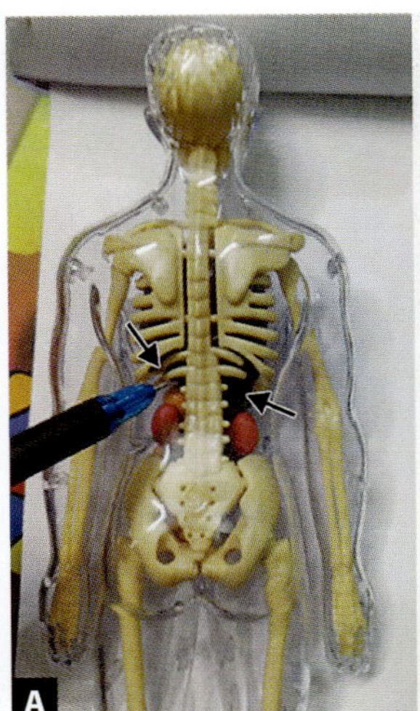

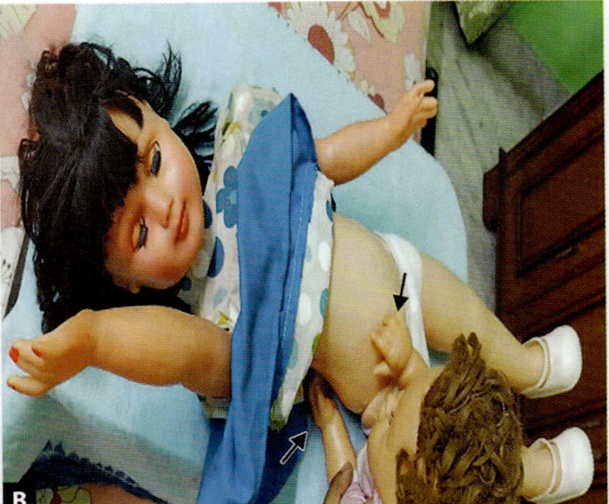

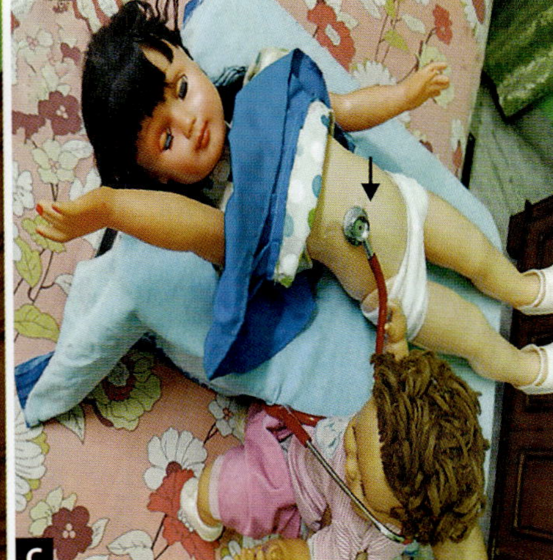

Figs. 6A to C: Genitourinary system examination: (A) Renal angle tenderness; (B) Bimanual palpation of right kidney; (C) Renal bruit over renal artery.

for renal vessel and may originate from any nearby vessels too.

After a complete genitourinary systemic examination, one may have to complete other systems examination to finally reach at a provisional diagnosis. We may always revisit out history once more and rectify it if we find some suggestions during examination related to the same disease in question.

SUGGESTED READING

1. Allan C, Stephen P. System Examination, The renal system. Macleod's Clinical Examination, 13th edition. Edinburgh: Elsevier Health Sciences; 2013. pp. 195-210.
2. Cendron M, Gearhart JP. The Mitrofanoff principle. Technique and application in continent urinary diversion. Urol Clin North Am. 1991;18(4):615-21.
3. Chow KM, Li PK, Cho Y, Abu-Alfa A, Bavanandan S, Brown EA, et al. ISPD Catheter-related Infection Recommendations: 2023 Update. Perit Dial Int. 2023; 43(3):201-19.
4. Keays MA, Dave S. Current hypospadias management: Diagnosis, surgical management, and long-term patient-centred outcomes. Can Urol Assoc J. 2017;11 (1-2Suppl1): S48-S53.
5. Simel DL, Rennie D. Abdominal Bruits. The Rational Clinical Examination: Evidence-Based Clinical Diagnosis. New York: McGraw-Hill Education; 2009.

PART D: APPROACH TO A CASE OF NEPHROTIC SYNDROME

A 3-year-old boy presented with puffy face for 5 days, decrease in urine output with frothy urine for 3 days, and generalized edema for 1 day. How to evaluate the child?

Q1. What is nephrotic syndrome?

Ans. Nephrotic syndrome (NS) happens due to increased permeability of glomerular filtration barrier of the kidney causing huge protein leak. It is classically characterized by massive proteinuria (nephrotic range: urine dipstick 3+/4+), hypoalbuminemia (serum albumin <3 g/dL), and edema. Hyperlipidemia (cholesterol >200 mg/dL) is no longer an essential criterion to diagnose NS as per recent Indian guideline (ISPN, SSNS Guideline 2021).

Q2. How much and what protein is being lost in urine in NS?

Ans. NS is characterized by selective albuminuria at least to start with; in huge amount, also called nephrotic range proteinuria. It is defined by (a) urine dipstick 3+/4+ (normal negative/trace) for 3 consecutive days *or* (b) spot urine protein creatinine ratio (Up:Uc) >2.0 (mg/dL)/(mg/dL) (normal <0.2) *or* (c) 24 hours urine protein excretion >1,000 mg/m^2/day (normal <100) *or* (d) urine protein 40 mg/m^2/hour (normal <4). It is also called glomerular proteinuria. Focal segmental glomerulosclerosis (FSGS) a variety of NS may have add-on tubular damage hence high molecular weight, nonselective, tubular proteinuria may happen too.

Q3. How common is this condition?

Ans. NS is a rare/orphan disease (when affected persons <50/100,000 population) with an incidence of 2–7 per 100,000 children per year and prevalence of around 16 per 100,000 children/year. The hospital-based prevalence seems to be bit more as relapsing disease keep on attending OPD and IPD repeatedly.

Q4. Which is the common age group affected with NS?

Ans. Idiopathic NS (iNS) is mostly a disease of childhood and majority of children have their onset of disease at 2–6 years and onset of classical disease is less common once teenage is achieved where secondary NS are more prevalent [lupus nephritis (LN), IgA vasculitis (IgAV), membranoproliferative glomerulonephritis (MPGN), idiopathic membranous nephropathy (IMN)]. Onset <3 months denotes congenital NS, mostly genetic abnormality in background, hence not amenable to immunosuppression. Onset less than 12 months denotes infantile onset NS where also a significant proportion are either due to genetic mutations or syndromic in nature.

Q5. Any gender preference for NS?

Ans. Among younger children, males have predominance, with ratio of boys to girls of 2:1, reason being unknown. In older kids, both the genders are equally affected.

Q6. How this kid usually presents?

Ans. (1) Children with NS present most commonly with edema. Puffiness starts from face and gradually progresses to limbs and trunk. As this is a dependent pitting edema so facial puffiness might decrease a bit as day progresses but for smaller children sacral edema may be prominent (to note anasarca of heart failure usually starts from leg and ascends upwards gradually).

Edema is obvious only when 3–5% of body weight of fluid is retained in the body mostly in the 3rd space (to note edema in AGN is associated with fluid accumulation mostly in the intravascular space too). Mechanism of edema in NS is through underfill theory though overfill mechanism or both may coexist in same patient sequentially. In severe cases, there may be ascites, pleural and pericardial effusion which are mostly transudate. Genital edema (scrotal in boys, vulvar in girls) denotes severe anasarca.

(2) Patients also complain of frothy urine and decrease in urine output.

(3) Many a time, these children have a trigger of upper respiratory tract infection of gastroenteritis to start a disease onset or a relapse.

Q7. What may be the unusual presentations?

Ans. Less often, children may present with red urine (hematuria), generalized rash, oral ulcer, arthritis, and hypertension at onset. These often exclude idiopathic NS (iNS) that denotes a secondary nephrotic state or nephrotic-nephritic picture like IgAV, MPGN, IMN, LN, and collagenopathy (Alport syndrome).

Q8. What negative history to look for?

Ans. (1) *Negative history regarding target organ*: Jaundice, vomiting, GI bleed (liver failure due to hepatitis); cyanosis, effort intolerance, sweating during feeding (heart failure); heat/cold intolerance, constipation (hypothyroid); itchy rashes tongue and lip swelling (angioedema)

(2) *Regarding etiology*: As mentioned in previous question and also abnormal hearing (suspected Alport), prior

sore throat or skin boils 2–4 weeks prior [suspected postinfectious GN (PIGN)], lower urinary tract symptoms like dysuria, incontinence, straining (reflux nephropathy may present with huge proteinuria and nephrotic state), or superadded UTI.

(3) *Regarding complication*: Existing cough cold respiratory distress (pneumonia bacterial/viral/PCP); diarrhea, vomiting (AGE); pain abdomen [spontaneous bacterial peritonitis (SBP)/mesenteric ischemia due to hypovolemia]; redness in abdomen, scrotum, thigh (cellulitis); unilateral limb swelling (venous thromboembolism); seizure [meningitis, cortical sinus venous thrombosis (CSVT), HTN (hypertension)]; anuria, hematuria [acute kidney injury (AKI), renal vein thrombosis (RVT)]

(4) *Regarding previous course of disease*: Onset, pattern, therapy, and management (how many relapses per year, prior drug used, prior hospitalization due to complication/renal biopsy)

Q9. What family history we need to ask for?

Ans.

1. Any family history of NS or renal failure, dialysis, kidney transplant in family members/siblings. Familial NS are mostly steroid resistance (SRNS) and not amenable to immunosuppressive therapy though familial steroid sensitive (SSNS) cases are also reported with good outcomes.
2. History of tuberculosis in family members or in close contacts in last 5 years (Mantoux test and sputum/gastric lavage CBNAAT may be required) as this kids will be requiring long-term immunosuppressions.
3. History of early onset diabetes mellitus (DM) in parents (long-term steroid or tacrolimus may put the kid at risk of DM). One may prefer cyclosporine (CsA) over tacrolimus (Tac) in such scenario if CNI (calcineurin inhibitors) is planned for.

Q10. What we can find in examination of such kid?

Ans. Examination of a nephrotic child has been explained in detail in previous Sections of this Chapter 8 [*Section B: General Survey and Section C: Examination of Genitourinary System*]. (a) Edema may vary from subtle/mild (only palpable when deep pressure given on shin or in sacrum) to severe anasarca (genital edema), usually pitting in nature. (b) Edema has to be differentiated from cushingoid features swelling of cheek and tummy with inverted umbilicus, but no eyelids or foot; cushingoid feature can be due to prolong steroid effect and it may coexist with skin striae in abdomen or inner thigh, bull neck, hirsutism, hair loss, etc.; hirsutism and gum hypertrophy may be due to CsA effect too. (c) Cold extremities, tachycardia, thready pulse may denote hypovolemia. (d) Altered sensorium may be due to HTN, PRES (posterior reversible encephalopathy syndrome) or CSVT or hyponatremia. (e) Child may look pale despite normal Hb or elevated Hb (marker of hypovolemia) due to subcutaneous edema. Jaundice may be present in viral hepatitis-induced nephrotic syndrome of nephrotic nephritic state (e.g., MPGN, MN). (f) Dysmorphism may be present in congenital or infantile onset NS (microcoria, iliac horn, Galloway–Mowat syndrome). (g) BP to be checked on every visit as per HTN guidelines (Flynn 2018); HTN may be due to disease process per se or drug induced (steroid, CNI).

Q11. What is the etiopathogenesis behind the whole story?

Ans. Idiopathic steroid sensitive nephrotic syndrome, especially MCD, is hypothesized to be mediated by a permeability factor produced by *T-cells*, potentially a cytokine. The hypothesis is backed by observations that NS is associated with lymphoma and atopy; induction of remission by immunosuppressive agents that inhibit T-cell function (corticosteroids or cyclophosphamide); prolonged remission of disease after infection with measles that depresses cell-mediated immunity; absence of immunoglobulins in kidney biopsies. On the other hand, pathogenesis of primary FSGS has been attributed to *B cell* activities as a putative circulating permeability factor [cardiotrophin-like cytokine-1 (CLC-1), vascular endothelial growth factor (VEGF), hemopexin, podocyte-derived angiopoietin-like-4 (ANGPTL4), IL-13, the soluble urokinase plasminogen activator receptor (suPAR), etc.] causing proteinuria recurrence immediately post-transplant in 30–50% of patients with idiopathic FSGS and therapeutic reduction in proteinuria by plasmapheresis or immune-adsorption. The glomerular filtration barrier consists of capillary endothelial fenestrations, GBM, and interdigitating podocyte foot processes communicating through signaling at the slit diaphragm. Proteinuria in NS is thus also attributed to structural abnormalities and loss of anionic charges of the GBM leading to ultrastructural changes, chiefly foot process effacement. Various genes, if mutated, cause recessive or dominant monogenic forms of steroid resistant nephrotic syndrome (described under genetic NS).

Q12. How we can classify NS?

Ans. NS can be classified as per *treatment outcomes* **(Fig. 7)**:

- Steroid-sensitive NS *(SSNS)*—attainment of remission (urine neg/trace for 3 consecutive days) in maximum 6 weeks of daily steroid
- Steroid resistance NS (*SRNS*)—failure to attain remission in maximum 6 weeks of daily steroid (approximately 15% of all NS).

Steroid-sensitive NS can be again subclassified as:

- Infrequent relapsing NS (*IFRNS*)—<4 relapses in any given year
- Frequent relapsing NS (*FRNS*)—≥2 relapses in first 6 months (date starts from steroid stoppage after 1st episode) *or* ≥4 relapses in any given year *or ≥3 relapses in any given 6 months*
- Steroid-dependent NS (*SDNS*)—relapses while already on alternate day steroid or within 14 days of omission of steroid and 2 such consecutive incidences. If relapse happens when the patient is on steroid dose >1 mg/kg on alternate day then it is a *high threshold SDNS*, below which is a *low threshold SDNS*. Many a time, there is an overlap between FRNS and SDNS unless patients maintain a very good uristix daily diary records for all the relapses.

If SRNS patient does not attain remission (partial or complete) with 6 months of CNI (calcineurin inhibitors) therapy (tacrolimus or cyclosporin) then they are labeled as CNI resistance (*CNI-R*).

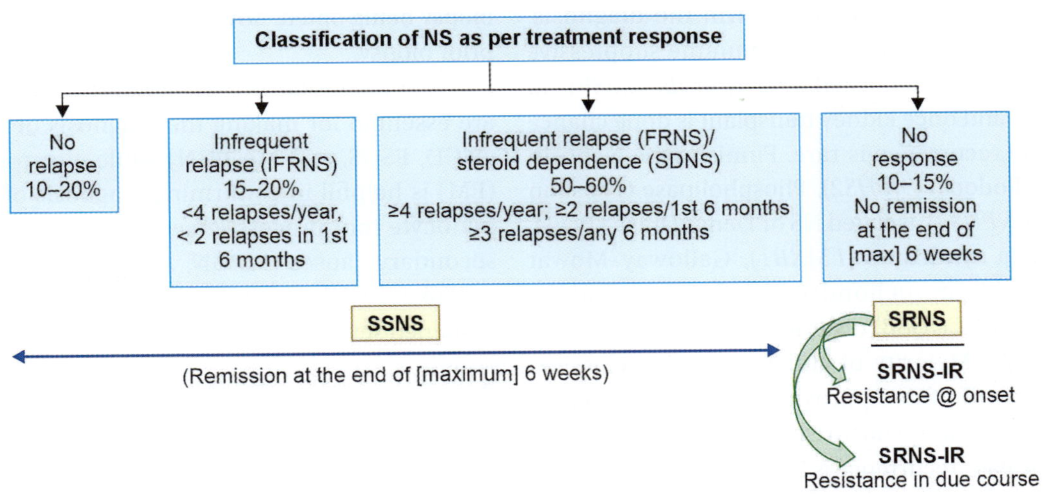

Fig. 7: Classification of NS as per treatment response. (NS: nephrotic syndrome).

Nephrotic syndrome can be also classified as per *age of onset* as:

- Congenital NS (CNS)—age of onset <3 months (majority have genetic mutation abnormality)
- Infantile onset NS—age of onset <12 months (fair number will have genetic mutation abnormality)
- Childhood onset NS—classical age of onset 2–5 years, most common variety
- Adolescent onset NS—age of onset after 12 years (may have underlying steroid resistance nature of secondary pathogenesis)

Nephrotic syndromes can be also classified as per their *histopathology* examination (HPE) as:

- *Minimal change disease (MCD)*: Light microscopy (LM) and immunofluorescence (IF) nearly normal and electron microscopy (EM) if done show diffuse (>50%) effacement of foot process (FPE) of podocytes. It happens in majority of NS (90% of SSNS and 45% of SRNS).
- *Focal segmental glomerulosclerosis (FSGS)*: <50% of all sampled glomeruli (focal) showed sclerosis in <50% of each glomerular capillaries (segmental). It occurs in 5–10% of all SSNS but 48% of SRNS.
- *Mesangial proliferative GN (MesPGN)*: 2–4% of all SRNS
- *Diffuse mesangial sclerosis (DMS)*: Leads to early and rapid end-stage kidney disease. It happens with *WT1* or *PLCE1* gene variants or with Denys–Drash syndrome.

Nephrotic syndromes can be also classified as per their *pathogenesis* as:

- *Primary/idiopathic NS*: Majority (90%) of NS with classic presentation, that includes MCD, FSGS, and MesPGN
- *Secondary NS*: It may present with some atypical presentation like microscopic hematuria, renal dysfunction, etc. and renal biopsy shows different glomerulonephritis (GN) like membranous nephropathy, MPGN, IgA nephropathy, lupus nephritis, hepatitis B related, etc.

Nephrotic syndromes can be also classified as per their *genetic etiology* as:

- *Genetic*: Majority of congenital NS and fair number of infantile and syndromic NS have genetic basis. We may opt for genetic testing (karyotyping, Sanger sequencing, clinical/whole exome sequencing) rather than renal biopsy to confirm the diagnosis. They usually do not respond to immune suppressive therapy hence not indicated. Mostly leads to ESRD in due course and once kidney transplant is done chance for disease recurrence is rare. Finnish type Nephrin (*NPHS1*), Podocin (*NPHS2*), Phospholipase C epsilon (*PLCE1* or *NPHS3*), isolated NS or Denys Drash (*WT1*), Nail patella syndrome (*LMXB1*), Galloway-Mowat syndrome, or mitochondrial CoQ10 cytopathies (*COQ2, COQ6, COQ8B*) disorders are few of them.
- *Acquired NS*: Majority of childhood onset classical nephrotic syndrome. Approximately 85% are steroid sensitive. They rarely end up with ESRD but if transplant is done, disease recurrence is 30–50% depending upon the histopathology.

Q13. What are the tests needed to come to a diagnosis of NS?

Ans. Routine urine test showing 3+/4+ proteinuria is the key to diagnose NS. Urine RBCs and WBCs are rarely found and may be due to underlying inflammation or FSGS pathology but not necessary infection/UTI. Nephrotic range proteinuria can be quantified in spot urine sample or timed collection as describes in Q2 above.

Documentation of low serum albumin (<3.0 g/dL) is essential while cholesterol of >200 mg/dL is supportive. Renal function is normal in most of the cases.

Atypical presentation like microscopic hematuria, skin rash, and older age of presentation may need serum C3, viral markers (hepatitis B, C, HIV serology). Mantoux test can be done prior prolong steroid therapy in TB endemic country like India and if positive may need to do chest X-ray, sputum or gastric lavage cartridge-based nucleic acid amplification test (CBNAAT) to rule out tuberculosis disease state. Kidney USG may be done as routine test in some centers to rule out underlying reflux nephropathy causing proteinuria.

Q14. When do we need renal biopsy in NS?

Ans. Renal biopsy is *not* required in majority of cases in NS in children as compared to adults. It is indicated if patients present with (1) gross hematuria, (2) persistent microscopic hematuria, low C3, (3) renal failure without hypovolemia, nephrotoxic drug use, (4) suspected secondary NS due to skin rash, arthritis, family history of secondary NS, higher age of onset (>14–16 years), (5) sustained severe HTN, and (6) steroid resistance. Suspected congenital NS, syndromic NS, Alport syndrome where previously renal biopsy being opted, now genetic testing is being preferred prior biopsy.

Light microscopy (LM) and immunofluorescence (IF) are essential for making the diagnosis of idiopathic NS (MCD, FSGS, and MesPGN) while electron microscopy (EM) is helpful in confirming diagnosis of MCD (to see podocyte foot process effacement) or to rule out other secondary causes (MPGN, Alport, etc.). LM also helps to look for CNI toxicity and renal vessel changes due to sustained severe HTN.

Q15. How to treat the condition at onset?

Ans. Idiopathic NS is treated with definite immune-suppressive therapy along with supportive therapy.

Steroid therapy [prednisolone 2 mg/kg/day (60 mg/m^2/day maximum 60 mg) in 1–2 divided doses daily in 1st phase and 1.5 mg/kg (40 mg/m^2 maximum 40 mg) in single morning dose on alternate day in 2nd phase] is the key drug and >85% patients respond to therapy and behave as SSNS. In 1st episode, the 1st phase is for 6 weeks and 2nd phase is also for 6 weeks (P6+6), whereas in subsequent episode, the 1st phase is for 2 weeks or till remission (urine neg/trace for 3 consecutive days) and 2nd phase is for 4 weeks (P2+4). On successful daily steroid therapy, child usually enters into remission [defined as free of edema and urine protein dipstick negative/trace for 3 consecutive days *or* Up:Uc < 0.2 (mg/dL)/(mg/dL) *or* 24 hours urine protein <100 mg/m^2/day (serum albumin >3.0 g/dL if done)]. Relapse is defined as further episodes with urine dipstick 3+/4+ for 3 consecutive days *or* Up:UC >2.0 *or* 24 hours urine protein >1,000 mg/m^2/day with or without edema once the child has entered into remission from previous episode. So, before jumping from daily dose to alternate day dose of prednisolone, it is prudent to document remission. There is very limited role for IV methylprednisolone pulse therapy in iNS as compared to AGN.

Q16. What are the nonpharmacological measures?

Ans. Supportive therapy is required for treating NS as well as to treat its various complications. Mild edema may not need any separate diuretics as prednisolone may cause diuresis by the virtue of disease remission in an average of median 8–12 days. Moderate to severe edema may require oral or IV diuretics (frusemide, thiazide, metolazone, spironolactone, or combination) for short period. In case of hypovolemia, diuretics to be preceded by volume (albumin) infusion. Fluid restriction may be needed in severe anasarca in hospitalized children. Calcium and antacids are not routine prescriptions but may be needed if steroid dose are prolonged (oral calcium with vitamin D) or steroid-induced gastritis happens (antacids). Salt zeroing is not advocated but restriction to free salt can be done. Protein-rich food like egg, etc. are promoted. For SRNS or CNS if TSH is found high, thyroxin supplements can be judicially used. Recurrent infections particularly URTI may precipitate a relapse so patients are advocated to use mask during outdoor activity and take age appropriate respiratory vaccines (flu, pneumococcal).

Q17. How to manage further course of relapses?

Ans. Subsequent course of relapses is treated with shorter course of prednisolone therapy (P2+4) as discussed earlier. If patient progresses to FRNS/SDNS then long-term agent has to be chosen as per ISPN 2021 guidelines. FRNS with no steroid toxicity can be treated with long-term alternate day prednisolone 0.5–0.7 mg/kg for 12 months. SDNS or patients with steroid toxicities (cataract, glaucoma, obesity, HTN, diabetes, and low BMD) need steroid-sparing agents.

Q18. What are the different steroid-sparing agents used in NS?

Ans. The different steroid-sparing agents to be used in FRNS/SDNS in increasing order of efficacy are levamisole, cyclophosphamide (CP) versus mycophenolate mofetil (MMF), CNI (Tac vs. CsA), and monoclonal antibody (rituximab).

- In FRNS or SDNS with steroid threshold for relapse <1 mg/kg: Levamisole, MMF
- In SDNS with steroid threshold for relapse >1 mg/kg: MMF, CP (>7 years age preferable)
- If patients fails (relapses despite 2nd agents) levamisole, MMF, and CP: May use CNI (for SDNS, doing renal biopsy prior CNI is not mandatory)
- *If CNI fails:* Rituximab or combination drugs

Q19. How to monitor side effects of various 2nd agents?

Ans. Adverse events of 2nd agents have to be monitored periodically:

- *Levamisole:* CBC, LFT, ANCA antibody, rash, flu like symptoms
- *MMF:* CBC, LFT, GI upset
- *CNI:* Nephrotoxicity, neurotoxicity, HTN, diabetes (Tac), hirsutism and gum hypertrophy (CsA); CNI trough level to be monitored (Tac 4–8 ng/mL, CsA 50–150 ng/mL)
- *Rituximab:* Infusion reaction, LRTI, hepatitis B reactivation, low IgG level; CD19 to be monitored

Q20. What are the common complications in children faced during the disease course?

Ans. As mentioned in history part above, various infective and noninfective complications have to be monitored.

Infective:

- *Chickenpox:* Varicella infection may have fatal outcome in NS; to be treated with varicella zoster immuneglobulin if available, else acyclovir prophylaxis/therapy; varicella vaccine to be given to NS patients when they are off all immune-suppressions for at least 4 weeks
- *Pneumonia:* Typical bacterial pneumonia, atypical organism (PCP, fungal, and CMV)
- *Spontaneous bacterial peritonitis (SBP):* Pneumococcal, Enterobacteriaceae
- *Cellulitis:* Anterior abdominal wall, inner thigh, preseptal in eyes

Proper antimicrobial agents for 7–10 days usually cause resolution.

Noninfective:

- *Thrombosis:*
  - Cerebral sinus venous thrombosis (CSVT)—headache, seizure, paresis
  - Pulmonary thromboembolism (PTE)—respiratory distress with silent chest
  - Renal vein thrombosis (RVT)—hematuria, oligoanuria, flank pain
  - Deep vein thrombosis (DVT)—lower limbs, redness, asymmetric leg swelling, pain

Heparin followed by oral anticoagulation (warfarin) for 3–6 months in CSVT, duration might be less in other cases.

- HTN and (posterior reversible encephalopathy syndrome) PRES: Headache, seizure; ACE inhibition (enalapril) > CCB (amlodipine) is drug of choice, PRES need IV anti-HTN (nitroprusside vs. labetalol)
    - *Hypovolemia and AKI*: NS may have 3rd space edema and hypovolemia at same time, judicious use of diuretics and prior volume (albumin) treatment will be required at that point
    - Adverse event of drugs used in NS including pancreatitis, gastritis: Periodic monitoring and symptomatic management

Q21. What are the causes of hematuria in NS?

Ans.

- Hemorrhagic cystitis due to cyclophosphamide therapy (due to acrolein component)
- Low platelets due to CP, MMF
- UTI (bacterial vs. adenoviral)
- Renal vein thrombosis

Q22. What are the causes of generalized tonic-clonic (GTC) seizure in NS?

Ans.

- PRES due to HTN
- CSVT
- Meningitis
- Hyponatremia

Q23. How to monitor these children in short term and medium term at home?

Ans. Parents to be taught to do daily uristix for home urine protein monitoring. To start with it helps to know day to remission (longer time may indicate future FRNS course), early diagnosis of relapse (prior to appearance of edema), and to assess the disease course in long run.

Q24. Any special vaccine care for this kids?

Ans. NS children should be well vaccinated with all the UIPs. To stress on *hepatitis B vaccine* [double dose (1 mL up to 18 years of age) at 0, 1, and 6 months to keep anti-HBsAb titer >10 IU/mL], annual *Flu* shots, *PCV-13* followed by PPSV-23 and *varicella* 2 doses. Live vaccine to be given when patient is off all immune-suppressions for at least 4 weeks and killed vaccine to be given while prednisolone dose is <0.5 mg/kg even if patient may be on 2nd agent.

Q25. When to refer to a pediatric nephrologist?

Ans. Most of the NS patients are well managed by general pediatricians. Referral to pediatric nephrologist is required if:

- Complicated relapse
- SDNS/FRNS course to choose 2nd agent
- SRNS course to plan for renal biopsy
- Familial/congenital NS

Q26. How to counsel the parents regarding the natural history of such children?

Ans. NS is a disease with prolong course with multiple relapses though majority (>90%) will outgrow the disease by adolescence and only few (<10%) will carry forward the disease through adulthood. If 2nd agents are wisely chosen and adverse events are well monitored, majority will have a normal renal function in adulthood. ESRD is rare (<2–5%) in overall cohort.

SUGGESTED READING

1. Churg J, Habib R, White RH. Pathology of the nephrotic syndrome in children: a report for the International Study of Kidney Disease in Children. Lancet. 1970;760(1):1299-302.
2. Eddy AA, Symons JM. Nephrotic syndrome in childhood. Lancet. 2003;362:629-39.
3. Hodson EM, Knight JF, Willis NS, Craig JC. Corticosteroid therapy in nephrotic syndrome: a meta-analysis of randomised controlled trials. Arch Dis Child. 2000; 83(1):45-51.
4. Sinha A, Bagga A, Banerjee S, Mishra K, Mehta A, Agarwal I, et al.; Expert Group of Indian Society of Pediatric Nephrology. Steroid Sensitive Nephrotic Syndrome: Revised Guidelines. Indian Pediatr. 2021;58(5):461-81.
5. Veltkamp F, Rensma LR, Bouts AHM, LEARNS consortium. Incidence and Relapse of Idiopathic Nephrotic Syndrome: Meta-analysis. Pediatrics. 2021;148:e2020029249.

PART E: APPROACH TO A CASE OF NEPHRITIC SYNDROME

A 9-year-old boy Ramu presented with puffy face for 5 days, decrease in urine output with red urine for 3 days. He had some skin boils in lower legs 2–3 weeks prior. How to evaluate the child?

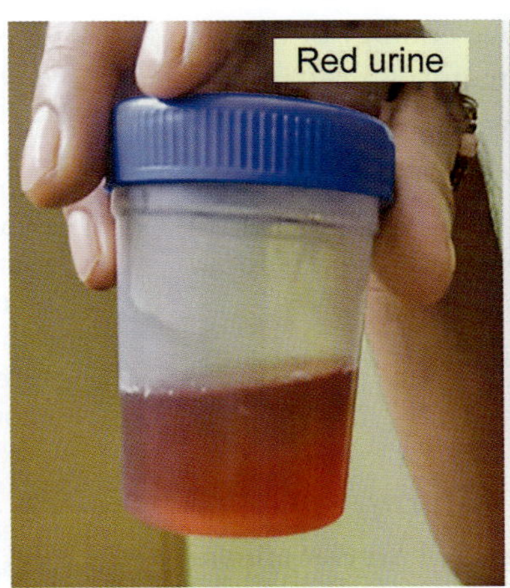

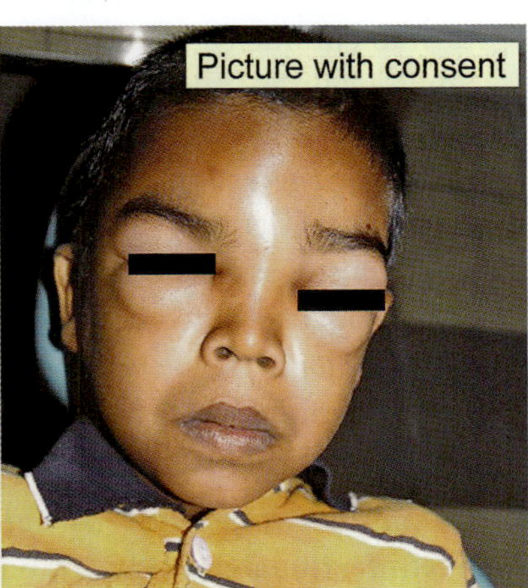

Q1. What is nephritic syndrome?

Ans. Nephritic syndrome or acute glomerulonephritis (AGN) is characterized by inflammation of the glomerulus due to diverse group of immune-mediated disorders that present with abrupt onset of:

Hematuria [gross/microscopic (>5 RBCs/HPF)]

- Proteinuria [nephritic range; Up 1+/2+ or Up:Uc = 0.2–2.0; 24-hours Up 100–1,000 mg/m^2]
- Hypertension (>95th centile age, height-related Flynn chart, 2018)
- Oliguria (<0.5 mL/kg/min)
- Low GFR [eGFR: (height × 0.42)/serum creatinine]
- Salt fluid retention, leading to vascular congestion

All features may not be present in a same patients or at same time.

Q2. How common is AGN in children and what is the common age group affected?

Ans. AGN is a prominent cause of renal impairment across all age group. The incidence of PIGN (most common prototype of AGN) in children is approximately 0.1–0.2% of all hospitalization though overall it is considered as an uncommon disease as affecting approximately 10–15 per 100,000 people (5–10 times common than nephrotic syndrome). Rates are higher in developing countries, with a prevalence of 50–90% of acute nephritis cases in low-socioeconomic societies. Whereas other primary glomerulonephritis is less common in children than in adults, with a global incidence of approximately 0.1 per 100,000 people per year. Common age group of PIGN being 3–12 years and rare in <2 years and >20 years. It is commoner in boys than girls. 97% of cases are seen in the low-socioeconomic world.

Q3. What are the differential diagnoses of AGN?

Ans. Similar phenotypes of red urine, proteinuria, deranged renal function, and puffy eyes may be found in:

- *Nephrotic syndrome*: Nephrotic range proteinuria (Up:Uc >2.0 or Up 3+/4+), low albumin, may be high cholesterol; hematuria is rare and renal failure occurs only if complications (see *Section D: Approach to a Case of Nephrotic Syndrome*)
- *Nephrotic-nephritic overlap*: Hematuria, renal failure, nephrotic range proteinuria, and low albumin
- *Collagenopathy*: Alport syndrome (type 4 collagen defect, X-linked, males are more affected, hematuria, adolescent onset renal failure, deafness, anterior lenticonus), thin basement membrane disease (TBMN) (familial hematuria, mostly benign condition, renal failure rare)
- *Tubulopathy*: Dents disease (tubular proteinuria, early onset renal failure, hematuria, and negligible acidosis)
- *Acute tubular necrosis (ATN)*: Hypovolemic, septic, drugs, and obstructive lesion are the common etiologies; mostly reversible. Hematuria is uncommon and proteinuria is rare at onset.
- *Acute interstitial nephritis (AIN):* Drugs or infection induced; hematuria, proteinuria may occur in 40–80% cases. Urine shows plenty of WBCs (eosinophil, if stained by Hansel's stain)

Q4. What are the different types of GN?

Ans. GN can be classified as per rapidity of *onset, etiology, histopathology, pathogenesis, and complements* level.

As per *onset*, it may be:

- *Acute glomerulonephritis (AGN)*: Onset within days to weeks, mostly <3 weeks; resolution by a month unless turn to chronicity; mostly infective etiology or trigger. Some features (microscopic hematuria, proteinuria) may continue for few months to years
- *Rapidly progressing glomerulonephritis (RPGN)*: In setting of AGN, worsening of renal function within days, mostly associated with crescent on renal biopsy and bit adverse outcome
- *Chronic glomerulonephritis (cGN)*: Onset over months; mostly immunologic etiology

As per *etiology*, it may be:

- *Commonly infection associated GNs*: May be postinfectious GN (PIGN), e.g., 2–4 weeks after a streptococcal skin infection (most common type of AGN in children worldwide) or sore throat (PSGN) (non-synpharyngitic) or concurrent with any bacterial infections, e.g., infection-related GN (IRGN), (IgA dominant lesion following staphylococcal infection) **(Box 1)**.

As per *pathogenesis*, it may be:

- *Primary*: PIGN, MPGN, MN, IgAN, primary MN, and anti-GBM disease
- *Secondary*: Lupus nephritis, ANCA vasculitis, HSP nephritis, and secondary MN due to malignancy

As per *histopathology*, it may be:

- *Subepithelial deposit*: PIGN, mostly IgG deposits
- *Subendothelial deposit*: MPGN (membranoproliferative GN, lupus): mostly C3, IgG

BOX 1: Etiology wise classification of AGN.

- *Postinfectious:*
  - Streptococci, staphylococci, pneumococci, meningococci, *Treponema pallidum, Salmonella typhi, Leptospira*
  - *Plasmodium malariae, P. falciparum, toxoplasma, filaria*
  - Hep B and Hep C, CMV, parvovirus, EBV, coxsackie virus, echo virus, varicella
  - Severe infections; infection of shunts, prosthesis, bacterial endocarditis
- *Autoimmunity-related GNs:*
  - Lupus nephritis, anti-MPO-Ab (ANCA-associated nephritis)
  - IgA nephropathy (most common noninfective cause in children in Western world and Japanese cohort; may be triggered with a sore throat within a week—synpharyngitic]
  - Anti-PLaR$_2$ Ab (membranous nephropathy)
- *Alloimmunity-related GNs:*
  - Allograft—solid organs, bone marrow or cells
- *Autoinflammation-related GNs:*
  - Inborn error of immunity—cytokines or complements; e.g., C3GN, MPGN (may need a second hit for onset)
- *Monoclonal gammopathy-related:*
  - Nephrotoxic immunoglobulin from B-cell/plasma cell: less common in children

(ANCA: antineutrophil cytoplasmic antibody; CMV: cytomegalovirus; EBV: Epstein-Barr virus)

- *Intramembranous deposit*: Membranous nephropathy (MN), mostly IgG
- *Pauci-immune*: No deposit, ANCA-associated nephritis

As per *complement (C3, C4) level*, it may be:

Low C3 is common in PIGN (the common garden variety AGN) at onset but it normalizes within 8–12 weeks, whereas persistent low C3 happens in lupus nephritis, C3G **(Flowchart 1)**.

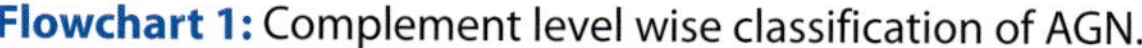

Flowchart 1: Complement level wise classification of AGN.

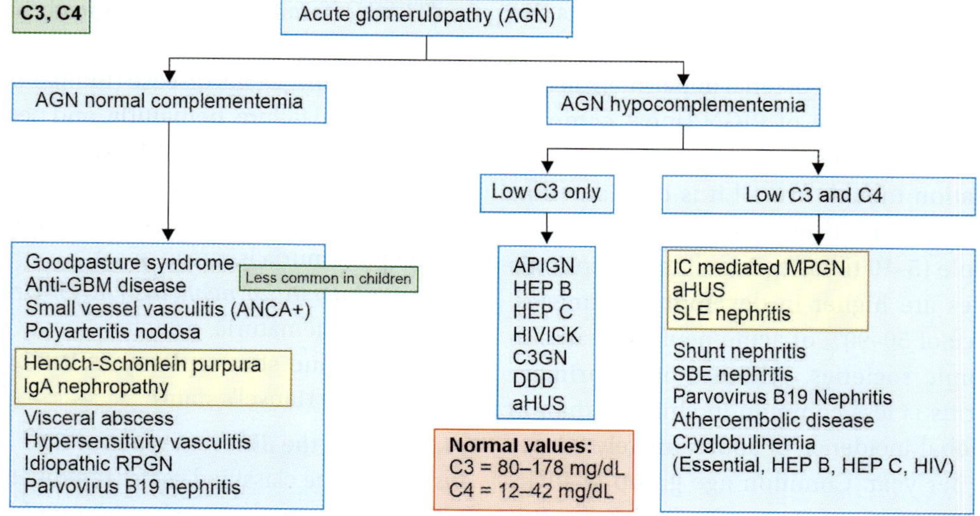

Q5. What is the pathogenesis behind AGN?

Ans. Following group A beta hemolytic streptococcal infection (nephritogenic strain) either a pyoderma or sore throat, the M protein, endostreptosin, strep pyrogenic exotoxin B (SPEB) like antigens trigger antibody production in patient. Due to mimicry of such streptococcal Ag with glomerular basement membrane and also due to some unknown genetic factor, Ab form against streptococcal components interacts with GBM or Ag-Ab complex circulates and later gets trapped in glomerular filter, stimulating complement activation and cytokines production subsequently leading to inflammation of the glomerular tufts. Risk of PSGN for nephritogenic strain is 15% and with B-hemolytic type 4 is approximately 25%. Repeat attacks are rare.

Q6. What are the clinical features in AGN?

Ans. At least 50% of AGN children are asymptomatic. Edema (60–70%), gross hematuria (30–50%), hypertension (50–90%), and oliguria are the major presenting features. Few patients may directly present with complications such as GTCS or CCF due to HTN or AKI without gross puffiness or red urine making initial diagnosis delayed. Boils or sore throat is mostly passive during presentation. Need to look for skin rash, purpura, arthritis, oral ulcers to rule out secondary causes of AGN.

Q7. What investigations we need to do in a case of Ramu as typical AGN and to rule out other DDs?

Ans. Urine analysis is the key test for AGN to document hematuria and subnephrotic range proteinuria **(Fig. 8)**. For typical PIGN, low C3 documentation is prudent. RFT to diagnose AKI and its repetition in case of worsening symptoms to diagnose RPGN which is a medical renal emergency. If secondary features are present, some other serology is also required. Renal biopsy is usually not required for Ramu as a typical PIGN but probably essential in all other variety to guide treatment.

Urinalysis:
- Microscopic or gross hematuria
- WBCs, RBCs, RBC cast, Dysmorphic RBCs (> 25%)
- Proteinuria [dipstick, spot urine protein: creatinine ratio, 24 hours Up]
- ASO titer levels: >200 IU, anti DNAse B-streptococcal markers
- CBC, CRP, ESR, C3, C4

Biochemistry:
- S.Creatinine, S.electrolytes, S.Albumin, S.Cholesterol

Selective conditions:
- ANA, dsDNA, ANCA
- Anti GBM IgM Ab, Anti PLaR Ab
- Hepatitis B, C and HIV serology
- Chest X-ray, paranasal sinus X-ray/CT scan, **Kidney biopsy**
- LDH, CBC, schistocytes

Imaging:
- USG KUB
- Echocardiography for ejection fraction in CCF, IVC fullness for fluid overload
- MRI brain in suspected PRES

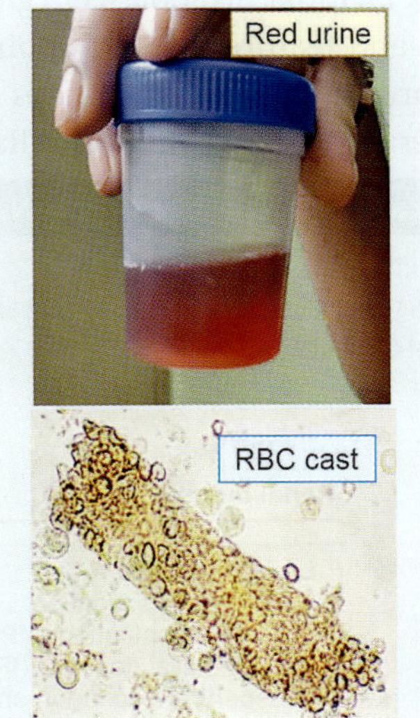

Fig. 8: Investigations in a case of AGN. (AGN: acute glomerulonephritis; ANCA: antineutrophil cytoplasmic antibody; LDH: lactate dehydrogenase; PRES: posterior reversible encephalopathy syndrome).

Q8. What is the main key complement which helps in diagnosis?

Ans. C3 is the key complement which helps to diagnose PIGN, rule out other DDs (as stated above). Repeat C3 after 8–12 weeks is also essential to reconfirm the diagnosis of PIGN. If repeat C3 is still low then C3G or lupus can be the alternate diagnosis and less likely PIGN. Hence, further course of treatment will also get changed.

A 10-year-old girl Rima presented with puffy face for 5 days, decrease in urine output with red urine for 3 days. He had some skin boils in lower legs 2–3 weeks prior. How to evaluate the child?

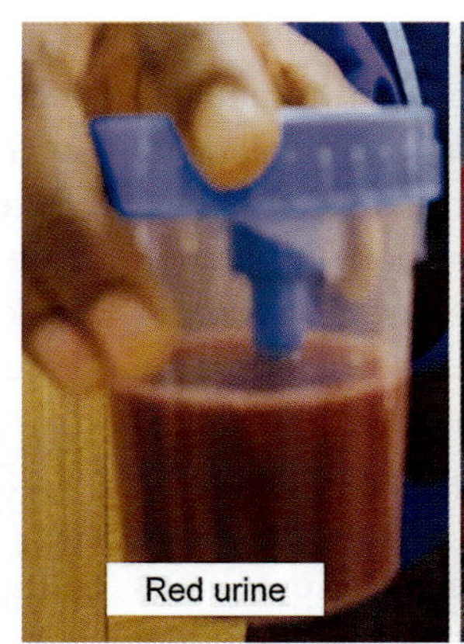

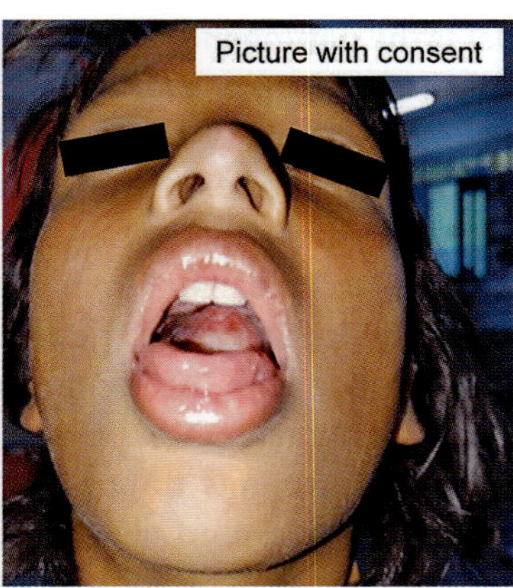

Q9. How renal biopsy can help us in diagnosis for Rima? Do we need a renal biopsy for all children with suspected AGN or typical PIGN?

Ans. Renal biopsy is *not* required in case of typical PIGN (most common cases of AGN). However, renal biopsy is essential for guiding therapy if some atypical features are there at onset or nonresolution of typical symptoms in due course **(Box 2)**. Rima, an adolescent girl with oral ulcer and malar rash and features of AGN, points toward SLE and lupus nephritis. Renal biopsy here is mandatory at onset to guide therapy for Rima but *not* for Ramu, a typical PIGN.

BOX 2: Indications of renal biopsy in AGN.

- *At the onset:*
  - *Systemic features:* Fever, rash, joint pain, and oral ulcers
  - Normal C3 level

Contd...

Contd...

  - *Atypical presentation:* mixed nephrotic–nephritic presentation, RPGN
- *Delayed resolution:*
  - Persistent oliguria, hypertension, or reduced kidney function >10–14 days
  - Gross hematuria >3–4 weeks
  - Persistent low C3 >12 weeks
  - Persistent subnephrotic range proteinuria >6 months
  - Persistent microscopic hematuria >12–18 months

(AGN: acute glomerulonephritis)

Q10. What are the key renal biopsy findings in RPGN cases?

Ans. RPGN patients reveal crescent formation on renal biopsy; underlying glomerular damage may manifest disease-specific changes (IRGN, MPGN, MN, and IgAN) as discussed in classification above **(Fig. 9)**.

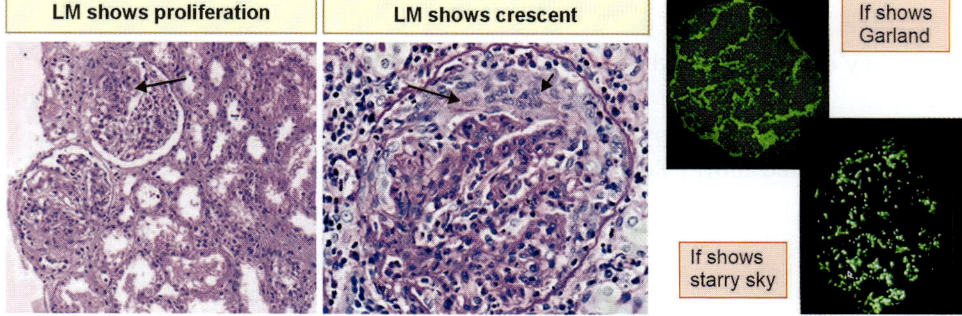

Fig. 9: Renal biopsy images of RPGN showing crescent in light microscopy. (RPGN: rapidly progressing glomerulonephritis)

Q11. How to manage a children with AGN?

Ans. Most AGN children need symptomatic management at home, at risk children require admission for volume overload, CCF, HTN, and uremic assessment **(Box 3)**. Most of them are managed conservatively. Few patients particularly RPGN cases require renal replacement therapy (RRT: peritoneal dialysis or hemodialysis as per feasibility). On stabilization, these children require renal biopsy on urgent basis and proper immunosuppressive therapy as per biopsy findings.

BOX 3: Outline of management in case of AGN.

- *Symptomatic:*
  - *Mild case:* Home management
  - *Mild edema:* Diuretics, fluid restriction
  - *Antibiotics:* Only if active lesions
- *HTN:*
  - *Oral:* Diuretics (furosemide/thiazide), amlodipine, enalapril once RFT and K^+ are stable on follow-up (overfill > underfill)
  - *Parenteral:* In HTN emergency—IV nitroprusside, labetalol (nitroglycerin if CCF)
- *Monitor:*
  - Weight, BP, intake, output → daily
  - RFT, Na^+/K^+, pH/HCO_3
- *Underlying cause:*
  - If treatable (IgAN, LN, RPGN, Hepatitis B, C); immune-suppression in specific cases
- *AKI:*
  - *Fluid restriction:* AKI regimen = insensible water loss (200–300 mL/m^2/day) + urine output → 4–6 hourly prescription, as urine output may be variable
- *CCF:* Injection furosemide → RRT in refractory cases
- *Electrolytes:*
- *Hyperkalemia (K^+):* Salbutamol nebulization → Injection calcium gluconate → Injection $NaHCO_3$ → calcium polystyrene resin [K-bind sachet (oral or per rectal, with lactulose]; STOP K^+in IV fluids/diet
- *Acid–base balance:*
  - Injection $NaHCO_3$ → if refractory or unable to treat → RRT
- *Nutrition:*
  - Resting energy 40–60 kcal/kg/day
  - Protein 10%, 2.5–3.5 g/kg/day (not to restrict protein in children)
- *Drug dosage:*
  - eGFR > 50 vs. < 50 vs. < 10 ml/1.73 m^2/min—nephrotoxic antibiotics dosage need to modify

(AGN: acute glomerulonephritis; AKI: acute kidney injury; CCF: congestive cardiac failure; eGFR: estimated glomerular filtration rate; HTN: hypertension; RFT: renal function test; RRT: renal replacement therapy)

Q12. When Rima will require renal replacement therapy (RRT)?

Ans. Patients with AGN particularly RPGN will require RRT in following situations:

A—Acidosis; refractory or unable to treat due to hypernatremia

E—Electrolytes abnormalities; refractory hyper-/hypokalemia; hyper-/hyponatremia

O—Overload; congestive heart failure, refractory to frusemide and fluid restriction

U—Uremic symptoms; uremic seizure, pericarditis

Mere high creatinine value is usually not a standalone indication for RRT in AGN.

Q13. What immune-suppressants we need for AGN?

Ans. Atypical AGN such as MPGN, MN, IgAN, lupus nephritis, ANCA nephritis, IRGN with or without RPGN presentation usually requires immune-suppressant. In case of RPGN:

- *Steroid:* Methylprednisolone pulse @10–30 mg/kg for 3–5 days (if patients is not infected) → followed by oral steroid in tapering dose for 6–12 months as per underlying pathology
- IV cyclophosphamide pulses 500–750 mg/m^2 3–4 weekly for 6 doses followed by oral mycophenolate (MMF) @800–1,200 mg/m^2 *or* azathioprine @1–2 mg/kg for 12–24 months
- *Monoclonal antibodies*: Rituximab (anti-CD-20) or newer agents like eculizumab (C5 inhibitors) may be required in special situations (e.g., MN, MPGN, and aHUS)

Q14. How to follow-up a child with AGN?

Ans. AGN child has to be followed up for a long duration with periodic assessment of growth (height), BP, proteinuria (urine spot PCR), renal function, and, if required, C3 and other serology. BP if elevated to be controlled with ACE inhibitor (enalapril, ramipril) or ARBs (losartan, telmisartan).

Q15. Do we need to give penicillin prophylaxis to patients with PIGN recovery just like rheumatic fever?

Ans. No. PIGN is caused commonly 2–6 weeks following a pyoderma by nephritogenic strains of Group A β-hemolytic streptococcal (GABHS strains 49, 55, 57, and 60) infection, occasionally by Group C or G and less commonly 1–2 weeks following sore throat by GABHS strain 1, 2, 4, 12, 18, and 25. Only handful of strains make recurrence uncommon, hence prophylaxis is unnecessary.

Q16. How to approach a child with suspected AGN?

Ans. After proper history and examinations to rule out atypical features; and after urine routine examination, blood biochemistry, serology once AGN is confirmed, we need to proceed as per serum C3 level as discussed earlier and need to direct our therapy accordingly **(Flowchart 2)**.

Flowchart 2: Approach to a case of AGN stepwise.

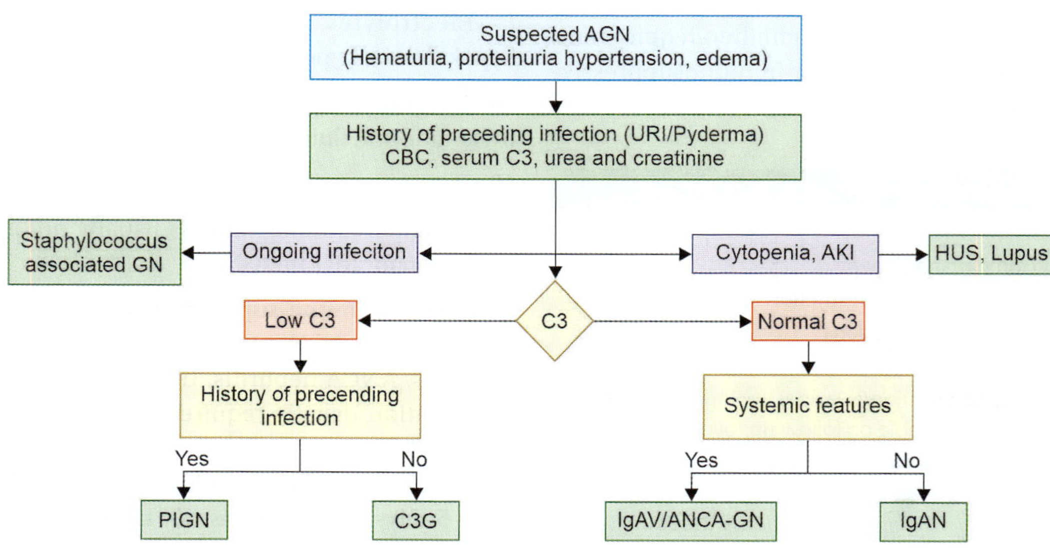

Q17. How is the prognosis for Ramu and Rima?

Ans. AGN patients particularly PIGN have excellent prognosis (95% complete recovery), ~1% develop RPGN, ~1–2% develop cGN; risk of CKD is <1%. Factors predicting poor outcome are crescent on renal biopsy, severe AKI at onset, and nephrotic-nephritic overlap. Hence, Ramu is expected to have good outcome.

SUGGESTED READING

1. Carapetis JR, Steer AC, Mulholland EK, Weber M. The global burden of group A streptococcal diseases. Lancet Infect Dis. 2005;5(11):685-94.
2. Ong LT. Management and outcomes of acute post-streptococcal glomerulonephritis in children. World J Nephrol. 2022;11(5):139-45.
3. Rodriguez-Iturbe B, Musser JM. The current state of poststreptococcal glomerulonephritis. J Am Soc Nephrol. 2008;19(10):1855-64.
4. Romagnani P, Kitching AR, Leung N, Anders HJ. The five types of glomerulonephritis classified by pathogenesis, activity and chronicity (GN-AC). Nephrol Dial Transplant. 2023;38:ii3-ii10.
5. Zahir Z, Wani AS, Jain M, Agrawal V, Jain S. Pediatric Glomerular Diseases in North India-Epidemiology and Clinicopathologic Correlation. Indian J Nephrol. 2023;33(1):28-34.

PART F: APPROACH TO A CASE OF URINARY TRACT INFECTION

Case 1: Misti, a 2-year-old girl, presented with 102°F fever for 2 days (January 23), cry during urination, and no cough and cold. There was no such prior history in this girl. Her primary pediatrician has asked for a urine routine and microscopic examination (RE/ME) which revealed Up trace/RBC 2–3 per HPF/WBC 4–5 per HPF and on day 3 urine culture (C/S) on clean catch sample revealed *Escherichia coli* with colony count 5×10^4/cc which was sensitive to amikacin.

Q1. What is the provisional diagnosis? In this present status of urine WBC count and colony count in urine CS report support the diagnosis of urinary tract infection (UTI)? Was the clean catch urine sample collection technique OK for a 2 years old girl?

Ans. Yes, this girl was suffering from UTI.

Urinary tract infection (UTI): Infection of the urinary tract is diagnosed based on the growth of a single uropathogen with a significant colony count in the presence of age-related symptoms.

As per ISPN 2023 guideline, presence of pus cell in urine is supportive but not essential to diagnose UTI. On a slight different tone, the American Academy of Pediatrics (AAP) defines an UTI in children with presence of both leukocytouria (WBC >5/ HPF in centrifuged sample; >10/HPF in uncentrifuged sample) and a positive urine culture with significant colony-forming units (CFUs) in presence of specific symptoms. Leukocytouria has only 76% sensitivity and 90% specificity to diagnose UTI and in non-*E. coli* UTI, pyuria is more often absent.

Significant colony count: As per ISPN 2023 guideline, significant colony count will vary as per sample collection method: clean catch: $>10^4$–10^5 CFU/mL, $>10^4$ CFU/mL in catheterized sample, and any growth (i.e., $>10^3$ CFU/mL) in a suprapubic specimen in the presence of symptoms. Previous convention for clean catch sample was $>10^5$ CFU/mL but infants with symptoms of UTI particularly with non-*E. coli* UTI may show lesser colony count so there has been a recent change in the colony count by clean-catch method.

Contamination rate of clean-catch (5%) is acceptable and comparable with specimens obtained from catheterization (8%) in young infants and it further reduces if perineal cleaning is done by soap and avoiding first-stream urine. Being noninvasive, ease of use, cost-effective, and acceptable, the clean-catch is the most preferred method of sample collection for toilet-trained children **(Fig. 10A)**. While it is challenging to secure urine specimens by clean-catch in nontoilet trained children, it should be attempted wherever feasible. Suprapubic aspiration and catheterization are reserved for sick infants and in patients where clean-catch has failed to obtain urine for culture. Warm and cold suprapubic stimulation (Quick-Wee method) may increase the yield of clean catch even further in infants. Once collected, the sample has to be processed fast within 2–4 hours else may be kept in fridge 4°C for 4–24 hours or in boric acid container. Culture sample to be sent prior starting/upgrading antibiotics. Urine bag sample or nappy pad sample is not at all recommended. *Staphylococcus epidermidis, Lactobacillus,* and *Corynebacterium* are considered nonuropathogen, so even if reported to be ignored.

Q2. How common is UTI?

Ans. UTI is a common infection in childhood especially in girls throughout pediatric age group except uncircumcised boys in first 3 months where the prevalence peaks up to 20.1%. Prevalence of UTI in various age group are as follows:

Infants: Boys < girls = 1.7% < 8.3%

Toddlers: Boys < girls = 1% < 2.1%

U-19 with fever/symptoms = 7.8%

2% of boys and 7% of girls experiencing at least one episode of UTI before 6 years of age.

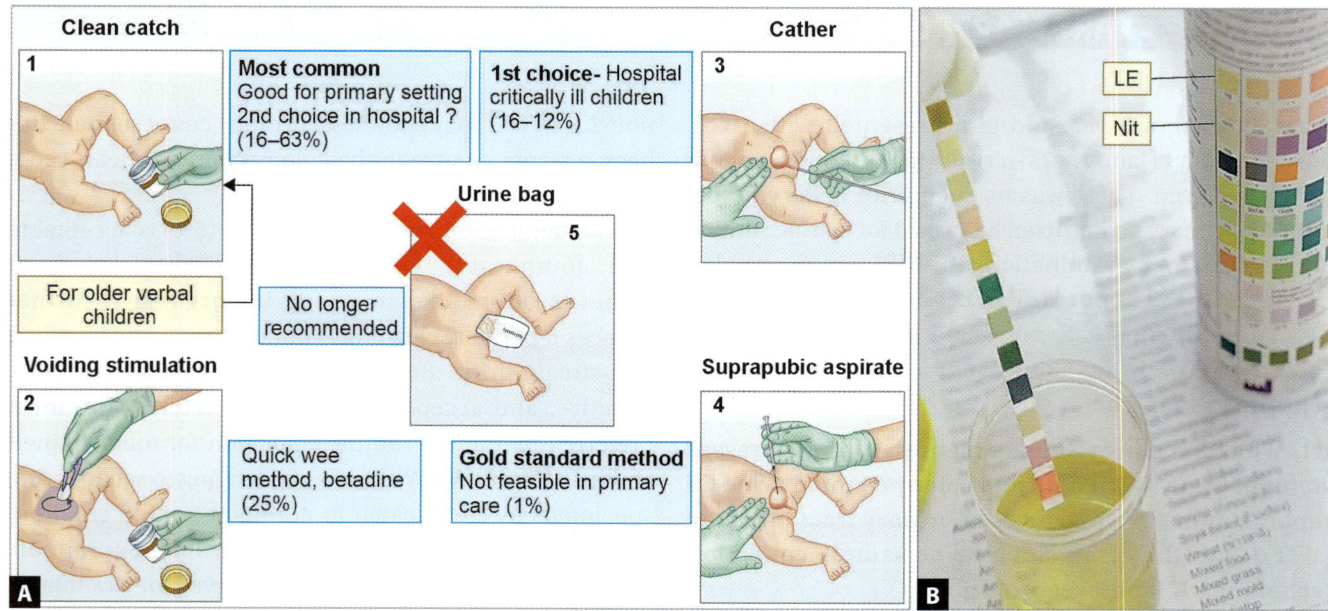

Figs. 10A and B: (A) Various methods of urine collections. (B) Urine multistix examination.

Case 2: Bristi, a 2-year-old girl, presented with 102°F fever for 2 days (January 23); cough and cold 5 days; no urinary symptoms. Her primary pediatrician has asked for a urine RE/ME which revealed Up trace/RBC 2–3 per HPF/WBC 14–15 per HPF and on day 3 urine culture (C/S) on clean-catch sample revealed *E. coli* with colony count 10^5/cc sensitive to cefixime and child was treated with the same just after sending the sample.

Q3. Is this also an UTI episode? What is asymptomatic bacteriuria (ABU)? Do we actually need to treat the girl for UTI?

Ans. NO, this is not an UTI episode. Asymptomatic bacteriuria (ABU): Presence of positive urine culture $>10^{4-5}$ CFU/mL of a single uropathogen in clean-catch urine specimen in *absence* of age-related UTI symptoms. Treatment of asymptomatic bacteriuria is not warranted under normal circumstances, not even in nephrotic syndrome or in other immune compromised state; unless child is planned for urinary tract instrumentation or child is an early renal transplant recipient. To be exact urine cultures should not be performed in asymptomatic children or if sent by mistake should be ignored. ABU may be also associated with leukocytouria. Leukocytouria without UTI may occur in any febrile condition, inflammatory state like Kawasaki disease, glomerulonephritis, foreign body/stone in urinary tract, AIN (acute interstitial nephritis) or in presence of UTI with urine CS negative as in tubercular, viral UTI or post-antibiotics sample (sterile pyuria).

Q4. What are the age-specific symptoms of UTI?

Ans. <3 months: Nonspecific, sepsis, vomiting, lethargy, prolong jaundice, poor feed, poor growth, and red urine

3 months: 2 years: Fever without focus, vomiting, lethargy, frequency, and hematuria

Older than 2 years and verbal children:

Complicated UTI: Fever, chills, abdominal/flank pain, renal angle tenderness

Uncomplicated UTI/cystitis: Dysuria, urgency, frequency, incontinence (recent), red urine, and suprapubic tenderness

Dirty urine or malodourous urine is neither sensitive nor specific for UTI.

Q5. What is the simple bedside test to diagnose UTI?

Ans. Urine multi-dipstick **(Fig. 10B)** testing for leukocyte esterase (LE) and nitrite reductase are two simple and effective point of care tests which may be done when UTI is suspected instead of or in addition to urine RE/ME (which is time taking and needs expertise to report). The sensitivity and specificity of either LE or nitrite are 84 and 88% and both LE and nitrite are 64 and 98%, respectively.

Q6. What other tests are required to manage UTI?

Ans. In uncomplicated UTI mere urine multi-dipstick, routine examination and CS are adequate. In complicated UTI, toxic child, and recurrent UTI, one may need additional blood tests like complete hemogram, CRP/procalcitonin, blood culture, urea, creatinine, G6PD (if planning to start prophylaxis with co-trimoxazole/nitrofurantoin specially in Asian boys), thyroid function, X-ray abdomen, USG for transverse rectal diameter (in case of constipation).

Q7. What are the prior history suggestive of risk factor for having UTI or its recurrence?

Ans. Other than the symptoms during an UTI episode, we need to ask the parents about the interim period symptoms like incontinence (primary/secondary), poor stream (self-check or ask parents to take few voiding videos), prior straining, frequency, urgency, urine holding maneuvers (Vincent curtsy posture), and most importantly constipation and child's potty habits/timings/sitting posture **(Fig. 11)** to rule bowel bladder dysfunction (BBD).

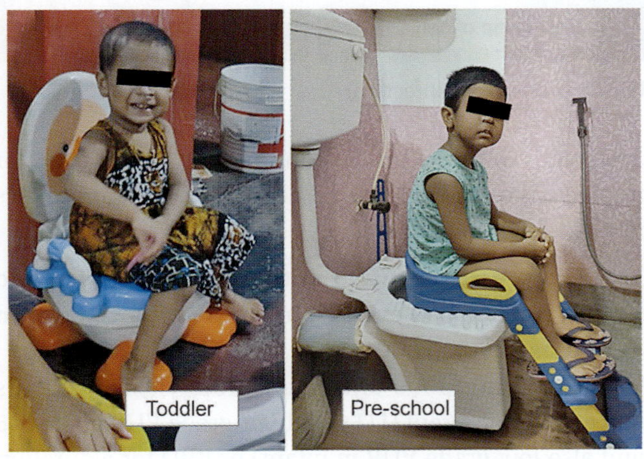

Fig. 11: Potty seat posture in various age group.

Q8. What are special examination points in a case of (recurrent) UTI?

Ans. Renomegaly (palpable kidney, ballotable and bimanually palpable) (also see *Chapter 8: Section C: Examination of Genitourinary System)* can be found in hydronephrosis **(Fig. 12)**. One may need to differentiate it from splenomegaly in left side (finger may be insinuated between rib cage and kidney lump but not in case of spleen). Renal angle tenderness suggests pyelonephritis/renal abscess. Genitals to be checked for phimosis and hypospadias for boys and vaginal synechiae in girl which may cause recurrent UTI if unresolved. Lower back to be checked for anorectal malformation, stigma for constipation (rectal prolapse), and marker of occult meningomyelocele (and tuft of hair, sacral pit/sinus) leading to neurogenic bladder and thus precipitating *recurrent UTI* (more than 1 episode of febrile UTI). Loaded colon or fecolith may be found in severe constipation. Privacy and consent during examining genitals to be kept in mind especially in case of older children in busy OPD. Blood pressure has to be checked and vesicoureteric reflux (VUR) or post-UTI scar in kidney may cause renin mediated hypertension. This kid may have normal clinic BP and high home BP (masked HTN) and may need 24 hours ambulatory blood pressure monitoring (ABPM) to diagnose that.

Case 1A: Misti, a 2-year-old girl, presented with 1st febrile UTI. Her primary pediatrician has started syrup cefixime for 7 days after sending urine routine and CS sample. Urine RE revealed Up trace/RBC 2–3 per HPF/WBC 4–5 per HPF and on day 3 urine culture (C/S) on clean-catch sample revealed *E. coli* with colony count 5×10^4/cc sensitive to amikacin but resistant to cefixime. Misti was already symptom free and well by day 3.

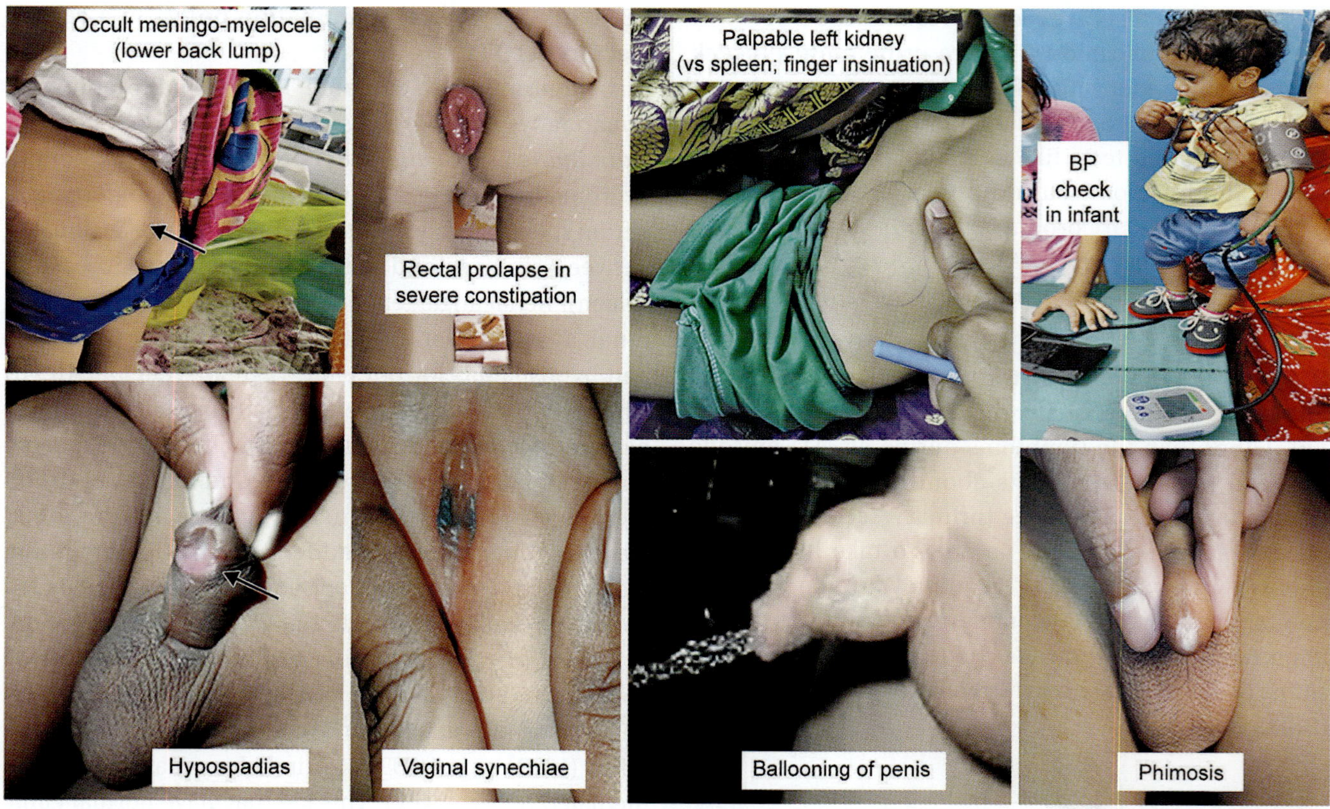

Fig. 12: Examination in a case of UTI. (UTI: urinary tract infection)

Q9. Was the choice of antibiotics, duration, and route were OK? Do we need to upgrade her therapy to amikacin on day 3?

Ans. Yah the choice of antibiotics was OK as in uncomplicated UTI oral route if preferred than IV and third-generation cephalosporin or amoxyclav (or as per local antimicrobial policy) is the first line choice. For UTI with systemic symptoms or fever, the duration of therapy is 7–10 days if the baby becomes well versus for lower tract symptoms like urgency, frequency, etc., only 5–7 days of therapy is fine. If child improves clinically by day 3 then same antibiotics may be continued till recommended duration irrespective of CS report. If child is not well by day 3 or worsens then antibiotics is upgraded to aminoglycoside, quinolones, carbapenem, or as per the CS report. If child is toxic or having repeated vomiting due to UTI or in case of young infants, hospitalization and IV third-generation cephalosporin, aminoglycoside, or quinolones may be indicated from day 1. Some drugs such as azithromycin or nitrofurantoin (NFT) are not drug of choice for treatment of UTI even if CS report reveals so though NFT may be used in lower tolerable dose for prophylaxis of UTI if needed. Early initiation of antibiotics may prevent renal scarring.

Q10. Does Misti requires antibiotics prophylaxis to prevent further UTI even if she does not have interim symptoms?

Ans. No. Continuous antibiotic prophylaxis (CAP) is indicated in recurrent UTI with high-grade VUR grade 3–5 (and also low-grade VUR in infant) or BBD for a duration till child is toilet trained, absence of BBD and no febrile UTI in the preceding 1 year. Narrow spectrum drug (in fear of drug resistance) like co-trimoxazole (2 mg/kg of trimethoprim) or NFT (1–2 mg/kg) is the prophylaxis of choice given at bedtime. For young infants, cephalexin is preferred (10 mg/kg). Prior G6PD deficiency, testing may be prudent before starting co-trimoxazole or NFT.

Q11. What are the supportive therapy required during UTI episode?

Ans. Adequate hydration is the key factor. Recurrent vomiting may warrant hospitalization and IV hydration. Constipation if any to be treated aggressively for a prolong period to prevent UTI recurrence by adequate water intake, proper potty posture and timings and osmotic agents or purgatives (lactulose, polyethylene glycol, and sodium picosulfate). Role of alkalization (Uriliser), steroid, etc. is dubious hence not recommended. Any voiding dysfunction to be treated with proper urotherapy (Kegel maneuver or other relaxation exercise) or drug therapy (alpha blocker, anticholinergics, mirabegron) as per urodynamic study findings. Neurogenic bladder or patients with high post void residue with difficult voiding may require clean intermittent catheterization (CIC) 3–4 times a day at home.

Case 3: Sristi a 4-month-old girl, presented with 1st febrile UTI. Urine CS revealed *E. coli* with 10^5 CFU/mL.

Q12. What radiological investigations she merits and at what time point?

Ans. A detail ultrasound of kidney-ureter-bladder (USG-KUB) including renometry is required in every case of UTI irrespective of age group, severity or recurrence to rule out some underlying congenital or acquired defect which may cause recurrent UTI or kidney damage in future. USG may be avoided in first few days of UTI as it may lead to overdiagnosis or underdiagnosis of hydronephrosis due to transient adhesion by the inflammation of UTI. But if a patient is not well by day 3, an early USG is warranted to rule out any renal abscess or pyonephrosis where add-on surgical steps will be required. Points to be covered on a post UTI renometry are kidney sizes, position, CAKUT (congenital anomalies of kidney and urinary tract; e.g.: horseshoe kidney, duplex system) cortical thickness in upper, middle, and lower pole, echogenicity, probable scarred area, AP diameter of pelvis if hydronephrosis (HDN) in pre-void and post-void condition, calyx dilatation, hydroureter (HU), urinary bladder (UB) wall, post void residue (PVR), urethra if dilated and additional comment on transverse rectal diameter (TRD) as a marker of constipation. Various abnormal ultrasound findings post-UTI are depicted in **Figure 13**.

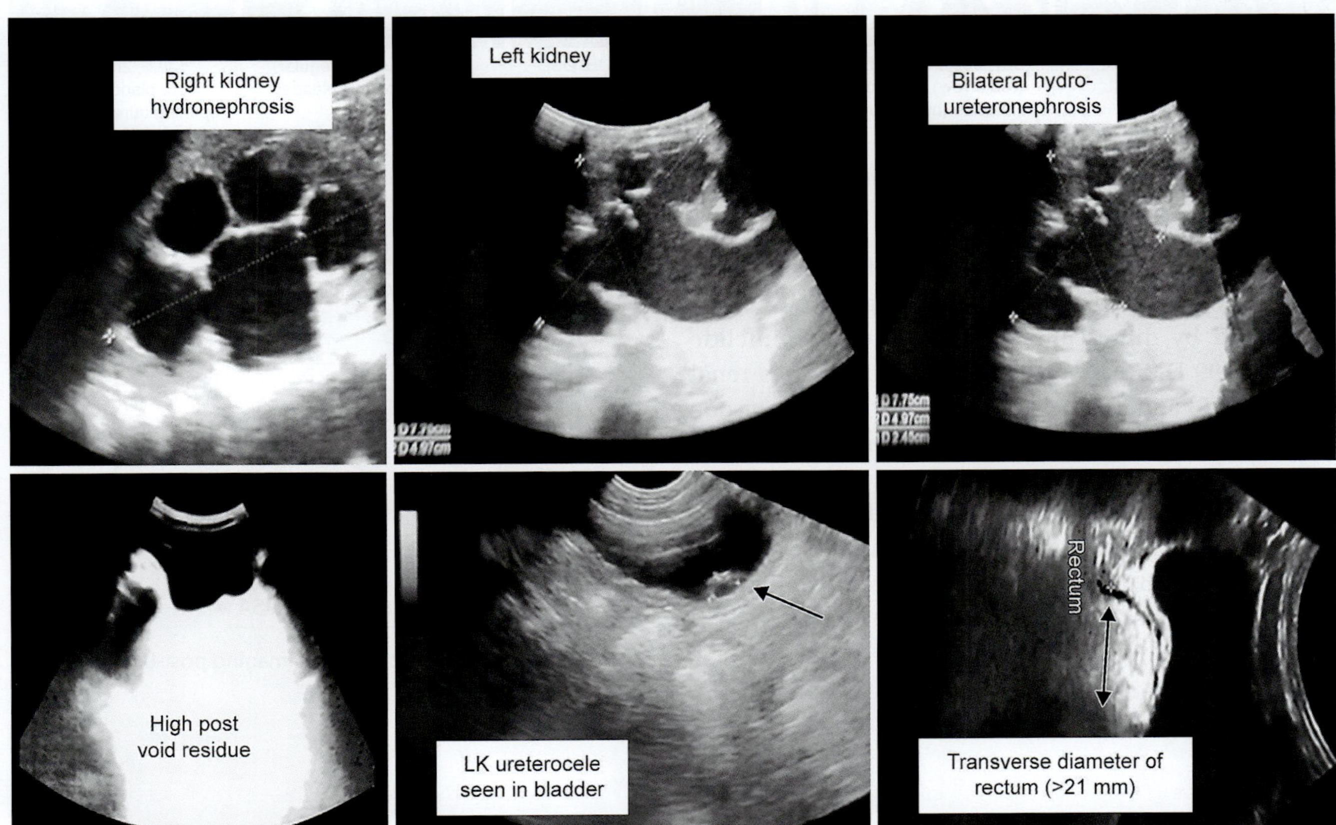

Fig. 13: Abnormal findings in USG-KUB.

The next radiological investigation required in UTI is a micturating cystourethrogram (MCUG/VCUG). It is indicated if USG-KUB shows any HDN or HDUN, abnormal bladder/urethra, or if the baby has prior poor stream or straining (especially boy child) or continuous urine leak or recurrent UTI even with a normal USG-KUB. Point to be covered in MCUG is urinary bladder wall and its volume during filling, any vesicoureteric reflux (VUR) grade 1–5 during voiding, proximal urethral abnormal dilatation or PUV (in male) or inappropriate contraction of urethra during voiding suggestive of detrusor sphincter dyssynergia (DSD), bladder neck inappropriate opening during voiding (dysfunction voiding), high PVR or any filling defects in UB like ureterocele. The initial control film also shows any spinal bony defects (neurogenic bladder) or bowel shadow of constipation. MCUG requires temporary catheterization, hence prior clean urine RE and 3–5 days antibiotics prophylaxis are practiced and it is prudent to do an MCU after 7–10 days of an UTI episode and not at onset. To lessen the radiation exposure during screening of VUR in siblings or for FU scan to see VUR resolution status, one may opt for DRCG (direct radionuclide cystography). Various MCUG abnormalities in post-UTI children are described in **Figure 14**.

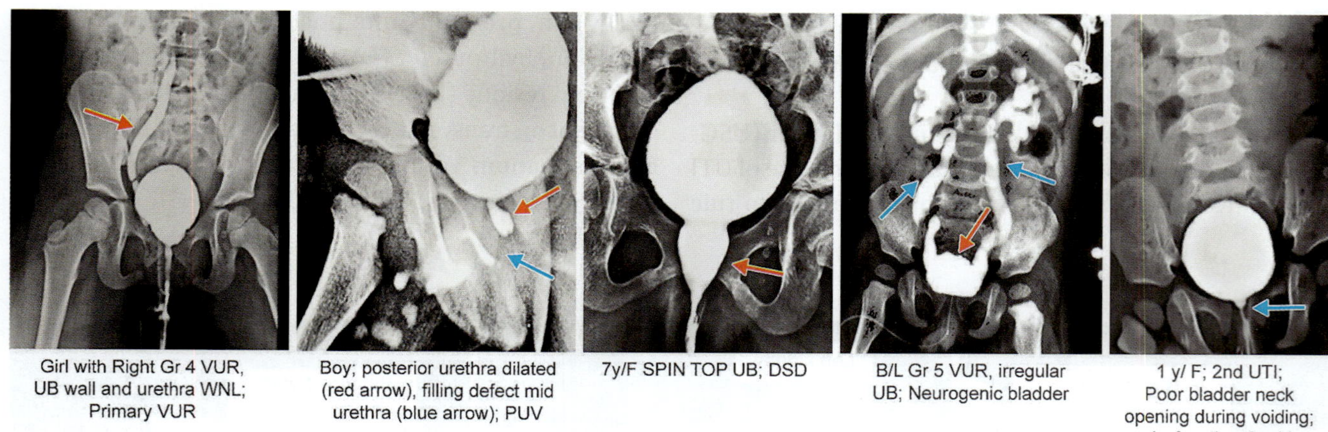

Figs. 14A to E: Various MCUG abnormalities post-UTI.

The UTI specially complicated, or delayed initiation of therapy may lead to kidney scarring which can be diagnosed by dimercaptosuccinic acid radionuclide scan (TC-99 DMSA). This static agent bounds to renal tubule (PCT) and if done 4 months after an UTI episode any abnormal/decrease uptake of radioactive material may suggest permanent renal cortical scar. DMSA is indicated if MCUG is showing high-grade VUR or USG-KUB has suspicion of scar or in recurrent UTI even with normal USG-KUB/MCUG. The decision tree of doing the 3 investigation post-UTI is shown in **Figure 15**.

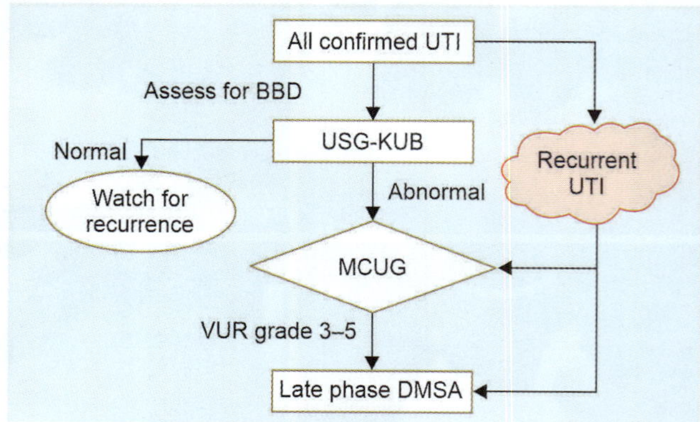

Fig. 15: Approach to radioimaging post-UTI.

Case 3A: Sristi at 12 months developed 2nd febrile UTI and mom also complains of intermittent straining in between. Her MCUG showed poor bladder neck opening as in **Figure 14E**.

Q13. What other investigations she merits now? What other investigations may be required during follow-up of UTI?

Ans. Sristi's MCUG shows inadequate bladder neck opening while voiding, she also has straining due to that, likely dysfunctional void. It may lead to recurrent UTI with or without high PVR. Diagnosis can be confirmed by urodynamic study (UDS) which may show high pressure and normal to low volume. Alpha blocker like prazosin, terazosin might help in such situation with age appropriate bowel care. Some patients with CAKUT may require CT KUB or MRI KUB with MR urography for more structural details. Toilet trained child with DSD (detrusor sphincter dyssynergia) may need uroflowmetry with EMG to confirm the perineum muscle contraction during voiding and the voiding flow may be staccato in nature. Boys with interrupted stream with recurrent UTI and doubtful urethral dilatation in MCUG may merit a cystoscopy examination.

Q14. What are the follow-up plans in a case of (recurrent) UTI and for how long?

Ans. Child with recurrent UTI may be followed up initially every 3–6 months during early childhood (up to 5 years) and thereafter every 6–12 months till transition of care to adult physicians. Points to be looked for are proper bowel, bladder habits, and early markers of renal injury like growth, blood pressure, and proteinuria (urine spot albumin creatinine ratio and renal function test). Boy infant with UTI may get benefit from circumcision. If USG and MCUG suggest PUV, patient may need cystoscopic fulguration. VUR with recurrent UTI may need antibiotics prophylaxis and if the UTI is still refractory, child may need VUR correction by endoscopic injection or ureteric re-implant by laparotomy.

Q15. When to refer to a pediatric nephrologist?

Ans. Uncomplicated UTI is well managed by primary pediatrician. Pediatric nephrologist referral is needed if UTI occurs along with underlying signs of urinary obstruction (HDN, HDUN), recurrent UTIs, significant underlying renal or urologic abnormalities (duplex system, VUR, solitary kidney), UTI with complications (AKI, renal abscess), and features of CKD (impaired kidney function, raised blood pressure, proteinuria, and cortical scar). Joint disciplinary care by pediatric nephrourology, physiotherapy, and other specialty may be required in some cases of complex renal anatomy diagnosed post-UTI. With regular follow-up by the pediatrician/pediatric nephrologist along with proper bowel and bladder habits, most of the children with (recurrent) UTI remain well with good renal function throughout their childhood and beyond. Early diagnosis of any such next UTI episode is of priority.

SUGGESTED READING

1. Hari P, Meena J, Kumar M, Sinha A, Thergaonkar RW, Iyengar A, et al.; Indian Society of Pediatric Nephrology. Evidence-based clinical practice guideline for management of urinary tract infection and primary vesicoureteric reflux. Pediatr Nephrol. 2024;39(5):1639-68.
2. Herreros ML, Tagarro A, García-Pose A, Sánchez A, Cañete A, Gili P. Accuracy of a new clean-catch technique for diagnosis of urinary tract infection in infants younger than 90 days of age. Paediatr Child Health. 2015;20:e30-2.
3. Roberts KB; Subcommittee on Urinary Tract Infection, Steering Committee on Quality Improvement and Management. Urinary tract infection: clinical practice guideline for the diagnosis and management of the initial UTI in febrile infants and children 2 to 24 months. Pediatrics. 2011;128:595-610.
4. Shaikh N, Morone NE, Bost JE, Farrell MH. Prevalence of urinary tract infection in childhood: a meta-analysis. Pediatr Infect Dis J. 2008;27:302-8.
5. Yun KW, Kim HY, Park HK, Kim W, Lim IS. Virulence factors of uropathogenic Escherichia coli of urinary tract infections and asymptomatic bacteriuria in children. J Microbiol Immunol Infect. 2014;47:455-61.

CHAPTER 9

Blood Disorders

Sudip Saha

APPROACH TO ANEMIA

Chief Complaints

- Looks pale
- Generalized weakness
- Decreased appetite

History of Present Illness

Once you are dealing with a case of anemia, it is important to find out the type of anemia or the etiology of anemia:

- History of (H/O) pain abdomen and pica (wall scrapings and mud eating).
- H/O walking barefoot or using ponds for bathing.
- H/O trauma leading to loss of blood.
- Enquire about any chronic illness like tuberculosis, recurrent diarrhea, renal problems, and glucose-6-phosphate-dehydrogenase deficiency.
- H/O drug intake that can lead to gastritis or gastric erosion, leading to blood loss and occult blood in stool.
- Is there any H/O recurrent blood transfusion for ruling out aplastic anemia, thalassemia, hereditary persistence of fetal hemoglobin, sickle cell anemia, or congenital dyserythropoietic anemia or leukemia?

  Find out the type of blood transfusion. If all three types (packed cell, fresh frozen plasma, and platelets) then the case may be leukemia or aplastic anemia.

History of Past Illness

- Any H/O blood transfusion that can lead to aplastic anemia.
- Any treatment with drugs that can cause bone marrow depression, such as chloramphenicol and phenytoin.
- Any specific hepatic-like illness that can lead to aplastic anemia.
- Any previous treatment for leukemia.

Nutritional History

Ask whether they are vegetarians (Vitamin B_{12} deficiency) or consuming goat's milk (folic acid deficiency).

Socioeconomic History

Enquire the source of water and the per capita income to understand the quality of food intake **(Flowchart 1)**

Flowchart 1: General survey.

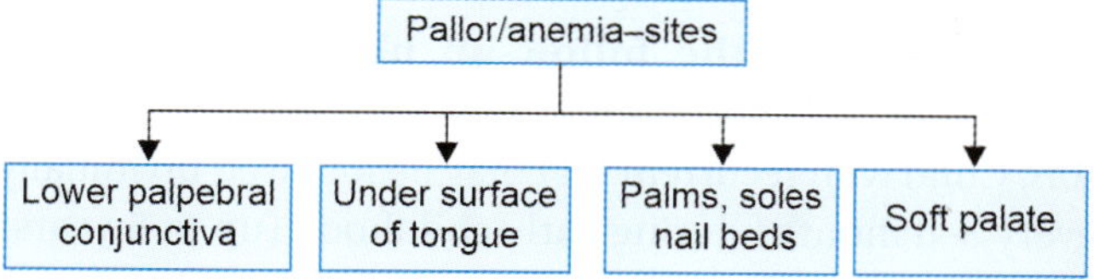

Q1. How to understand mild, moderate, and severe anemia?

Ans.

In the lower palpebral conjunctiva: If the vessels are pale along with the surrounding area, it is severe anemia. If the vessels are slightly better red than the surrounding it is moderate pallor.

In palms and soles: it is mountains and valleys. If mountains are pale along with the valley (creases), then severe pallor, and if the creases are slightly better colored than the mountains, then it is moderate pallor.

Q2. Definition of anemia.

Ans. The concentration of hemoglobin in the peripheral blood is below the normal range of values for the age and sex **(Table 1)**.

TABLE 1: Normal hemoglobin values in children.

Birth	*13.5 to 24.0 g/dl (mean 16.5 g/dl)*
<1 month	10.0–20.0 g/dL(mean 13.9 g/dL)
1–2 months	10.0–18.0 g/dL(mean 11.2 g/dL)
2–6 months	9.5–14.0 g/dL(mean 12.6 g/dL)
0.5–2 years	10.5–13.5 g/dL(mean 12.0 g/dL)
2–6 years	11.5–13.5 g/dL(mean 12.5 g/dL)
6–12 years	11.5–15.5 g/dL(13.5 gm/dL)
Females	
Age 12–18 years	12.0–16.0 g/dL(mean 14.0 g/dLl)
Age > 18 years	12.1–15.1 g/dL(mean 14.0 g/dL)
Males	
12–18 years	13.0–16.0 g/dL(mean 14.5 g/dL)
>18 years	13.6–17.7 g/dL(mean 15.5 g/dL)

Q3. Discuss the etiology of anemia.

Ans.

- Increased destruction by the spleen.
- Decreased production, i.e., bone marrow suppression.
- Blood loss—visible or occult.

Q4. Discuss anemia of infancy.

Ans. In healthy term infants, hemoglobin levels are high(>14 g/dL) at birth and then rapidly decline, reaching a nadir of approximately 10-11 g/dL at 6-9 weeks of age, which is called "Physiologic anemia of infancy."

Q5. Why are preterms prone to have lower hemoglobin levels or anemia of prematurity?

Ans.

- Born with lower hematocrit or iron levels.
- Shorter red blood cell life span.
- Impaired erythropoietin production due to immature liver function.
- *General survey:*
  - *Jaundice*: May be present in hemolytic anemia, like thalassemia. So always enquire about the color of urine.
  - Cyanosis, clubbing, and Lymph nodes are absent. Neck veins are not engorged. Edema may be present in severe anemia.
- *Systemic examination:* For anemia, the approach starts with gastrointestinal system (GI) examination.
- *Gastrointestinal system:* Upper GI may indicate paleness of the tongue, soft palate.
  - *Gastrointestinal proper*:
    - Inspection is usually normal
    - *Palpitation*: Liver just palpable in some cases-soft nontender unless there is heart failure due to severe anemia.

The spleen may be palpable in 10% of cases of iron deficiency anemia. (Where as in thalassemia, there is hepatosplenomegaly)

- *Cardiovascular system (CVS):* There is tachycardia with a high-volume pulse if there is severe anemia.
  - *Cardiovascular system proper*: Cardiomegaly may be present, i.e., apex beat is down and out (fifth intercostal space outside midclavicular line). Heart sounds S1 loud, S2 loud with a flow murmur in the new aortic area.
- *Respiratory system*: Usually not affected except if there is severe anemia leading to heart failure, then there may be basal crepitations.
- *Nervous system*: Normal.

Q6. What is the method for blood transfusion in severe anemia?

Ans. The method is: 5 g/dL 12-hourly.

Q7. What are the symptoms of iron deficiency anemia?

Ans. The symptoms of iron deficiency anemia are as follows:

- Dizziness, tachycardia, lethargy, lightheadedness, or malaise.
- Inability to concentrate, somnolence.
- Giddiness
- Eating disorder characterized by the persistent, compulsive consumption of non-food items

Q8. What are the investigations for anemia?

Ans.

- Complete blood count—microcytic, hypochromic anemia.
- Reticulocyte index <1.5%
- *Serum ferritin and serum iron:* Low
- Serum total iron binding capacity—will be high or normal.
- Transferrin saturation is decreased below 10%. Normal is 15–50%
- Free erythrocyte protoporphyrin is increased (normal 30–40 µg/dL).

Q9. Treatment of anemia

Ans.

- Iron-rich food containing less phytates—*fenugreek seeds, jiggery, dates,* and *Bengal gram.*
- Iron supplementation—various salts are present with some side effects.

- Sulphate causes constipation, blackening of the tongue, metallic taste along with gastritis. Other salts are:
  - Ferrous fumarate and gluconate.
  - Dosage: 3–6 mg/kg/day in two to three divided doses.

Q10. What are the factors affecting oral iron absorption?

Ans. Factors affecting oral iron absorption **(Table 2)**.

TABLE 2: Enhancers and inhibitors of iron absorption.

Enhancers	*Inhibitors*
Vitamin C	Phosphates in milk
Ferrous salts	Phytates in cereals
Bedtime—decreases the motility of the gut during sleep	Ferric salts—to be converted to ferrous salts
	Oxalates

Q11. What is the response to iron therapy?

Ans. Response to iron therapy **(Table 3)**.

TABLE 3: Duration of iron response to treatment.

Hours/days	*Response*
12–24 hours	Decreased irritability, feeling of well-being, increase in appetite
36–48 hours	Bone marrow response, i.e., erythroid hyperplasia
48–72 hours	Reticulocytosis
4–30 days	Hemoglobin level increases
90 days	Replenishment of iron stores in marrow

Parental Iron Therapy

Indications

- Poor patient compliance
- Persistent blood loss
- Impaired intestinal absorption
- Associated infections
- Malabsorption syndromes

Q12. Parental iron requirement—iron requirement includes the iron required for replenishment of iron stores. Explain.

Ans.

Iron requirement = Weight (kg) × hemoglobin deficit (g/dL) × 4.4

Preparation: >Iron dextran > Ferric gluconate

Red Cell transfusion 5 mg/kg 12 hourly with diuretics @mid of transfusion

Q13. Discuss Anemia Mukht Bharat.

Ans.

- *Beneficiaries:*
  - Children 6–59 months
  - Children 5–9 years
  - Adolescents 10–19 years
  - Women of reproductive age group 15–49 years.

Launch Date March 2018

Interventions: Prophylactic Iron and Folic acid supplementation and deworming. Intensified year-round behavior, change, and communication campaign (solid body and smart mind).

APPROACH TO APLASTIC ANEMIA

Chief Complaints

- Paleness and fatigue
- Bleeding spots
- Ecchymotic patch
- Fever

History of Present Illness

Everything occurs within a short duration. The closest differential diagnosis is leukemia. Both have the same manifestations with a history of red and white blood transfusions. Preceding history is very important. Enquire about the history of viral illness and drug history.

List of infections and drugs causing aplastic anemia:

- *Infection:* Hepatitis, Epstein–Barr virus, cytomegalovirus, parvovirus B19, herpes simplex, human immunovirus.
- *Autoimmune disorders:* Lupus
- *Drugs:* Chloramphenicol, phenytoin, tolbutamide, and chlorpropamide
- *Miscellaneous:* Gold compounds and chemotherapy
- Pregnancy

On Examination

- *General survey:* Pallor/anemia ++, skin and appendages (bleeding spots and ecchymosis), Jaundice, cyanosis, clubbing, neck veins, neck glands, and edema are absent.
- *Vitals:* Temperature ±, blood pressure (BP) may be low, heart rate—tachycardia usually due to fever/anemia.
- *Systemic examination:*
  - GI—usually hepatomegaly may be present, but the spleen is not palpable.

- CVS—same features of severe anemia.
- Respiratory system—same features of severe anemia.
- Nervous system—same features of severe anemia.

Q1. What are the investigations for Anemia without splenomegaly

Ans.

Aplastic anemia:

- Complete Blood count—anemia, leucopenia, and thrombocytopenia.
- Reticulocyte count—low.
- Bone marrow studies—aspiration shows dry tap. Bone marrow biopsy shows hypocellular or acellular marrow.
    - *Chromosomal studies*: Fanconi anemia and myelodysplastic anemia.
    - Flow cytometric analysis of erythrocytes for CD55 and C59 [paroxysmal nocturnal hemoglobinuria (PNH)].

Q2. What are the types of aplastic anemia?

Ans. Types of aplastic anemia are as follows:

- Acquired
- Inherited—gene defects

Q3. What is the treatment for aplastic anemia?

Ans.

- Supportive care—removal of offending agent/drugs control of bleeding—platelets and packed cell
- Specific treatment—bone marrow transplantation (BMT) using allogenic hematopoietic stem cells.
    - Methyl prednisolone
    - Antilymphocytic globulin dose 40mg/kg/day once daily for 4 days with methylprednisolone
    - *Cyclosporin A*: Dose 8 mg/kg/day for 14 days
    - Tacrolimus with antithymocyte globulin (ATG) can be given to patients who cannot tolerate cyclosporine.
    - Haemopoietic colony-stimulating factor. Recombinant human granulocyte macrophage colony-stimulating factor (GM-CSF). Dosage: 8–32 μg/kg/day along with cyclosporine A or ATG.
    - Intravenous immunoglobulin (IVIG) is useful in collagen vascular disorders, PNH, and infections, such as Parvovirus.
    - Cyclophosphamide is useful in newly diagnosed cases or patients not responding to immunosuppression.

APPROACH TO HEMOLYTIC ANEMIA

- Chief complaints*:* (1) Low-grade fever, (2) weakness, and (3) paleness.
- *History of present illness:* Most of the cases will have a history of blood transfusion. Some cases may be presenting for the first time. Those having a history of blood transfusion will give a history of low-grade fever [increased basal metabolic rate (BMR)], paleness, and weakness due to anemia and hypoxia. There may be a history of recurrent infections. Some complain of increasing abdominal size due to organomegaly. Some may present with mild jaundice. So do not forget to ask about urine color and stool color.
- *Past history:* Enquire about any history of complications due to blood treatment, i.e., reactions or infections due to blood transfusion.
- *Treatment history:* Enquire about iron chelation. Enquire about the frequency of blood transfusions.
- *Family history:* Find out how many children are affected with thalassemia. Find out if parents have been diagnosed with thalassemia trait/carrier.
- *Socioeconomic history:* As thalassemia treatment is costly and also causes wage loss, it is important to understand the per capita income and the household.
- *Examination:*
    - General survey: Anthropometry: there could be moderate to severe malnutrition, and also the height can be affected in thalassemia.

Q1. Why is there growth failure in thalassemia?

Ans. If there is improper iron chelation, there is iron deposition in the pituitary and thyroid gland, resulting in a deficiency of growth hormone and abnormalities in thyroid-releasing hormone (TRH). The pathogenesis of growth failure is multifactorial and is mainly due to chronic anemia and hypoxia, chronic liver disease, zinc and folic acid deficiency, iron overload, and excessive use of chelating agents, endocrinopathies (hypogonadism, delayed puberty, and hypothyroidism), and growth hormone–insulin-like growth factor I axis (GH-IGF-1 axis) dysregulation.

Vitals: There may be tachycardia with a water hammer pulse due to severe anemia. There may be respiratory distress due to chronic heart failure.

- Anemia/pallor has already been discussed in anemia.
- Jaundice ±

Q2. What are the causes of jaundice in hemolytic anemia?

Ans.

- Hemolytic anemia—excessive breakdown by the spleen
- *Hepatocellular jaundice*: Iron deposition in the liver leading to cirrhosis >> hepatic sclerosis >> portal fibrosis >> cirrhosis. Also, due to blood transfusion—hepatitis B and hepatitis C.
- *Facies—typical chipmunk facies*: Changes in facial and cranial bones have been identified as the overexpansion of bone marrow:
    - Box-shaped cheekbone.
    - Depressed nasal bridge.
    - Protruding maxilla.
- Clubbing, cyanosis, and neck glands are absent unless there are secondary causes.
- Edema—secondary due to heart failure or due to severe anemia.
- Skin—due to hemosiderosis, there may be slight tanning of the skin.

Systemic examination of thalassemia usually affects the reticular endothelial system, which is examined by the GI:

- BP + anemia + pallor
- Lymph nodes not palpable
- Bone marrow/sternum tenderness
- Neck veins

The liver is palpable X centimeter below right coastal margin in mid clavicular line, left lobe palpable, margins round or sharp, consistency soft to firm, tender or non-tender, surface smooth/nodular in cirrhosis span.

The spleen is usually palpable unless splenectomy is done, X centimeter from the left coastal margin in the splenic axis; notch is palpable.

Q3. What are the causes of hepatomegaly?

- Increase erythropoiesis
- Increase iron deposition
- Hepatitis due to infection
- Hepatomegaly due to heart failure

Q4. What are the causes of splenomegaly?

Ans.

- Increase the destruction of red blood cells (RBCs).
- Increase extramedullary hematopoiesis.
- Increase iron overload.
- Other systems are usually normal if no complication occurs due to severe anemia or hemosiderosis.

Diagnosis: A Case of Chronic Hemolytic Anemia, Most Likely Beta Thalassemia

Q5. Why it is Hemolytic anemia?

Ans.

- Thalassemic facies
- Repeated blood transfusion
- Hepatosplenomegaly

Q6. Classify hemolytic anemia.

Ans. Hemolytic anemia **(Table 4)**

- Sickle cell disease
- Thalassemia (alpha and beta)
- Hereditary spherocytosis, elliptocytosis, and pyropoikilocytosis
- Pyruvate kinase deficiency

TABLE 4: Hemolytic anemia classification.

Inherited hemolysis (Intrinsic)	*Acquired hemolysis (Extrinsic)*
Defects in RBCs result when one or more genes that control RBCs' production do not function properly. RBCs destroyed early	Factor outside the RBC's
	Antibodies from an autoimmune disorder
	Immune hemolytic are: • Autoimmune hemolytic anemia • Alloimmune • Drug-induced • Paroxysmal nocturnal hemoglobinuria

Q7. What is the diagnosis of chronic hemolytic anemia?

Ans.

- Complete blood count with indices.
    - Low hemoglobin, low RBC, packed cell volume (PCV), decreased mean corpuscular volume (MCV), mean corpuscular hemoglobin concentration (MCHC), and increased platelets.
    - Reticulocyte count corrected reticulocyte count is high >1% in child >5% in infants.
    - *Peripheral smear:* RBC normal to microcytic, hypochromic with anisocytosis (abnormal size) and poikilocytosis (abnormal shape) target cells, teardrop cells. There will be marked basophilic stippling and variable polychromasia. Fragmented red cell nuclear remnants such as hall jolly bodies and Heinz bodies may be seen

- Hemoglobin electrophoresis of child and parents—HbF raised disease—HbF > 3.4% carrier
- Liver function test-May show an increase in unconjugated bilirubin initially or conjugated bilirubin due to hemosiderosis or infection.
- Naked Eye Single Tube Red Cell Osmotic Fragility Test (NESTROF): Naked eye single tube red cell osmotic fragility test) is done on a mass scale to screen for thalassemia osmotic fragility test is increased as the cell wall is thinner and can absorb more water.
- Serum ferritin levels are done after 10 transfusions.
- Radiology—medullary portion of the bone is widened, and the bone cortex is thinned out with a core trabecular pattern in the medulla. X-ray of the metacarpals, ribs, and vertebrae show the thinning of the cortex. X-ray of the skull shows a hair-on-end appearance.

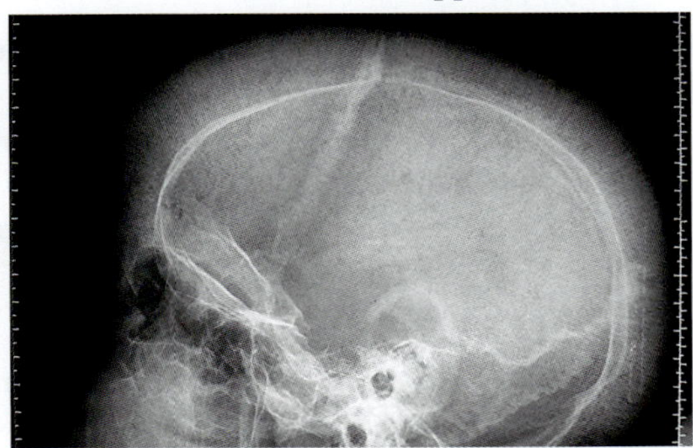

In doubtful cases also genetic analysis or if blood transmission has to be given at a very early age.

Q8. Types

Ans. Beta thalassemia—mutation in the beta gene resulting in decreased production of beta chains. Alpha thalassemia- mutation in the alpha genes resulting in decreased production of alpha chains **(Flowchart 2)**.

Flowchart 2: Classification of beta thalassemia.

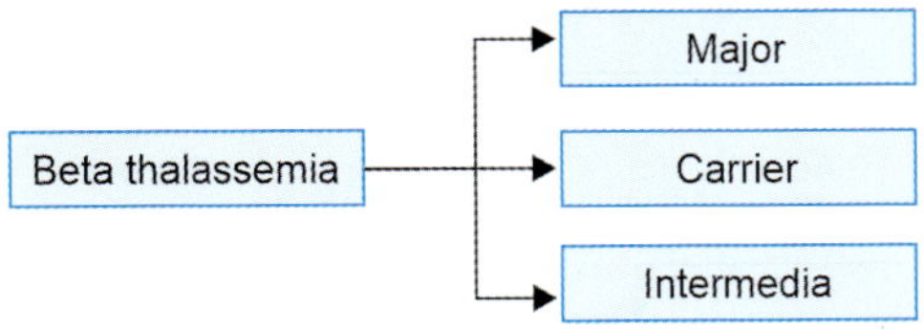

These variants are designated as follows.

- Beta—normal beta globulin chains
- Beta zero—no beta globulin change
- Beta ± demonstrable beta chain production

Q9. Sometimes, it is asked how to approach this case. How?

Ans. The approach includes investigations, counseling, and treatment.

Q10. What are the treatment options?

Ans. Counseling to parents about definitive treatment options:

- Bone marrow transplant
- Stem cell transplant—in this method, the source of stem cells is a healthy, compatible sibling. Sources of stem cells are cord blood, peripheral blood, bone marrow, and fetal liver.

In this procedure, the patient's bone marrow is destroyed with large doses of radiation and chemotherapy. The patient is kept in isolation with broad-spectrum antibiotics and antifungals. Then the patients' defective stem cells are replaced with normal stem cells from an immunologically compatible donor.

Treatment of Anemia

Blood Transfusion

Type of blood: Triple saline washed leukodepleted RBCs.

Regimens: Hyper transmission is done for cosmetic reasons and normal growth. It prevents anemia and its complications, suppresses erythropoiesis, prevents skeletal changes, prevents gastrointestinal iron absorption, and inhibits extramedullary hematopoiesis, thus preventing splenomegaly and hypersplenism.

Hypertransmission requires more blood at diagnosis (to get a rise of 3–4 g. transmission done at 15 mL/kg). Pretransmission level should be maintained at 10 g/dL or more to inhibit the marrow activity. Problems of super transmission are high viscosity, as the post-transmission target is 16 g/dL, so that next transmission can be done after 3–4 weeks

Q11. What are complications of blood transmission?

- Mismatch
- Graft versus host disease
- Infections, such as hepatitis B, hepatitis C, cytomegalovirus, malaria, and human immunodeficiency virus (HIV).
- Nonhemolytic febrile reactions due to leucocytes. It is prevented by the use of leucocyte filters.
- Iron overload.

Chelating agents: These are indicated when serum ferritin levels are >1,000 μg/L or at least 10 transfusions.

- Deferoxamine—is given subcutaneously as continuous infusion over a period of 8–12 hours per day for 5–6 weeks.
  - Side effects—thinning of retinal vessels.
    - Sensorineural hearing loss
    - Metaphyseal dysplasia

- Deferiprone (Kelfar)—oral iron chelating agent dose 75–100 mg/day in two to three divided doses.
  - Side effects—arthropathy.
    - Agranulocytosis.
    - Idiosyncratic reactions—increased liver enzymes.
- *Deferasirox:* Another oral iron chelating agent, it binds iron with high affinity in a ratio of 2:1
  - Side effects—abdominal pain.
    - Nausea increased
    - Liver enzymes

APPROACH TO LEUKEMIA

Chief Complaints

- *Sudden onset of pallor*:
  - Fever high grade
  - Loss of appetite
  - Weight loss
  - Lymphadenopathy
  - Neck swelling
  - Bleeding spots or bleeding from gums or any other site bleeding
  - Arthralgia or arthritis
  - Recurrent infections—fever and respiratory tract infection

History of Present Illness

All the features of leukemia are not present at one moment. As because due to bone marrow involvement, resulting in pallor or decreased hemoglobin, bleeding spots due to thrombocytopenia, and recurrent infection due to a decrease in white blood cell (WBC) and neutrophil count.

Parlor results in weakness, loss of appetite, and easy fatigability.

History of Past Illness

- History of infection such as HIV, Epstein–Barr virus, cytomegalovirus, and human herpes virus 6, varicella zoster due to preexisting immunodeficiency.
- *Treatment history:* Supportive treatment for pallor and bleeding manifestations and antibiotics for infection.

Clinical Examination

- General survey pallor +, jaundice, cyanosis, clubbing, and edema absent.
- Lymph nodes cervical, axillary, inguinal, as well as epitrochlear.
- Skin and appendages, bleeding spots, and ecchymotic spots.
- Vitals temperature, BP normal to low, pulse tachycardia, respiration plus minus toxic look.

Systemic Examination

Reticular endothelial system:

- Bone tenderness—put mild pressure on the sternum or any long bones.
- Vitals and generals will already be done.
- *GI:* Liver is palpable and enlarged; spleen is enlarged and palpable. Palpation of the abdomen may sometimes reveal a mass due to lymph nodes.
- Palpation of the genitalia to exclude any testicular involvement.

Provisional diagnosis—a case of hepatosplenomegaly with lymphadenopathy with anemia, with bleeding spots due to acute lymphoblastic leukemia.

Q1. Enumerate other causes of hepatosplenomegaly with lymphadenopathy.

Ans. Causes of hepatosplenomegaly with lymphadenopathy **(Table 5)**.

TABLE 5: Causes of hepatosplenomegaly with lymphadenopathy.

Infectious causes	*Noninfectious causes*
Enteric fever	Acute leukemia
Scrub typhus	Chronic myeloid leukemia
Disseminated tuberculosis	Hodgkin's lymphoma
Infectious mononucleosis	Histiocytosis
Toxoplasmosis	Juvenile rheumatoid arthritis
Human immunodeficiency virus (HIV)	Niemann–Pick disease
	Hurler disease

Classification of Leukemia (Flowchart 3)

Flowchart 3: Leukemia classification.

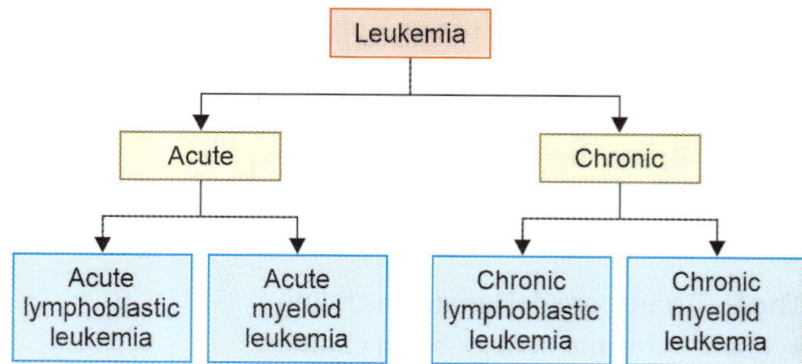

French-American-British (FAB) classification of ALL **(Table 6)**: The malignant cells in the bone marrow are classified into the following types based on morphological features such as cell size, nuclear cytoplasmic ratio, nuclear shape, and number of nucleoli.

TABLE 6: French-American-British (FAB) classification of ALL.

Cytologic features	*L1*	*L2*	*L3*
Cell size	Small cells predominate, homogenous	Large, heterogeneous in size	Large, homogenous
Cytoplasm	Scanty	Variable, often moderately abundant	Moderately abundant
Nucleoli	Small	One or more, often large	One or more prominent
Nuclear shape	Homogenous	Variable, heterogeneous	Stippled, homogenous
Nuclear shape	Regular	Irregular clefts	Regular
Cytoplasmic basophilia	Variable	Variable	Intensely basophilic
Cytoplasmic vacuolation	Variable	Variable	Prominent

- Classification based on immunophenotyping, based on surface markers present on the abnormal lymphoblastic cells in most cases, all can be classified as discussed in **Table 7**.

TABLE 7: Classification based on immunophenotyping.

	Classification based on immunophenotyping	
	B: Acute lymphoblastic leukemia	
	B: Lymphopoiesis	*B: All phenotype*
BONE MARROW ↓	Pro-B	Pro- B (I)
	CD34, CD19, CD79a	CD34, CD19, CD79a
	Pre-B I	Common-B (II)
	CD34, CD19, CD10	CD10
	Pre-B II	Pre-B (III)
	CD19, CD10, CD20, cyu	cyu
	Immature B cell	Mature B (IV)
	CD19, CD20, sIgM	sIg
	T: Acute lymphoblastic leukemia	
	T lymphopoiesis	*T: ALL phenotype*
THYMUS ↓	T progenitor	Pro-T (I)
	CD34, CD7, and cyCD3	CD7, cyCD3
	Subcapsular zone	Pre-T (II)
	CD2, CD5	CD2, CD5, CD1a neg
	Cortical zone	Cortical T (III)
	CD1a, CD4, and CD8	CD1a pos
	Immature T cell	Mature T (IV)
	sCD3, CD4 or CD8	sCD3

- *Cytogenetics:*
  - Various abnormalities in chromosome numbers and structure may be associated with ALL.
  - A hyperdiploid chromosome number is >50, which carries a good prognosis.
  - Hypodiploid chromosome number is <45.
  - Pseudodiploidy—normal chromosome number with abnormalities such as translations.
  - Near haploid chromosome number approximately equal to the number of haploid cells in most of the blast cells; some cells may show hyper diploid. It carries the worst prognosis.

Q2. What are the prognostic factors of acute lymphoblastic leukemia?

Ans. Prognostic factors of ALL **(Table 8)**.

TABLE 8: Prognostic factors of ALL.

Determinants	*Favorable*	*Unfavorable*
WBC counts	<10,000	>200,000
Age	2–10 years	<1 year, >10 years
Gender	Female	Male
Ethnicity	White	Black
Node, liver, and splenomegaly	Absent	Massive
Testicular enlargement	Absent	Present
CNS involvement	Absent	CSF blast and pleocytosis
FAB type	L1	L2
Cytogenetics	T(12;21) (TEL-AML1), trisomies 4,10,17	t(9;22) (BCR-ABL), t(4;11)(MLL-AF4)
Ploidy	Hyperdiploidy	Hypodiploidy
Time to remission	<14 days	>28 days

(ALL: acute lymphoblastic leukemia; CNS: central nervous system; CSF: colony-stimulating factor)

Q3. What investigations are needed to confirm your diagnosis?

Ans.

- Complete blood count (CBC) showing anemia, normocytic, normochromic, with increased total leukocyte count, with thrombocytopenia; occasionally leucocyte count may be low. Blast cells of >20% indicate leukemia.
- Activated partial thromboplastin time (aPTT) and prothrombin time.
- Increased serum levels of uric acid, potassium, calcium, and lactate dehydrogenase
- Chest X-ray mediastinal mass, ultrasonography (USG) hepatosplenomegaly with abdominal masses.
- Bone marrow examination for psychology, phyto-chemistry, blast immunology, chromosomal analysis. Marrow is hypercellular and shows >25% lymphoblasts
- CSF increases cell count.

Q4. Discuss its treatment.

Ans. The cornerstone of treatment is a combination chemotherapy for the control of the active disease, together with central nervous system (CNS) profile access for the prevention of CNS relapses.

Chemotherapy: Induction of remission 4 to 6 weeks defined as the absence of blast cells in the peripheral smear and the presence of less than 5% blast cells in the marrow.

- Vincristine 1.5 mg/m^2/week intravenous
- Prednisolone 40 mg/kg/m^2/day orally

  Maintenance therapy for 2–3 years to prevent relapses
  - 6 Mercaptopurine at 50 mg
  - Methotrexate

  Intermittent doses of vincristine and Prednisolone may be given if required.

Central nervous system profile—given to eradicate the leukemic cells that have crossed the blood-brain barrier.

- Radiation and/or intrathecal therapy (triple therapy)
- Methotrexate 15 mg/m^2
- Hydrocortisone 15 mg/m^2
- Cytosine arabinoside 30 mg/m^2
- Supportive therapy
- Blood transmission
- Antibiotics for infections
- Treatment for hyperuricemia or tumor lysis syndrome

Treatment of relapse: Bone marrow relapse is common. Marrow ablative chemotherapy followed by allogenic transplantation of stem cells for early bone marrow relapse.

Intensive chemotherapy for late bone marrow relapse.

Q5. What are the complications of treatment?

Ans.

- Secondary malignancy
- Endocrinal dysfunction
- Cardiomyopathy
- Neurophysiological changes

APPROACH TO LYMPHOMA

Chief Complaints

- *Fever:* Periodic and/or unexplained.
- Neck swelling or groin or axilla.
- Unexplained weight loss.

History of Present Illness

- Prolonged fever not responding to antibiotics.
- Loss of appetite and weight.
- Generalized pruritus.
- Pressure symptoms
  - Chest pain
  - Dysphagia
  - Airway obstruction (cough and dyspnea)
  - Swelling of the neck or face due to superior vena cava obstruction.

History of Past Illness

Same as leukemia.

- *Examination:*
  - *General examination:*
    - Pallor +
    - Lymph nodes
- *Sites*:
  - Cervical all groups
  - Axillary all groups
  - Inguinal all groups
  - Consistency—feel rubbery
  - Tenderness absent
- *GI*:
  - Hepatosplenomegaly
  - Abdominal mass
  - Ascites

Q6. What are the types of lymphoma?

Ans. Types of lymphoma **(Flowchart 4)**

Flowchart 4: Lymphoma types.

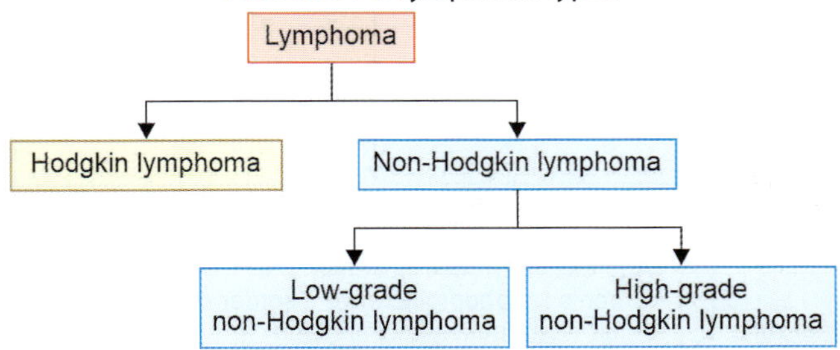

Q7. What investigations are needed to confirm the diagnosis?

Ans.

- Complete blood count low hemoglobin with occasional neutropenia and thrombocytopenia.
    - Erythrocyte sedimentation rate (ESR)—increased.
    - Lactate dehydrogenase (LDH)—raised.
- *Radiology*:
    - Chest X-ray mediastinal widening.
    - Computed tomography (CT) chest and abdomen to reveal masses.
- *Lymph node biopsy diagnosis*: Reed–Sternberg cells.
- Bone marrow examination.

Classification of Hodgkin's and non-Hodgkin's Lymphoma (Boxes 1 and 2)

BOX 1: Hodgkin lymphoma (Hodgkin disease).

- Nodular lymphocyte-predominant Hodgkin lymphoma (5%)
- Classical Hodgkin lymphoma (95%)
- Hodgkin lymphoma, nodular sclerosis (grades I and II)
- Classical Hodgkin lymphoma, lymphocyte-rich
- Hodgkin lymphoma. Mixed cellularity
- Hodgkin lymphoma. Lymphocytic depletion (includes most Hodgkin-like anaplastic large-cell lymphomas)

BOX 2: St Jude staging classification of non-Hodgkin lymphoma.

Stage	*Description*
Stage I	A single tumor (extranodal) or single anatomical area (nodal) with the exclusion of the mediastinum or abdomen
Stage II	• A single tumor (extranodal) with regional node involvement • Two or more nodal areas on the same side of the diaphragm • Two single (extranodal) tumors with or without regional node involvement on the same side of the diaphragm • A primary gastrointestinal tract tumor, usually in the ileocecal area, with or without involvement of associated mesenteric nodes, only, grossly completely resected
Stage III	• Two single tumors (extranodal) on opposite sides of the diaphragm • Two or more nodal areas above and below the diaphragm • All the primary intrathoracic tumors (mediastinal, pleural, and thymic) • All extensive primary intra-abdominal disease, and unresectable • All paraspinal or epidural tumors, regardless of other tumor site(s)
Stage IV	Any of the above with initial central nervous system and/or bone marrow involvement

- New World Health Organization (WHO)/Revised European American Lymphoma (REAL).
- Ann Arbor staging classification **(Table 9)**

TABLE 9: Ann Arbor staging.

Stage	*Involvement*	*Extranodal (E) Status*
Limited		
Stage I	One node or a group of adjacent nodes	Single extranodal lesion without nodal involvement
Stage II	Two or more nodal groups on the same side of the diaphragm	Stage I or II, by nodal extent, with limited contiguous extranodal involvement
Stage II bulky	Stage II as above with "bulky" disease	Not applicable
Advanced		
Stage III	• Nodes on both sides of the diaphragm • Nodes above the diaphragm with spleen involvement	Not applicable
Stage IV	Additional noncontiguous extralymphatic involvement	Not applicable

Classification of non-Hodgkin Lymphoma (Flowchart 5)

Flowchart 5: Non-Hodgkin lymphoma (NHL) classification.

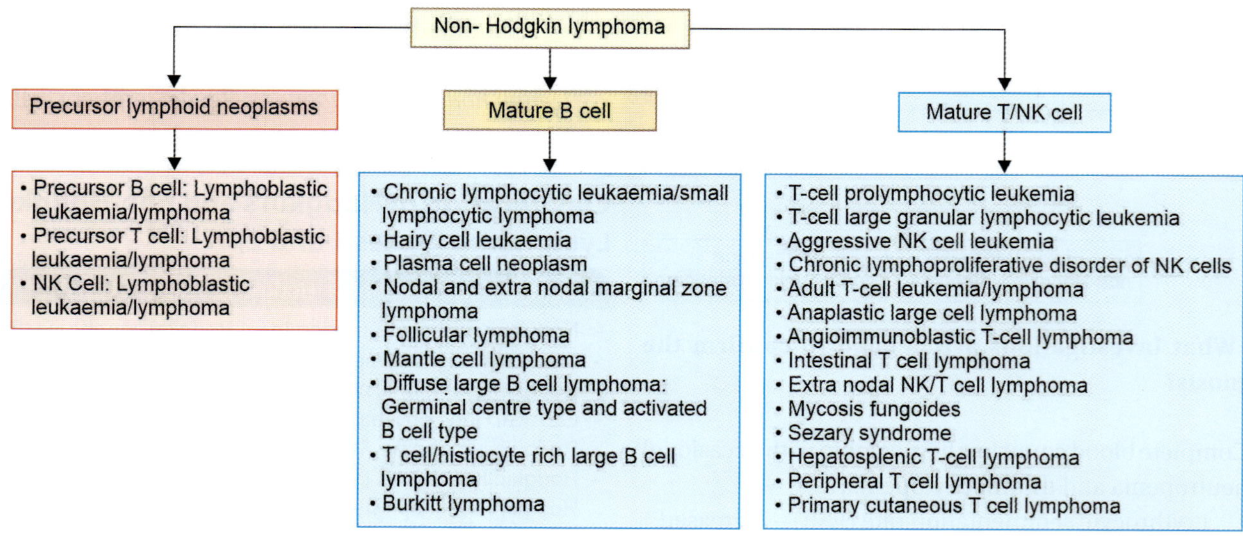

Treatment

Therapy based on the Ann Arbor staging of Hodgkin's disease

- Radiotherapy-indication:
  - Stage 1
  - Stage 2 disease
  - Post chemotherapy
  - Sites with pressure symptoms
  - *Complication*:
    - Growth retardation
    - Impaired organ failure, hard thyroid
    - Secondary malignancy
- *Chemotherapy—indication:*
  - All patients with B symptoms
  - Stage 2 disease
  - Stage 3 and stage 4 disease

Drugs

- Vinblastine 6 mg/m^2
- Procarbazine 100 mg/m^2
- Prednisolone 40 mg/m^2
- Cyclophosphamide 650 mg/m^2
- Adriamycin 25 mg/m^2
- Etoposide 100 mg/m^2
  - Vincristine 0.42—1.4 mg/m^2
  - Bleomycin 10 mg/m^2
  - Dacarbazine 37.5 mg/m^2

Complications:

- Myelodysplasia
- Adult leukemia
- Azoospermia
- Secondary malignancy

Relapse: Mostly occurs within the first year or 1–3 years after diagnosis. Treatment of relapse that occurs within 12 months after chemotherapy or in refractory cases is done by myeloblastic autologous stem cell transplant.

Prognostic Indicators of Hodgkin's Lymphoma

- *Being male:*
  - 45 years or older, stage 4 disease.
  - Albumin level below 4 g/dL.
  - Hemoglobin level below 10.5 g/dL.
  - Leucocytes, white blood cell count >15,000/UL
  - Lymphocytopenia: Lymphocyte count <8% of the white blood cell count
- Early-stage favorable—stage 1 to stage 2 with no unfavorable risk factors
- Early-stage unfavorable—stage 1 to 2 with one or more of the following unfavorable risk factors.
  - Bulky disease—a mass in the chest that is 1/3 the width of the chest or any lymph node node mass >10 cm.
  - Involvement of three or more nodes.
  - B symptoms: Fever, drenching night sweats, and/or unexplained weight loss >10% of body weight over 6 months.

- Extra Nodal disease involvement of an organ outside the lymphatic system
- ESR 50 or high.
- *Advanced stage*: Stage 3 to 4.

Treatment of non-Hodgkin's lymphoma: The primary modality of treatment of NHL is a systemic combination of chemotherapy. Radiotherapy is used only in specific cases, such as CNS involvement and Superior mediastinal syndrome.

New cases and those at risk of tumor lysis syndrome require maintenance of good hydration and either an xanthine oxidase inhibitor or recombinant urate oxidase.

CHAPTER 10

Endocrine System and Its Disorders

Sumana Kundagrami

PART A: HISTORY TAKING AND GENERAL SURVEY

INTRODUCTION

The common conditions, complaints the child or an adolescent, come to us to clinic who need endocrinology assessment are short stature, obesity, hypothyroidism or thyroid disorders, precocious puberty, and Cushing syndrome. In such common cases, the important points in history taking and general survey are discussed below. A good focused history and good general survey will help us come to reach to a diagnosis earlier without doing unnecessary expensive investigations.

HISTORY TAKING AND GENERAL SURVEY

History Taking

- Birth weight—important for assessing short stature, obesity
- Perinatal history—pregnancy-related issues
- Family history for obesity cases, thyroid disorders, short stature, history of early, or delayed puberty in parents for assessing cases of precocious and delayed puberty. A pedigree chart is very helpful for genetic cases of obesity or short stature disorders of sex development (DSD).
- Drug history for obesity, short stature, thyroid disorders precocious puberty, and delayed puberty
- History of fetal loss in mother/death of sibling
- History of any headache, visual disturbances, and features suggestive raised intracranial tension in cases of precocious puberty
- Nutritional history for obesity and short stature cases, coeliac disease (wheat intolerance)
- Lifestyle history for obesity cases
- Chronic complaints should point out to a chronic cause leading to failure to thrive.

General Survey

This is the basis of examination of a child/adolescent who presents to us in our clinic. We have to observe the child from head to toe and look for pointers.

- Head—macrocephaly and microcephaly
- Face—characteristics facies as in Turner syndrome, Down syndrome, Noonan syndrome, and Russell Silver syndrome
    - Also we can find cataract, squint, high-arched palate low set ears, and asymmetry of face (Russell Silver syndrome in some cases).
    - There may be asymmetric unilateral overgrowth of face and body in Beckwith-Weidman syndrome.
    - Protruded tongue (macroglossia) may be spotted in cretins.
- Neck—Goiter may be present in pubertal children or cases of dyshormonogenesis in thyroid disorders.
    - Webbing of neck should be picked up in Turner syndrome.
    - Acanthosis nigricans is very important finding in obese children with insulin resistance.
- Chest—shielded chest, wide spaced nipples in Turner syndrome
    - Precordial bulge in a short child may point toward congenital heart disease in the child to be the cause of short stature.
- Abdomen may be distended in coeliac disease. Lax abdominal wall may point toward Prader Willi syndrome as a cause of obesity.
- *Body proportions*—US:LS ratio is very important parameter to be calculated in any child presenting with short stature.
    - Digital abnormalities, e.g., polydactyly in Laurence-Moon-Bardet-Biedl syndrome

- *Genitalia:* In cases of DSD, a good survey of the genitalia is the most important examination.
    - Undescended testis, macroorchidism, etc., may be picked up in cases of obesity, hypothyroidism, etc.
- Skin—striae (violaceous in Cushing syndrome), café au lait spots (neurofibromatosis), and naevi (Turner syndrome) should not be missed.
- *Back and spine:* A survey of spine to look for spinal deformities is important in short stature cases specially.

SUGGESTED READING

1. Bajpai A, Agarwal N. Growth failure. In : Bajpai A, Patel R, Dave C, Agarwal N, editors, MedEclasses. Pediatric Endocrinology. Kanpur; Growth Society Publications; 2019. p 49-53.
2. Bajpai A, Patel R . Multiple pituitary hormone deficiency. Mere classes Online Course in Pediatric Endocrinology. learning.growsociety.in
3. Banerjee S, Bajpai A. Precocious Puberty. Indian J Pediatr. 2023 Jun;90(6):582-589.
4. Desai MP, Sharma R, Riaz I, et al. Newborn screening guidelines for congenital hypothyroidism in India: recommendations of the Indian Society for Pediatric and Adolescent Endocrinology (ISPAE) -Part I : Screening and confirmation of diagnosis. Indian J Pediatr. 2018;85:440-7.
5. Jain V, Menon RK, Case based reviews in Pediatric Endocrinology. 2nd ed. New Delhi, India: Jaypee Publications; 2024.
6. Kaiser U, Ho K.Pituitary physiology and diagnostic evaluation. In: Williams Textbook of Endocrinology. Eds:Melmed S, Auchus R, Goldfine A, Koenig R, Rosen C. 14th Edition, Elsevier, Manesar. Pp 184-235.
7. Khadilkar V, Khadilkar A, Choudhary P, et al. Revised IAP growth charts for height, weight and body mass index for 5-to-18-year-old Indian children. Indian Pediatr. 2015; 52:47-55.
8. Khadilkar V, Kondpalle S, Normal growth. In: Khadilkar V, Bajpai A, Prasad HK, editors .IAP Textbook on Pediatric Endocrinology. New Delhi, India: Jaypee Publications; 2019. p.37.
9. Krebs NF, Himes JH, Jacobson D, et al. Assessment of child and adolescent overweight and obesity. Pediatrics. 2007;120:S193-228
10. Murray PG, Clayton PE.Disorders of growth. In: Dattani M, Brook C.G.D, editors.Brook's Clinical Pediatric Endocrinology, 7th ed. Oxford, UK: Wiley; 2020. p.201.
11. Nieman LK, Biller BM, Findling JW, et al. Treatment of Cushing's syndrome: an Endocrine Society Clinical Practice Guideline. J Clinic Endocrinol Metab. 2015; 100:2807-31.
12. Polidori N, Castorani V, Mohn A, Chiarelli F. Deciphering short stature in children. Ann Pediatr Endocrinol Metab. 2020;25(2):69-79.
13. Ranjani H, Mehreen TS, Pradeepa R, et al. Epidemiology of childhood overweight and obesity in India: a systemic review. Indian J Med Res. 2016;143:160-174.
14. Rosenfield RL, Cooke David M, Radovik S. Puberty in the female and it's disorders.In: Sperling Pediatric Endocrinology.Sperling MA (Eds). Elsevier 2021, Philadelphia. 5th Edn, pp 528-626.
15. Shah NS, George J, Acharya SV, et al.Cushing disease in children and adolescents: twenty years' experience in a tertiary care center in India. Endocr Pract. 2011;17:369-76.
16. Stratakis CA. Diagnosis and clinical genetics of Cushing's syndrome in pediatrics. Endocrinol Metab Clinic N Am. 2016;45:311-28
17. Styne DM, Arslanian SA, Connor EL, Farooqi IS, Murad MH, Silverstein JH, Yanovski JA. Pediatric Obesity - Assessment, Treatment, and Prevention: An Endocrine Society Clinical Practice Guideline. J Clin Endocrinol Metab. 2017; 102:709-757
18. Unnikrishnan AG, Vyas U. Congenital hypothyroidism – An Indian perspective. Thyroid Res Pract. 2017;14:99-105.

PART B: SMR—HOW TO ASSESS?

INTRODUCTION

Sexual maturity rating or Tanner scale (after the British pediatrician) as it is better known as, is an objective classification of the sexual characteristics development in children and adolescents as they grow older.

It is a five point scale. Where 1 is prepubertal, stage 2 indicates changes at the onset of puberty, stage 3 indicating changes at mid puberty, and 5 is adult like/adult stage **(Fig. 1)**.

Tanner divided the processes of breast development in girls, genitalia development in boys, and pubic hair development in both sexes into five stages and axillary hair development in both sexes into three stages.

The accepted terminology is to describe breast development in stages B1–B5, genitalia development in stages G1–G5, pubic hair development in stages PH1–PH5 and axillary hair development in stages Al–A3.

As the descriptions are given in pictorial and descriptive form, the health professionals usually use the method of comparison to identify the pubertal stage of the child or adolescent.

Maintain privacy while examining. *Consent* of the child and their parents should be taken prior to assessment and a *chaperone* needs to be present.

BOYS—EXTERNAL GENITALIA

- *Stage 1:* Prepubertal
- *Stage 2:* Enlargement of scrotum and testes; scrotum skin reddens and changes in texture
- *Stage 3:* Enlargement of penis (length at first); further growth of testes
- *Stage 4:* Increased size of penis with growth in breadth and development of glans; testes and scrotum larger, scrotum skin darker
- *Stage 5:* Adult genitalia

GIRLS—BREAST DEVELOPMENT

- *Stage 1:* Prepubertal
- *Stage 2:* Breast bud stage with elevation of breast and papilla; enlargement of areola
- *Stage 3:* Further enlargement of breast and areola; no separation of their contour

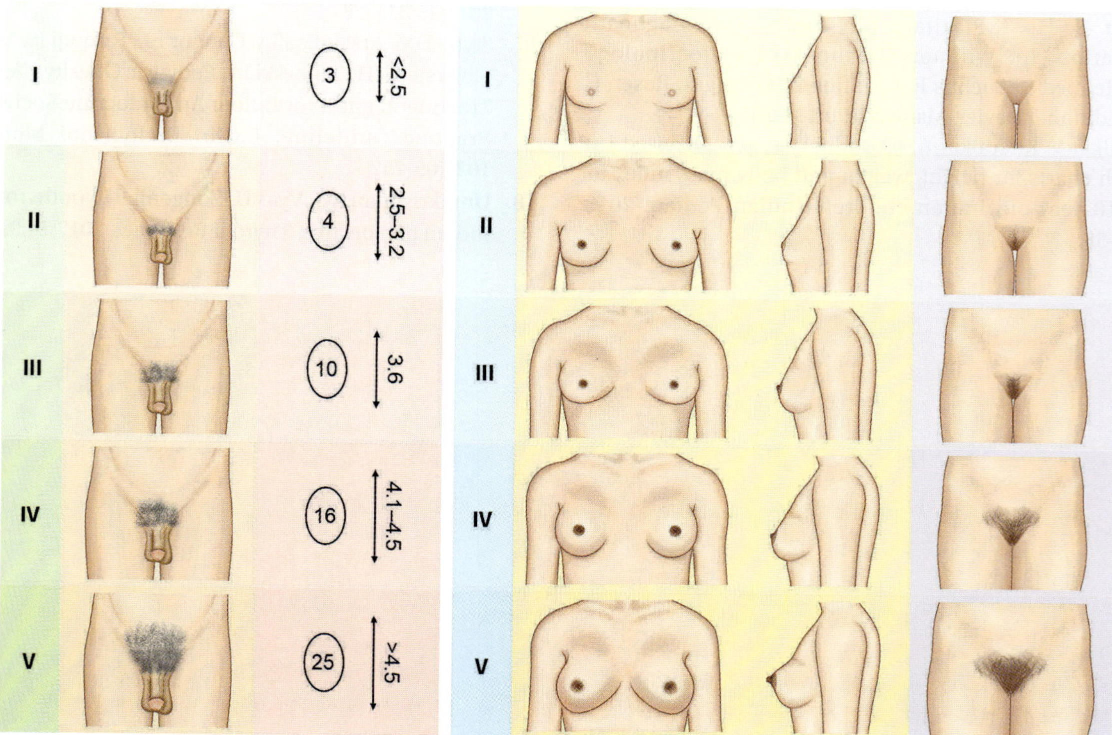

Fig. 1: Tanner staging in boys and girls.

- *Stage 4:* Areola and papilla form a secondary mound above level of breast
- *Stage 5:* Mature stage: projection of papilla only

BOYS AND GIRLS—PUBIC HAIR

- *Stage 1:* Prepubertal (can see vellus hair similar to abdominal wall)
- *Stage 2:* Sparse growth of long, slightly pigmented hair, straight or curled, and at base of penis or along the labia
- *Stage 3:* Darker, coarser and more curled hair, and begins to extend laterally.
- *Stage 4:* Hair adult in type, but covering smaller area than in adult; no spread to medial surface of thighs
- *Stage 5:* Adult in type and quantity, with horizontal distribution

Ideally, the examiner should examine the child and assign the stages of puberty. Sometimes, the child/adolescent may be shown the following pictures or the orchidometer **(Fig. 2)**. and asked to assign his or her own pubertal stage if they are not ready to let the examiner examine. These should be recorded and documented properly for future follow-up.

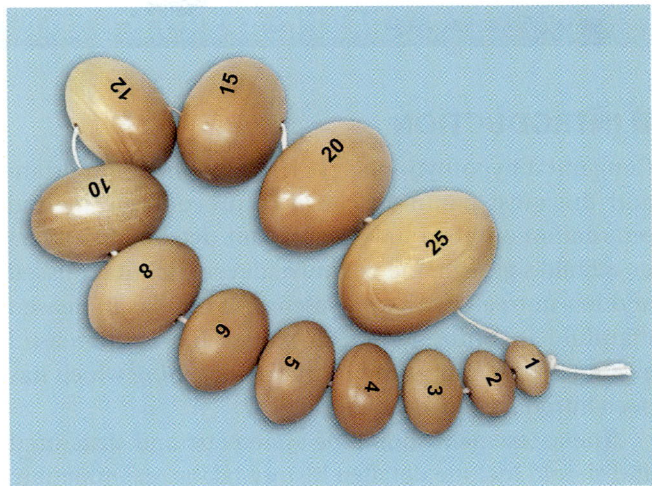

Fig. 2: Orchidometer.

PART C: APPROACH TO A CASE OF HYPOTHYROIDISM

INTRODUCTION

Congenital hypothyroidism (CH) is the most important and the most common cause of preventable mental retardation and can have significant detrimental effect on a child's growth and cognitive development if missed and left untreated. The prevalence of CH has increased manifold in India across all states due to increased awareness, reporting, and newborn screening which has been introduced in few states.

The assessment should be systematic and structured and should include detailed history taking, examination, and rational investigations.

It is to be remembered that <10% of infants are symptomatic. So, it is very important to do blood investigations in babies to diagnose CH as symptoms will take time to manifest.

ETIOLOGY

Etiology is listed in **Table 1**.

TABLE 1: Etiologies of hypothyroidism.

Thyroidal CH (permanent)	
Defect in thyroid gland development (thyroid dysgenesis) 80%	• Almost always sporadic or nonhereditary • Mutations in genes responsible for thyroid gland development (the TSH receptor or the transcription factors PAX8, NKX2-1, or FOXE1) 2–5%
Defect of thyroid hormone biosynthesis (dyshormonogenesis) 20%	
Thyroidal CH (transient)	
	• Transplacental passage of maternal antithyroid medications (methimazole or propylthiouracil) • Maternal thyroid blocking antibodies (in a mother with autoimmune thyroid disease) • Iodine deficiency or excess
Central CH	
	Pituitary or hypothalamic abnormality (secondary/tertiary hypothyroidism)

HISTORY TAKING

- Antenatal—maternal history of taking anti thyroid drugs or exposure to Iodine
- Birth weight and gestation with significant history of perinatal asphyxia, neonatal jaundice
- Family history of hypothyroidism in parents or siblings

CLINICAL EXAMINATION

- To look for stigmata of hypothyroidism such as goiter and lingual thyroid
- To look for other anomalies weight and height assessment
- Look for squint, hearing loss
- Congenital anomalies such as cleft lip/palate

INVESTIGATIONS

- *Free T3, T4, and TSH* to be done. The values should be interpreted carefully using appropriate age specific cut offs.
  - Low FT4 and high TSH indicate primary CH, normal FT4 with high TSH indicates subclinical hypothyroidism and low FT4 with low or inappropriately normal TSH indicates central hypothyroidism, transient hypothyroxinemia of prematurity.
- *X-ray of knees* may show absence of epiphyses of lower femur and tibia indicating severe hypothyroidism with poor neurocognitive outcome.
- *Thyroid scan:* In a confirmed case of primary hypothyroidism, it is important to know the etiopathogenesis of hypothyroidism. USG of thyroid gland or Tc 99m pertechnetate scan therefore has to be done to know the presence of the gland or if it is hypoplastic or located elsewhere. This will guide the duration of treatment and outcome.
  - USG is available easily in most hospital settings and is relatively cheaper than Tc 99 scan. Thyroid scan should be ideally done before starting treatment or within 1 week but not later. Therapy with thyroxine should be started without delay even when thyroid scan cannot be done.

TREATMENT

Levothyroxine is the medicine in case of hypothyroidism. Treatment should be started as early as possible after confirming by a venous blood sample. Earlier diagnosis and treatment ensure good neurodevelopmental outcome and optimum growth.

Dose is usually 10–15 μg/kg/day for neonates and infants depending on the severity of the condition which is reflected by FT4 levels.

The tablet may be mixed with expressed breast milk and taken at a fixed time every day in the morning at least 1 hour before the feed. The age wise therapeutic doses of thyroxine are as follows:

- *Newborn:* 10–15 μg/kg/day
- *1-6 months:* 8–10 μg/kg/day
- *6-12 months:* 6–8 μg/kg/day
- *1-5 years:* 5–6 μg/kg/day
- *6-12 years:* 4–5 μg/kg/day
- *12 years onwards:* 1–3 μg/kg/day

FOLLOW-UP

The newborns started on thyroxine should be called back after 2 weeks and then at 1 month to see if serum TSH has normalized. The dose should be titrated to maintain FT4 in higher range of normal for age. The sample should be taken in the morning before taking the medicine.

Further follow-up will be done every 2 months till 6 months of age, then 3 monthly until the infant is 3 years old. It can then be spaced to 4–6 monthly from 3 years to puberty.

After every dose modification, a repeat thyroid profile should be done after 4–6 weeks.

Babies with ectopic thyroid have permanent hypothyroidism and need to have lifelong supplementation. Those with transient hypothyroidism (needed very little dose, TSH is borderline at diagnosis) can be asked to stop thyroxine for 4–6 weeks after 3 years of age and reevaluated. Many a time, these children have normal height velocity and cognitive development. These parents need to be counseled well.

Generally, parents need to be thoroughly educated regarding dose, blood tests, and follow-up to improve compliance and good outcome.

Genetic counseling may be important in cases of dyshormonogenesis.

PART D: APPROACH TO A CASE OF CUSHING SYNDROME

ETIOLOGY

Etiology of Cushing's syndrome could be exogenous or endogenous. This is shown in **Table 2**.

CLINICAL POINTERS

Generalized obesity, growth failure, hirsutism, and pigmentation

ASSESSMENT HISTORY

- Assessment history of intake of oral, topical, or inhaled corticosteroids and alternative medicines
- *Age of onset:* Infantile onset suggests adrenal neoplasm, ACTH-independent causes more likely in younger children, Cushing s disease after 8 years. Ectopic Cushing's will present in adolescents.

PRESENTATION—GRADUAL—CUSHING'S DISEASE

Virilization (precocious puberty ion boys, and clitoromegaly, voice change, and increased features of masculinity in girls) indicates adrenal carcinoma, whereas rapid progression, pigmentation, and hypertension suggest ectopic Cushing's.

INITIAL EVALUATION

Exogenous Cushing's to be excluded by a morning cortisol of 138 nmol/L.

The diagnosis requires two or more positive screening tests (24-hour urinary free cortisol more than three times the normal limit, midnight cortisol above 50 nmol/L or levels above 50nmol/L after overnight dexamethasone suppression test.

CONFIRMATORY TEST

Low dose dexamethasone suppression test involves oral dexamethasone (1.25 mg/m^2 up to 2 mg/day given in four divided doses for 2 days, starting at 8 AM). Serum cortisol is measured on the third day at 8 AM with levels above 50 nmol/L (1.8 μg/dL) confirming hypercortisolism.

8 AM plasma ACTH levels will guide investigations to find out the etiology of Cushing's syndrome.

If ACTH levels are >15 pg/mL, it is ACTH dependent and if ACTH levels are below 5 pg/mL, it is ACTH independent. ACTH-dependent causes are the more common and include pituitary adenoma or hyperplasia and ectopic secretion from cancer cells (extremely rare in children).

TABLE 2: Etiology of Cushing's syndrome.

Type	*Source*	*Mechanism*
Exogenous		
	Iatrogenic	Exogenous administration of supraphysiologic doses of glucocorticoids or ACTH
Endogenous		
ACTH-dependent	Pituitary	Corticotroph pituitary neuroendocrine tumor
		Pituitary blastoma
	Ectopic	Neuroendocrine tumors secreting ACTH and/or CRH
ACTH-independent	Unilateral adrenal (except in metastatic disease)	Cortisol-secreting adrenocortical adenomas and carcinomas
	Bilateral adrenals	• Bilateral micronodular adrenocortical disease • Primary pigmented nodular adrenocortical disease (PPNAD), isolated or in the context of carney complex • Isolated micronodular adrenocortical disease (iMAD)
		Bilateral macronodular adrenocortical disease

Accordingly, MRI of hypothalamic-pituitary region may be done. In other cases, adrenal CT scan may help in reaching the diagnosis.

MANAGEMENT

It will depend upon the diagnosis.

Transsphenoidal resection is done in pituitary adenomas. Recurrence is common in 30–40% of cases.

Laparoscopic resection is done for adrenal adenomas. Adrenal carcinomas may be difficult to operate and have poor prognosis.

The management of ectopic lesions is very complicated. Medical management often leads to various side effects and is therefore unsatisfactory. Steroidogenic inhibitors such as ketoconazole and metyrapone may be used.

To treat exogenous causes, we have to do physiological hydrocortisone replacement (8–10 $mg/m^2/day$) to avoid adrenal crisis with gradual reduction over a period of 3–6 months. Discontinuation of steroids will improve the patient's clinical condition and growth eventually.

PART E: APPROACH TO A CASE OF PRECOCIOUS PUBERTY

QUESTIONS

1. Define precocious puberty.
2. How to determine whether it is central puberty or peripheral puberty or central puberty secondary to peripheral precocity?
3. Explain investigations for precocious puberty.
4. How to interpret laboratory investigation to differentiate central puberty or peripheral puberty or central puberty secondary to peripheral precocity

Precocious puberty is defined as appearance of secondary sexual characters (appearance of breast buds in girls) before 8 years and or menarche before 9 years and testicular enlargement in boys before 9 years.

APPROACH

- Assess if it is *truly a case of breast enlargement* or fat deposition (lipomastia)
  This can be done by slowly trying to feel the breast bud by apposing the index finger and thumb. If a resistance is felt, it is breast bud or else it is lipomastia.
- We have to see whether it is an isolated case of thelarche or are there other true features of puberty too. In boys, we should look for testicular enlargement with maturation of external genitalia. The children may have sudden increase in height known as the growth spurt and features of mood swings.
- *Age of presentation:* The younger the child (<6 years), the greater is the chance of it being pathological.

However isolated thelarche is a benign condition.

- Girls older than 6 years will most likely have idiopathic precocious puberty whereas boys have higher chance of having pathological precocity.
- Rate of progression is very important to note. It may help us to take the decision of starting treatment. Slow progressors may have normal age of menarche and wait and watch policy may be just the right approach.
- *History taking:* Birth weight is an important predictor as small for gestational age children are known to have early pubarche and precocious puberty.

Family history of precocious puberty may be important.

- To determine whether it is central puberty or peripheral puberty or central puberty secondary to peripheral precocity.

In central precocity, the progression maintains the usual sequence of events like thelarche followed by pubarche followed by menarche in girls.

Children who have peripheral causes of precocity with significantly advanced bone age may develop secondary central precocity with treatment. Treatment of peripheral precocity leads to suppression of sex steroids which will then activate the hypothalamo-pituitary gonadal axis leading to central precocity.

In peripheral precocious puberty, on the other hand, will have discordant and inappropriately rapid progression. For example, menarche without advanced breast enlargement in girls.

CLINICAL EXAMINATION

A goiter or short stature in the child may point toward hypothyroidism.

Café au lait spots, bony deformities may point toward McCune-Albright syndrome.

Visual disturbances, squint, nystagmus may point toward features of raised intracranial tension.

History of ingestion or application of medicines or lotions and creams may point toward exogenous exposure of steroids.

INVESTIGATIONS

- *Hormonal test:* LH, FSH, estradiol, and testosterone. If early morning:
  - LH is >0.2 IU/L, it is an indicator of central precocity.
  - Suppressed levels of LH, FSH, and high estrogen/testosterone will confirm peripheral causes of precocity.
- If LH is prepubertal but clinical features are suggestive of progressive precocious puberty, GnRH stimulation test should be done to confirm diagnosis.
  - LH > 5 IU/L with LH: FSH ratio > 1 is diagnostic of central precocious puberty.
- Other supportive tests such as serum prolactin is high is suprasellar tumors, or prolactinomas or primary hypothyroidism with high TSH.
  - 17-hydroxyprogesterone may be high in 21 hydroxylase deficiency.

- *Radiological tests:*
    - X-ray of left hand (nondominant) and wrist and calculating bone age by comparison with Greulich–Pyle charts or other validated apps. Advanced bone age is a strong indicator of precocity.

      Skeletal survey may be required in cases of suspected McCune–Albright syndrome.
    - *USG of abdomen:* Length and size of uterus, endometrial thickness, and ovarian volume should be noted in girls. In boys, USG scrotum is needed to rule out masses or tumors in asymmetric testes or to look for adrenal rest tumors in cases of suspected peripheral precocity.
    - USG and CT scan of abdomen may be rarely required for excluding tumors of adrenal glands or ovarian cysts and tumors in girls.
    - MRI of brain is to be done in all children <6 years presenting with central precocious puberty, all boys with central precocity and in any child with neurological signs or deficit.

CT scan may be done as an alternative in resource poor settings.

MANAGEMENT

The main goal of treatment is to postpone the puberty to the age where it is acceptable to the child, family, and society, to preserve the growth potential and ensure psychological wellbeing in the child.

Treatment is done with GnRH analogs injections monthly or 3 monthly. Treatment should be continued till 10/11 years of age. Pubertal progression will restart after 3/6 months of discontinuation of treatment. Leuprolide acetate and triptorelin are commonly given.

Treatment should be offered in cases with significantly advanced bone age, compromised final adult height, complete central precocity, high LH values, and for psychological reasons.

Growth hormone therapy in addition to GnRH therapy may be needed in cases with suboptimal growth.

The treatment in peripheral precocity is the treatment of the cause, e.g., supplementation of steroids in CAH, treatment with letrozole in McCune–Albright syndrome, etc.

Regular monitoring and follow up are needed to look for optimum growth, puberty assessment, adequate suppression of axis by hormonal assessment, etc.

PART F: APPROACH TO A CASE OF OBESITY

DEFINE OBESITY

According to World Health organization (WHO), overweight and obesity are defined as excessive fat accumulation that is detrimental to health and wellbeing.

Children <2 years are diagnosed as obese if the weight for length is >97.7th percentile of WHO growth charts. Children >2 years are diagnosed as obese if the BMI is >95th percentile for age and sex.

CALCULATE BMI

Weight in kg/Height in meter^2

Obesity in children can be caused by a combination of factors. Here are some of the most common causes:

- *Poor diet choices*:
  - *High-calorie, low-nutrient foods:* Diets rich in processed foods, sugary snacks, sodas, and fast food can lead to weight gain.
  - *Overeating*: Eating large portions, especially of high-calorie foods, can contribute to obesity.
- *Lack of physical activity:*
  - *Sedentary lifestyle:* Increased screen time (TV, video games, and smartphones) and reduced physical activity can lead to weight gain.
  - *Limited outdoor play:* Fewer opportunities for outdoor activities and exercise can decrease calorie expenditure.
- *Genetics:*
  - *Family history:* Children with obese parents are more likely to become obese themselves, as genetics can play a significant role in how the body stores fat and processes calories.
- *Environmental factors:*
  - *Access to unhealthy foods:* Living in "food deserts" with limited access to healthy food options can contribute to poor dietary choices.
  - *Marketing of unhealthy foods:* Children are often targeted by advertisements promoting unhealthy, calorie-dense foods.
- *Socioeconomic factors:*
  - *Limited resources:* Families with fewer financial resources may struggle to buy healthy foods or may have to rely on cheaper, less nutritious options.
  - *Stress and food insecurity:* Economic hardship and lack of access to healthy foods can also lead to overeating or poor nutrition.
- *Psychological factors:*
  - *Emotional eating:* Stress, anxiety, depression, or boredom can lead children to eat for comfort, rather than for hunger.
  - *Low self-esteem:* Some children may cope with emotional issues through overeating.
- *Sleep patterns:*
  - *Inadequate sleep:* Lack of sleep or poor-quality sleep can disrupt hormones that regulate appetite, leading to overeating.
  - *Sleep apnea:* Sleep disorders such as sleep apnea can interfere with weight management.
- *Medical conditions:*
  - *Hormonal imbalances:* Conditions such as hypothyroidism or polycystic ovary syndrome (PCOS) can contribute to weight gain.
  - *Medications:* Certain medications, such as corticosteroids or antidepressants, can lead to weight gain as a side effect.
- *Lack of parental guidance or support:*
  - *Parental influence:* Parents who model unhealthy eating habits or who don't encourage physical activity can contribute to their child's obesity risk.
  - *Limited supervision:* Without guidance on nutrition and healthy lifestyle habits, children may adopt unhealthy behaviors.

CLASSIFICATION OF OBESITY

Obesity is classified into different categories based on BMI as follows:

1. *Normal weight:* BMI 18.5–24.9
2. *Overweight:* BMI 25–29.9
3. *Obesity:*
   - *Class 1 (Moderate obesity):* BMI 30–34.9 or above the 95th percentile to 119% of the 95th percentile
   - *Class 2 (Severe obesity):* BMI 35–39.9 or BMI 120–139% of the 95% percentile
   - *Class 3 (Very severe or morbid obesity):* BMI 40 and above

Peripheral obesity and central obesity refer to two different patterns of fat distribution in the body. Here's a breakdown of each:

Peripheral Obesity

- *Description:* In peripheral obesity, excess fat is primarily stored in the *arms, legs, and hips*. The fat tends to accumulate around the limbs and outer parts of the body.
- *Appearance:* People with peripheral obesity often have a "pear-shaped" body, where the lower body is larger than the upper body.
- *Health risks:* Although it can lead to discomfort or mobility issues, peripheral obesity is generally considered less risky in terms of heart disease and metabolic disorders compared to central obesity.

Central Obesity

- *Description:* Central obesity, also known as *visceral obesity*, involves fat accumulation around the *abdomen and internal organs*, particularly around the waist and stomach. This type of fat is often referred to as visceral fat.
- *Appearance:* People with central obesity often have an "apple-shaped" body, where the waistline is larger than the hips.
- *Health risks:* Central obesity is associated with *higher risks* for serious health conditions such as heart disease, type 2 diabetes, hypertension, and metabolic syndrome. This is because visceral fat can release hormones and chemicals that increase inflammation and affect the body's metabolism.

ASSESSMENT

- *History:*
  - Age of onset, duration, rapidity of progression of weight gain
  - Perinatal history—history of maternal gestational diabetes, birth weight (small for gestational age or large for gestational age)
  - Developmental history—delays if any
  - Family history—diabetes, obesity, hypertension, and lipid disorders
  - Dietary pattern—quality, quantity of food, snacking habits, and junk food habits
  - Physical activities if any and sleeping habits
  - Drug history—history of any chronic medication if any
  - Pubertal history—wherever appropriate
  - Comorbidities if any—snoring, headache, hip pain, abdominal pain, increased hair growth, and menstrual irregularities
- *Physical examination:*
  - Weight, height, waist circumference, BMI
  - Dysmorphism if noted
  - Blood pressure measurement with appropriate sized cuff
  - Acanthosis nigricans in neck
  - General condition of skin and hair
  - Systemic examination (hepatomegaly may be there)
  - Pubertal assessment should not be missed.
- *Investigations:*
  - No special investigations are required for exogenous obesity. We can screen for comorbidities in children with BMI >85th centile with 2 or more risk factors and those with BMI >95th percentile.
  - Risk factors include strong family history of type 2 diabetes, early cardiovascular disease, familial dyslipidemias, etc., sedentary lifestyle, low birth weight, genetic or syndromic obesity, and signs of insulin resistance such as acanthosis, hirsutism, PCOS, etc.
  - The usually ordered investigations are fasting blood glucose, HbA1C, lipid profile, SGPT, and USG abdomen to rule out fatty liver.

PREVENTION AND MANAGEMENT OF OBESITY

Prevention of Obesity in Children

- *Promote healthy eating habits:*
  - *Balanced diet:* Encourage a diet rich in fruits, vegetables, whole grains, lean proteins, and low-fat dairy products.
  - *Portion control:* Teach children about appropriate portion sizes to avoid overeating.
  - *Limit sugar and processed foods:* Reduce the consumption of sugary drinks, snacks, and highly processed foods high in fats and sugars.
  - *Family meals:* Eating together as a family encourages healthier eating and allows for better portion control.

- *Increase physical activity:*
  - *Regular exercise:* Encourage at least 60 minutes of physical activity each day, such as walking, running, biking, or playing sports.
  - *Active play:* Encourage outdoor play and limit screen time (television, video games, etc.) to no >1–2 hours per day.
  - *Engage in family activities:* Participate in physical activities together as a family, such as hiking or biking, to make exercise fun and engaging.
- *Create a positive environment:*
  - *Role models:* Parents and caregivers should model healthy behaviors, as children often mimic the habits of adults.
  - *Healthy home environment:* Keep nutritious foods readily available, and try to minimize unhealthy snacks at home.
  - *Encourage self-esteem:* Help children feel confident in their bodies and avoid focusing on weight in a negative way. Emphasize health over appearance.
- *Adequate sleep:*
  - *Consistent sleep routine:* Ensure children get enough sleep (9–12 hours per night depending on their age). Sleep deprivation can contribute to weight gain and unhealthy eating patterns.
  - *Limit screen time before bed:* Avoid screens for at least an hour before bedtime to help improve sleep quality.

MANAGEMENT OF OBESITY IN CHILDREN

- *Early intervention:*
  - *Regular check-ups*: Regular pediatric visits can help identify early signs of obesity and allow for timely intervention.
  - *Body mass index monitoring*: Keep track of BMI to identify children at risk of obesity and to develop appropriate management strategies.
- *Behavioral changes:*
  - *Goal setting:* Set realistic and achievable goals for weight management, focusing on gradual changes rather than rapid weight loss.
  - *Positive reinforcement:* Use praise and reward to reinforce healthy behaviors, such as trying new fruits or vegetables or engaging in physical activities.
  - *Behavioral therapy:* Cognitive-behavioral therapy (CBT) and family-based programs can help children and families address eating behaviors and attitudes towards food and body image.
- *Medical and nutritional support:*
  - *Dietitian consultation:* A pediatric nutritionist or dietitian can help create a customized meal plan to ensure that the child is receiving adequate nutrition while managing calorie intake.
  - *Medication:* In some cases, healthcare providers may recommend medication for children who are severely obese, though this is typically combined with lifestyle changes.
- *Surgical intervention (for severe cases):*
  - *Bariatric surgery:* In rare cases, for children who have severe obesity and related health complications, bariatric surgery (such as gastric bypass) may be considered, usually after other options have been explored.
- *Parental involvement:*
  - *Support at home:* Parents should actively participate in the child's weight management plan by providing healthy meals, encouraging physical activity, and offering emotional support.
  - *Education and advocacy:* Parents should be educated about the importance of healthy behaviors and how to navigate social pressures, food advertising, and other external factors that might contribute to obesity.

PSYCHOSOCIAL SUPPORT

- *Address emotional eating:* Emotional or stress-related eating can contribute to weight gain. Providing support for children experiencing stress or emotional challenges is essential.
- *Promote a positive body image:* Ensure that the child feels accepted and valued regardless of their weight. Encourage self-esteem and body positivity.
- *Social support:* Engaging in community-based programs or support groups can provide additional resources and motivation for families facing obesity challenges.

SYNDROMES ASSOCIATED WITH OBESITY

Obesity is associated with a variety of syndromes and health conditions. Some of these syndromes are directly caused by obesity, while others may be exacerbated or triggered by it. Below are some of the key syndromes associated with obesity.

Metabolic Syndrome

- *Description:* A cluster of conditions that increase the risk of heart disease, stroke, and type 2 diabetes.
- *Key features:*
  - Abdominal obesity (excess fat around the waist)
  - High blood pressure
  - High blood sugar levels
  - High triglyceride levels
  - Low HDL (good cholesterol) levels

Sleep Apnea Syndrome

- *Description:* A sleep disorder where breathing repeatedly stops and starts during sleep, often due to fat accumulation around the neck and throat area.
- *Key features:*
  - Loud snoring
  - Interrupted sleep
  - Excessive daytime sleepiness
  - Difficulty concentrating

Prader–Willi Syndrome

- *Description:* A rare genetic disorder characterized by insatiable hunger (hyperphagia), leading to overeating and obesity.
- *Key features:*
  - Severe obesity beginning in early childhood
  - Developmental delays
  - Hypotonia (muscle weakness)
  - Cognitive impairment

Bardet–Biedl Syndrome

- *Description:* A genetic disorder that can cause obesity along with other symptoms such as retinal degeneration and polydactyly (extra fingers or toes).
- *Key features:*
  - Obesity, often beginning in childhood
  - Vision problems
  - Intellectual disabilities
  - Kidney issues

Cushing's Syndrome

- *Description:* A hormonal disorder caused by high levels of cortisol, often resulting in weight gain and fat accumulation, especially in the abdomen and face.
- *Key features:*
  - Rapid weight gain, particularly in the face, abdomen, and upper back
  - Thinning skin, bruising, and purple stretch marks
  - High blood pressure
  - Diabetes
  - Weak muscles

Hypothyroidism (Underactive Thyroid)

- *Description:* A condition in which the thyroid gland does not produce enough thyroid hormones, leading to a slower metabolism and weight gain.
- *Key features:*
  - Weight gain
  - Fatigue
  - Depression
  - Dry skin and hair
  - Cold intolerance

Polycystic Ovary Syndrome

- *Description:* A hormonal disorder that can affect women and often leads to weight gain, insulin resistance, and infertility.
- *Key features:*
  - Irregular periods
  - Excessive hair growth (hirsutism)
  - Cysts on the ovaries
  - Weight gain and difficulty losing weight
  - Acne

Lipoedema

- *Description:* A chronic condition involving the abnormal accumulation of fat in the lower body (hips, thighs, and legs), often mistaken for obesity.
- *Key features:*
  - Symmetrical fat deposition, mainly in the legs and buttocks
  - Painful legs and bruising easily
  - Swelling in the legs
  - Disproportionate body shape

Nonalcoholic Fatty Liver Disease

- *Description:* A condition where excess fat builds up in the liver without alcohol consumption, which is commonly associated with obesity and metabolic syndrome.
- *Key features:*
  - Fatigue
  - Abdominal discomfort
  - Liver enlargement
  - Elevated liver enzymes

Gastroesophageal Reflux Disease (GERD)

- *Description:* Obesity increases the risk of gastroesophageal reflux disease (GERD), a chronic digestive condition where stomach acid or bile irritates the food pipe.
- *Key features:*
  - Heartburn
  - Regurgitation of food or sour liquid
  - Chest pain
  - Difficulty swallowing

Osteoarthritis

- *Description:* Excess weight can put additional strain on joints, particularly weight-bearing joints such as the knees and hips, leading to osteoarthritis.
- *Key features:*
  - Joint pain and stiffness
  - Decreased mobility
  - Swelling around the joint

Cardiovascular Disease

- *Description:* Obesity is a major risk factor for heart disease, including coronary artery disease, heart failure, and stroke.
- *Key features:*
  - High blood pressure
  - High cholesterol
  - Increased risk of heart attack or stroke
  - Shortness of breath and fatigue

Type 2 Diabetes

- *Description:* Obesity, especially abdominal obesity, is a major risk factor for developing insulin resistance, which can lead to type 2 diabetes.
- *Key features:*
  - Increased thirst
  - Frequent urination
  - Fatigue
  - Blurred vision
  - Slow healing of wounds

PART G: APPROACH TO A CASE OF SHORT STATURE

- What is short stature?
- What are the causes of short stature?
- What is proportionate and disproportionate short stature?
- How to measure height?
- What is correlation of upper limb and lower limb measurements?
- Explain investigations of short stature.
- Explain management of short stature.

INTRODUCTION

It is very common to find children coming with the problem of not gaining height or short stature to pediatric outdoor. Although most of these children have physiological causes of short stature, at least 20% of them may have underlying pathological causes.

Short stature in children can be caused by a variety of factors, ranging from genetic influences to medical conditions. Here are the most common causes.

GENETIC FACTORS

- *Family history:* If the parents or close relatives are shorter in stature, it is likely that the child will also be shorter, though they will usually follow their own growth curve.
- *Constitutional growth delay (delayed growth):* Some children experience a slower rate of growth, but they often catch up during adolescence. This condition is sometimes referred to as "late bloomers."

NUTRITIONAL DEFICIENCIES

- *Inadequate nutrition:* Poor intake of essential nutrients such as protein, vitamins (particularly vitamin D), and minerals (calcium, iron, and zinc) can stunt growth.
- *Malnutrition:* Conditions such as anorexia nervosa or chronic undernutrition can significantly affect growth.
- *Celiac disease:* This autoimmune disorder, when untreated, can interfere with nutrient absorption, leading to growth failure.

ENDOCRINE (HORMONAL) DISORDERS

- *Growth hormone (GH) deficiency:* A lack of GH can result in slow growth and short stature.
- *Hypothyroidism:* An underactive thyroid gland can affect growth and development.
- *Cushing's syndrome:* This condition results from excessive cortisol, which can inhibit growth.
- *Precocious puberty:* Early onset of puberty can lead to early closure of growth plates, limiting further growth.

CHRONIC MEDICAL CONDITIONS

- *Chronic kidney disease:* Children with kidney problems may experience growth delay due to the body's difficulty in processing nutrients or maintaining the correct balance of hormones.
- *Asthma and respiratory diseases:* Children with chronic lung conditions, especially if on long-term corticosteroid treatment, may experience growth delays.
- *Congenital heart disease:* Some children with heart conditions may grow slowly due to inadequate oxygen and nutrient supply to tissues.
- *Rheumatic diseases:* Conditions such as juvenile arthritis may interfere with normal growth.

GENETIC SYNDROMES

- *Turner syndrome:* A chromosomal disorder in girls where one of the X chromosomes is partially or completely missing, leading to short stature and other developmental issues.
- *Down syndrome:* A genetic condition causing intellectual disability and often associated with short stature.
- *Noonan syndrome:* A genetic disorder that affects many parts of the body, including growth and development.
- *Prader-Willi syndrome:* A genetic disorder that can lead to short stature, developmental delays, and obesity.

BONE DISORDERS

- *Dysplasia:* Conditions such as osteogenesis imperfecta (brittle bone disease) or other skeletal dysplasias can result in short stature due to abnormal bone development.
- *Rickets:* Caused by a vitamin D deficiency, rickets affects bone development, leading to short stature and skeletal deformities.

PSYCHOSOCIAL FACTORS

- *Emotional stress:* Prolonged psychological stress, such as from abuse, neglect, or family instability, can have a significant impact on growth, especially if it affects appetite or sleep.
- *Severe anxiety or depression:* In some cases, these conditions can manifest physically by impairing growth.

INFECTIONS AND INFLAMMATORY CONDITIONS

- *Chronic infections:* Long-standing infections (e.g., tuberculosis or chronic viral infections) can interfere with growth by diverting the body's resources toward fighting infection.
- *Inflammatory bowel disease (IBD):* Conditions such as Crohn's disease or ulcerative colitis can impair nutrient absorption, leading to growth failure.

PREMATURITY AND LOW BIRTH WEIGHT

- *Premature birth:* Babies born prematurely may experience delays in growth during infancy and early childhood, although many catch up over time.
- *Intrauterine growth restriction (IUGR):* Babies who experience growth restriction in the womb may have slower growth in the early years of life.

OTHER RARE CAUSES

- *Idiopathic short stature:* In some cases, no clear cause can be found for a child's short stature, even after thorough evaluation. This is considered a diagnosis of exclusion when all other conditions have been ruled out.
- *Another way of classification is:*
  - *Proportionate short stature (PSS):*
    - *Definition:* In PSS, the individual's body parts grow at a uniform rate, meaning all body parts are shorter than average, but their proportions remain normal.
    - *Cause:* This type of short stature is often caused by general growth delays or conditions that affect overall growth but do not disproportionately affect specific body parts. Examples include:
      - *Genetic short stature:* Inherited shorter stature without underlying medical conditions
      - *GH deficiency:* The body does not produce enough GH, leading to a general slowing of growth.
      - *Chronic illnesses:* Conditions such as malnutrition, chronic kidney disease, or hormonal imbalances may lead to PSS.
      - *Constitutional growth delay:* A temporary delay in growth that resolves over time.
    - *Appearance:* The individual looks smaller than others, but the body's proportions (head, trunk, arms, and legs) are in balance and follow typical growth patterns.
  - *Disproportionate short stature (DSS):*
    - *Definition:* In disproportionate short stature, the individual's body parts are not proportionally sized. Some parts of the body (such as the trunk, limbs, or head) may be shorter or longer than others, creating noticeable discrepancies in body proportions.
    - *Cause:* Disproportionate short stature is often caused by skeletal dysplasias (genetic conditions that affect bone development) or other conditions that affect the growth of specific body parts. Some common causes include:
      - *Achondroplasia:* A form of dwarfism where the limbs are shorter than average, but the trunk and head may be of normal size or relatively larger.
      - *Hypochondroplasia:* Another form of dwarfism with similar characteristics to achondroplasia, though often less severe.
      - *Turner syndrome:* A genetic disorder in females where the X chromosome is missing or partially missing, leading to short stature and other characteristic features like a webbed neck and low-set ears.
      - *Morquio syndrome:* A metabolic disorder where short stature is accompanied by disproportionate shortening of the limbs.
      - *Primordial dwarfism:* A rare condition where individuals are extremely small in stature and have disproportionate features.
    - *Appearance:* Individuals with disproportionate short stature may have features such as a larger-than-average head with shorter limbs or a longer trunk relative to their limbs. The specific proportions depend on the underlying cause.

APPROACH TO A SHORT STATURE

A detailed history taking and proper systematic examination and investigations will help us to come to a correct diagnosis without doing irrational investigations.

Constitutional delay of growth and puberty (CDGP) and familial short stature are the most common causes of physiological short stature whereas pathological causes may vary from systemic illness, skeletal dysplasia, or endocrinological diseases such as hypothyroidism and GH deficiency.

- Assessment starts with the *confirmation* of short stature first by plotting the child's weight and height on age and gender appropriate IAP (5–18 years) or WHO (for <5 years) growth charts.
- Evaluation is required only if child's height is <1st centile, that is if the child is very short, or short and not growing which is height between 1st and 3rd centiles but the height velocity is below 25th centile, or not growing at all that is those who have crossed 2 or more major centiles between the age of 2 years and puberty.
- *History taking:* It should include:
  - Birth weight
  - Duration since when growth faltering has been noticed
  - Family history of diseases
  - Detailed nutritional history
  - History to rule out chronic diseases such as coeliac (diarrhea, constipation, abdominal pain, and intolerance to wheat products and rice preference), respiratory Illness such as asthma, cystic fibrosis, heart diseases (recurrent chest infection), hematological (blood transfusion in chronic hemolytic anemias), renal problems(use of steroids for prolonged period suggestive of nephrotic syndrome), etc.
  - Other history of past hospitalization
  - Perinatal history: Episode of hypoglycemia/jaundice (hypopituitarism/GHD)
  - Use of any chronic medicines for any reason
  - Difficulties in hearing may suggest Turner syndrome.
- *Examination:*
  - Pallor—chronic renal failure, malnutrition, coeliac disease, chronic hemolytic anemia, etc.
  - Clubbing—liver disease, coeliac disease, and cystic fibrosis
  - Brachymetacarpia (short 4th metacarpal) and brachymetatarsia (short 4th toes)—Turner and pseudohypoparathyroidism (PHP)
  - Rickets or rachitic changes—renal failure, coeliac disease, or renal tubular acidosis
  - Body proportion (US: LS ratio)—skeletal dysplasia
  - Facies for Turner/Noonan/Russell silver syndrome
  - Micropenis/undescended testis/midline defects—panhypopituitarism
  - Puberty assessment
  - Particular pointers to diagnosis—facies/digits/asymmetry of face/skin findings, etc.
- *Investigations:*
  - There are some screening tests which must be done first to rule out common and physiological causes before going for more sophisticated and expensive endocrinological tests.
  - Screening tests include CBC, ESR, serum urea and electrolytes, liver function test, calcium, phosphorus, blood sugar, and FT4 and TSH.
  - Chest X-ray should be done to rule out tuberculosis.
  - Children who show nutritional pattern of growth failure should have blood gas done and blood for tissue transglutaminase levels to rule out renal tubular acidosis and coeliac disease, respectively.
  - Karyotype (30 metaphase) should be done in a short girl with no apparent abnormality in screening tests as Turner syndrome cannot be missed.
- *To decide whether it is nutritional or endocrine/other cause:*
  - Only after exclusion of common causes such as malnutrition, malabsorption, chronic systemic illness such as congenital heart disease, and infection (tuberculosis), should we think of endocrine causes such as hypothyroidism, GH deficiency, panhypopituitarism, Cushing syndrome, or pseudohypoparathyroidism.
  - If weight is more affected than height (weight age < height age), it is most likely nutritional or due to systemic illness.
  - If height age is less than weight age, then it is most probably endocrinological.
- *Assessment of GH-IGF1 axis:* It is the last investigation to be done only after excluding all other commoner causes of growth failure. Normal values of thyroid and cortisol hormones are essential before assessing the GH axis.
  - There is *no role* of doing isolated GH levels. IGF1 and IGFBP3 levels may be done as screening test. GH stimulation test with clonidine or insulin or glucagon is the gold standard test for diagnosing GH deficiency.

  - A peak stimulated GH value < 5 ng/mL is defined as complete GHD whereas levels between 5 and 10 ng/mL will be defined as partial GH deficiency (GHD).
- *Management:*
  - Dietary modification and supplements—protein rich diet, iron, zinc, and calcium supplementation
  - Physical activity
  - Gluten-free diet in coeliac disease
  - Thyroxine supplementation in hypothyroidism
  - Alkali in renal tubular acidosis
  - Creons and antibiotics in cystic fibrosis
  - GH therapy is indicated in GHD, Turner syndrome, and small for gestational age children who haven't had catch up by 3–4 years, chronic kidney disease, Prader-Willi syndrome with growth failure.
  - GH therapy has been also used in idiopathic short stature.
- *Follow-up:* It is very important to follow these children closely every 4–6 months depending on the cause to see the trend and height velocity. This will help better compliance and reassurance to parents.
- *Psychological counseling:* This should not be forgotten as many children and adolescents may suffer from low self-esteem and anxiety/depression because of short stature and addressing these issues will help in long term wellbeing and good mental health of these children and adolescents.

CHAPTER 11

Chromosomal Disorders

Joydeep Das

Identifying dysmorphism is a difficult subject which needs experience over the years. We have few major or minor dysmorphic signs. An anomaly is a structural defect and can be categorized as minor or major. A major anomaly may need structural, surgical, or cosmetic correction but minor anomaly may not. Examples of few major and minor anomaly are given in **Table 1**.

TABLE 1: Major and minor anomaly.

Major malformation:	
Neurologic	• Severe hydrocephalus • Lissencephaly • Schizencephaly • Megalencephaly • Neural tube defect • Meningomyelocele • Encephalocele
Abdominal wall	• Gastroschisis • Omphalocele
Craniofacial	• Craniosynostosis • Facial cleft • Cleft lip and palate • Structural eye defect • Coloboma • Aniridia • Structural ear defect • Microtia • Aplasia of the auditory canal
Cardiovascular	• Various congenital malformation • Cardiomyopathy • Genetic arrhythmia syndrome
Genitourinary	• Ambiguous genitalia • Kidney malformation • Urachal defect
Respiratory	• Congenital pulmonary airway malformation • Tracheoesophageal malformation
Limb	• Amelia • Split/hand foot malformation
Minor malformation:	
Hand	• Simian crease • Bridged upper palmar crease • 5th finger clinodactyly • Joint hypermobility (hyperextension of thumb) • Cutaneous syndactyly • Polydactyly • Short broad thumb • Narrow or hyperconvex thumb • Hypoplastic nails • Camptodactyly • Short fourth metacarpal
Foot	• Syndactyly of 2nd/3rd toe • Asymmetric toe length • Clinodactyly of second toe • Overlapping toe • Nail hypoplasia • Wide gap between hallux and 2nd toe • Deep planter crease between hallux and 2nd toe
Craniofacial	• Large fontanel • Flat or low nasal bridge • Saddle nose, upturned nose • Micrognathia • Cutis aplasia of the scalp
Eye	• Palpebral fissure • Telecanthus or epicanthus up or down slanting • Hypertelorism • Brushfield spots
Ear	• Posteriorly rotated pinna • Lack of helical fold • Preauricular with or without auricular skin tag • Small pinna • Auricular (preauricular) pit or sinus • Folding of helix • Darwinian tubercle • Crushed (crinkled) ear • Asymmetric ear sizes • Low-set ears

Contd...

Contd...

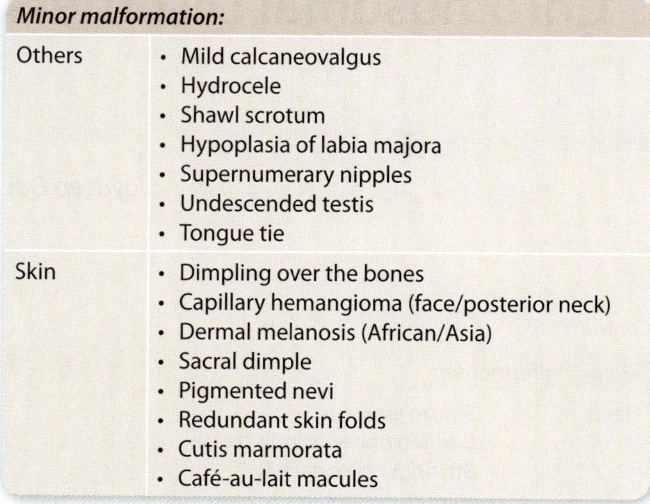

Minor malformation:	
Others	• Mild calcaneovalgus • Hydrocele • Shawl scrotum • Hypoplasia of labia majora • Supernumerary nipples • Undescended testis • Tongue tie
Skin	• Dimpling over the bones • Capillary hemangioma (face/posterior neck) • Dermal melanosis (African/Asia) • Sacral dimple • Pigmented nevi • Redundant skin folds • Cutis marmorata • Café-au-lait macules

Flowchart 1: Four types of structural defects that can result in a chain of defects (sequence) by the time of birth.

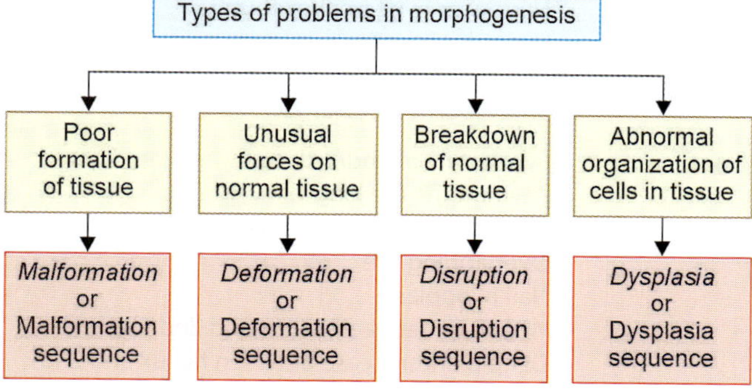

To level a major dysmorphic syndrome, we need 2 major or 3 minor criteria **(Flowchart 1)**.

In malformation, there is structural defect arising out of intrinsically abnormal process of embryogenesis. Examples are cleft lip and palate and ventricular septal defect.

In deformation sequence, there is no inherent problem in the embryo or fetus, but mechanical force inside or outside the uterus results in altered morphogenesis or molding. Examples are oligohydramnios sequence and breech presentation sequence.

In disruption sequence, a normal fetus is subjected to destructive process or its consequences. It may be vascular, infection, or amniotic band. Examples are intestinal atresia due to vascular insult, limb reduction defect in amniotic band.

In dysplasia, there is disorderly growth and maturation of cells within a tissue or atypical organization of cells.

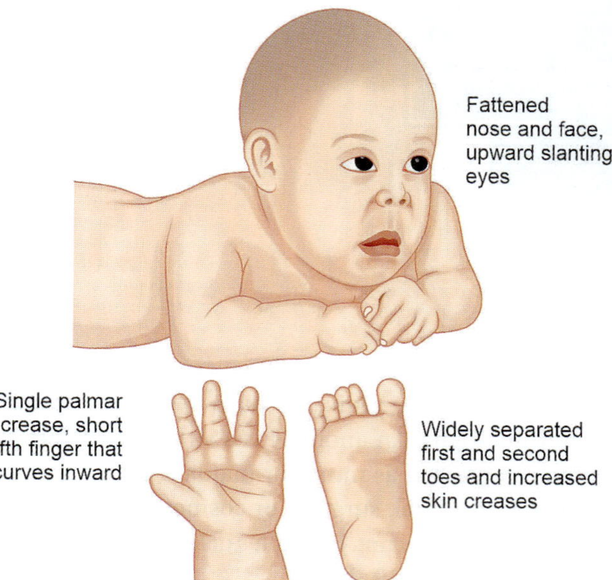

Fig. 1: Clinical features of trisomy 21 (Down syndrome) in an infant.

Examples are neurocutaneous melanosis sequence, multicystic dysplasia of kidney, and capillary malformation like port-wine stain.

For beginners, we will discuss a few common syndromes.

Trisomy 21 (Down syndrome) **(Fig. 1)***:*

Keylines:

- Incidence is 0.5% or 1 in 200 in all live births.
- Incidence increases with increasing maternal age.
- 3.95–97% non-disjunction, 2–3% translocations, 1% mosaic
- Mother or father may be carrier of balanced translocation (Robertsonian translocation)
- Most common translocation is 14:21 **(Fig. 2)**.
- If a baby has translocation Down syndrome then 25% chance that parents have balanced translocation, and 75% chance it is de-novo translocation during formation of gamete (where parents are normal).
- No trisomy 21 cannot be discharged from postnatal ward until baby has passed meconium and an echocardiography is done.

You are in busy OPD and 5-year-old down syndrome baby has come to you for follow-up:

- Assessment of growth/obesity
- Assessment of hearing as conductive as well as sensorineural is 10 times more prevalent.
- Assessment of vision for early cataract

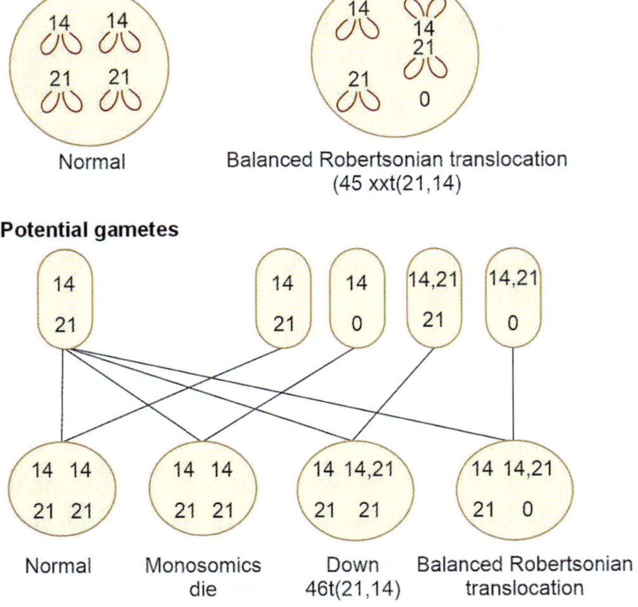

Fig. 2: A genetic description of how a Down syndrome translocation may occur.

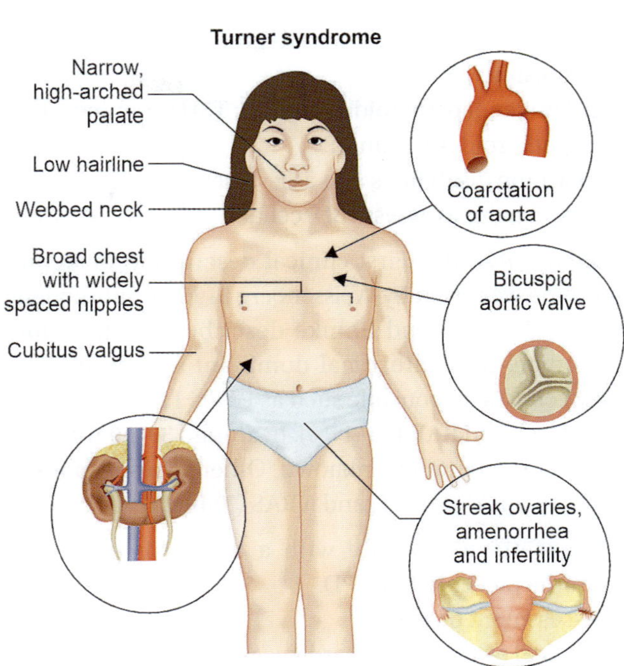

Fig. 3: Clinical features associated with Turner syndrome.

- Atlantoaxial dislocatibility by cervical MRI
- Assessment of celiac disease early dietary restrictions
- Assessment of behavior as autism and attention-deficit/ hyperactivity disorder (ADHD) is more prevalent.
- Clinical assessment of pulmonary hypertension
- Echocardiography at least once in a year
- Peripheral blood smear for early leukemia screening
- Evaluation of Hirschsprung disease

Turner syndrome: Incidence is 1 in 5,000 live female births. Maternal age is not a predisposing factor in turner. 75% of cases loss of X chromosome is from father.

Dictum: Any short stature female who has no menarche is Turner until proved otherwise **(Fig. 3)**.

Small for gestational age, edema of hands and feet, and excess nuchal skin fold are present at birth. Congenital heart defect is common in 40% of cases out of which bicuspid aortic valve is most common. Any accidental finding of horseshoe kidney in ultrasonography can be turner **(Table 2)**.

Latest American Academy of Pediatrics Guidelines say all 45XO Turner must be evaluated with metaphase FISH for remnants of Y chromosome for future gonadoblastoma.

You are in busy OPD and an 8-year-old child with Turner syndrome has come for follow-up.

- Anthropometric assessment using Turner syndrome-specific growth chart

TABLE 2: Signs of Turner syndrome.

Signs of turner syndrome:	
Face	Low posterior hairline
Eye	Cataract, strabismus
Ear	Sensorineural hearing loss, recurrent otitis media
Chest	Wide spread nipples, shield chest
Skeletal	Short stature, increase carrying angel of elbow, dislocation of patella, congenital hip dislocation, scoliosis
Cardiac	Bicuspid aortic valve, coarctation of aorta, cardiac conduction disturbance, hypoplastic left heart
Gonad	Gonadal dysgenesis (infertility, primary amenorrhea), gonadoblastoma (if Y chromosome material)
Endocrine	Hypothyroidism, type 2 DM
GIT	Celiac disease, inflammatory bowel disease

- Clinical assessment of preexisting cardiac lesion (bicuspid aortic valve which is most common in Turner is a progressive disease causing stenosis of aortic valve) and yearly echocardiography
- Assessment of hearing (recurrent otitis media, sensorineural hearing loss is common, perceptive hearing impairment in more than 50% of cases)

and vision (cataracts, red-green color blindness, strabismus)
- Assessment of thyroid status (T4, TSH) as autoimmune hypothyroid is common.
- Learning disabilities and assessment of behavior
- Bowel habit to assess IBD/celiac

Noonan syndrome: First clinical description of Noonan syndrome was given by Weissenberg in 1928. Subsequently in 1963, Noonan and Ehmke described the full blown phenotype. It is autosomal dominant and mutation of many genes is responsible such as PTPN 11 (40–50%), SOS 1 (10–20%), and RAF 1 (3–17%). In around 30–40% of cases, the mutation remains unknown. Other genes responsible are KRAS, BRAF, MEK 1, and NRAS **(Table 3)**.

A 5-year-old male child with a diagnosis of Noonan syndrome presented to OPD.
- Assessment of growth
- Clinical evaluation of cardiac lesion if any
- Confirmation and yearly review by echocardiography
- Thyroid profile at least yearly
- Platelet count for thrombocytopenia
- If any history of easy bruise, coagulation profile

Fragile X syndrome (FXS): This is the most frequent form of inherited intellectual disability.

There are fragile sites on some chromosomes that show a tendency for separation, breakage, or attenuation. The faulty gene of FXS lies on the fragile site of x chromosome. In FXS, CGG repeat expansion silences the gene producing fragile x mental retardation protein (FMRP), lower levels of FMRP appear to have a major impact upon the severity of the FXS phenotype. Individuals with nearly normal levels of FMRP may have mild or no symptoms, while those with very little or no normal FMRP may have more severe phenotypes **(Table 4)**.

Key lines:
- School complaints for ADHD or poor scholastic performance with large soft pinna, think of fragile X syndrome
- Prominent forehead elongated face macrocephaly with large testes during puberty with poor intelligence, rule out fragile X syndrome
- Any autistic child with IQ <70 with or without classical phenotype, rule out fragile X syndrome
- Any schoolgoing child with hypermobility with less IQ with features of mitral valve prolapse, think of fragile x syndrome

TABLE 3: Characteristic findings in Noonan syndrome.

IQ	Varies from 48 to 130 with a mean of 86, verbal IQ is always higher
Face	Ptosis of eyelid, hypertelorism, down slanting palpebral fissure, myopia, keratoconus, strabismus, nystagmus, anterior dental malocclusion, prominent protuberant upper lip
Neck	Low posterior hairline, short webbed neck
Skeletal	Shield chest, pectus excavatum or carinatum or both, cubitus valgus, scoliosis with thoracic lordosis, winging of scapula, cervical ribs
Heart	Pulmonary valve stenosis due to dysplastic or thickened valve, hypertrophic cardiomyopathy, ASD, TOF, CoA
Genitalia	Small penis, cryptorchidism
Bleeding diathesis	Partial factor XI:C, XII:C, VIII:C deficiencies, Von Willebrand disease, platelet dysfunction and thrombocytopenia occurring between 50 and 89% of patients
Hands and feet	Rarely edema of dorsum of hands and feet, lymphatic vessel dysplasia

TABLE 4: Characteristic findings in fragile X syndrome.

Growth	• Macrocephaly in early childhood, accelerated linear growth in childhood subsequently growth velocity slows • A subset of patient are obese mimics PWS
Performance	Mild to moderate intellectual disability with IQ 30–55. Deficit in executive function with age
Speech	Cluttered speech in mildly affected male, short bursts of repetitive speech in moderate cases. Complete lack of speech in severely affected males
Eye	Strong gaze avoidance, pale blue iris with epicanthic fold
Ear	Large ear with soft cartilage
Skeletal	Hyperextensible finger, mild cutis laxa, pectus excavatum, kyphoscoliosis
Face	Prominent forehead elongated face, prognathism during puberty, thickened nasal bridge, high arched palate
CVS	Mitral valve prolapse, aortic dilatation
Genital	Testicular size is large and common during pubertal years

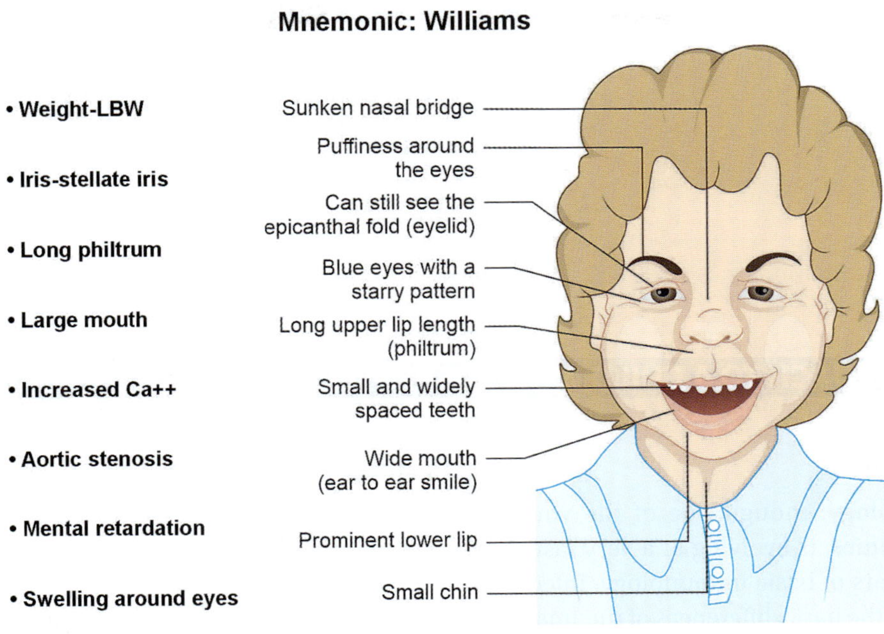

Fig. 4: Distinctive facial features in William's syndrome.

TABLE 5: Characteristic findings in William's syndrome.

Features	*Description*
Growth	Mild prenatal growth deficiency, postnatal growth approximately 75% or normal
Face	Medial eyebrow flare, short palpebral fissure, depressed nasal bridge, epicanthal fold, anteverted nares, long philtrum, prominent lips with open mouth
Dentition	Partial anodontia, microdontia, enamel hypoplasia, malocclusion
Skeleton	Joint hypermobility, contracture, lordosis, scoliosis, kyphosis
Kidney	Nephrocalcinosis, asymmetry in kidney size, small solitary or pelvic kidney
Skin	Soft lax skin, premature graying of the hair, hypoplastic nails
Eye	Amblyopia, refractive error, tortuosity of retinal vessel
CVS	Supravalvular aortic stenosis, pulmonary valvular stenosis, renal artery stenosis with hypertension, peripheral artery pulmonary stenosis, other arterial anomalies
Genetics	Deletion at 7q11.23, a region that includes 17 genes, elastin gene is responsible for vascular stenosis

William's syndrome **(Fig. 4 and Table 5)**:

Key lines:

- Any child with ADHD with aortic systolic murmur, rule out William
- Infantile hypercalcemia with or without classical facial phenotype, rule out William
- Prominent lips with open mouth (fish mouth) with long philtrum, think of William.

SUGGESTED READING

1. Kliegman RM, St Geme JW, Blum NJ, Shah SS, Tasker RC, Wilson KM. Nelson Textbook of Pediatrics. 22nd ed. Philadelphia: Elsevier; 2023.
2. Smith DW, Jones KL. Smith's Recognizable Patterns of Human Malformation. 4th ed. Philadelphia: W.B. Saunders; 1988.

CHAPTER 12

Muscular and Rheumatic Disorders

Madhumita Nandi

PART A: APPROACH TO A CHILD WITH SUSPECTED RHEUMATOLOGICAL DISORDER

INTRODUCTION

Pediatric rheumatology, though one of the youngest pediatric subspecialities, is evolving at a very fast pace, standing on the pillars of basic immunology, infections, and genetics. One of the basic differences of rheumatology from other subspecialities is that instead of involvement of a single organ system, rheumatic diseases are a diverse group of chronic diseases characterized by the presence of inflammation in multiple organs. Sometimes we, as clinicians, find ourselves not very conversant with elicitation and interpretation of history and clinical examination in a patient with suspected rheumatological disorder, probably because our current curriculums do not give as much importance to rheumatology as a system as is done to other organ systems. Although a thorough knowledge of examination of all organ systems is essential for elicitation and interpretation of rheumatological symptoms and signs, we need to develop our clinical acumen and temperament specific to rheumatology.

SYMPTOMS AND SIGNS: INTERPRETING THE OBSCURE

Rheumatology is often considered "gray area" of medicine as there are only a few useful diagnostic tests, sparse pathognomonic physical tests, controversies even in nomenclature which is ever evolving and therapy that often lacks specificity. This is the reason why we have "classification criteria" for almost all rheumatological conditions unlike the usual "diagnostic criteria" for other conditions in medicine. Hence, a detailed history and thorough physical examination of the whole child with careful observation over time are mandatory with an overall objective of arriving at a diagnosis based on "pattern recognition". Common mimickers of rheumatologic disorders should also be considered.

Although there is no single classic symptom which would guide a physician to a definite rheumatologic etiology with confidence, the common symptoms include *joint pain and swelling, fever, fatigue, joint pain and swelling.*

Chronic, recurrent, persistent or intermittent *pain* is a primary symptom of many rheumatic diseases but is often difficult to assess objectively especially in children. Nonverbal clues are more important. Face rating scale is useful **(Fig. 1)**. Pain without any other physical finding is a frequent reason for referral to pediatric rheumatological specialists. Arthralgias without physical findings for arthritis could suggest a myriad of conditions including infection, malignancy, orthopedic conditions, benign

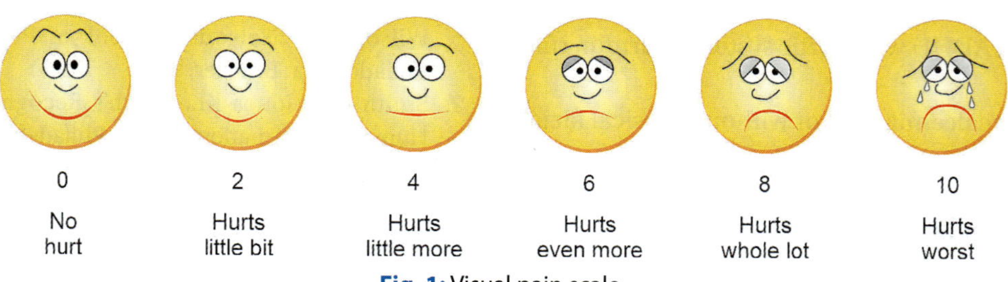

Fig. 1: Visual pain scale.

hypermobility syndromes, or even pain syndromes such as fibromyalgia. Arthralgia may also be a presenting symptom of pediatric systemic lupus erythematosus (SLE) and juvenile idiopathic arthritis (JIA), though children with JIA may not complain of joint symptoms at presentation.

Rheumatic diseases may manifest as arthralgias only, but, objective features of arthritis such as swelling, heat, and restriction of movement are stronger predictor to the presence of rheumatic disease. Whenever a swelling is encountered, it is important to assess that swelling is arising from which structure around the joint namely, skin, bursa, tendon, bone tissue, or synovial effusion/blood.

Fatigue is a nonspecific pointer to a rheumatic disease but is also common in non-rheumatic causes, such as viral infections, pain syndromes, and malignancy. Fatigue is a common presenting complaint in juvenile dermatomyositis (JDM). It may also be frequently associated with vasculitis and JIA. Overwhelming fatigue with inability to do daily activities is more suggestive of chronic fatigue syndrome, fibromyalgia, or other amplified pain syndromes. **Table 1** summarizes the typical symptoms of some rheumatological conditions seen in children.

A complete physical examination is essential in any child with suspected rheumatic disease. Many diseases have associated subtle physical findings that may help us in delineating the differential diagnosis. In addition, many rheumatic diseases have multisystem involvement, and a systematic assessment should focus on delineating the degree and extent of organ system involvement (e.g., skin, joints, muscle, renal, cardiovascular, hepatic) **(Fig. 2)**. **Table 2** gives a summary of common signs of rheumatologic disorders.

Raynaud phenomenon may be a primary benign disorder or could be a presenting complaint of scleroderma, SLE, mixed connective tissue disease (MCTD), or an overlap syndrome.

Diffuse lymphadenopathy is present in many rheumatic diseases, including SLE, pJIA, and sJIA.

TABLE 1: Common symptoms of some rheumatological conditions.

Symptom	*Rheumatic disease(s)*	*Possible nonrheumatic disorders with similar complaints*
Fever	Systemic JIA, SLE, vasculitis, ARF, MCTD, sarcoidosis	Malignancies, infection and postinfectious, inflammatory bowel disease, periodic fever (autoinflammatory), Kawasaki disease, HSP
Arthralgias	JIA, SLE, JDM, ARF, scleroderma, sarcoidosis	Hypothyroidism, trauma, malignancies, growing pain, pain syndrome, overuse syndrome
Weakness	JDM, myositis secondary to SLE, MCTD, deep localized scleroderma	Muscular dystrophy, metabolic and other myopathies, hypothyroidism
Chest pain	JIA, SLE (associated with pericarditis or costochondritis)	Isolated costochondritis, rib fracture, viral pericarditis, anxiety disorder
Back pain	ERA, Juvenile AS	Spinal SOL, vertebral compression fracture, osteomyelitis, spondylosis, spondylolisthesis, pain syndrome
Fatigue	JIA, SLE, JDM, MCTD, vasculitis	Pain syndrome, chronic fatigue syndrome, depression

(JIA: Juvenile idiopathic arthritis; JDM: Juvenile dermatomyositis; SLE: systemic lupus erythematosus; MCTD: mixed connective tissue disease; ERA: enthesitis-related arthritis; ARF: acute rheumatic fever)

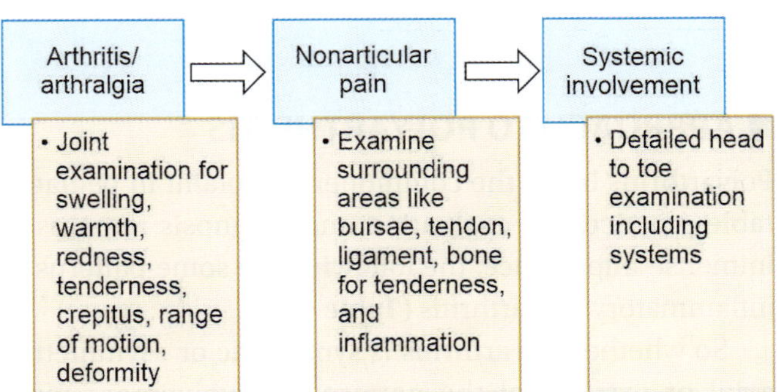

Fig. 2: Physical examination depends on the presenting complaints.

■ APPROACH TO MONOARTHRITIS

Acute pain or swelling of a single joint requires immediate attention for exclusion septic arthritis. Delay may rapidly destroy the joint if left untreated. It is important to differentiate pain originating from periarticular structures like tendons, bursa, etc. from pain due to joint pathology **(Table 3)**. Referred pain in shoulder may be due to peritonitis or heart disease. History taking should exclude trauma. Also, clues like tick bites (Lyme disease), sexual risk factors (giant cell arthritis), and triads like colitis, uveitis, urethritis (reactive arthritis) should be sought.

TABLE 2: Common and typical physical signs of some rheumatological disorders.

Sign	*Rheumatic*	*Comments*	*Nonrheumatic*
Malar rash	SLE, JDM	SLE spares nasolabial fold	Sun burn, fifth disease, Kawasaki disease
Oral ulcers	SLE, Behcet	Behcet's disease is associated with genital ulcer	HSV infection, PFAPA
Purpuric rash	ANCA-positive vasculitis, HSP	HSP rash affects lower limbs and buttocks	Meningococcemia, thrombocytopenia, clotting disorder
Gottron papules	JDM	Associated heliotrope rash, periungual telangiectasias	Psoriasis, eczema

(ANCA: antineutrophilic cytoplasmic antibody; HSV: herpes simplex virus; PFAPA: periodic fever, aphthous stomatitis, pharyngitis and adenitis; HSP: Henoch–Schonlein purpura)

TABLE 3: etiology of joint-related conditions.

Entity	*Etiology*
Infectious arthritis	Bacterial (staphylococcal), viral (HIV), Lyme's, *Mycobacterium*, fungi
Trauma	Fracture, hemarthrosis
AVN bone	Trauma, corticosteroid use
Tumors	Primary or metastatic
Systemic disease	Rheumatoid arthritis, reactive arthritis, SLE, and psoriatic

(AVN: avascular necrosis; SLE: systemic lupus erythematosus)

APPROACH TO POLYARTHRITIS

Polyarthritis being the commoner complaint in pediatric table practice, the evaluation and diagnosis remains of immense importance, the following are some patterns of inflammatory polyarthritis **(Table 4)**.

So whether the arthritis is symmetric or asymmetric, axial or extra-axial the pattern of involvement must be delineated first, regarding the etiology, the causes remain vast but majority of them can be snuffed out from a meticulous history taking **(Table 5)**.

Polyarthritis could be a self-limiting illness or the beginning of a serious chronic illness like JIA or an emergency requiring urgent intervention. The differential diagnosis can be very broad. A probable etiological diagnosis can often be made by meticulous attention to the history and physical examination.

TABLE 4: Approach to polyarthritis.

Pattern	*Etiology*
Polyarticular peripheral (usually symmetric)	Rheumatoid arthritis (additive), SLE, viral arthritis, and psoriatic arthritis
Oligoarticular; axial involvement (usually asymmetric, peripheral joints)	Seronegative spondyloarthropathy (ankylosing spondylitis, reactive arthritis, psoriatic arthritis)
Oligoarticular without axial involvement (usually symmetric joints)	Rheumatic fever (migratory), Lyme disease, enteropathic arthritis

(SLE: systemic lupus erythematosus)

TABLE 5: Causes of polyarthritis.

Etiology	*Causative agent*
Viral	Parvovirus B19, *Enteroviruses*, Adenoviruses, mumps, rubella, varicella zoster virus, hepatitis B, Coxsackie virus, *Cytomegalovirus*, EBV, HIV
Bacterial	Staphylococcal and streptococcal infections, *Neisseria gonorrhoeae*, *Haemophilus influenzae*; bacterial endocarditis
Other infections	Tuberculosis, leptospirosis, fungal infections, brucellosis
Parainfectious (reactive)	HIV, Group A streptococcal infections, *Salmonella, Shigella, Yersinia, Campylobacter, Mycoplasma, Chlamydia*
Rheumatological	Juvenile idiopathic arthritis (JIA), systemic lupus erythematosus (SLE), Juvenile dermatomyositis (JDM), Behcet syndrome
Systemic vasculitides	Henoch-Schonlein purpura (HSP), Kawasaki disease (KD), polyarteritis nodosa (PAN), Wegener's granulomatosis
Spondyloarthropathies	Juvenile ankylosing spondylitis (JAS), psoriatic arthritis Enteropathic arthritis
Miscellaneous	Sarcoidosis, drug/serum sickness reactions

EXAMINATION AND INVESTIGATION

Broadly 80% of rheumatological diagnoses come from clinical history, 15% from examination and only 5% need investigation for confirmation. So apart from the history taking, examining the patient is also important just to differentiate between a chronic disease in early phase or just a pain syndrome requiring symptomatic treatment. Few areas need to be given special emphasis during clinical examination like checking the vitals including the blood pressure with an appropriate size cuff, detailed anthropometry which will give us an idea about the duration of the disease, and thorough examination of hair (alopecia), skin (heliotropic rash, Gottron's papule, discoloration, calcinosis), nail (pitting, periungual telangiectasia), nose and mouth (oral ulcers, red tongue, cracked lips), genitals (ulceration), and back (spinous process, paraspinal and surrounding muscle, sacroiliac joint).

Detailed systemic examination would include examination of cardiovascular and respiratory systems (pericardial and pleural rub, decreased breath sound due to pulmonary fibrosis) and examination of abdomen for ischemic pain, hepatosplenomegaly, and ascites. It is the constellation of physical signs rather than a single finding that provide clues for diagnosis on the basis of preset disease specific diagnostic criteria.

There are two systems available in examining a patient of presumed rheumatic disorders i.e.:

1. pGALS (pediatric gait, arms, legs, spine) as screening test
2. pREMS (pediatric regional examination of musculoskeletal system) as detailed examination

pGALS is a simple screening approach to musculoskeletal (MSK) examination which can be done in a very short time (within 2 minutes) in school-aged children and even in younger children as well **(Table 6)**. It is a simple and quick test having an excellent sensitivity of 97% to detect abnormality. Also the acceptability by children and their parents is good.

The sequence of pGALS is same as adult GALS with some extra maneuvers to screen the foot and ankle like walk on heels and then on tiptoes, wrists like palms together and then hands back to back and temporomandibular joints like opening the mouth and inserting three of the child's own fingers. It has some amendments at screening the elbow like reach up and touch the sky and neck like asking to look at the ceiling. These additional maneuvers were included because when adult GALS was originally tested in school-aged children, it failed to detect abnormalities at these sites **(Fig. 3)**.

TABLE 6: pGALS—A musculoskeletal screening assessment for school-aged children.

Section	*Assessment/instructions*
Screening questions	• "Do you have any pain or stiffness in your joints, muscles, or back?" • "Do you have any difficulty getting yourself dressed without any help?" • "Do you have any difficulty going up and down stairs?"
Gait	• Observe the child walking • "Walk on your tip-toes/walk on your heels"
Arms	• "Put your hands out in front of you" • "Turn your hands over and make a fist" • "Pinch your index finger and thumb together" • "Touch the tips of your fingers with your thumb" • Squeeze the metacarpophalangeal joints • "Put your hands together/put your hands back to back" • "Reach up and touch the sky" • "Look at the ceiling" • "Put your hands behind your neck"
Legs	• Feel for effusion at the knee • "Bend and then straighten your knee" (check active movement of knees and feel for crepitus) • Passive flexion (90°) with internal rotation of hip
Spine	• "Open your mouth and put 3 of your (child's own) fingers in your mouth" • Lateral flexion of cervical spine—"Try and touch your shoulder with your ear" • Observe the spine from behind • "Can you bend and touch your toes?" Observe curve of the spine from side and behind

(pGALS: pediatric gait, arms, legs, spine)
Source: Foster HE, Kay LJ, Friswell M, et al. Musculoskeletal screening examination (PGALS) for school-age children based on the adult GALSscreen. Arthritis Rheum. 2006;15(55):981.

When to perform pGALS:

- Child with bone, muscle, or joint pain
- Unwell child with fever
- A limping child
- Delay or regression of *motor milestones*
- "*Clumsy*" child in the absence of neurological disease
- Child with *chronic disease* and known association with MSK presentations

Some practical tips for pGALS include:

- Get the child to *copy you* doing the maneuvers
- Look for verbal and nonverbal *clues of discomfort* (e.g., facial expression, withdrawal)

Documentation of the pGALS screen

Documentation of the pGALS screening assessment is important and a simple pro forma is proposed with the following example — a child with a swollen left knee with limited flexion of the knee and antalgic gait.

pGALS screening questions		
Any pain?	*Left knee*	
Problems with dressing?	*No difficulty*	
Problems with walking?	*Some difficulty on walking*	
	Appearance	Movement
Gait		×
Arms	✓	✓
Legs	×	×
Spine	✓	✓

Fig. 3: Documentation of the pGALS screen. (pGALS: pediatric gait, arms, legs, spine)
Source: Foster HE, Jandial S. pGALS - paediatric Gait Arms Legs and Spine: a simple examination of the musculoskeletal system. Pediatr Rheumatol Online J. 2013;11(1):44.

- Do the *full screen*
- Look for *asymmetry* (e.g., muscle bulk, joint swelling, and ROM)
- Consider *clinical patterns* and association of leg-length discrepancy and scoliosis

Those with abnormal findings in pGALS must undergo:

pREMS (pediatric regional examination of musculoskeletal system) which is a detailed local examination based on principles of "look, feel, and move".

POINTS TO REMEMBER

- In a child presenting with symptoms suggestive of musculoskeletal system, first do pGALS.
- This gives clues to sites requiring further detailed examination.
- Identify rheumatological from nonrheumatological illness.
- Identify inflammatory from noninflammatory etiology.
- Identify articular from nonarticular causes.
- Identify pattern of joint affection.
- Detail systemic examination is essential.
- Constellation of signs and symptoms and disease evolution over time help clinch diagnosis and order appropriate investigations.

SUGGESTED READING

1. Canadian Rheumatology Association. (2011). A Resident's guide to Pediatric Rheumatology. [online] Available from https://reumaped.es/images/site/pdf/locomotor/Resident_Guide_to_Pediatric_Rheumatology_2011.pdf.
2. Coté CJ, Lerman J, David TI. A practice of anesthesia for infants and children. Amsterdam: Elsevier Health Sciences; 2009. p. 940.
3. Foster HE, Jandial S. pGALS - paediatric Gait Arms Legs and Spine: a simple examination of the musculoskeletal system. Pediatric Rheumatol Online J. 2013;11:44.
4. Foster HE, Kay LJ, Friswell M, Coady D, Myers A. Musculoskeletal screening examination (PGALS) for school-age children based on the adult GALSscreen. Arthritis Rheum. 2006;15(55):981.
5. González-Mayda MC. Washington Manual of Rheumatology Subspecialty Consult, 3rd edition. Massachusetts: Wolters Kluwer Health; 2020. chapter 1, p. 18-35.
6. Hakim A, Clunie G, Haq I. Oxford handbook on rheumatology, 3rd edition. London: Oxford University Press; 2012. chapter 1, p. 10.
7. Kliegman R. Nelson Textbook of Pediatrics, 21st edition, volume 2. Amsterdam: Elsevier Health Sciences; 2019. chapter 153. P. 1151
8. Singh S. Approach to Polyarthritis. Indian J Pediatr. 2010;77:1005-10.

PART B: APPROACH TO A CASE OF JUVENILE IDIOPATHIC ARTHRITIS

Frequently asked in examination:

1. *Define Juvenile idiopathic arthritis (JIA)*
2. *Classify JIA*
3. *PRINTO classification criteria of JIA*
4. *Clinical features of JIA*
5. *What is arthritis and arthralgia*
6. *Characteristics of systemic onset Juvenile idiopathic arthritis (SOJIA)*
7. *Mimickers of JIA*
8. *Investigations for JIA*
9. *MRI findings in septic arthritis, leukemic arthritis, and JIA*

Juvenile idiopathic arthritis (JIA) is a homogeneous group of chronic arthritis in children of <16 years of age where the symptoms persist for >6 weeks and where all other known causes of arthritis have been excluded. Hence, that qualifies the nomenclature of "juvenile" and "idiopathic" respectively.

Several attempts have been made in the past to classify various group of such chronically persistent arthritis in children and adolescents without any known cause. Previously grouped under various names such as Juvenile rheumatoid arthritis (ACR) and Juvenile chronic arthritis (EULAR) with widely differing criteria which made it difficult to interpret research and compare results from different centres. Finally, International league against Rheumatism (ILAR) made an effort to find a consensus for classification and nomenclature and this leads to the current classification and to use the common term JIA. Classification is based on the symptoms present during the initial 6 months of the disease **(Box 1, Table 7)**. The main principle underlying ILAR classification is that all categories of JIA are *mutually exclusive*. Each category has, therefore, a list of *exclusion criteria*. First brought out in 1997, it has undergone modifications from time to time as ILAR classification was itself conceived as an *evolving* process. Recently, in 2019, the Pediatric Rheumatology International Trials Organization (PRINTO) has suggested a newer classifications, the important points of which are highlighted in **Table 7**. In this new classification, ANA and RF positivity have been given more emphasis rather than joint count.

BOX 1: ILAR classification of JIA.

- *Age:* <16 year at time of onset
- *Duration:* At least 6 weeks
- Arthritis in one or more joints
- Exclusion of other rheumatologic conditions
- Subgroup named after 6 months
  - *Systemic:* Arthritis with fever
  - *Pauciarticular:* 4 or fewer joints
  - *Polyarticular:* 5 or more joints

(ILAR: International league against Rheumatism; JIA: Juvenile idiopathic arthritis)

TABLE 7: JIA ILAR category, frequency, age distribution, and exclusion criteria.

ILAR category	*Frequency*	*Preferential onset age*
Oligoarthritis	30–60%	Early childhood
Rheumatoid factor positive polyarthritis	3–7%	Late childhood or adolescence
Rheumatoid factor negative polyarthritis	10–25%	Biphasic distribution: early peak <6 years and late peak >6 years
Systemic arthritis	5–15%	Any pediatric age
Psoriatic arthritis	3–10%	Biphasic distribution: early peak <6 years and late peak >6 years
Undifferentiated arthritis	10–20%	

(ILAR: International league against Rheumatism; JIA: Juvenile idiopathic arthritis)

EXCLUSION CRITERIA

a. Psoriasis or a history of psoriasis in the patient or first-degree relative
b. Arthritis in an HLA-B27 positive male beginning after the 6th birthday
c. Ankylosing spondylitis, enthesitis-related arthritis, sacroiliitis with inflammatory bowel disease, Reiter's syndrome, or acute anterior uveitis, or a history of one of these disorders in a first-degree relative
d. The presence of IgM rheumatoid factor on at least 2 occasions at least 3 months apart
e. The presence of systemic JIA in the patient

OLIGOARTHRITIS

Arthritis affecting one to four joints during the first 6 months of disease. Two subcategories are recognized:

1. *Persistent oligoarthritis:* Affecting not more than 4 joints throughout the disease course

2. *Extended oligoarthritis:* Affecting a total of more than 4 joints after the first 6 months of disease

Exclusions: a, b, c, d, e

POLYARTHRITIS (RHEUMATOID FACTOR POSITIVE)

Arthritis affecting 5 or more joints during the first 6 months of disease; 2 or more tests for RF at least 3 months apart during the first 6 months of disease are positive.

Exclusions: a, b, c, e

POLYARTHRITIS (RHEUMATOID FACTOR NEGATIVE)

Arthritis affecting 5 or more joints during the first 6 months of disease; a test for RF is negative.

Exclusions: a, b, c, d, e

SYSTEMIC ONSET

Arthritis in one or more joints with or preceded by fever of at least 2 weeks' duration that is documented to be daily ("quotidian") for at least 3 days, and accompanied by one or more of the following:

1. Evanescent (nonfixed) erythematous rash
2. Generalized lymph node enlargement
3. Hepatomegaly and/or splenomegaly
4. Serositis

Exclusions: a, b, c, d

ENTHESIS-RELATED ARTHRITIS

Arthritis and enthesitis, or arthritis or enthesitis with at least 2 of the following:

1. The presence of or a history of sacroiliac joint tenderness and/or inflammatory lumbosacral pain
2. The presence of HLA-B27 antigen
3. Onset of arthritis in a male over 6 years of age
4. Acute (symptomatic) anterior uveitis
5. History of ankylosing spondylitis, enthesitis-related arthritis, sacroiliitis with inflammatory bowel disease, Reiter's syndrome, or acute anterior uveitis in a first-degree relative

Exclusions: a, d, e

PSORIATIC ARTHRITIS

Arthritis and psoriasis, or arthritis and at least 2 of the following:

1. Dactylitis
2. Nail pitting or onycholysis
3. Psoriasis in a first-degree relative

Exclusions: b, c, d, e

UNDIFFERENTIATED ARTHRITIS

Arthritis that fulfils criteria in no category or in two or more of the above categories.

The ILAR classification, which was conceived as an evolving process, has been recently criticized since there is evidence that while some categories identify quite definite disease entities, others still represent heterogeneous conditions. The newly proposed PRINTO classification takes care of this issue to some extent **(Table 8)**.

OLIGOARTHRITIS

In Western Countries, where oligoarthritis represents up to 50% of all JIA cases, the large majority of patients belong to a well-defined disease entity observed only in children and characterized by several common features: an asymmetric arthritis (meaning an asymmetric pace in joint involvement), an early onset (before 6 years of age), a female predilection, positive antinuclear antibodies (ANA), a high risk for developing chronic iridocyclitis, and consistent HLA associations (HLA-DRB1*08 in particular). Oligoarthritis is predominantly a disease of the lower limbs, with the knee joint being most commonly affected followed by the ankles. Acute phase reactants are usually normal or moderately increased; although in some instances ESR may be quite high. Except uveitis, other extra articular manifestation are absent.

TABLE 8: Highlights of new proposed PRINTO classification criteria of JIA.

a	Systemic arthritis: Allows inclusion of patients with fever but without arthritis
b	RF-positive arthritis: Anti-CCP antibodies have been added to the definition
c	Enthesitis/spondylitis-related JIA: Definition and nomenclature have been made similar to the adult counterpart
d	Early onset ANA positive JIA: This is the major novelty
e	Other JIS: Does not fit the disorders a to d. Arthritis ≥6 weeks
f	Unclassified JIA: Fits >1 disorder a to d. Arthritis ≥6 weeks

(CCP: cyclic citrullinated peptide; JIA: Juvenile idiopathic arthritis; PRINTO: Pediatric Rheumatology International Trials Organization; RF: rheumatoid factor)

According to ILAR classification, there are two categories: persistent oligoarthritis in which the disease remains confined to 4 or less joints and extended oligoarthritis in which arthritis extends to more than 4 joints after the first 6 months of disease. It has been shown in **Figure 4**, however that ANA-positive patients with persistent or with extended oligoarthritis share the same features, strongly suggesting that they represent the same disease differing just in the spread of arthritis. Involvement of an upper limb joint and higher sedimentation rate at onset have been identified as predictors for an evolution to the extended phenotype, which may occur in up to 50% of patients. While children with persistent oligoarthritis have in general a good long-term articular outcome, those with extended oligoarthritis may have a less favorable long term prognosis.

Iridocyclitis in oligoarticular arthritis is asymptomatic in its early stages as compared to acute iridocyclitis of enthesis-related arthritis which is very painful. About 30% of patients develop a chronic, nongranulomatous, anterior uveitis that involves the iris and the ciliary body (iridocyclitis) and can cause severe visual impairment.

POLYARTHRITIS (RHEUMATOID FACTOR POSITIVE)

It accounts for just a small (≤5%) percentage of patients with JIA. It primarily affects girls and usually presents in late childhood or adolescence. It can be rapidly progressive and destructive. Rheumatoid factor (RF) is by definition positive; also antibodies to cyclic citrullinated peptides (CCP) are present in some cases.

Fig. 4: Both knees involved in a child with oligoarthritis
Source: Picture M Nandi.

The usual presentation is a symmetric polyarthritis of the small joints of the hands and feet **(Fig. 5)**. The large joints, usually knees and ankles, can also be involved early but usually in association with small joint involvement **(Fig. 6)**.

Low-grade fever and lymphadenopathy are rarely present. Rheumatoid nodules are observed in this JIA category while they are rare in the others. They should not be confused with pseudo-rheumatoid nodules which

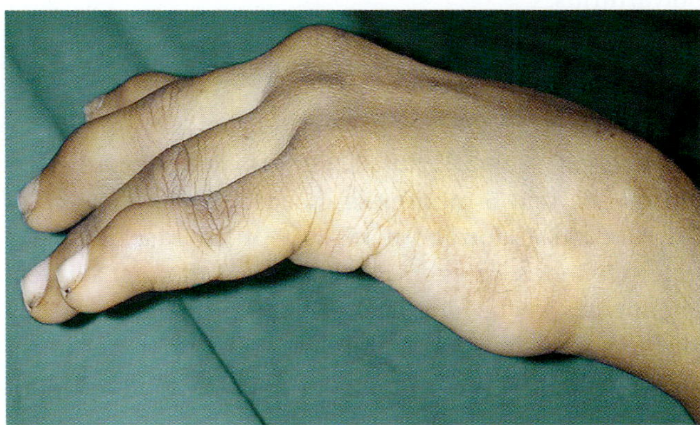

Fig. 5: Swan neck deformity in hand (hyperextension of PIP and flexion of DIP) in a child with pJIA
Source: Picture M nandi.

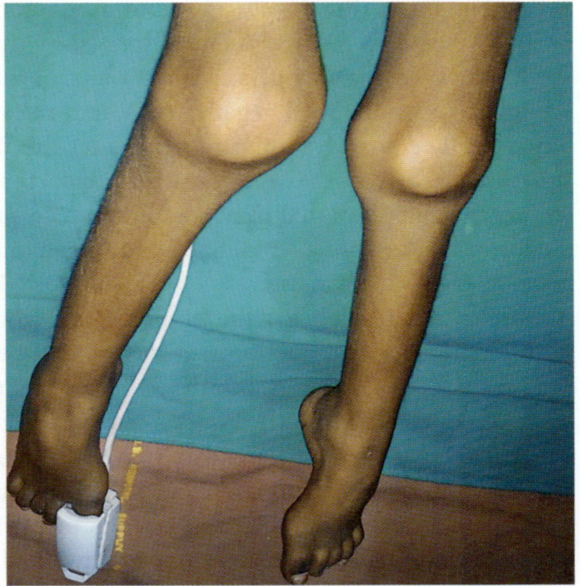

Fig. 6: Fixed deformity of joints genu valgum with fixed flexion deformity of both knees and equinus deformity of both ankles
Source: Picture M Nandi.

represent a form of granuloma annulare: they are observed mainly in children, especially on the lower legs and scalp, have a similar histological appearance (acellular central areas surrounded by palisading histiocytes) and a favorable prognosis. Severe extra-articular manifestations may be present in some cases. These include aortic valve regurgitation and lymphocytic interstitial pneumonitis.

Erythrocyte sedimentation rate and C-reactive protein are elevated and a moderate normochromic and normocytic anemia may be present. Antinuclear antibodies may be present but are not associated with an increased risk of developing chronic iridocyclitis, a complication that is not characteristic of RF-positive polyarthritis.

POLYARTHRITIS (RHEUMATOID FACTOR NEGATIVE)

It is defined as an arthritis that affects five or more joints during the first 6 months of disease in the absence of RF. It accounts for about 15–20% of JIA cases and is a heterogeneous category. At least two distinct clinical phenotypes can be identified:

- First one that resembles ANA-positive early onset oligoarthritis in any respect (early age at onset, ANA positivity asymmetric arthritis, female predominance, elevated incidence of chronic iridocyclitis, association with HLA-DRB1*08) except the number of joint involved during the first 6 months of disease
- Second a form that is closely similar to adult-onset RF-negative RA and is characterized by overt symmetric synovitis of large and small joints, onset in school age, elevated ESR, negative ANA, and variable outcome. The strong similarities between the first subset and early onset, ANA-positive oligoarthritis led to the suggestion that they are the same disease, the former representing a rapid arthritis spread in the latter. The hypothesis is also very strongly supported by studies on the prevalence of the various JIA categories in different ethnic populations. It has indeed been shown that early onset, ANA-positive, iridocyclitis-associated oligoarticular arthritis is seldom observed in countries such as Costa Rica, India, New Zealand, and South Africa. In these same countries, the RF-negative polyarthritis subset characterized by ANA positivity, early onset and risk of developing chronic iridocyclitis is also rare.

The long-term prognosis of ANA-positive, early onset, RF-negative polyarthritis is worse than that of persistent oligoarthritis and similar to that of extended oligoarthritis. ANA-positive patients carry a high risk of chronic iridocyclitis and have to be checked every 3 months with slit lamp examination.

SYSTEMIC ARTHRITIS

Systemic arthritis (sJIA) is a category that sets well apart from all the others because of the presence of prominent systemic features. The disease does not show a preferential age at onset and occurs as often in boys as in girls. It accounts for 10–15% of children with JIA.

Characteristic of sJIA is the presence of a quotidian, high spiking fever with one or two fever peaks, usually in the late afternoon or evening, and a rapid return to normal value. Myalgias and abdominal pain may be intense during fever peaks. On the contrary and characteristically, patients feel quite well in the absence of fever. Fever peaks are very often associated with an evanescent, nonfixed, erythematous rash most commonly on the trunk and proximal extremities **(Fig. 7)**. Sometimes, the rash can be pruritic and urticaria-like. It can be induced by rubbing or scratching the skin (Koebner phenomenon). Splenomegaly, hepatomegaly, and generalized lymphadenopathy are often detectable and occasionally can be very marked. Serositis (pericarditis and pleuritis) is not rare if looked for with imaging techniques but is rarely symptomatic. Myocarditis may occur but is very uncommon. Arthritis is more often symmetrical and polyarticular; it may be absent at onset and develop during disease course.

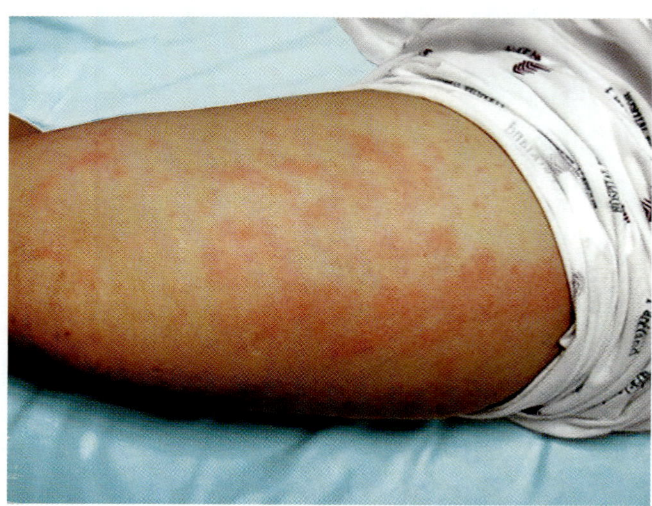

Fig. 7: Evanescent rash of sJIA
Source: Picture M Nandi.

Laboratory examinations show a prominent inflammatory response characterized by leukocytosis (with neutrophilia), high erythrocyte sedimentation rate (ESR), and C-reactive protein (CRP) concentration, hyperferritinemia, thrombocytosis, very high serum levels of S100A8/S100A9 and S100A12. A microcytic anemia is common and is due to a marked iron sequestration in the reticuloendothelial system induced by inflammation.

For unknown reasons, children with sJIA are uniquely susceptible to develop macrophage activation syndrome (MAS), a form of reactive hemophagocytic lymphohistiocytosis (HLH) that occurs in about 5–8% of patients. It should be promptly recognized and treated.

The presence of a marked activation of the innate immune system has led to consider sJIA a polygenic autoinflammatory disease. It is probable that rather than representing a disease, sJIA is a syndrome, the common endpoint of several different diseases all causing a marked and persistent activation of the innate immune system. This potential heterogeneity is suggested by differences in disease outcome as well as by a differential sensitivity to the treatment with interleukin-1 blockers.

The clinical course of sJIA is indeed highly variable. In about half of patients, the disease is either monocyclic or characterized by relapses with intervals of remission; in these patients, the arthritis usually remits when systemic features are controlled and the long-term prognosis is usually good since the disease tends to go into spontaneous remission with time. In the other half of patients, the disease follows an unremitting course; often systemic symptoms tend to disappear with time and a severe persistent arthritis remains the major long-term problem.

ENTHESITIS-RELATED ARTHRITIS

The concept of spondyloarthritis includes a heterogeneous group of chronic inter-related inflammatory arthritides associated with enthesitis that often affect the spine and/or sacroiliac joints. These diseases are associated with the HLA-B27 gene, although the degree of association shows important variation depending on the type of spondyloarthritis and ethnicity.

The disease typically begins after the age of 6 years and affects boys more often than girls. It is characterized initially by lower limb arthritis; arthritis is more often asymmetrical and oligoarticular but around one quarter of patients may have a polyarticular onset. Often there is involvement of intertarsal joints and bones, overlying tendons, entheses, and soft tissue with swelling, pain and restriction of movement (tarsitis) in the midfoot. Hip involvement at disease presentation is quite frequent (while it is exceptional in the other JIA categories). Arthritis is often accompanied by an enthesitis (inflammation of the point where a tendon, ligament or fascia inserts into the bone) which is the most characteristic features of this JIA category. Palpation and/or medical history often reveal sign of enthesitis. The most common sites of enthesitis are at the insertions of the plantar fascia (the calcaneum, the base of the fifth metatarsal and the metatarsal heads), the insertion of the Achilles tendon into the calcaneum, the tibial tuberosity, and around and below the patella (2, 6, and 10 o'clock positions). Other less common sites include the greater trochanter of the femur, iliac crest, pubic symphysis, ischial tuberosity, and costochondral junctions.

PSORIATIC ARTHRITIS

The diagnosis of juvenile psoriatic arthritis by ILAR criteria requires the simultaneous presence of arthritis and a typical psoriatic rash or, if the latter is absent, the presence of arthritis and any two of the following: family history of psoriasis in a first-degree relative, dactylitis (swelling of one or more digits that extends beyond the joint margins), and nail pitting. The Vancouver criteria are other previously designed criteria to diagnose juvenile psoriatic arthritis. These include: (1) Arthritis plus psoriasis or (2) arthritis plus at least 2 of: Dactylitis; Nail pits; Family history in a first- or second-degree relative psoriasis-like rash. They are very similar but, at variance with the ILAR criteria, they do not incorporate exclusion criteria. Psoriatic arthritis represents about 5–10% of all JIA cases and also appears to be markedly heterogeneous.

The association of psoriasis with arthritis leads to the identification of two very different groups of patients, one that is similar to adult PsA and the other that has the same characteristics of ANA-positive early onset oligoarthritis.

If the ILAR classification is used to define psoriatic arthritis, most of those patients that have a form of PsA similar to that observed in adults are excluded because of the presence of the exclusion criterion which include patients with enthesitis-related arthritis. These patients usually fall in the category of undifferentiated arthritis.

The long-term prognosis of PsA is not well defined, due to its heterogeneity and the lack of available information.

ANA-positive patients have to be checked every 3 months with slit lamp examination.

UNDIFFERENTIATED ARTHRITIS

This category does not represent a defined entity; it includes patients who do not fulfil inclusion criteria for any category, or fulfil the criteria for more than one category. About 10–15% of all JIA cases are included in this category.

CLINICAL APPROACH

Answers to the following questions need to be attempted when dealing with a child of chronic arthritis:

1. Is the pain inflammatory or noninflammatory: Early morning worsening of pain and stiffness which improves as the day progresses in contrast to growing pains and joint hypermobility syndromes where pain is more at the end of the day.
2. Is it one joint or more which may not be obvious at presentation but has to be discerned by meticulous examination?
3. Are there any extra-articular manifestations?

It should be remembered that joints in JIA are not acutely painful or red which is a characteristic finding of infective arthritis or a joint bleed. Severe growth failure, hypertension, and nonevanescent vasculitic rashes are also pointers of non-JIA etiology.

DIFFERENTIAL DIAGNOSIS (JUVENILE IDIOPATHIC ARTHRITIS MIMICKERS)

The following should be carefully excluded by thorough history and meticulous examination and, if needed, by appropriate laboratory tests.

- Leukemia and neuroblastoma and other malignancies
- Oligoarthritis in children living in endemic areas—Lyme disease
- Large joint swelling and bleeding tendencies—hemophilia
- Acute fever, painful, erythematous, hot joint—septic arthritis
- Monoarticular involvement, unresponsive to anti-inflammatory treatments—*Mycobacterial* infections
- Metabolic conditions such as Farber's disease, mucopolysaccharidosis
- Acute hip pain with decreased ROM: Perthes disease, slipped capital femoral epiphysis, toxic synovitis, osteomyelitis, suppurative arthritis, chondrolysis of hip

INVESTIGATIONS IN JUVENILE IDIOPATHIC ARTHRITIS

Laboratory Tests

- *Complete blood count (CBC):* Anemia is common in JIA, as well as elevated white blood cell count (WBC) due to inflammation.
- *Erythrocyte sedimentation rate (ESR):* A nonspecific marker of inflammation. It is typically elevated in active disease.
- *C-reactive protein (CRP):* Another marker of inflammation, often elevated during disease flare-ups.
- *Rheumatoid factor (RF):* A positive RF test is often associated with the *polyarticular* form of JIA but is not specific to JIA and can be found in other diseases.
- *Anti-citrullinated protein antibodies (ACPA):* These antibodies can be present in a small proportion of JIA patients, particularly in those with the polyarticular or RF-positive subtype.
- *Antinuclear antibodies (ANAs):* ANA testing is useful, especially in systemic onset JIA (so-called Still's disease) and in children with oligoarticular JIA, as a positive result may indicate a higher risk of uveitis (inflammation of the eye).
- *HLA-B27:* Testing for HLA-B27 is especially relevant in cases of *enthesitis-related arthritis* (ERA), which is a subtype of JIA associated with axial disease, sacroiliitis, and sometimes inflammatory bowel disease.

Imaging Studies

- *X-rays:* Plain radiographs of the affected joints are used to assess for joint damage, such as erosion or joint space narrowing. Early in the disease, X-rays may appear normal, but over time, they can show signs of joint destruction in chronic cases.
- *Ultrasound:* This can detect synovitis (inflammation of the synovial membrane) and effusions (fluid in the joints), often earlier than X-rays.
- *MRI:* Magnetic resonance imaging can be used to evaluate both soft tissue involvement (such as synovitis) and bone changes, including erosions, in more complex cases of JIA.
- *Bone scintigraphy (bone scan):* This can be used in cases where the diagnosis is unclear, to assess for active inflammation or infection in the joints.

Synovial Fluid Analysis

If the diagnosis is uncertain, synovial fluid analysis obtained through joint aspiration can help distinguish JIA from other causes of arthritis, such as infections or crystal-induced arthritis (e.g., gout). The fluid in JIA is typically inflammatory with a high white blood cell count, but without the presence of infection.

Other Specialized Tests (If Required)

- *Urinalysis:* To monitor for kidney involvement, particularly in systemic-onset JIA, where renal abnormalities can occasionally occur.
- *Liver function tests:* For monitoring systemic involvement, especially in systemic JIA, where liver inflammation or dysfunction may be a concern.

Assessment of Uveitis Risk

Children with *oligoarticular JIA* are at higher risk for uveitis (inflammation of the eye). Regular eye examinations by an ophthalmologist are recommended, particularly in children who are ANA-positive.

SEPTIC ARTHRITIS

Septic arthritis is an infection of the joint, usually caused by bacteria. The MRI findings are typically related to joint effusion, soft tissue inflammation, and bone changes. Key findings include:

- *Joint effusion:* This is one of the earliest and most common findings. It can be seen as fluid collection in the joint space.
- *Synovial thickening:* Inflammation of the synovium leads to thickening, which may be visible on MRI.
- *Bone marrow edema:* In the early stages, bone marrow edema may appear in the adjacent bone. This reflects inflammation and possible bone infection.
- *Abscess formation:* In more advanced cases, localized abscesses can form around the joint, often showing as areas of fluid collection outside the joint capsule.
- *Cortical bone changes:* In severe or untreated infections, erosion of the cortical bone or even osteomyelitis can occur, which would be visible on MRI.
- *Soft tissue swelling:* Soft tissue around the joint may be swollen due to inflammatory changes.
- *Enhancement after contrast:* The synovium, joint capsule, and periarticular tissues often enhance after contrast injection due to inflammation.

LEUKEMIA ARTHRITIS

Leukemia can involve the joints due to either direct infiltration of leukemic cells or secondary changes like infection or inflammation. The MRI findings often reflect joint inflammation, bone involvement, and possible infiltration by leukemic cells.

- *Joint effusion:* Similar to septic arthritis, joint effusion is commonly present.
- *Periarticular soft tissue swelling:* Swelling around the joint due to inflammation or infiltration by leukemic cells can be seen.
- *Bone marrow edema:* Bone marrow involvement can manifest as edema in the affected bones, often with a patchy appearance.
- *Osteopenia:* A generalized decrease in bone density can be noted on MRI, reflecting the systemic nature of leukemia.
- *Osteolytic lesions:* In advanced cases, osteolytic lesions or focal areas of bone destruction may be visible, especially in the context of leukemia infiltration.
- *Synovial thickening:* The synovium may appear thickened and heterogeneous due to leukemic infiltration or inflammatory changes.
- *Absence of classic infection features:* Unlike septic arthritis, there is no significant abscess formation or localized pus collection in leukemia arthritis.

JUVENILE IDIOPATHIC ARTHRITIS

Juvenile idiopathic arthritis is a chronic inflammatory arthritis that can involve multiple joints, and MRI findings are related to synovitis, bone changes, and cartilage involvement. MRI features include:

- *Synovial thickening:* A hallmark of JIA, synovial thickening is often seen and may lead to joint space narrowing over time.
- *Joint effusion:* Fluid accumulation within the joint is commonly seen in active disease.
- *Bone marrow edema:* This can be seen in the affected joints and may be associated with subchondral bone involvement, reflecting inflammation.
- *Cartilage damage:* In advanced disease, cartilage thinning or destruction may be evident, leading to joint deformities.
- *Joint space narrowing:* Chronic inflammation in JIA can result in progressive narrowing of the joint space over time.
- *Erosions:* In long-standing cases, erosions of the joint margins may develop, although this is more common in adult rheumatoid arthritis.
- *Enhancement of synovium after contrast:* The synovial tissue will typically enhance with contrast due to active inflammation.

- *Soft tissue edema:* The soft tissues around the joint can show swelling as a result of inflammation.
- *Tendon involvement:* Tendons around the joint may also be thickened or edematous due to inflammation, particularly in cases with enthesitis.

MRI is a valuable tool for diagnosing these conditions and assessing the extent of joint involvement, and it helps in differentiating between infection, malignancy, and chronic inflammatory diseases like JIA. **(Table 9)**.

TABLE 9: Distinguishing imaging features of septic arthritis, leukemia arthritis, and juvenile idiopathic arthritis.

Feature	*Septic arthritis*	*Leukemia arthritis*	*JIA (Juvenile idiopathic arthritis)*
Joint effusion	Common, usually large	Common, variable size	Common, moderate to large
Synovial thickening	Present, can be marked	Mild to moderate	Prominent, often marked
Bone marrow edema	Present, near joint or in adjacent bone	May be patchy, can involve metaphysis	Present, may be focal or diffuse
Abscess formation	May be seen in advanced cases	Rare, usually no abscess	None
Cortical bone erosion	May occur with osteomyelitis	Possible, due to leukemia infiltration	May occur in long-standing cases
Cartilage destruction	Not usually prominent	Rare	Can occur in advanced disease
Soft tissue swelling	Present, can be severe	Present, may have infiltration	Present, usually mild to moderate
Enhancement after contrast	Present, especially in synovium and soft tissue	Mild to moderate, if infiltration present	Present, especially in synovium

SUGGESTED READING

1. Barnes MG, Grom AA, Thompson SD, Griffin TA, Luyrink LK, Colbert RA, et al. Biologic similarities based on age at onset in oligoarticular and polyarticular subtypes of juvenile idiopathic arthritis. Arthritis Rheum. 2010;62:3249-58.
2. Clarke SL, Sen ES, Ramanan AV. Juvenile idiopathic arthritis-associated uveitis. Pediatr Rheumatol Online J. 2016;14(1):27.
3. Kimura Y, Weiss JE, Haroldson KL, Lee T, Punaro M, Oliveira S, et al. Pulmonary hypertension and other potentially fatal pulmonary complications in systemic juvenile idiopathic arthritis. Arthritis Care Res. 2013;65:745-52.
4. Martini A, Ravelli A, Avcin T, Beresford MW, Burgos-Vargas R, Cuttica R, et al. Pediatric rheumatology international trials organization international consensus. J Rheumatol. 2019;46(2):190-7.
5. Martini A. Are the number of joints involved or the presence of psoriasis still useful tools to identify homogeneous disease entities in juvenile idiopathic arthritis? J Rheumatol. 2003;30:1900-3.
6. Martini A. It is time to rethink juvenile idiopathic arthritis classification and nomenclature. Ann Rheum Dis. 2012; 71:1437-9.
7. Martini A. Systemic juvenile idiopathic arthritis. Autoimmun Rev. 2012;12:56-9.
8. Prakken B, Albani S, Martini A. Juvenile idiopathic arthritis. Lancet. 2011;377:2138-49.
9. Ramanathan A, Srinivasalu H, Colbert RA. Update on juvenile spondyloarthritis. Rheum Dis Clin North Am. 2013;39:767-88.
10. Ravelli A, Davì S, Minoia F, Martini A, Cron RQ. Macrophage Activation Syndrome. Hematol Oncol Clin North Am. 2015;29:927-41.
11. Tse SM, Laxer RM. New advances in juvenile spondyloarthritis. Nat Rev Rheumatol. 2012;8:269-79.
12. Vastert S, Prakken B. Update on research and clinical translation on specific clinical areas: From bench to bedside: How insight in immune pathogenesis can lead to precision medicine of severe juvenile idiopathic arthritis. Best Pract Res Clin Rheumatol. 2014;28:229-46.

PART C: APPROACH TO A CASE OF SYSTEMIC LUPUS ERYTHEMATOSUS

FREQUENTLY ASKED IN EXAMS

1. *Why the diagnosis of SLE?*
2. *What is the most common age and sex affecting the disease?*
3. *Diagnostic criteria for SLE*
4. *Describe the rashes of SLE:*
5. *Describe the renal involvement in SLE.*
6. *Histopathological classification of lupus nephritis*
7. *What are the neurological and cardiological manifestations of SLE?*
8. *How will you diagnose the case?*
9. *False positive and false negative causes of ANA test:*
   - *Malar rash (butterfly rash):* Red raised rash over the cheeks and the bridge of the nose. It spares the nasolabial folds
   - *Discoid rash:* Thickened scaly and hyperpigmented plaques that may cause scarring. Affects face, scalp, and ears
   - *Photosensitivity:* Rash or exacerbation of existing lesions in sun-exposed areas
   - *Livedo reticularis:* A lace like purplish discoloration of the skin commonly seen in legs associated with antiphospholipid syndrome which may coexist with SLE.
   - Alopecia
   - Vasculitis rash—purpura, petechiae, or ulcerations resulting small vessel inflammation over lower extremities

False positive:

- Healthy individuals up to 15%
- *Infections*: Viral infections (hepatitis, Epstein-Barr virus) or chronic bacterial infections
- *Medications*: Certain drugs like procainamide or isoniazid
- *Other conditions*: Liver and thyroid disorders or chronic inflammatory conditions

False negative:

- Dilution effects
- *Test variability:* ELISA versus immunofluorescence
- Seronegative autoimmune diseases, e.g., certain cases of lupus or Sjogren's syndrome may not produce detectable ANA

Systemic lupus erythematosus (SLE) is the classic prototype of a multisystem disease of autoimmune origin caused by tissue damage resulting from antibody and complement fixing immune complex deposition. This disease is typically characterized by remissions and exacerbations and has a wide range of severity of clinical manifestation varying from a condition well under control to a severely debilitating state to even death.

Why the name?

Lupus means "wolf". How the name of this animal came to be associated with a multisystem disease is not exactly known. There is evidence that the medical use of this word appeared for the first time in 10th century. The earliest workers used this term mostly for skin manifestations of lupus erythematosus. The knowledge that lupus is primarily a collagen disease affecting mainly the connective tissues as a result of the organism reacting against its' own constituents became evident in the 1940s'. Initially, with a few exceptions, SLE remained in the domain of dermatologists. Gradually, it became evident that it may occur in various other systems without the involvement of skin, thereby shifting it slowly to the domain of medical specialists. And, now, it is placed firmly in the domain of rheumatology.

Who can get it?

Systemic lupus erythematosus affects population throughout the globe but there are geographical and ethnic differences in incidence due to various factors. Although classically the disease has been described most common in women of reproductive age group where the F:M ratio is 9:1 (mostly due to the role of female reproductive hormones in pathogenesis), we should not forget that it occurs in male also especially in pediatric age group. In children, the F:M ratio comes down to around 4:1. But, younger the age of presentation, more are the chances of monogenic SLE.

CLASSIFICATION CRITERIA/DISEASE ACTIVITY/DISEASE FLARE/DAMAGE INDEX

A disease having such a varied presentation, valid, agreed upon diagnostic criteria was necessary for further epidemiologic and therapeutic research. But, as with most other rheumatological conditions, it was difficult to arrive at so-called "diagnostic criteria" because of various reasons. So it was gradually accepted to have a set of "classification criteria" based on a pattern of certain clinical and laboratory features. For diseases where there is no "gold standard" of diagnosis, it is necessary to have "classification" criteria for homogeneity of research and reporting. These sets of criteria have evolved over the years. First, it was 1971 ACR criteria, from an extraordinarily large list of 74 clinical and laboratory items, 14 were included in the classification criteria. This was revised in 1981 and the number of criteria was reduced to 11 which was again revised in 1997. Later in 2012, the Systemic Lupus International Collaborating Clinics (SLICC) came up with a set of clinical and laboratory criteria. With advancements in laboratory techniques, greater emphasis is being on placed on the serologic findings rather than just clinical criteria. Later, with better availability of kidney biopsy facilities, sole histopathological and immunofluorescence staining pattern consistent with SLE is sufficient to classify as SLE.

The latest are 2019 EULAR/ACR criteria where a positive ANA report by an appropriate method has been made an obligatory entry criterion, followed by additive weighted criteria in some clinical and immunological domains **(Table 10)**. A score of 10 or more is classified as SLE.

All said and done about the evolution of criteria over the years, one should not forget the caveat that the features may appear serially over a time, even years, rather than all at presentation **(Table 11)**. And so, if one waits for full set of criteria to occur before diagnostic confirmation and initiating treatment, a valuable window period of opportunity will be lost with consequent irreversible organ damage.

TABLE 10: 2019 ACR/EULAR classification criteria for SLE.

Entry criterion: Antinuclear antibodies (ANAs) at a titer of ≥1:80 on HEp-2 cells or an equivalent positive test (ever)

↓

- If absent, do not classify as SLE
- If present, apply additive criteria

↓

- *Additive criteria:*
  - Do not count a criterion if there is a more likely explanation than SLE
  - Occurrence of a criterion on at least one occasion is sufficient
  - SLE classification requires at least one clinical criterion and ≥10 points
  - Criteria need not occur simultaneously
  - Within each domain, only the highest weighted criterion is counted toward the total score[9]

Clinical domains and criteria	*Weight*	*Immunology domains and criteria*	*Weight*
Constitutional: Fever	2	• *Antiphospholipid antibodies:* – Anti-cardiolipin antibodies *or* – Anti-β2GP1 antibodies *or* – Lupus anticoagulant	2
• *Hematologic:* – Leukopenia – Thrombocytopenia – Autoimmune hemolysis	 3 4 4	• *Complement proteins:* – Low C3 *or* low C4 – Low C3 *and* low C4	 3 4
• *Neuropsychiatric:* – Delirium – Psychosis – Seizure	 2 3 5	• *SLE-specific antibodies:* – Anti-dsDNA antibody *or* – Anti-Smith antibody	6
• *Mucocutaneous:* – Nonscarring alopecia – Oral ulcers – Subacute cutaneous *or* discoid lupus – Acute cutaneous lupus	 2 2 4 6		
• *Serosal:* – Pleural or pericardial effusion – Acute pericarditis	 5 6		

Contd...

Contd...

Musculoskeletal: Joint involvement	6	
• *Renal:* – Proteinuria >0.5 g/24h – Renal biopsy Class II or V lupus nephritis – Renal biopsy Class III or IV lupus nephritis	 4 8 10	
Total score:		
↓		
Classify as systemic lupus erythematosus with a score of 10 or more if entry criterion fulfilled.		

(ACR: American College of Rheumatology; EULAR: European Alliance of Associations for Rheumatology; SLE: systemic lupus erythematosus)
Note: Additional criteria items within the same domain will not be counted.
Source: Aringer M, Costenbader K, Daikh D, Brinks R, Mosca M, Ramsey-Goldman R, et al. 2019 European League Against Rheumatism/American College of Rheumatology Classification Criteria for Systemic Lupus Erythematosus. Arthritis Rheumatol. 2019;71(9):1400-1412.

TABLE 11: Comparison of classification criteria of SLE evolved over the years.

Suspicion of SLE:		
ACR	***SLICC***	***EULAR/ACR***
Any 4 of 11	Histology compatible with lupus nephritis and ANA or anti-dsDNA *Or* Any 4 of 17 (at least one immunological)	ANA positive and 10 points weighted items (highest in each domain counted only)
The overall structure for classification according to the ACR 1982 and 1997, the SLICC 2012, and the EULAR/ACR 2019 classification criteria for SLE		

(ACR: American College of Rheumatology; EULAR: European Alliance of Associations for Rheumatology; SLE: systemic lupus erythematosus; SLICC: Systemic Lupus International Collaborating Clinics)

After a diagnosis of SLE has been made and treatment initiated, some disease activity scores are essential to quantify changes in patients, standardize differences between patients, to evaluate clinical responses to therapy and for research purposes. Some 60 systems exist to assess disease activity in SLE. Some of these systems are:

- British Isles Lupus Assessment Group (BILAG)
- Systemic Lupus Erythematosus Disease Activity Index (SLEDAI)
- Systemic Lupus Activity Measure (SLAM)
- University of California, San Francisco/Johns Hopkins University Lupus Activity Index (LAI)

AUTOANTIBODIES

The humoral immune response protects an organism from environmental pathogens by producing antibodies that mediate destruction or inactivation of microbial organisms or their toxins. The immune system generates antibodies to a wide array of foreign antigens without generating pathogenic antibodies to self. But, the production of antibodies that react against self-determinants is a hallmark of SLE and other autoimmune diseases. Some antibodies are simply markers for disease like anti-RNP, ANA while others play an active role in the tissue damage like anti-DNA, anti-cardiolipin, and anti-Ro. Anti-cardiolipin antibodies are associated with fetal wastage and thrombosis. Anti-Ro antibodies are responsible for manifestations of neonatal SLE and cardiac conduction defects. In such scenarios, where autoantibodies are directly responsible for the pathogenesis of a clinical feature of SLE, treating the disease with the primary target of lowering the titer of specific autoantibodies becomes a therapeutic goal with clear physiologic rationale.

ANTINUCLEAR ANTIBODY

Antinuclear antibody (ANA) is often used as a marker of autoimmune rheumatic disease (ARD) such as SLE or a related disorder. It is thus a serologic indicator of autoimmune disease and further immunological investigations are required to make a specific diagnosis. Identification of the presence and pattern of staining of ANA on IFM of HEp2 cells is an essential first step in the diagnosis of SLE. The pattern of staining may be homogenous, rimmed, speckled, or nucleolar.

Anti-DNAs are the classic autoantibodies that characterize SLE. High avidity IgG antibodies to double-stranded DNA (dsDNA) play a major role in the pathogenesis of some of the manifestations of SLE (especially nephritis). They are also relative specific for the disease and are good markers of the disease activity. It can be detected in the serum by different methods such as precipitation, hemagglutination, complement fixation, and ELISA.

These tests vary in their sensitivity and specificity. Anti-dsDNA by precipitation and complement fixation are highly specific but less sensitive whereas ELISA, hemagglutination, and PEG assays are more sensitive but correlate less well with the disease activity.

Other antibodies associated with SLE are anti-histone, anti-Ro and La, anti-SM, antiphospholipid, coombs antibodies, lupus anticoagulant, antithyroid, and antiribosomal P antibody.

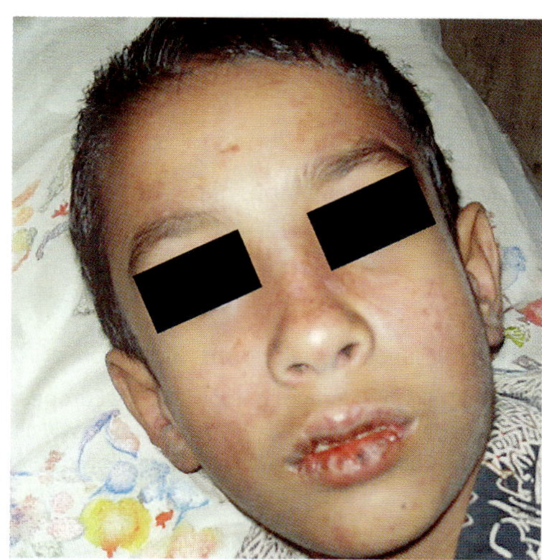

Fig. 8: An 8-year-old male child presenting with typical butterfly rash subsequently diagnosed with lupus nephritis.

PATHOGENESIS

In SLE, there is breakdown of the self-tolerance and the reasons for this could be many like excess generation of self-antigen, defects in pathways of clearance of self-antigens, defects in deletion of autoreactive T cells, etc. The presence of the triggering antigen is often required for the development of autoimmunity. In lupus patients, this initiating stimulus is not clear. The most plausible ones are apoptotic cells and pathogens. Apoptosis, or programmed cell death, is a process that leads to the ordered destruction of cells. The rate of apoptosis is increased in patients with SLE. The increased apoptosis and possibly some infections initiate the immune dysregulation. There is development of autoreactive T cells and autoantibody producing B-cells. These autoreactive cells mediate tissue injury leading on to various clinical manifestations.

Autoantibodies probably are important for pathogenesis of SLE but they alone are not sufficient. Antibody binding to antigen and resulting immune complexes activate complement and other mediators of inflammation, with subsequent release of cytokines, chemokines, and proteolytic enzymes, resulting in organ inflammation and damage.

CLINICAL FEATURES

Systemic lupus erythematosus is a chronic disorder of pleomorphic nature. No classic pattern exists. The diagnosis is based on the overall clinical picture, serologic and laboratory investigations, and, in some cases, biopsies and other procedures.

Meticulous history-taking is important including the family history. Seemingly unimportant events may also provide a clue to the diagnosis. The patient may come to the physician for a variety of complaints relating to diverse systems of the body. The classical presentation of butterfly rash **(Fig. 8)** and arthritis is present only in a minority of patients. Any system may be affected or heal. The same or any other system may be involved months or years later. At the Mayo Clinic, 101 children with SLE were followed up which showed that presentation in children is similar to that of adults. But, children and adolescents with SLE present with more severe manifestations than adults and early age of onset has been correlated with a worse prognosis.

Unexplained fever, malaise, and weight loss are the most common manifestations of SLE in children and adolescents. In such cases, the physician should actively seek evidence of joint involvement, photosensitive rash, hematuria, proteinuria, hypergammaglobulinemia, and hypocomplementemia. The following table lists the cumulative percentage of clinical manifestations of SLE in two large pediatric series.

Most children with SLE present with chronic illness, presentation may also be in the form of acute severe illness like seizures, psychosis, uremia, severe anemia, pulmonary hemorrhage, and sepsis. It often happens that the diagnosis is not suspected until it is noted that the child is not recovering as expected despite adequate therapy for the presenting illness. Confirmation of diagnosis is based on the criteria developed for use in adults. While these criteria are useful guidelines, fulfillment of four criteria does not exclude other diagnoses; likewise failure to fulfill

TABLE 12: ISN/RPS histopathological staging of lupus nephritis.

International Society of Nephrology/Renal Pathology Society 2003 classification of LN:	
Class	*Description*
Class I	Minimal mesangial LN
Class II	Mesangial proliferative LN
Class III	• Focal LN (≤50% of glomeruli) • III (A): Active lesions • III (A/C): Active and chronic lesions • III (C): Chronic lesions
Class IV	• Diffuse LN (≥50% glomeruli) • Diffuse segmental (IV-S) or global (IV-G) LN • IV (A): Active lesions • IV (A/C): Active and chronic lesions • IV (C): Chronic lesions
Class V	Membranous LN
Class VI	Advanced sclerosing LN (≥90% globally sclerosed glomeruli without residual activity)

(ISN: International Society of Nephrology; LN: lupus nephritis; RPS: Renal Pathology Society)

TABLE 13: Modified National Institutes of Health indices of activity and chronicity.

Index	*Score*[a]
Modified activity indices:	
Endocapillary hypercellularity	0–3
Neutrophils/karyorrhexis	0–3
Fibrinoid necrosis	(0–3) × 2
Hyaline deposits	0–3
Cellular/fibrocellular crescents	(0–3) × 2
Interstitial inflammation	0–3
Modified chronicity indices:	
Total glomerulosclerosis[b] score	0–3
Fibrous crescents	0–3
Tubular atrophy	0–3
Interstitial fibrosis	0–3

Note:
[a]1, <25%; 2, 25%–50%; 3, >50% glomeruli/tubules/cortical interstitium involved
[b]Global and/or segmental sclerosis

criteria does not exclude SLE. ANA-positive children who fall short of criteria should be periodically reevaluated. Full-fledged disease may manifest even decades after the initial presentation.

Rates of organ involvement are higher in the child compared to adult patients. Signs and symptoms of renal disease occur in two-thirds of the children with SLE, but renal biopsy without regard to the clinical manifestations demonstrates varying degrees of renal involvement in nearly all the cases. Although renal disease may be mild, severe diffuse proliferative glomerulonephritis remains a leading cause of morbidity in childhood SLE. The ISN/RPS histopathological staging is mainly based on glomerular features **(Table 12)** but tubules and interstitium may also be involved in the disease process. In addition to the staging, it is also important to discern how much active the disease **(Table 13)**. More the activity index, more aggressive immunomodulation therapy may help but once markers of chronicity are high, probably no more immunosuppression will help, one has to opt for only renal replacement therapy.

Neurological manifestations involve both the central and peripheral nervous system.

All CNS manifestations described in adults also occur in children, but behavioral disturbance and chorea are seen more commonly in children. Headache is a common symptom and may have a multitude of causes. It is most commonly due to tension or fatigue but may also be a manifestation of intracranial pathology. A type of severe unremitting headache, the so-called "lupus headache" may be secondary to cerebral vein thrombosis associated with presence of antiphospholipid antibodies. Many patients with lupus experience memory loss or other cognitive dysfunction in their disease course.

Pulmonary involvement may occur in the form of pleurisy, pleural effusion, pulmonary fibrosis, and pulmonary hemorrhage. Diaphragmatic dysfunction is common and may be the predisposing cause of recurrent episodes of pneumonia.

Musculoskeletal manifestations like arthritis and myopathy may be the predominating features at presentation, but these seldom contribute to long-term morbidity. But, avascular necrosis may occur with or without steroid therapy which may require joint replacement. Dermatologic involvement is common in childhood; SLE is rarely a cause for concern, except when the face is prominently disfigured. DLE is unusual in childhood and its incidence is 2–3%.

Cardiac manifestations include pericarditis, myocarditis, and pericardial effusion. Valvular involvement may predispose to bacterial endocarditis. Premature myocardial infarctions have occurred in young adults with significant atherosclerosis following prolonged steroid therapy. Gastrointestinal manifestations are varied ranging from nonspecific findings such as chronic abdominal pain and anorexia to bowel infarction and pneumatosis intestinalis.

Infections are a major cause of morbidity and mortality in childhood SLE. Predisposition to sepsis may be due to combined effects of SLE and immunosuppressive effects of the drugs that are used to treat it. In addition to the bacterial infections, viral, fungal, and opportunistic infections occur with an increasing frequency. Often it becomes unclear if the rapid clinical deterioration is due to an infection or disease exacerbation.

Hematological manifestations are common, but, most are nonspecific. Thrombocytopenia is a frequent presenting complaint and it may be the cause of menorrhagia in adolescent females. Presence of anti-cardiolipin antibodies predisposes to bleeding diathesis and stroke in children.

LABORATORY EVALUATION

The different laboratory tests may be divided into:

- Tests for detection of different types of autoantibody
- Tests for detection of other immunological derangements like hypergammaglobulinemia, hypocomplementenimia, etc.
- Tests for detection of individual organ involvement
- Tests for detection of complications like MAS, infections, and disease flare

Diagnosis of SLE is strongly suggested by the constellation of hypergammaglobulinemia, leukopenia, anemia, and thrombocytopenia. IgA deficiency and even panhypogammaglobulinemia may also be seen. C3 levels correlate with disease activity. Reduced C4 level may correlate with C3 level or it may also occur in isolation. Reduced C4 levels may also be found in relatives of children with SLE which may be the evidence of C4 null allele, a manifestation of subclinical disease or both.

Elevated ANA is an excellent screening tool, although ANA can be found without any disease or can be associated with rheumatic and other conditions. ANA has a sensitivity of 95% in titers of 1:80 or more but the specificity is on 40%. Anti-dsDNA antibodies are both specific and sensitive and are the hallmark of SLE. Anti-Sm antibodies are more specific but less sensitive.

Anticardiolipin antibodies (aCLs) are present in up to 65% of pediatric patients. The levels may vary with disease activity, high titers are often associated with the presence of neurological features and deep venous thrombosis.

CONCLUSION

Systemic lupus erythematosus is an autoimmune disease that manifests as a chronic inflammatory disorder with multisystem involvement. The presentation is highly variable, the disease follows a relapsing and remitting course, and although standardized treatment has improved the short- and medium-term outlook, long-term prognosis remains poor in children with lupus with major organ involvement.

SUGGESTED READING

1. Aringer M, Costenbader K, Daikh D, Brinks R, Mosca M, Ramsey-Goldman R, et al. 2019 European League Against Rheumatism/American College of Rheumatology Classification Criteria for Systemic Lupus Erythematosus. Arthritis Rheumatol. 2019;78(9):1151-9.
2. Bajema IM, Wilhelmus S, Alpers CE, Bruijn JA, Colvin RB, Cook HT, et al. Revision of the International Society of Nephrology/Renal Pathology Society classification for lupus nephritis: clarification of definitions, and modified National Institutes of Health activity and chronicity indices. Kidney Int. 2018;93:789-96.
3. Bongu A, Chang E, Ramsey-Goldman R. Can morbidity and mortality of SLE be improved? Best Pract Res Clin Rheumatol. 2002;16(2):313-32.
4. Grossman JM, Kalunian KC. Definition, classification, activity and damage indices. In: Wallace D, Hahn BH (eds). Dubois' Lupus Erythematosus, 7th edition. Philadelphia, PA: Lippincott, Williams & Wilkins; 2007. pp. 16-31.
5. King K, Kornrich HK, Bernstein BH. The clinical spectrum of systemic lupus erythematosus. Proceedings of the conference of rheumatic diseases of childhood. Arthritis Rheum. 1977;20(supple2):287294.
6. Kumar A. Indian guidelines of management of SLE. J Indian Rheumatol Assoc. 2002;10:80-96.
7. Mondal R, Nandi M, Ganguli S, Ghosh A, Hazra A. Childhood lupus: experience from Eastern India. Indian J Pediatr. 2010;77(8):889-91.
8. Samanta M, Nandi M, Mondal R, Hazra A, Sarkar S, Sabui T, et al. Childhood lupus nephritis: 12 years of experience from a developing country's perspective. Eur J Rheumatol. 2017;4(3):178-83.
9. Vaidya S, Samant RS, Nadkar MY, Borges NE. Systemic lupus erythematosus - a review of 220 patients. J Indian Rheumatol Assoc. 1997;5:14-8.
10. Weening JJ, D'Agati VD, Schwartz MM, Seshan SV, Alpers CE, Appel GB, et al. The classification of glomerulonephritis in systemic lupus erythematosus revisited. J Am Soc Nephrol. 2004;15:241-50.

"Lead us to understand more about this mysterious disease, and one day, to conquer it."

CHAPTER 13

Newborn

Saugata Chaudhuri

HOW TO PRESENT A CASE IN AN EXAMINATION

OPENING STATEMENT

Start by discussing biological risk factors, gestational age, birth weight, and the method of delivery along with the reason for it. Conclude the opening statement with your current situation and concerns, such as respiratory distress requiring mechanical ventilation. Note the postnatal age in hours, particularly if the infant is under 5 days old.

For instance, my baby is named Sharmila, a single male infant born at 34 weeks of gestation, weighing 1,754 grams, and delivered via emergency cesarean section. The reason for the delivery was pregnancy-induced hypertension (PIH). Presently, the infant is 96 hours old with a postnatal age of 34 weeks and 4 days, and has been admitted due to severe perinatal asphyxia and is currently on noninvasive ventilatory support.

ANTENATAL HISTORY

A 36-year-old gravida 2 has given birth to a baby after experiencing a prior abortion at 14 weeks. After that, she encountered secondary infertility and pursued in-vitro fertilization, during which she took peri-conceptional folic acid. During her first trimester, she did not report any symptoms of fever, rash, or vaginal bleeding. Throughout her second and third trimesters, she received calcium and iron supplements as well as two doses of tetanus toxoid. There was no history of gestational hypertension, gestational diabetes, postpartum vaginal bleeding, late postpartum vaginal bleeding, decreased fetal movements, or either excess or insufficient amniotic fluid. She experienced preterm premature rupture of membranes (PPROM) 1 week prior to delivery and was treated with antibiotics (if labor occurred around 24 hours, include labor details). During her second and third trimesters, she continued taking calcium and iron supplements and received two doses of tetanus toxoid. There was no documented history of gestational hypertension, gestational diabetes, postpartum vaginal bleeding, late postpartum vaginal bleeding, decreased fetal movements, or issues with amniotic fluid levels. A week before delivery, she dealt with PPROM and was administered antibiotics (if labor occurred around 24 hours, include details). HIV ELISA, Hepatitis B, and VDRL tests all returned normal results. If a TORCH profile was performed, include that as well.

NATAL HISTORY

Information on labor and delivery is provided. She received two doses of antenatal steroids before delivery, with the first given 48 hours prior and the second 24 hours prior. After a 24-hour period of PPROM, she went into spontaneous or induced labor. The fetal heart rate was monitored using cardiotocography (CTG) and intermittent auscultation, showing clear signs of fetal well-being. The delivery was completed via cesarean section due to the indication of antepartum hemorrhage (APH). The newborn needed initial resuscitative measures and was given an APGAR score of 7 and 8 at 1 and 5 minutes, respectively.

POSTNATAL CARE IN NEONATAL INTENSIVE CARE UNIT

The infant was transferred to the neonatal intensive care unit (NICU) and received treatment with surfactant/continuous positive airway pressure (CPAP). In the past 24 hours, the baby has been on ventilatory support or CPAP. If consulted, I would like to know the maximum level of ventilatory support given to the baby, any extubation attempts made, whether feeding has commenced, and if supplementation has begun with the feeds. If the baby is stable, I would like to hear about the skin-to-skin care session. I also want to understand the family's demographic profile, as well as the social and psychological support available to the mother. A better-organized postnatal history should categorize clinical systems into respiratory, cardiovascular, neurological, gastrointestinal, and nutritional aspects, ensuring all information is captured. It concludes with the discussion on supportive care and the mother's perception of her infant. I will compile a list of relevant examinations, I would like to perform based on the provided history. The baby is currently being cared for under a radiant warmer at a set temperature of 36.5°C, with a measured temperature of 36.3°C and a heater output of 20%. There are three infusions being administered, including dextrose, TPN, and inotropes, totaling 11 mL/h, which amounts to 100 mL/kg/day. There is also a LED phototherapy unit turned off. The baby is placed supine under the warmer, wearing a cap, with the endotracheal tube secured firmly at 8 cm, showing no signs of leakage, and 2 cm in length from the mouth to the adapter. An NG tube measuring 6F is fixed at 18 cm. The baby has central/peripheral lines in place, with continuous pulse oximetry and temperature monitoring. She is being ventilated in synchronized intermittent mandatory ventilation (SIMV) mode with pressures set to 16/5 at a rate of 30 breaths per minute, and the FiO_2 is at 40%. The tidal volume is delivering 5 mL/kg. The humidification chamber displays a temperature of 37°C, with adequate water levels and minimal condensation observed in the expiration limb. Heart rate is continuously monitored, and there are no activated alarms. The pulse oximeter readings show a saturation of 95% with the probe positioned on the right hand, within a saturation range of 85–100. The heart rate is noted at 144, with limits between 100 and 180. During the examination, there have been no episodes of desaturation or bradycardia. (Alternatively, if on CPAP, state: The baby is on bubble CPAP at 4 cm of water and 50% FiO_2, with a flow rate of 4 L/min, demonstrating adequate bubbling in the chamber.)

VITAL

- *Pulse/heart rate:* Rate, volume, regularity, and femoral pulses. Alarm limits of pulse oximeter
- Respiratory rate and pattern
- Color, CRT (capillary refill time)
  How to check capillary refill time:
  Gentle pressure is applied over the sternum for 5 seconds, observe how fast the blanched area refills. CRT >3 seconds indicates poor perfusion. However, in case of hypothermia, it can be prolonged also.
- *Blood pressure:* SBP, DBP, MBP, PP, and centiles
- *Temperature:* set, measured, and axillary temperature
- *Saturation:* reading with FiO_2. Limits: Pre- and postductal difference
- Perfusion index (PI)
- Pleth variability index (PVI)
- *Neonatal sickness score:* SNAPPEII score and CRIBII score

Heart rate:

- Tachycardia can indicate tube blockage, pain, shock, sepsis, use of inotropes, or paralytic agents.
- Bradycardia may result from sedation, vagal stimulation, increased intracranial pressure, or hypo-/hyperkalemia.

The baseline heart rate varies by newborn. For instance, a baby with a baseline heart rate of 120 beats/minute that suddenly rises to 160 beats/minute is considered tachycardia. Conversely, another newborn may normally have a baseline of 180/min.

Respiratory rate: Count for 1 minute. Observe patterns of respiration as they are crucial. Utilize respiratory distress scoring (Downe/Silverman) and exclude periodic breathing.

Blood pressure: Dependent on gestational and postnatal age (see Zubrow Chart). A general rule is that mean blood pressure is equivalent to the gestational age in weeks.

A wide pulse pressure (PP) in newborns indicates a difference between systolic and diastolic blood pressure exceeding 15–25 mm Hg for premature infants and greater than 25 mm Hg for term infants. A narrow PP is defined as being <25% of the systolic pressure and can signify PDA, anemia, fluid overload, or warm shock. A narrow pulse pressure might suggest hypovolemia or cold shock.

Hypothermia is a frequent issue among newborns, arising from several factors:

- *Environmental factors:* Being born in cooler conditions or in an inadequately warm room
- *Newborn care practices:* Being placed on a cold surface after birth, improper drying or wrapping, or bathing in cool water.
- *Maternal factors:* Maternal hypertension, low maternal temperature, or insufficient antenatal care
- *Birth factors:* Prematurity, low birth weight, cesarean delivery, or multiple gestation
- *Other factors:* Chorioamnionitis, prolonged rupture of membranes, or need for resuscitation
- *Delayed breastfeeding:* Not starting breastfeeding within the first hour after birth can heighten the risk of hypothermia.

Normal axillary temperature ranges from 36.5 to 37.5°C.

- *Cold stress*: 36.4–36°C (cold feet, warm abdomen)
- *Moderate hypothermia:* 35.9–32°C
- *Severe hypothermia:* <32°C

Temperature measurement: Axillary temperature is as effective as rectal temperature and poses less risk of injury or infection.

The three primary causes of fever in newborns and infants include infections, overheating, and dehydration.

OXYGEN SATURATION (TABLES 1 AND 2)

Oxygen saturation target after birth:

- At 1 minute of life 60–65%
- At 2 minutes of life 65–70%
- At 3 minutes of life 70–75%
- At 4 minutes of life 75–80%
- At 5 minutes of life 80–85%
- At 10 minutes of life 85–95%

TABLE 1: Table of saturation targets and limits.

Gestation	*Air/oxygen*	*Target*	*Alarm limit*
Preterm <37 weeks or birth weight <1.5 kg	Air	91–95%	90–96%
	Oxygen	91–95%	90–100%
Term infant ≥37 weeks	Air	≥95%	94–99%
	Oxygen	≥95%	94–100%
Risk of PPHN/ Established PPNH	Air/oxygen	>95%	95–100%

(PPHN: persistent pulmonary hypertension of the newborn)

TABLE 2: Oxygen saturation in various congenital heart disease.

Congenital heart disease (unrepaired)	*SpO_2*	*Special consideration*
VSD	Normal saturation	SpO_2 may come down to 80% if the patient develops pulmonary hypertension causing Rt to Lt shunt
ASD	Normal saturation	SpO_2 may come down to 80% if the patient develops pulmonary hypertension causing Rt to Lt shunt
Coarctation of aorta	90–100%	If PDA remains open, preductal > postductal (differential cyanosis)
Interrupted aortic arch	70–100%	Preductal > postductal, in the presence of large VSD, may result in higher saturation due to Lt to Rt shunt
Tetralogy of Fallot	80–100%	Desaturation depends on the degree of desaturation
Transposition of great arteries	75–95%	• If good mixing at the atrial septum or VSD (especially if the PDA is also open), may saturate higher • If additional coarctation or interrupted aortic arch, PDA shunting from pink pulmonary artery to blue aorta will lead to higher postductal saturation than preductal saturation (reverse differential cyanosis)
Hypoplastic left heart syndrome	75–95%	Mixing lesions; hence, higher saturation indicates more pulmonary venous components than the systemic venous component in the blood mixing in the heart (hence, more pulmonary over circulation)
Partial anomalous pulmonary venous connection	90–100%	If pulmonary hypertension develops, then right-to-left shunting through the ASD may reduce saturation
Total anomalous pulmonary venous connection	75–90%	All the oxygenated pulmonary venous return mixes with systemic venous return in the right atrium, and shunts right to left across the ASD to then be pumped by the left heart to the body
Tricuspid atresia/pulmonary atresia/ Ebstein anomaly with insufficient prograde flow through the pulmonary valve (functional pulmonary atresia)	75–95%	Pulmonary blood flow depends on PDA shunting from the aorta to the pulmonary artery; higher saturation indicates more pulmonary over circulation
Truncus arteriosus	85–95%	Higher saturation indicates more pulmonary over circulation
Pulmonary AVM	70–100%	Pulmonary AVMs bypass the normal gas exchange at the alveoli, leading to desaturation; they may occur with or without other CHD

(ASD: atrial septal defect; AVM: arteriovenous malformation; CHD: congenital heart disease; PDA: patent ductus arteriosus; VSD: ventricular septal defect; SpO_2: peripheral capillary oxygen saturation)

PERFUSION INDEX

The perfusion index (PI) reflects the fluctuations in pulsatility and is influenced by factors such as stroke volume, skin temperature, and vasomotor tone. A PI value below 1.24 has been utilized as a benchmark for diagnosing severe neonatal illnesses in infants. Typically, perfusion index values are represented as percentages (0.02–20%). The PI in newborns may vary based on their gestational age and age in days, with numerous influencing factors:

- *For preterm infants:* The median PI is 0.9% on the 1st day, 1.22% on the 3rd, and 1.35% by the 7th day. The PI range for preterm newborns in their initial week of life can span from 0.7 to 1.35%.
- *For term infants:* The median PI for asymptomatic term newborns after 24 hours of life is 1.8.

Altitude can lead to an increase in the PI.

The placement of the pulse oximeter sensor can impact the PI, particularly in very preterm newborns.

Postnatal development seems to stabilize the PI around the 5th day of life, likely due to the maturation of the sympathetic nervous system.

PLETH VARIABILITY INDEX

Pleth variability index (PVI) is a measurement used to assess fluid responsiveness. In various investigations, the median PVI value observed was 21. This parameter remains unaffected by gestational age, days of life, gender, or weight. Monitoring a series of PVI values provides more actionable insights than relying on a single reading when making clinical decisions. Increased variability suggests a stronger likelihood of the patient responding to fluid administration.

Clinical scores of sick neonate: SNAPPE II score and CRIB II score: **Table 3** and **Figure 1** describe the two standard clinical Score. **Figure 1** is applicable up to 32 weeks of gestation.

CRIBII chart included here with permission

TABLE 3: SNAPPE II score (Chart included after permission).

Variable	*Values*	*Points*
Mean blood pressure	≥30 mm Hg	0
	20–29 mm Hg	9
	<20 mm Hg	19
Temperature	>35.6°C	0
	35–35.6°C	8
	<35°C	15
PO_2 (mm hg)/FiO_2 (%)	>2.49	0
	1–2.49	5
	0.3–0.99	16
	<0.3	28
Lowest serum pH	≥7.2	0
	7.1–7.19	7
	<7.1	16
Multiple seizures	No	0
	Yes	19
Urine output (mL/kg/h)	≥1	0
	0.1–0.9	5
	<0.1	18

ANTHROPOMETRY

In a sick baby, it is not possible to check anthropometric parameters **(Table 4)**.

Growth charts to be plotted in Lubchenco/Fenton/intergrowth 21st century chart:

Weight: It is recommended to use a digital weighing scale for measuring an infant's weight.

Length: The infantometer should be situated on an even and sturdy surface. Position the baby supine and straight on the infantometer. Use a firm board-like structure (headpiece) to stabilize the head. Another board-like structure (footpiece) should be pressed securely against the feet and heel. Ensure the baby's body and legs remain straight, with one hand needed to firmly press the knee joint. The baby's eyes should be directed straight up. At least two individuals are required for this process.

Head circumference: Employ a flexible, narrow tape measure that does not stretch.

Position the tape measure just above the eyebrows, roughly 1–2 fingers above the supraorbital ridge. Encircle the tape around the widest section of the head, typically the back. Gently pull the tape to compress any hair present. Take three measurements, and compute the average.

Microcephaly: Defined as a head circumference that is more than 3 standard deviations below the normal range.

Macrocephaly: Identified as a head circumference that exceeds 2 standard deviations above the normal range.

Fontanels: The anterior fontanel typically measures around 2.5 cm × 2.5 cm but can be as large as 4 cm, particularly in the anterior-posterior direction. Immediately after birth, the anterior fontanel appears narrow due to overriding

Birthweight (g) and gestation (weeks):
The maximum (worst) score for birthweight and gestation is 15, which is obtained for a 22 weeks male infant of less than 501 g birthweight

Male infants

Birthweight (g)	22	23	24	25	26	27	28	29	30	31	32
2,751 to 3,000											0
2,501 to 2,750										1	0
2,251 to 2,500									3	0	0
2,001 to 2,250									2	0	0
1,751 to 2,000								3	1	0	0
1,501 to 1,750						6	5	3	2	1	0
1,251 to 1,500					8	6	5	3	3	2	1
1,001 to 1,250		12	10	9	8	7	6	5	4	3	3
751 to 1,000		12	11	10	8	7	7	6	6	6	6
501 to 755	14	13	12	11	10	9	8	8	8	8	
251 to 500	15	14	13	12	11	10	10				

Gestation (weeks)

Female infants

Birthweight (g)	22	23	24	25	26	27	28	29	30	31	32
2,751 to 3,000											0
2,501 to 2,750										1	0
2,251 to 2,500									2	0	0
2,001 to 2,250									1	0	0
1,751 to 2,000								3	1	0	0
1,501 to 1,750						6	4	3	1	1	0
1,251 to 1,500					7	5	4	3	2	1	1
1,001 to 1,250		11	10	8	7	6	5	4	3	3	3
751 to 1,000		11	10	9	8	7	6	5	5	5	5
501 to 755	13	12	11	10	9	8	8	7	7	7	
251 to 500	14	13	12	11	10	10	10				

Gestation (weeks)

Temperature at admission (°C)

Temperature	Score
≤29.6	5
29.7 to 31.2	4
31.3 to 32.8	3
32.9 to 34.4	2
34.5 to 36	1
36.1 to 37.5	0
37.6 to 39.1	1
39.2 to 40.7	2
≥40.8	3

Base excess (mmol/L)

Base excess	Score
< –26	7
–26 to –23	6
–22 to –18	5
–17 to –13	4
–12 to –13	3
–7 to –3	2
–2 to 2	1
≥3	0

Sex, birthweight (g) and gestation (weeks): ______
Temperature at admission (°C): ______
Base excess (mmol/L): ______

Total CRIB II score

The logistic regression equation relating CRIB II to mortality (CRIB II algorithm) is:
Log odds of mortality = G = –6.476 + 0.450 × CRIB II
Probability of mortality = exp(G)/[1+exp(G)]
The range of possible CRIB II scores is 0 to 27

Fig. 1: Clinical risk index for babies II (CRIB II) score.

TABLE 4: Anthropometric parameters.

	At birth	*Present*	*Centile*	*Comments*
Weight				% of weight loss/weight gain
Head circumference				
Length				
Ponderal index				Asymmetrical IUGR

(IUGR: intrauterine growth restriction)

tensions from molding. It is best evaluated when the infant is calm and placed upright, and it should typically be slightly depressed relative to the surrounding surface. The posterior fontanel is usually <1 cm in size.

Various head shapes: The cephalic index is calculated as head width multiplied by 100 and divided by head length. The length of the head refers to the maximum diameter through the sagittal plane, stretching from the glabella at the front to the most prominent point on the occiput at the back. Head width is determined by the maximum biparietal diameter.

A cephalic index of 81 or higher indicates brachycephaly (coronal synostosis), a normal range is between 70 and 80.9, while a cephalic index below 76 indicates dolichocephaly/scaphocephaly (a kneel-shaped head due to sagittal synostosis).

In cases of combined sagittal, coronal, and lambdoid synostosis, the head is characterized as acrocephaly/oxycephaly/turricephaly, with a cephalic index of 80 or above. In turricephaly, the head exhibits a relatively tall appearance compared to its width and length, while in acrocephaly/oxycephaly, the top of the skull takes on a cone shape.

Plagiocephaly refers to a head shape where the occipital area is flattened, causing the ipsilateral frontal region to protrude.

General physical examination:

- Emphasize important details and provide interpretation
- Anterior fontanel—dimensions, position, pulsation
- Posterior fontanel
- Sutures
- Any signs of birth-related head injuries
- Dimensions and contour of the head
- Eyes—cataracts, subconjunctival bleeding, periorbital swelling
- Facial anomalies, deformities
- Skin—jaundice, paleness, neurocutaneous lesions
- Umbilical area, genitals, anal opening, lower limb swelling
- *TIPS:* Employ a head-to-toe examination approach. Assess the oral cavity and back
- Head to toe examination is essential as early as 1–2 hours of life according to **Figure 2** to exclude congenital anomalies.

Pallor:

Skin pallor causes:

- Newborn may have slightly pale complexion than others
- Anemia of prematurity
- Baby may be having poor perfusion
- Hypothermia
- Mild jaundice newborn may look pale
- In case of heart failure, newborn may look pale

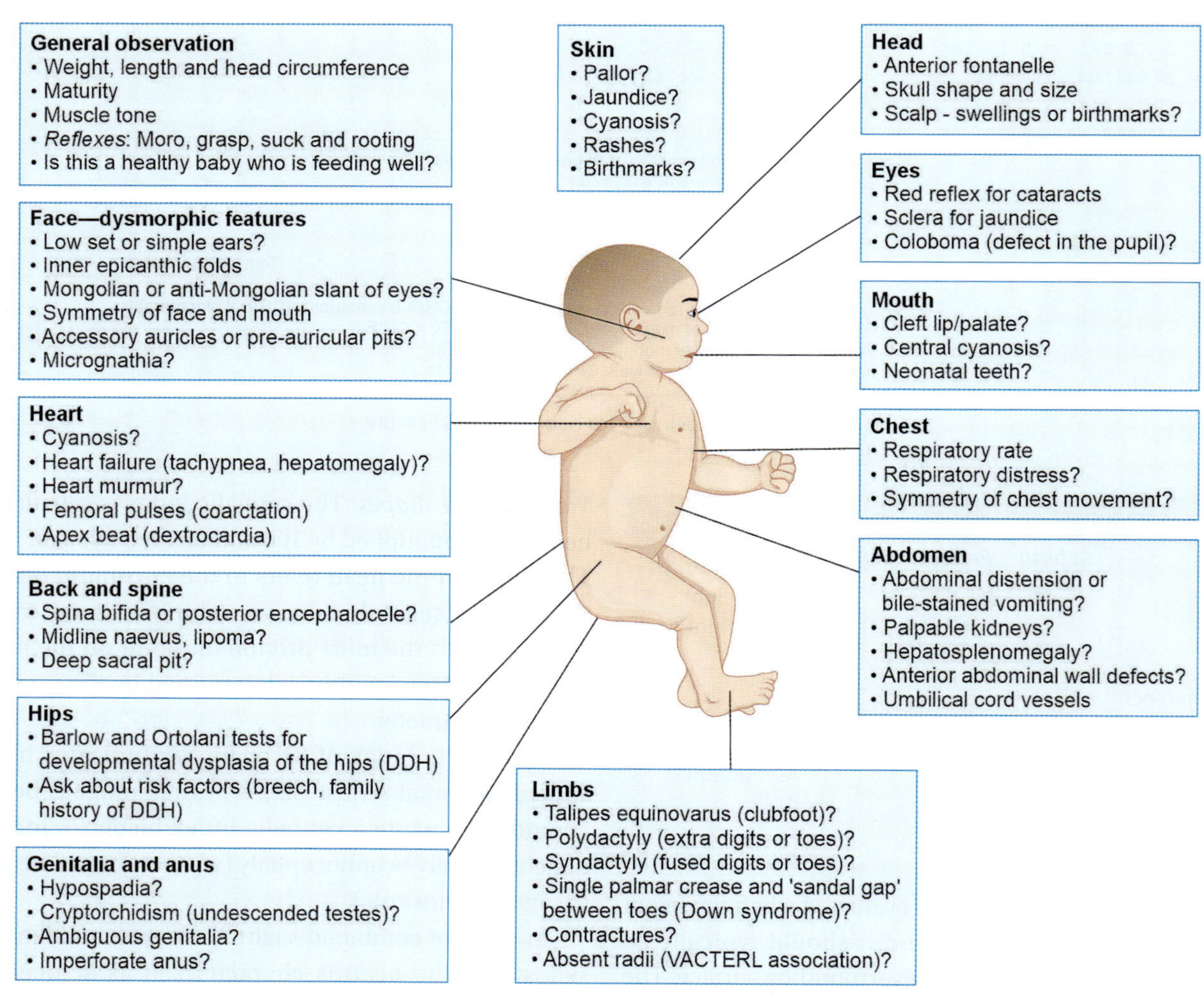

Fig. 2: Head-to-toe clinical examination to exclude congenital anomalies.

- Neonatal sepsis
- Hypoxia
- Bleeding neonate
- Hemolysis due to any cause
- Some genetic causes may cause paleness of skin.

Red flag signs: Pallor associated with poor feeding, lethargy, and respiratory distress warrants emergency medical attention.

Jaundice:

Classical pattern of physiological jaundice:

- Appearance between 24 and 72 hours
- Always ≤15 mg/dL
- On 7th day preterm and on 3rd day term, baby has maximum intensity of bilirubin
- Undetectable clinically after 14 days
- Close observation to identify the worsening of symptoms

Alert signs for jaundice:

- Jaundice within the first 24 hours of life
- Total serum bilirubin (TSB) ≥15 mg/dL
- TSB increasing by >5 mg/dL/day or 0.3 mg/dL/h in the first 24 hours and 0.2 mg/dL/h
- Conjugated serum bilirubin >1 mg/dL
- Clinical jaundice persisting >2 weeks in full term and >3 weeks in preterm

Causes of jaundice:

- *Appearing ≤24 hours of age:*
    - Hemolytic disease of newborn: Rh, ABO, and minor blood group incompatibility
    - Infections
    - G6PD deficiency
- *Appearing >24 hours of age:*
    - All the above
    - Physiological
    - Cephalohematoma
    - Intraventricular or subarachnoid hemorrhage
    - Sepsis
    - Hypothyroidism
    - Breastfeeding jaundice (inadequate feeding)
    - Breast milk jaundice
    - Sepsis
    - Inborn error of metabolism defects (tyrosinemia, etc.)
    - Neonatal cholestasis syndrome
    - Small or large bowel obstruction
    - Delayed feeding
    - Surgical conditions of liver
    - Hereditary hematological disorders

Clinical assessment:

- *Face and neck:* 6 mg/dL
- *Chest and back:* 9 mg/dl
- *Abdomen below the umbilicus to the knees:* 12 mg/dL
- *Arms and leg below the knees:* 15 mg/dL
- *Hands and feet:* 18–20 mg/dL

Color of the skin may be misleading without bright day light and also in some dark complexion newborn.

Always use 4 AAP charts

1. Phototherapy threshold by gestational age in hours for infants with no recognized hyperbilirubinemia neurotoxicity risk factors other than gestational age,
2. Phototherapy threshold by gestational age in hours for infants with any recognized hyperbilirubinemia neurotoxicity risk factors other than gestational age,
3. Exchange transfusion threshold by gestational age in hours for infants with no recognized hyperbilirubinemia neurotoxicity risk factors other than gestational age,
4. Exchange transfusion threshold by gestational age in hours for infants with any recognized hyperbilirubinemia neurotoxicity risk factors other than gestational age) and
5. NICE guidelines for <35 weeks gestation.

Edema:

- Generalized
- Local

Generalized edema causes:

- Physiological edema of newborn—may appear at 2–3 days life at the face, lower limb, face, and genitalia and disappear within a week.
- *Sclerema:* Diffuse hardening of subcutaneous tissue is known as sclerema, specifically referred to as sclerema neonatorum when it occurs in newborns and infants. This condition is characterized by widespread, firm hardening of the subcutaneous fat and skin, which binds the skin to the underlying muscles and bones, making it impossible to pinch or elevate the skin. Risk factors of developing sclerema are:
    - Prematurity
    - Sepsis
    - Hypothermia
    - Dyselectrolytemia
- *Neonatal fat necrosis:* Subcutaneous fat necrosis in newborns appears as a temporary region of swelling in the skin, which is then accompanied by

Flowchart 1: Causes of hydrops.

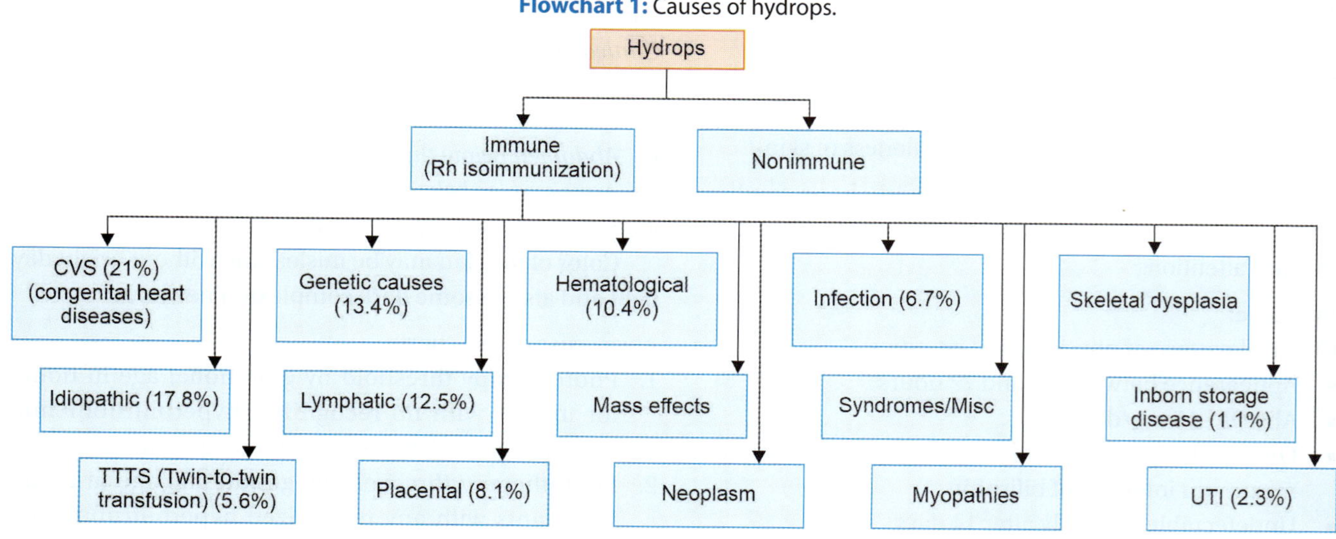

(UTI: urinary tract infection)

hardened subcutaneous plaques or painless, movable nodules, occasionally accompanied by changes in skin color. It is associated with asphyxia and other neonatal and maternal risk factors. It is a self-limiting condition.

- *Hydrops:* Presence of excessive fetal fluid in two or more of the following spaces: abdominal ascites, pleural effusion, pericardial effusion, skin edema, polyhydramnios, or placentomegaly. **Flowcharts 1 and 2** show the causes and pathophysiologies of hydrops fetalis.

COMMON SKIN FINDINGS OF NEWBORN

- *Salmon patch:* The macular pink red lesions tend to fade with time and those on the glabellum, eyelids, nose, and upper lip are rarely detected after the age of 6.
- *Portwine stain:* Usually found on the face, portwine stain is a permanent birthmark. On a newborn, it begins as smooth, flat, pink, or red patches. It might get bigger, thicker, and darker with time. Certain blood vessel syndromes, such as Sturge-Weber and Klippel-Trenaunay-Weber syndrome, are linked to certain portwine stains.
- *Erythema toxicum:* Eosinophil-containing flesh-colored papules with an erythematous base disappear within the 1st week.
- *Milia:* Neonatal milia are small, white cysts or bumps that frequently develop on the skin of newborns, particularly on or around the nose, cheeks, chin, forehead, and occasionally on the scalp or inside the mouth (palate or gums also known as Epstein pearls or Bohn nodules). The protein keratin solidifies into these tiny cysts when dead skin cells get trapped in tiny pockets close to the skin's surface. Up to 30–50% of newborns suffer from neonatal milia, which is benign and harmless.
- *Mongolian spots:* Mongolian spots are congenital birthmarks that usually manifest as flat, pigmented patches that range in color from bluish-gray to blue-black. They are most frequently found over a newborn's lumbosacral region, which includes the lower back and buttocks. They typically appear at birth or soon after, reaching their peak around the age of 1 year. By early childhood, they gradually diminish and frequently vanish entirely.
- *Cafe-au-lait spot:* Newborns frequently have pigmented birthmarks called café-au-lait spots, which show up as flat, light to dark brown patches on the skin. They can vary in size from a few millimeters to several centimeters, and they are typically round or oval with smooth edges. These spots, which are usually harmless and do not cause itching or pain, are either present at birth or may appear early in childhood. More than six spots could be a sign of a genetic disorder, such as neurofibromatosis type 1 (NF1).
- *Cutis marmoratum:* Cutis marmoratum is a common, benign skin condition that is typically brought on by exposure to cold temperatures. It is characterized by

Flowchart 2: Causes of nonimmune hydrops.

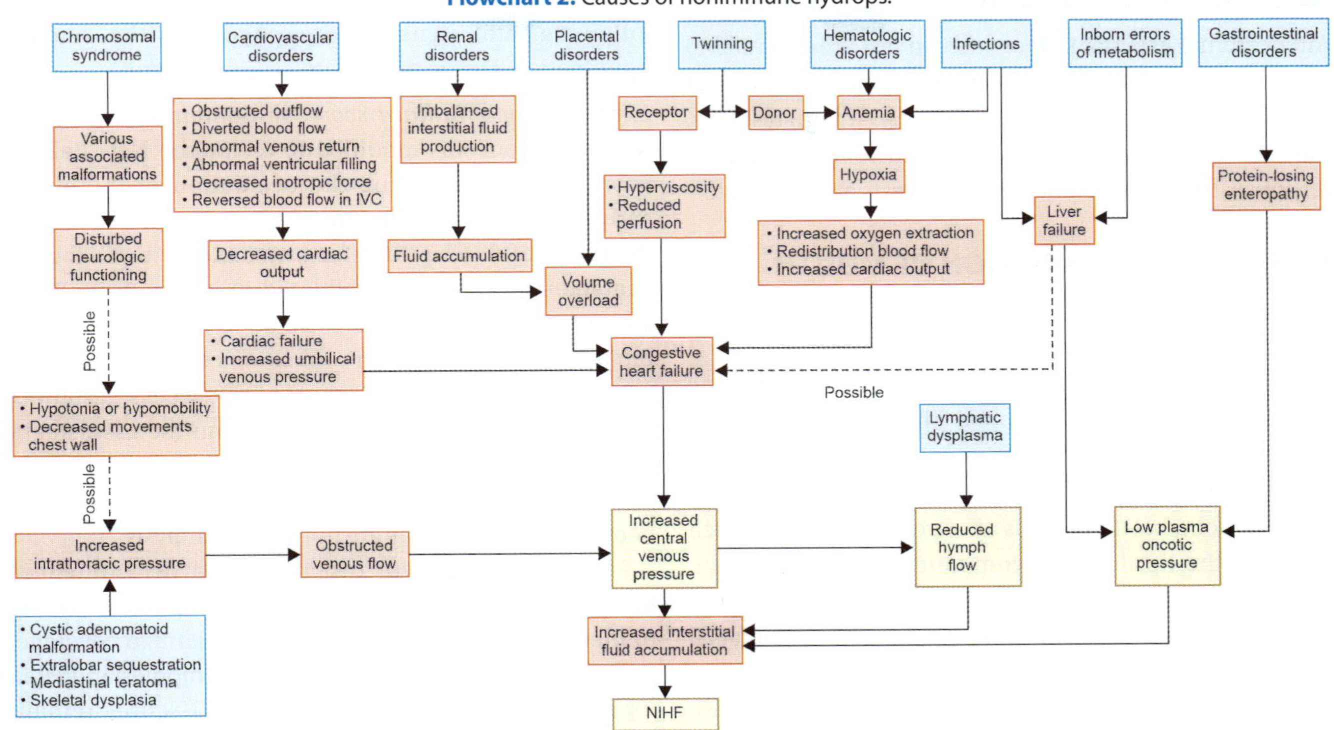

a pinkish-blue mottled or marbled appearance of the skin. Rewarming usually cures this condition, and as people age, it usually gets better.

- *Transient neonatal pustular melanosis:* Transient pustular melanosis, or transient neonatal pustular melanosis (TNPM), is a harmless and temporary skin disorder frequently observed in newborns. It appears at or soon after birth as delicate, shallow pustules measuring 1–3 mm that break easily, leaving a rim of scale and dark brown spots. These marks may show anywhere on the body, including the palms and soles. The condition usually clears up on its own within 3–4 weeks, although the dark spots can persist for up to 3 months.
- *Infantile acropustulosis:* It is a benign, self-limiting skin condition characterized by recurrent crops of small, itchy pustules and vesicles, primarily affecting the palms and soles of infants, typically in the first 2–3 years of life.

Key Features

- Presents with small, reddish, flat bumps that turn into raised blisters or pustules, often arranged in crops that recur periodically.
- The lesions are intensely itchy and may cause discomfort in affected infants.
- Usually resolves spontaneously within a few months to 3 years.
- *Harlequin color change:* It is a transient phenomenon that occurs in roughly 10% of healthy newborns. This unique condition is marked by a well-defined color change, with one side of the body exhibiting erythema and the other side showing pallor. It generally occurs between 2 and 5 days of age, although it can be observed as late as 3 weeks. The condition is benign, and the color change typically resolves within 30 seconds to 20 minutes.

EXAMINATION OF THE EYES

- *Ptosis:* Urgent referral to the pediatric ophthalmologist
- Large eye s/o congenital glaucoma or corneal
- *Eye discharge:* Mostly due to nasolacrimal duct blockage
- *Subconjunctival hemorrhage:* It is common. It does not require treatment.
- *Red reflex:* Presence of red reflex in both eyes—excludes congenital cataract.

EXAMINATION OF EAR OF A NEWBORN

After external examination of ear, two test are essential to exclude hearing defect. Otoacoustic emission (OAE) test is done in every babies before discharge. If OAE test fails, they should undergo augmented brainstem audiometric response. In high-risk newborn, both tests are indicated.

STEPWISE EXAMINATION OF MOUTH

- *Lips:*
    - Inspect symmetry, color, cleft, swellings
    - Callosities at normal newborn lips are sucking pads—normal, harmless thickened skin from feeding friction that resolves spontaneously without intervention.
    - Coloboma of the lips is a congenital fissure or notch in the lip due to incomplete embryonic fusion, distinct but related to cleft lip anomalies, and may occur alone or as part of broader craniofacial malformation syndromes.
    - Absence of the depressor anguli oris muscle is a congenital condition causing lower lip asymmetry due to failure to depress the mouth angle on one side, important for facial expression and oral function.
- *Oral mucosa:* Inspect both cheeks, under the lips for normal pink coloration, ulcers, and abnormal spots. Epstein pearls are common keratin-filled cysts found in the mouths of newborns that are benign, painless, and self-limiting.
- *Gums:* Check for neonatal teeth and Bohn's nodules. Bohn's nodules are common, benign cysts on newborn gums that are self-limiting and harmless.
- *Tongue:* Observe the size of the macroglossia. Identify macroglossia and pseudomacroglossia (due to small mouth). Observe for tongue tie.
- *Palate:*
    - *Hard palate:* Look for high-arched palate and cleft palate
    - *Soft palate:* Inspect for submucosal or overt cleft
- *Floor of the mouth and sublingual area:* Inspect for cyst (e.g., ranula), swelling, or other lesions
- Sucking, rooting, and swallowing reflex

EXAMINATION OF NECK

Inspect the neck for masses and lymphadenopathy.

Gestational age assessment: This can be documented following vital signs or integrated into the general examination. Utilize the Ballard scoring system.

Expanded new Ballard score: In September 1991, the Ballard system was modified to create the New Ballard Score (NBS), enhancing the evaluation of infants as early as 20 weeks gestation. This approach broadened the range of descriptions for physical and neurological characteristics and was validated in infants from 20 to 44 weeks of gestation. The correlation of the assessment remained consistent, with evaluations conducted within 96 hours after birth for neonates at 26 weeks gestation; however, it is recommended to perform the assessment within 12 hours for those under 26 weeks.

This scoring system can be applied to sick ventilated neonates, provided they are not under paralysis.

Intrauterine growth restriction (IUGR) influences both physical and neuromuscular development, leading to increased scores for skin condition, lanugo coverage, and skin crease counts, while scores for nipples and labia majora decrease; however, the overall scores remain unchanged.

Among the neurological assessments, posture shows the best correlation, while arm recoil correlates the least in cases of IUGR. In terms of genital development, IUGR infants show the best correlation, whereas plantar creases have the weakest relationship.

The Parkin score evaluates four physical attributes—skin color, skin texture, ear shape, and nipple development. It shows a correlation with the extended new Ballard score within a range of ± 2 weeks, even in critically ill neonates.

SYSTEMIC EXAMINATION

Respiratory System Examinations

Inspection: Count the respiratory rate. Normal respiratory rate is 40–60/min. Observe for nasal flaring, head bobbing, suprasternal retraction, intercostal recession, subcostal retraction, lower chest retraction, chest wall asymmetry, and mucosal cyanosis.

Auscultation: The apex, right axilla, and back correspond sequentially to the upper lobe, right middle lobe, and lower lobe.

Respiratory distress is characterized by any one of the following:

- Respiratory rate >60 breaths/min
- Severe chest indrawing

TABLE 5: Downe score.

Score	Respiratory rate	Cyanosis	Air entry	Grunt	Retraction
0	<60/min	Nil	Normal	None	Nil
1	60–80/min	In room air	Mild decrease	Audible with stethoscope	Mild
3	>80/min	In 40% FiO_2	Mild decrease	Audible without stethoscope	Moderate

TABLE 6: Silverman Anderson's score.

Features	Score 0	Score 1	Score 2
Upper chest movement	None	Respiratory lag	See-saw respiration
Lower chest retraction	None	Minimal	Marked
Xyphoid retractions	None	Minimal	Marked
Nasal flaring	None	Minimal	Marked
Grunting	None	Audible with stethoscope	Audible with unaided ear

- Grunting,
- Apnea/gasping

Tables 5 and 6 describe standard scorings to interpret the severities of respiratory distress. **Table 6** is mainly for preterm infant.

Downe's score and its interpretation:

Interpretation:
- *Score 1–3:* Mild respiratory distress
- *Score 4–6:* Moderate respiratory distress (may need CPAP)
- *Score >6:* Impending respiratory distress (may need CPAP or mechanical ventilation)

Silverman Anderson score (for preterm neonate):

Interpretation:
- Score 1–6 = Respiratory distress
- Score >6 = Impending respiratory failure

Respiratory system examination of newborn with respiratory support:

The account includes the interface, ventilation mode, and settings on the respirator, as well as humidification.

Sufficiency of ventilation—clinical, radiological, and blood gas analysis

Example 1: Neonate on conventional ventilation:
- The infant is intubated using an ET size of 3.5, secured at 9 cm with a lip-to-connector distance of 3 cm, receiving support from the Bear Cub ventilator.
- She is set to SIMV mode with parameters of PIP 18, PEEP 5, RR 35, Ti 0.4, Fio_2 of 30%, and is receiving warm humidified air. The water level in the chamber is adequate with the displayed temperature of 37°C. There is no condensation in the inspiratory limb.
- In these settings, the baby is well-synchronized with the ventilator and has adequate chest rise with minimal retraction: Baby's spontaneous respirator rate is 50/min and maintaining a saturation of 95% on the right upper limb.
- On auscultation, the air entry is equal on both sides and there are no added sounds.

Example 2: Baby on CPAP: The baby is on bubble CPAP with a mask as an interface, which is snugly fitted with no evidence of trauma. Baby is CPAP of 4 cm of water and fio_2 of 50% and flow of 2 l/min with adequate bubbling in the chamber. The water level in the chamber is sufficient with a displayed temperature of 37°C. There is no condensation in the inspiratory limb. The baby is comfortable on CPAP, has a respiratory rate of 44 per minute, and minimal intercostal retraction with a Silverman–Anderson score of 2. The saturation is 92% in the right upper limb.

On auscultation, air entry is equal on both sides.

Example 3: Baby on high-frequency oscillatory ventilation (HFOV) with nitric oxide: The baby is intubated with ET size 3.0 fixed at 8 cm with a lip-to-connector distance of 3 cm and is being provided HFOV.

She is receiving a MAP of 12 cm of H_2O at frequency 8 and amplitude of 25 with FiO_2 of 70%. The water level in the chamber is adequate with a displayed temperature of 37°C.

There is no condensation in the inspiratory limb.

With the above settings, the chest expansion is adequate, with no asynchrony or retractions and saturations of 95% in the right upper limb and 90% in the right lower limb receiving FiO_2 of 70% and iNO of 20 ppm.

Example 4: Baby on high-flow nasal cannula (HFNC): Baby is on heated humidified high-flow nasal cannula (HHHFNC) with prongs fixed appropriately and the leak is audible. There are no evidence of trauma due to interface.

Baby is on the flow of 4 L/min and FiO_2 of 40%. The water level in the chamber is adequate with the displayed temperature of 37°C. There is no condensation in the tubings.

The baby is comfortable, has a respiratory rate of 44 per minute, and has minimal intercostal retraction with a Silverman–Anderson score of 2. The saturation is 92% on the right upper limb.

On auscultation, air entry is equal on both side.

Cardiovascular examination of newborn: Key steps:

- Inspection
- Palpation
- Auscultation

Inspection:

- *General appearance:* Review the vitals again along with general appearance and comfort. Head-to-toe examination showing any stigmata or not. Note the oxygen saturation, peripheral and central pulses, capillary refill time, blood pressure of all the 4 limbs, PI, and PVI. Especially look for absent femoral pulse and bounding dorsal pedis. If facilities of NIRS (near infrared spectroscopy) is available mention that also.
- *Precordial examination:* Look for any bulging at the chest wall and also any visible pulsation along with the visible point of maximum impulse.

Palpation: Identify the point of maximum impulse and presence of thrill.

Always palpate the liver—mention the liver span, upper border of liver dullness, tenderness, pulsation, consistency, character of the liver border, and also the palpability of the left lobe of liver.

Auscultation:

- Auscultate throughout the precordium and search for abnormalities of heart sounds, and presence of murmur and also for additional sounds.
- Specially look for PDA murmur, diastolic part of this murmur may not be heard because of persistence of increased pulmonary pressure of intrauterine period.
- Search for bruits at the liver, and also at the fontanelles.

Approach to a newborn with cardiac murmur: Up to 1% of neonates have a murmur; 30–75% of murmurs in neonates are due to congenital heart disease, so vigilance is necessary.

All murmurs require a careful, systematic assessment.

Early detection and timely referral for echocardiography improves outcomes.

Innocent murmurs are typically soft, isolated, and found in otherwise healthy, asymptomatic infants; however, an echocardiogram is recommended to rule out disease before reassurance.

How to present the cardiovascular findings of a hemodynamically unstable newborn:

- Vital signs, precordial assessment, perfusion, inotrope support, and any additional drugs
- The infant is pink, has a heart rate of 150 beats per minute, and has regular, rhythmic, and normal-volume palpable peripheral pulses. You can feel the femoral pulse bilateral. The peripheries are warm, and the CRT is 2 seconds at the sternum. According to Zubrow's chart, the right upper limb's blood pressure is in the 50th percentile.
- No precordial impulse in sight. There is no murmur in the heart sounds.
- *End-organ perfusion*: Due to the baby's sedation, sensorium cannot be evaluated, and urine output is 1.5 mL/kg/h.
- Dobutamine is given to the infant at a rate of 8 μg/kg/min.

NEUROLOGICAL EXAMINATION OF THE NEWBORN

Higher function:

- *Level of alertness: Alertness levels are judged by* **Tables 7 and 8**.
- *High level: Nonstereotyped, definite latency and habituating*
- *Low level: Stereotyped, rapid onset, nonhabituating, or absent*

Neonatal behavioral states (Prechtl's): Assessment is best conducted during stage 3 or 4.

Habituation: It is well recognized in full-term infants.

- Visual assessment involves using a bright light at a frequency of about 1 per second.
- Observe for—blink/startle responses and halting of movement/breathing.
- A normal reaction consists of an initial response that diminishes after 3–5 exposures.
- An abnormal reaction is indicated by either an initial lack of response or an absence of habituation.
- Auditory assessment involves a similar response using a loud bell.

TABLE 7: Assessment of level of alertness.

Level		*Appearances*	*Arousal response*	*Motor response*	
				Quantity	*Quality*
Normal		Awake	Normal	Normal	High level
Stuper	Slight	Sleepy	Slight diminished	Slight diminished	Do
	Moderate	Asleep	Moderate diminished	Moderate diminished	Do
	Deep	Asleep	Absent	Marked diminished	Do
Coma		Asleep	Absent	Marked diminished/absent	Low level

TABLE 8: Neurobehavioral state (Prechtl's).

State	*Eyes open*	*Respiration regular*	*Gross movement*	*Vocalization*
1	–	+	–	–
2	–	–	±	–
3	+	+	–	–
4	+	–	+	–
5	+	–	+	+

Consolability: It should be evaluated after the infant has cried for 15 seconds:

- Whether the infant calms down spontaneously
- By talking to them
- By placing a hand on their abdomen
- By picking them up and holding them
- If they cannot be consoled at all
- *Cuddliness:* It involves assessing how the baby reacts to being held when they are alert.

Cranial nerves:

For the optic nerve:

- Response to light is needed.
  - *Reaction:* At 28 weeks, there should be a consistent blink response.
  - *At 32 weeks:* Persistent eye closure should occur until the light is removed.
- *Light reflex:* Observe the size and reaction of the pupils.
  - Preterm infants usually have pupil sizes of 2–3 mm; term infants may have slightly larger pupils
  - From 29–32 weeks, pupils begin to react to light.
- *Fixation and tracking:* A red cotton wool ball or optokinetic drum can be used.
  - At 32–34 weeks, visual fixation is expected.
  - At 37 weeks, the infant should turn their head and eyes toward the light
  - By term, they should follow objects and display optokinetic nystagmus

  (If the infant fails to follow objects, it suggests cerebral dysfunction instead of a primary optic tract issue.)
- *Fundoscopic examination:* The fundus may appear pale and gray-white; retinal hemorrhages are found in 20–40% of healthy newborns.

For the 4th and 6th cranial nerves:

- Perform the doll's eye maneuver by 25 weeks.
- Look for spontaneous roving eye movements at 32 weeks and any squint.

5th cranial nerve:

- *Motor:* evaluate rooting and sucking reflexes; assess muscle strength by allowing the baby to bite a finger
- Sensory assessment—test facial sensation through response

7th cranial nerve:

- Observe the vertical width of the palpebral fissure and the position of the mouth angle
- Evaluate the sucking reflex

8th cranial nerve:

- Test response with a bell; by 28 weeks, there should be a startle or blink response
- As development progresses, startle responses may involve cessation of breathing and changes in respiratory rate and heart rate.

For the 9th and 10th cranial nerves:

- Check for any pooling of secretions and the position of the soft palate
- Demonstrate breastfeeding and assessing the ability to swallow
- If swallowing difficulties arise, test the gag reflex

Cranial nerve XII (12th):

- Observe the size and symmetry of tongue movements; look for signs of fasciculation

Motor system:

Tone:

- *Passive tone:* Assessed by observing the resting posture and resistance to movement. Make sure the head is in the axis of the trunk while examining the tone **(Table 9)**.
- *Active tone:* Observe the alteration tone produced by changing the position of the head, trunk, and extremities about gravity **(Fig. 3)**.

Basis of these changes: Anatomically, the brainstem can be described in terms of two motor control systems:

1. The subcortical system includes pathways from the tectum, reticular formation, and vestibular nuclei and has connections to the cerebellum. It is known as the lower motor system or extrapyramidal system.
2. The corticospinal system consists of the motor zones of the cortex, the corticospinal pathways, and the basal ganglia. It is referred to as the upper motor system or pyramidal system.

TABLE 9: Neonatal tone assessment (28–40 weeks).

Maneuver	*28 weeks*	*32 weeks*	*36 weeks*	*40 weeks*
Posture	Head/trunk aligned; supine; head midline	Increased flexion; supine; mild flexion	Pronounced flexion; supine; limbs flexed	Optimal flexion; supine; strong flexion
Flapping of extremities	High flappability; hands/feet waving	Moderate flappability; hands/feet small waves	Reduced flappability; limbs stiffer	Absent flappability; limbs rigid
Ventral/dorsal incurvation	Mild incurvation; trunk mildly arched	Moderate incurvation; trunk moderately arched	Strong incurvation; trunk strongly arched	Maximal incurvation; trunk fully arched
Scarf sign	Arm easily crosses chest; arm across chest	Arm with resistance; arm partly flexed	Movement restricted; arm stopped halfway	Arm stops at midline; arm at chest midline
Arm recoil	Slow recoil; arm slowly returning	Moderate recoil; arm somewhat flexed	Fast recoil; arm quickly flexed	Immediate recoil; arm sharply flexed
Square window	>90° flexion; wrist large angle	60° flexion; wrist intermediate angle	30° flexion; wrist acute angle	0° flexion; wrist fully flexed

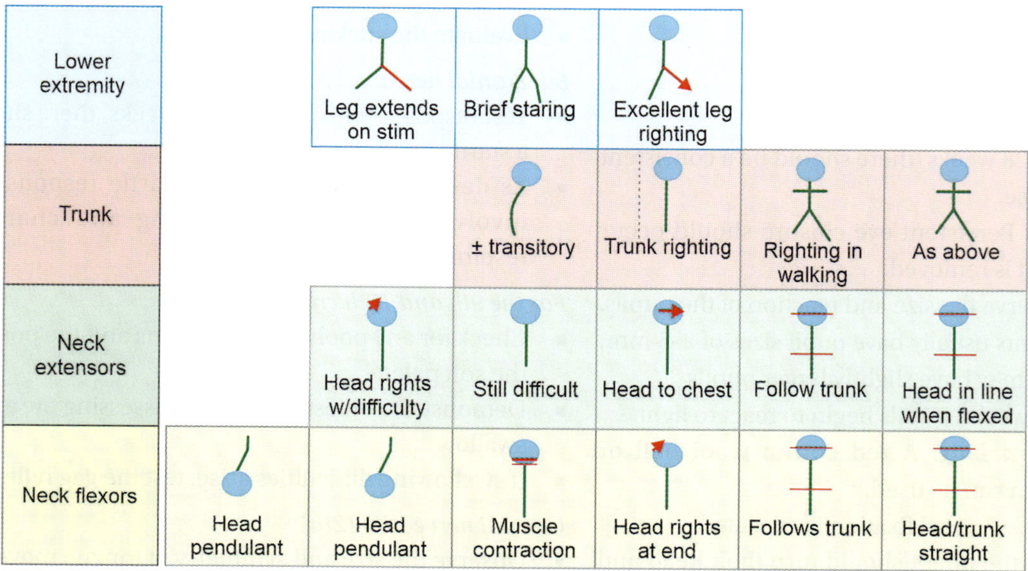

Fig. 3: Assessment of active tone. Figures drawn from the descriptions given in reference [15].

Functions of these systems: The subcortical system plays a crucial role in maintaining antigravity functions that regulate the postural tone of the body. It also oversees the flexor tone in both the upper and lower extremities as well as controlling primitive reflexes.

The corticospinal system matures later, allowing for increased cortical control over motor functions. Maintaining an upright posture is achieved through the balance of inhibitory and excitatory influences on motor neurons. This system fine-tunes postural responses and facilitates the gradual relaxation of passive muscle tone in the limbs, which is vital for independent finger movements, precision, and speed in tasks requiring fine motor skills. Additionally, it suppresses primitive reflexes.

The development of the subcortical system is completed by 24 weeks postmenstrual age. Maturation of the corticospinal tract commences at 32 postmaturation weeks. The first 2 years are marked by rapid growth of the corticospinal tract, while from ages two to twelve, development progresses at a slower pace **(Fig. 4)**.

The subcortical corticospinal tract displays an ascending pattern of control, while the corticospinal tract follows a descending pattern, meaning that control of the lower limbs is developed after that of the upper limbs.

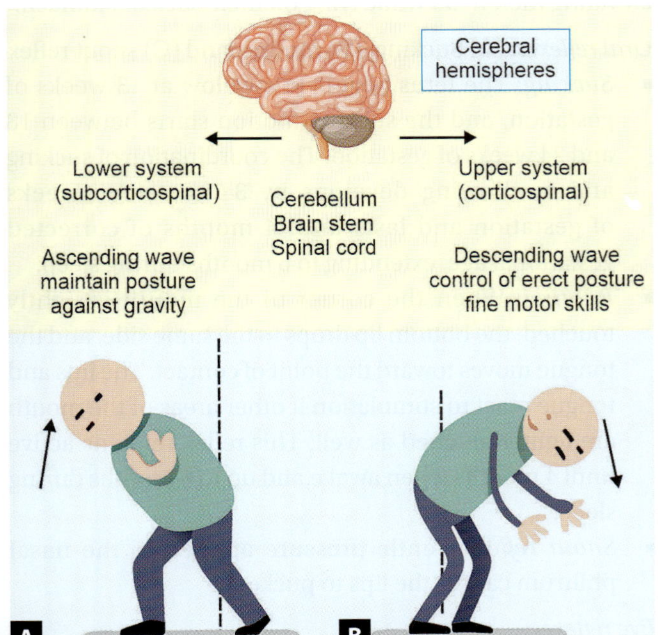

Fig. 4: Maturation of the central motor function: (A) Early ascending maturation of the lower system; (B) Later slower, descending maturation of the upper system.

Reflexes:

Moro reflex: This reflex is triggered by a sudden drop of the head relative to the trunk, prompting the response of catching the head as it falls. The components of this response include:

- Opening of the hand occurs by the 28th week.
- Extension and abduction of the arms happen by 32 weeks.
- Anterior flexion of the arms is observed by 37 weeks.
- An audible cry may also be present.
- The Moro reflex typically disappears between 3 and 6 months in most healthy infants.
- It may be diminished or absent in cases of CNS depression and can be exaggerated in cases of Bilirubin encephalopathy.
- Asymmetry in the reflex may indicate a brachial plexus injury or clavicle fracture.
- It is not connected with autonomic changes. Occasionally, a quick startle response may occur prior to the Moro reflex.
- If an object is being held in one hand, the reflex may be inhibited on that side.
- The neural center for this reflex is found in the lower pons region, with the vestibular system playing a significant role in its activation.

Startle reflex: The startle response is an immediate reaction characterized by flexion and adduction of the arms along with eye blinking in reaction to a sudden stimulus (for instance, a loud noise at 96 dB). Autonomic changes may accompany this reflex.

Grasp reflex: When a finger is placed into the palm from the ulnar side, the fingers first flex (catching phase) and then grip (holding phase). In full-term infants, this reflex is strong enough to allow for lifting from a bed. If the back of the hand is touched, the hand will open in response to this stimulus. This reflex emerges by 28 weeks and generally disappears between 2 and 3 months; persistence beyond 6 months may indicate a spastic/athetoid form of cerebral palsy.

Plantar grasp reflex: This reflex is triggered by gently stroking the sole of the foot behind the toe (the distal half of the outer side of the foot). The plantar grasp usually lasts until the baby reaches 9 months of corrected gestational age. It may be absent or weak in breech-born infants with extended legs. This reflex is often unobtainable in cases of myelomeningocele and may also be absent in the spastic type of cerebral palsy. The spinal reflex center for this plantar reflex is likely located at the L5-S2 level of the spine.

Crossed extension reflex: When one leg is held in an extended position while its sole is massaged, the opposite leg initially flexes, adducts, and then extends, with the toes fanning out. The final movement involves bringing that leg closer to the side that received stimulation. This reflex is generally not observed after the 1st month. The adduction element of the reflex does not become apparent until 37 weeks of gestation, and the final action is only seen in term infants. The neural center for the crossed extension reflex in newborns is located in the spinal cord, where afferent nerve fiber branches cross over and connect with interneurons. These interneurons then either excite or inhibit alpha motor neurons, which are responsible for controlling the muscles of the opposite limb.

Hip reflex: When one leg is bent at the hip, the opposite leg also flexes.

Placing reflex: When the front part of the tibia or ulna touches the edge of a table, the child either lifts the leg to step onto the table or raises the arm to place the hand on the table. The neural center responsible for the placing reflex is located at L5-S2. This reflex is present in full-term infants weighing over 1,800 g.

Stepping reflex: When the infant is held upright above a table and their foot presses against it, the baby will exhibit walking movements characterized by alternating flexion and extension of the legs. Preterm infants tend to walk on their toes. The stepping reflex diminishes by 5–6 weeks of age, though it can be observed for a few weeks if the baby's head is held back while their foot is flat on the surface. The spinal cord and brainstem circuitry are responsible for a newborn's stepping reflex.

Asymmetrical tonic reflex: When the head is turned to one side, the upper extremities extend on that side while flexing occurs on the opposite side. A similar, albeit less pronounced, reaction happens in the lower limbs. This reflex emerges by 18 weeks of gestation and becomes prominent by one month post-term, peaking at 2–3 months of age before disappearing by 6 months. This reflex is intricately connected to the vestibular system and plays a crucial role in visual fixation and visuomotor development. Its persistence can hinder rolling, the ability to bring hands together, and bringing hands to the mouth. Continued presence of this reflex may harm the developing joints and bones, potentially resulting in scoliosis or dislocation of the hip joint. In infants with spasticity, this reflex is more pronounced and tends to last longer.

Symmetrical tonic neck reflex: When the head is lifted, the tone in the upper limbs extends, and the tone in the lower limbs flexes. Conversely, when the head is flexed, the opposite occurs. This reflex prevents the child from crawling and aids in the formation of feeding habits. It is not typically observed but may be enhanced in specific forms of cerebral palsy.

Righting reflex: (A) The neck righting reflex is present at birth and is most robust at 3 months. Turning the head to one side prompts movement of the entire body. (B) The labyrinthine righting reflex, which affects the head, appears at 2 months and is strongest at 10 months. It allows the child to raise their head while lying on their stomach at 1–2 months and later while lying on their back. (C) The body-righting reflex, which affects the body, develops between 7 and 12 months. It modifies the neck righting reflex and is essential for a child's initial attempts to sit and stand. In cases of severe cerebral palsy, the righting reflex may be absent, leading to challenges in turning to one side. Here, the neck righting reflex is inhibited by the labyrinthine reflex, making it difficult for the child to roll over or sit upright, and they have significant trouble elevating their head while lying on their back or stomach.

Oral reflexes: (A) Sucking, (B) rooting, and (C) snout reflex

- *Sucking:* The fetus begins to swallow at 13 weeks of gestation, and the sucking motion starts between 18 and 24 weeks of gestation. The coordination of sucking and swallowing develops by 34 corrected weeks of gestation and lasts until 4 months of corrected gestational age, extending to 6 months during sleep.
- *Rooting:* When the corner of the mouth is lightly touched, the bottom lip drops to the same side, and the tongue moves toward the point of contact. The lips and tongue react to stimulation if other areas of the mouth are lightly touched as well. This reflex remains active until 4 months when awake and up to 6 months during sleep.
- *Snout reflex:* Gentle pressure applied to the nasal philtrum causes the lips to pucker.

Eye reflexes:

Blink reflexes:

- The visuopalpebral or dazzle reflex involves blinking in response to light.

- The cochleopalpebral reflex causes blinking in reaction to a loud noise.
- The cutaneous-palpebral reflex leads to blinking when there is painful touch.
- The nasopalpebral reflex results in blinking when the bridge of the nose is tapped.
- McCarthy's reflex triggers homolateral blinking when the supraorbital area is tapped.
- In newborns with abnormalities, this reflex can be elicited by stimulation at a distance from the supraorbital region.
- The corneal reflex is activated when the cornea is touched, causing blinking.

Galant's reflex: When a child is held in a prone position or ventral suspension, stimulation along the side of the spine with fingertips produces trunk flexion.

Perez reflex: While a child is in a prone position or ventral suspension, applying upward pressure along the spine from the sacrum to the head results in the infant flexing their arms and legs, extending the neck, and crying.

Landau reflex: When a child is suspended in a prone position, both the head, spine, and legs extend. If the head is pushed down, the hips, knees, and elbows flex. This reflex is typically present from around 3 months and usually vanishes after the 1st year. In cases of cerebral palsy and motor weakness, it remains absent past 3 months of age.

Parachute reflex: A sudden drop of the child toward the bed from the ventral suspension position causes the arms to extend for protection. This reflex emerges between 6 and 9 months and lasts throughout life. In cerebral palsy, it may be absent or incomplete.

Movement: Schematic diagram showing development of general movement **(Fig. 5)**

Prior to term, we refer to them as fetal or preterm general movements; at term age and until 6–9 weeks post-term, they are known as writhing movements. After 6–9 weeks post-term writhing, this movement pattern gradually fades while fidgety general movements begin to appear. After the first 6 months of life, intentional and antigravity movements become predominant.

Writhing movements are characterized by small to moderate amplitude and speed, presenting an ellipsoid shape that gives an impression of writhing.

Fidgety movements are small, moderate-speed actions with variable acceleration occurring in the neck, trunk, and limbs, happening in all directions and continuous during awake periods, except when the infant is fussing or crying.

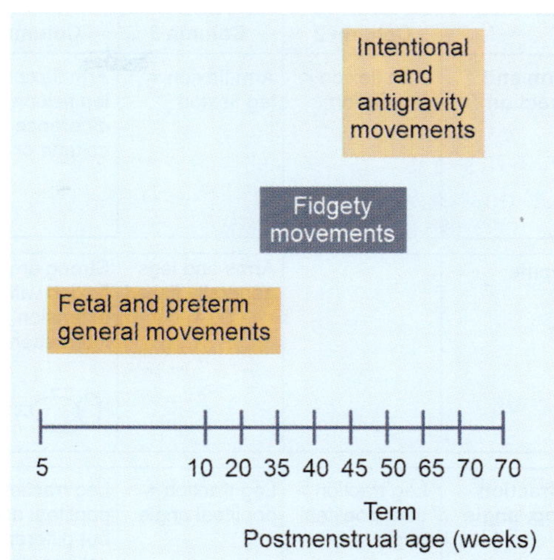

Fig. 5: Developmental course of general movement.

Fidgety movements can be categorized as continual (score 2), intermittent (score 1), or sporadic (score ±).

The following movement patterns are considered abnormal if:

- Fidgety movements are either absent or display abnormal quality.
- Swiping movements are prevalent.

Wiggling and oscillating movements are dominant. Saccadic arm movements are prominent. Kicking is repetitive in nature. Excitement bursts are consistent. Smiles appear frozen. Mouth movements involve synchronous opening and closing. Tongue protrusions are either repetitive or prolonged. Head rotations are repetitive in nature.

Hammersmith infant neurological examination: The Hammersmith infant neurological examination (HINE) is a simple and scorable standardized neurological examination developed by Dr Lilly Dubowitz and Professor Victor Dubowitz. It helps identify infants between 3 and 24 months of age who have a high probability of all types of CP **(Figs. 6 to 8)**.

Examination—abdomen:

Inspection: Check for abdominal distension and specially the visible gut loops. In case of preterm baby, abdomen looks distended and also some visible gut loops may be there even in normal condition. If doubt persist prefeed abdominal girth, >2 cm is suggestive of abdominal

		Column 2	Column 3	Column 4	Column 5
Flexor tone 1	**On arm and leg traction**	Arm flexion < leg flexion	Arm flexion = leg flexion	Arm flexion > leg flexion but difference 1 column or <	Arm flexion > leg flexion and difference > 1 column
Flexor tone 2	**In supine**		Arms and legs generally flexed	Strong arm flexion with extension intermittent	Strong arm flexion with strong leg extension continuos
Leg ext. tone	**Leg traction vs pop. angle**	Leg traction > than popliteal angle	Leg traction = popliteal angle	Leg traction < popliteal angle but difference 1 column <	Leg traction < popliteal angle but difference > 1 column
Neck ext. tone	**Neck in ext. vs neck in flexion**	Head extension < head flexion	Head extension = head flexion	Head extension > head flexion but difference 1 column <	Head extension > head flexion but difference > 1 column
Inc. ext. tone	**Vent susp vs head lag**	Ventral suspension < head lag	Ventral suspension = head lag	Ventr suspension > head lag but difference 1 column <	Ventr suspension > head lag and difference > 1 column

1	.5	2	.5	3	.5	4	.5	5	
0	0	29	0	69	0	2	0	0	**6w**
0	0	37	0	60	0	3	0	0	**10w**
0	0	3	0	94	0	3	0	0	**6w**
0	0	0	0	100	0	0	0	0	**10w**
0	0	20	0	54	0	26	0	0	**6w**
0	0	29	0	54	0	17	0	0	**10w**
0	0	3	0	88	0	9	0	0	**6w**
0	0	3	0	97	0	0	0	0	**10w**
0	0	37	0	43	0	17	0	3	**6w**
0	0	34	0	26	0	40	0	0	**10w**

Fig. 6: Tone pattern.

distension. Divarication of recti is common in a normal newborn.

After delivery, umbilical cord should be examined to look for one umbilical vein and 2 umbilical artery. Single umbilical artery may be associated with renal anomalies.

Umbilical hernia is common in case of normal newborn but must exclude hypothyroidism. Check for periumbilical erythema and foul smelling discharge from the umbilicus which indicates umbilical sepsis.

Umbilical granuloma with discharge should be treated with cauterization only.

In case of prolonged sterile (no foul smelling) umbilical discharge, not improved with cauterization—patent urachus should be excluded.

Palpation:

- Check for abdominal mass. Most of the cases abdominal masses are renal origin after hepatomegaly. Liver is normally palpable 1-2 cm from the right costal margin.
- In a newborn, spleen enlarges toward the left iliac fossa.

Percussion:

- Check for ascites in case of hydrops and neonatal cholestasis syndrome
- Inguinal areas to examined specially in a preterm newborn

Genitalia:

- Exclude genital anomalies, hypospadias and epispadias, and hydrocele
- Exclude disorders of sexual development

Anal examination:

- Check the buttocks and anal areas to exclude anomalies
- Sacral pits may be visible at the back suggestive of spina bifida occulta.

Examination of spine:

Inspection: Examine the spine is intact or not, exclude meningocele, myelomeningocele (ruptured/intact). Look for the curvature of the thoracic and lumbar spine.

	Column 1	Column 2	Column 3	Column 4	Column 5
Tendon	Absent	Felt, not seen	Seen	Exaggerated	Clonus
Suck/Gag	No gag/no suck	Weak irregular suck only No stripping	Weak regular suck Some stripping	Strong suck: • Irregular • Regular Good stripping	No suck but strong clenching
Palmar grasp	No response	Short, weak flexion of fingers	Strong flexion of fingers	Strong finger flexion, shoulder ↑	Very strong grasp: infant can be lifted off couch
Plantar grasp	No response	Partial plantar flexion of toes	Toes curve around the examiner's finger		
Placing	No response	Dorsiflexion of ankle only	Full placing response with flexion of hip, knee and placing sole on surface		
Moro reflex	No response or opening of hands only	Full abduction at shoulder and extension of the arms; no adduction	Full abduction but only delayed or partial adduction	Partial abduction at shoulder and arm extension followed by smooth adduction	• No abduction or adduction • Only forward extension of arms from the shoulders • Marked adduction only

	1	.5	2	.5	3	.5	4	.5	5	
Tendon	0	0	3	3	91	0	3	0	0	6w
	0	0	0	0	100	0	0	0	0	10w
Suck/Gag	0	0	0	0	0	0	100	0	0	6w
	0	0	0	0	0	0	100	0	0	10w
Palmar grasp	0	0	6	0	40	0	54	0	0	6w
	0	0	26	3	37	0	34	0	0	10w
Plantar grasp	0	0	3	0	97	0	0	0	0	6w
	0	0	3	0	97	0	0	0	0	10w
Placing	6	0	0	3	91	0	0	0	0	6w
	0	3	3	3	91	0	0	0	0	10w
Moro reflex	0	0	11	0	54	3	26	0	6	6w
	0	3	31	0	49	3	11	0	3	10w

Fig. 7: Reflexes.

Palpation: Dermal cyst and lipomas should be excluded.

Examination of the upper limbs: Look for birth trauma like erb's palsy or fracture. Fracture can occur subsequently in osteogenesis imperfecta and also in case of osteopenia of prematurity.

Examine the arm for the length, proportion and symmetry—exclude skeletal dysplasia.

Look for polydactyly (pre/post)—which may be associated with renal anomalies.

Clinodactyly and palmar crease abnormalities should be searched for.

Examination of the lower limb:

Leg: check the asymmetry, length, and proportions and also the spontaneous movement and pain and fracture.

Foot: Examine for Tallies

Examination of the hip joint:

Ortolani test: Flex the knees and secure the legs by placing the middle finger over the greater trochanter and the thumb along the inner thigh area. With the middle finger exerting upward force. The greater trochanter of the leg is abducted. Should the hip be dislocated, a "clunk" may be perceived?

Movements

	Column 1	Column 2	Column 3	Column 4	Column 5
Movement (Quantity)	No movement	Sporadic and short isolated movements	Frequent isolated movements	Frequent generalized movements	Continuous exaggerated movements
Movement (Quantity)	Only stretches	Frequent stretches and abrupt movements; some smooth movements	Fluent movements but monotonous	Fluent alternative movements of arms + legs: good variability	Cramped synchronized; mouthing jerky or other abn.mov.
Head raising prone	No response	Infant rolls head over, chin not raised	Infant rolls head over, raises chin	Infant brings head and chin up	Infant brings head up and keeps it up

	1	.5	2	.5	3	.5	4	.5	5	
Movement (Quantity)	0	0	0	0	9	0	91	0	0	6w
	0	0	0	0	0	0	94	3	3	10w
Movement (Quantity)	0	0	3	0	17	3	77	0	0	6w
	0	0	6	0	17	3	69	3	3	10w
Head raising prone	0	0	20	0	74	3	3	0	0	6w
	0	0	6	0	49	3	29	0	14	10w

Abnormal signs

	Column 1	Column 2	Column 3	Column 4	Column 5
Abn. hand of toe posture		Hands open, toes straight most of the time	Intermittent fisting or thumb adduction	Continuous fisting or thumb adduction; index finger flexion thumb opposition	Continuous big toe extension or flexion of all toes
Tremor		No tremor or tremor only when crying	Tremor only after Moro or occasionally when awake	Frequent tremors when awake	Continuous tremors
Startle	No startle, even to sudden noise	No spontaneous startle but reacts to sudden noise	2-3 spontaneous startles	More than 3 spontaneous startles	Continuous startles

	1	.5	2	.5	3	.5	4	.5	5	
Abn. hand of toe posture	0	0	6	0	94	0	0	0	0	6w
	0	0	29	3	63	0	6	0	0	10w
Tremor	0	0	46	3	46	0	6	0	0	6w
	0	0	63	0	31	0	6	0	0	10w
Startle	0	3	71	0	23	0	3	0	0	6w
	0	0	51	3	34	0	11	0	0	10w

Fig. 8: Hammersmith neonatal neurological examination.

Barlow test: Hold the legs in the same manner as for the Ortolani test.

Adduct the hip and apply slight downward pressure on the knee. If the hip is unstable, it will pop out of the acetabulum.

Generally, these test will be positive in case of developmental dysplasia of hip. However, ultrasound of hip is required to confirm the diagnosis even if these tests are negative in presence of risk factors (breech presentation/multiple birth) with strong suspicion.

How to write diagnosis in a newborn case:

- Single/twin/triplet
- *Conception:* Spontaneous/IVF
- Mode of delivery [indication: PIH/PROM (hours)/ others]
- Gestational age
- Cried at birth/cried after initial steps/cried after bag and mask—resuscitation
- Perinatal asphyxia/RDS(Respiratory Distress Syndrome)/TTNB (Transiet
- Sepsis/jaundice, etc.
- BPD/ROP/osteopenia of prematurity, etc.

So, complete diagnosis to be written keeping with those points.

SUGGESTED READING

1. Afroze F, Pietroni MA, Chisti MJ. Recurrent sclerema in a young infant presenting with severe sepsis and severe pneumonia: an uncommon but extremely life-threatening condition. J Health Popul Nutr. 2013;31(4):538-42.

2. Bellini C, Hennekam RC. Non-immune hydrops fetalis: a short review of etiology and pathophysiology. Am J Med Genet A. 2012;158A(3):597-605.
3. Cawley P, Talbot J, Mara CO, Mugrave E, Kapadia J. Clinical Guideline Saturation targeting in the infant admitted to the Neonatal Unit. NHS [Internet]. 2016 Jan; 1-21. [online] Available from https://econeonatalpccsicnetwork.nhs.uk/wp-content/upload/2024/02/EOE-Saturation-targetting_JK_18119.pdf. [Last accessed December, 2025]
4. Downes JJ, Vidyasagar D, Boggs TR, Jr, Morrow 3rd GM. Respiratory distress syndrome of newborn infants. I. New clinical scoring system (RDS score) with acid-base and blood-gas correlations. Clin Pediatr. 1970;9(6):325-31.
5. Dubowitz LM, Dubowitz V, Mercuri E. The Neurological Assessment of the preterm & Full-term Newborn Infant, 2nd edition. Bermondsey: Mac Keith Press; 1999. pp. 140-1 p. (Clinics in Developmental Medicine).
6. Einspieler C, Prechtl HF, Boss AF, Ferrari F, Cioni G. Prechtl's Method on the Qualitative Assessment of General Movements in Preterm, Term and Young Infants (Clinics in Developmental Medicine), 1st edition. Bermondsey: Mac Keith Press; 2008. p. 104.
7. Harsha SS, Archana BR. SNAPPE-II (Score for Neonatal Acute Physiology with Perinatal Extension-II) in Predicting Mortality and Morbidity in NICU. J Clin Diagn Res. 2015;9(10):SC10-2.
8. Illingworth RS. Illingworth's The Development of The Infant and Young Child: Normal and Abnormal, 11th edition. Philadelphia: Elsevier; 2021. p. 520.
9. Mandala VK, Mendu SB, Bollaboina SKY, Kotha R. Role of Perfusion Index and Pulse Variability Index in the Assessment of Neonatal Hemodynamics: A Systematic Review. Cureus. 2023;15(10):e48058.
10. Parry G, Tucker J, Tarnow-Mordi W; UK Neonatal Staffing Study Collaborative Group. CRIB II: an update of the clinical risk index for babies score. Lancet. 2003;361(9371):1789-91.
11. Prechtl HF. The behavioural states of the newborn infant (a review). Brain Res. 1974; 1974;76(2):185-212.
12. Restrepo R, Inarejos Clemente EJ, Corral G, Mas TR, Fenlon EP 3rd, Jaramillo D. Subcutaneous fat necrosis of the newborn: a pictorial essay of an under-recognized entity. Pediatr Radiol. 2023;53(2):313-23.
13. Silverman WA, Anderson DH. A Controlled Clinical Trial of effect of water mist on obstructive respiratory signs. Death rate and necropsy findings among premature infants. Pediatrics. 1956;17:1-10.
14. Tang J, Bergman J, Lam JM. Harlequin colour change: unilateral erythema in a newborn. CMAJ. 2010;182(17):E801.
15. Tison AT. Neurological assessment from birth to six years: Guide for examination and evaluation. Baltimore: The Johns Hopkins; 2001. p. 160.
16. Volpe JJ. Neurological Examination: Normal and Abnormal Features. In: Volpe JJ (Ed). Volpe's Neurology of the Newborn, 6th edition. Philadelphia: Elsevier; 2018. p. 205 Table no. 8.9.

CHAPTER 14

Radiology

Swapan Kumar Ray

INTRODUCTION

Pediatric radiology is a vast subject. In postgraduate examinations, a table will be there in oral and practical. All the students should learn radiology for clinical purpose as well as an aid to clinics. Routine roentgenogram interpretation is very important in daily practice as it is convenient to avail off. But there had been a paradigm shift in radiology with much access to ultrasound (USG), computed tomography (CT), magnetic resonance imaging (MRI), and radioisotope scan in nuclear medicine.

We will confine ourselves only to the important X-rays, CT, and MRI which may be asked in examination. But you need to know in details later. We will discuss how to interpret pediatric common conditions by a step-wise approach.

Still now 70% of radiological examinations are X-rays, among it chest X-ray constitutes almost 75–80%. Rest are USG (10–12%), CT (4–5%), MRI (2–4%), and nuclear medicine (1–2%).

So, we must learn chest X-ray thoroughly not only for examination, but also for day-to-day practice.

We will have a road map of learning:

- X-ray skull and neck
- X-ray chest
- Neonatal X-ray
- X-ray bones
- Barium studies
- IVP
- MRI brain

USG is a dynamic study and CT involves radiation, so these two modalities are not included in this chapter of radiology.

X-RAY OF SKULL (LATERAL VIEW)

X-ray Number 1

- See 4 "*S*" (Size, Shape, Suture, and Sphenoid to see pituitary fossa) **(Fig. 1A)**.
- Size should be measured by calculating the ratio of calvarium and facial bones.
- Size of skull is measured by maximum transverse diameter (A) **(Fig. 2B)**.

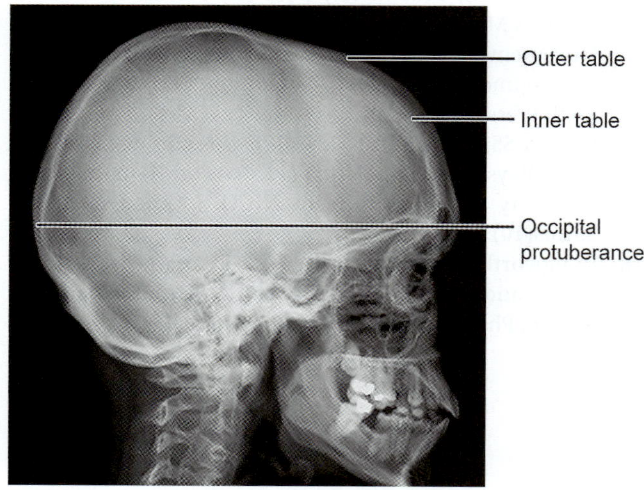

Fig. 1A: X-ray of skull in lateral view.

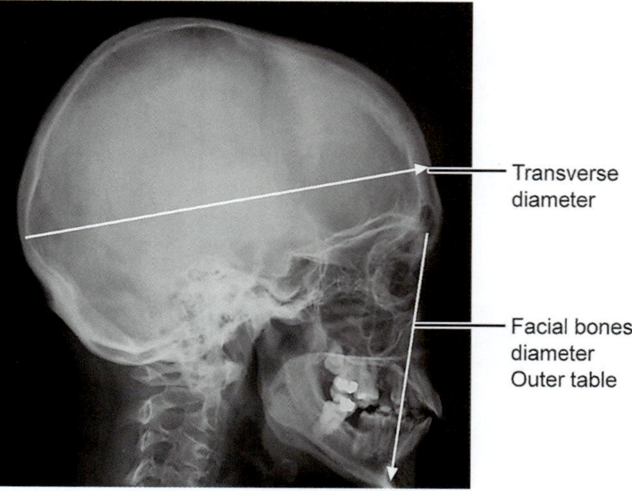

Fig. 1B: Method to measure the transverse diameter and facial bone diameter.

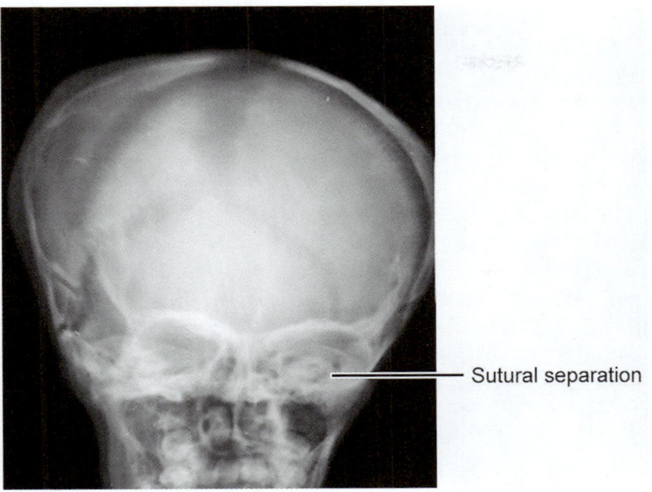

Fig. 2: Sutural diastasis/separation.

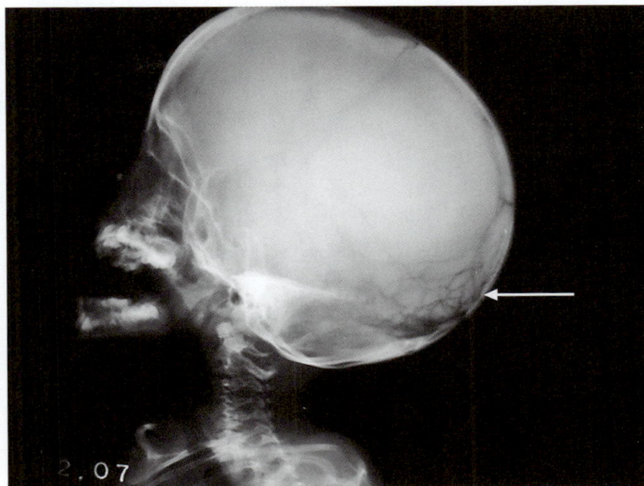

Fig. 3: Multiple intrasutural bones within the calvarium.

- Facial bones measured by distance from nasion to mentum with mouth closed. Normal value is 2.5.
- If the ratio is <2.5—it is microcephaly.
- If >2.5—it is macrocephaly.

X-ray Number 2

Interpretation:

- AP view of the skull showing sutural separation (sutural diastasis) **(Fig. 2)**
- *Most probable diagnosis is raised intracranial tension due to hydrocephalus.*

X-ray Number 3

- X-ray skull lateral view showing multiple intrasutural bones within the calvarium **(Fig. 3)**.
- *Impression:* Wormian bones

Causes of Wormian bones: Osteogenesis imperfecta, hypothyroidism, and pyknodysostosis. Down's syndrome, cleidocranial dysplasia, progeria, Zellweger syndrome, hypophosphatasia, and chondrodysplasia punctata.

X-ray Number 4

Interpretation: This is an X-ray lateral view of the skull showing:

- Increase in size of the cranial vault
- Diploic expansion
- Characteristic hair-on-end appearance **(Fig. 4)**

Diagnosis: Chronic hemolytic anemia

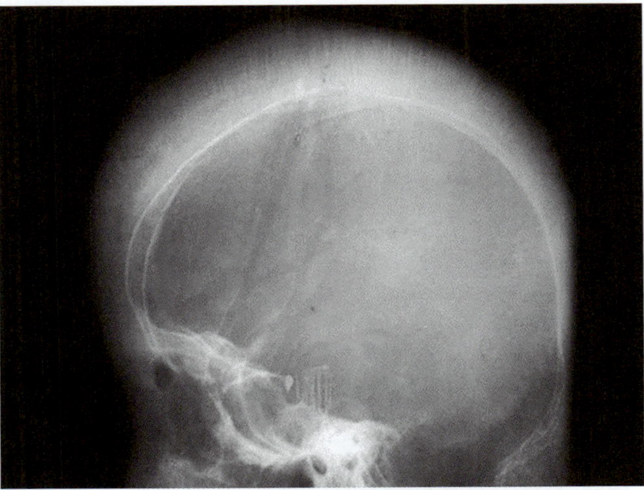

Fig. 4: Hair-on-end appearance.

X-ray Number 5

X-ray skull lateral view shows multiple radiolucent areas (Lytic lesions) over the calvarium **(Fig. 5)**.

Impression: Lytic lesions over skull bones

Causes of lytic lesions of skull bones: Infiltrative disorders like metastasis and eosinophilic granuloma. LCH, ALL, NF1, neuroblastoma, etc.

X-ray Number 6

X-ray skull lateral view showing symmetrical calcification (periventricular region) **(Fig. 6)**.

Impression: Cytomegaloviral infection in neonate

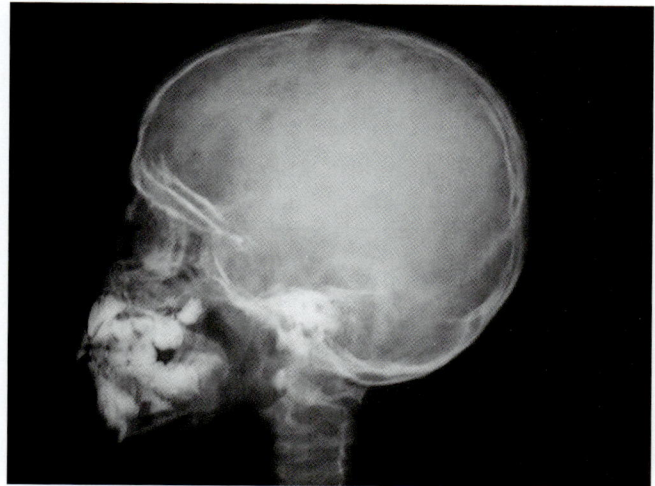

Fig. 5: Multiple radiolucent areas (Lytic lesions) over the calvarium.

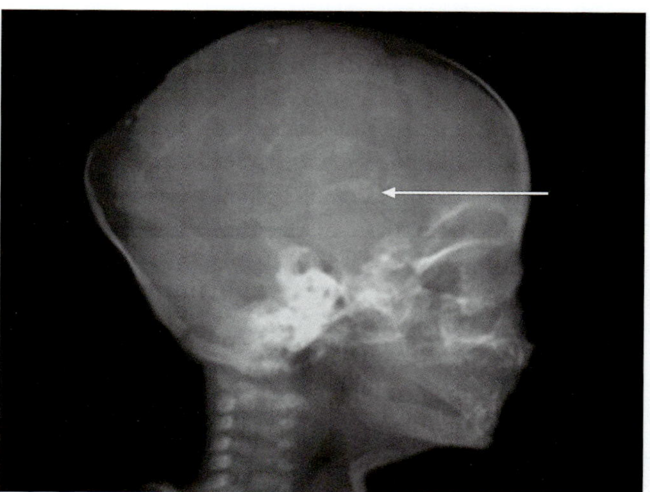

Fig. 6: Symmetrical calcification (periventricular region).

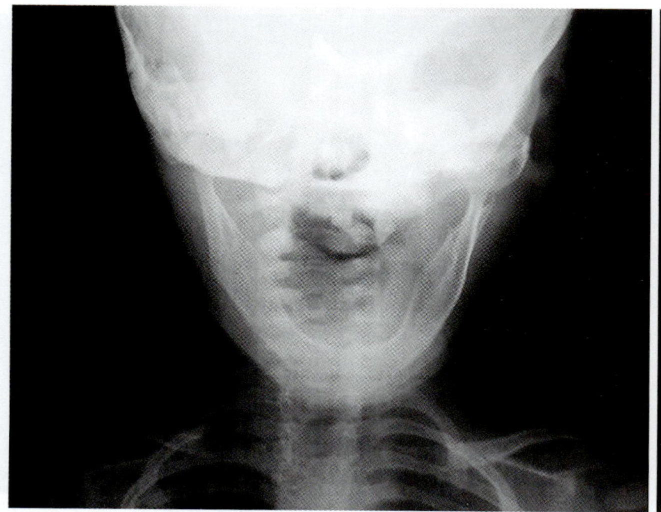

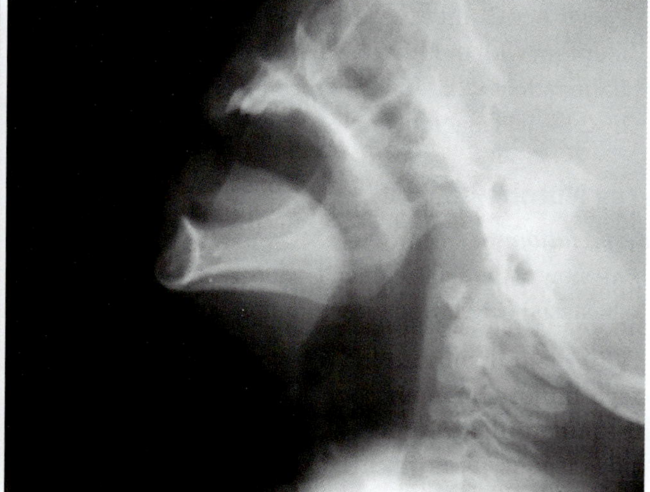

Fig. 7: Ectodermal dysplasia: No tooth socket on X-ray mandible.

X-ray Number 7

X-ray mandible AP and lateral views show no tooth socket **(Fig. 7)**.

Impression: Ectodermal dysplasia

X-ray Number 8

X-ray neck OM view showing increased soft tissues in front of neck with layers of bones over the mandible.

Impression: Infantile cortical hyperostosis (Caffey's disease) **(Fig. 8)**

X-ray Number 9

Interpretation: X-ray PA view of the neck and upper part of the thorax showing *steeple sign* (abrupt narrowing of upper part of trachea) **(Fig. 9)**.

Diagnosis: Acute laryngotracheobronchitis

X-ray Number 10

Interpretation: X-ray lateral view of the neck showing *thumb like* radiopaque shadow at the level of C2 and C3 **(Fig. 10)**.

Diagnosis: Acute epiglottitis

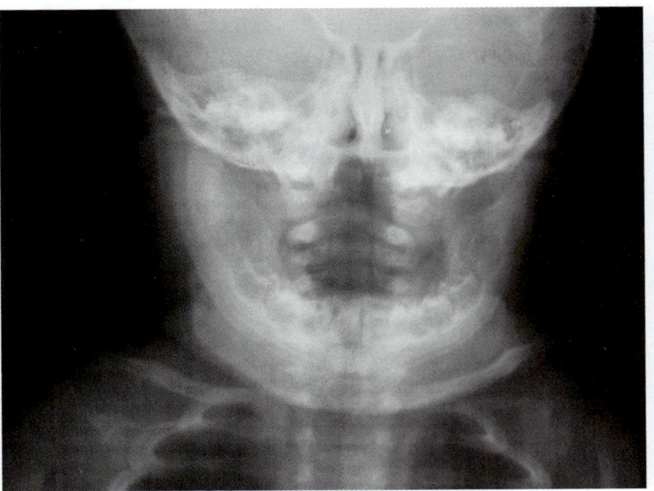

Fig. 8: X-ray of neck OM view: Infantile cortical hyperostosis.

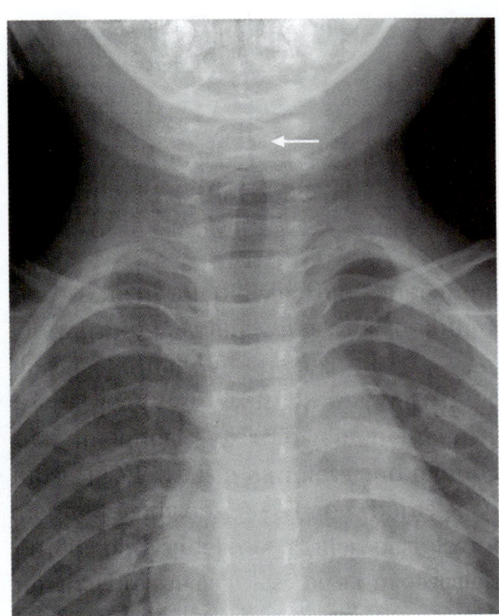

Fig. 9: X-ray PA view of the neck and upper part of the thorax showing steeple sign.

X-ray Number 11

X-ray nasopharynx lateral view showing increased prevertebral soft tissue shadows (retropharyngeal space) **(Fig. 11)**. The maximum distance of retropharyngeal soft tissue is greater than the AP diameter of C2 vertebra.

Impression: Retropharyngeal abscess.

Chest X-rays: All students must know how to interpret chest X-rays properly.

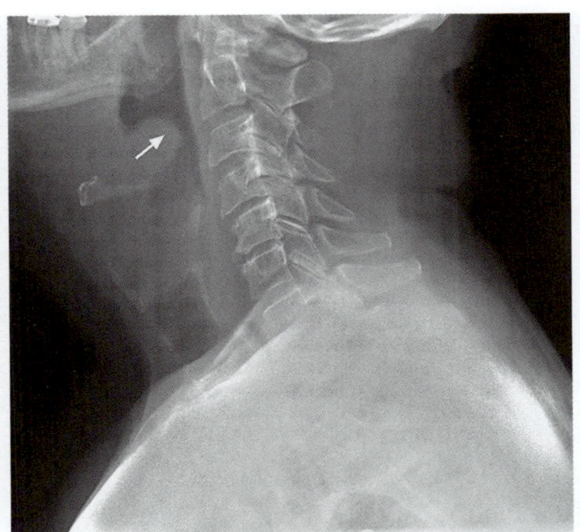

Fig. 10: X-ray lateral view of the neck showing *thumb sign—acute epiglottitis.*

A systematic approach may help to avoid missing any finding. You must look carefully the X-ray from outside inward.

Chest X-ray:

- Views—PA, lateral, AP, lateral decubitus
- *Steps of interpretation*:
  1. Soft tissue shadows
  2. Bones (ribs, clavicles, and sternum)
  3. Domes of diaphragm
  4. Trachea
  5. Cardiac silhouette
  6. Superior mediastinal and hilar shadows
  7. Costophrenic sulci
  8. Lung fields

You must also know three cardinal points for a good quality X-ray chest.

- *R*otation
- *I*nspiratory or expiratory
- *P*enetration (overexposed or underexposed)

A pneumonic *RIP* might be helpful.

X-ray Number 12

Interpretation: This is an X-ray chest PA view of the thorax with normal ribs and clavicles, trachea central in position showing radiolucent shadows within the soft tissue over chest wall and over the scapular region on both sides **(Fig. 12)**.

Diagnosis: Subcutaneous emphysema (surgical emphysema)

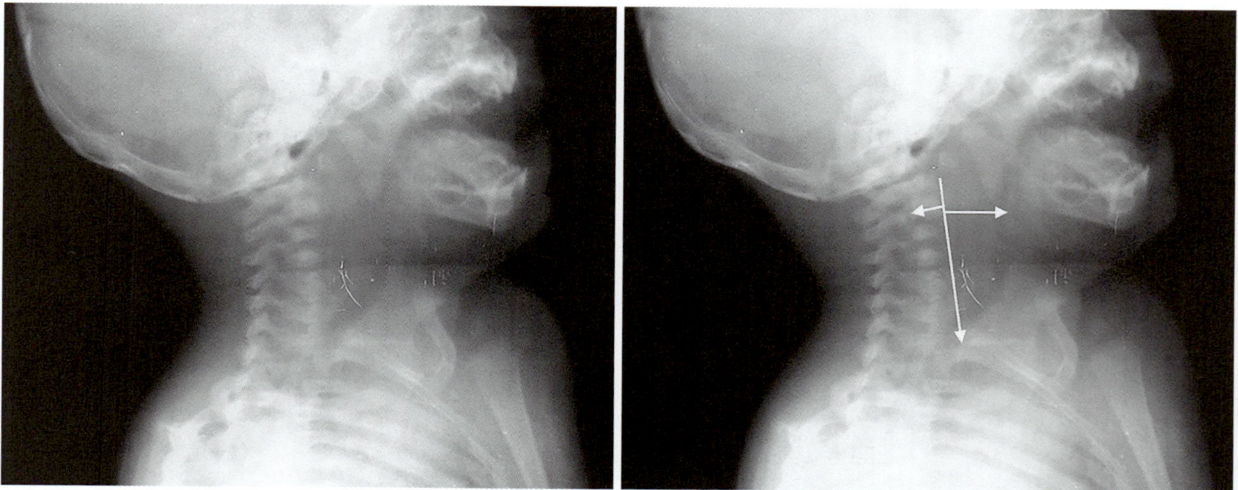

Fig. 11: X-ray nasopharynx lateral view showing increased retropharyngeal space—retropharyngeal abscess.

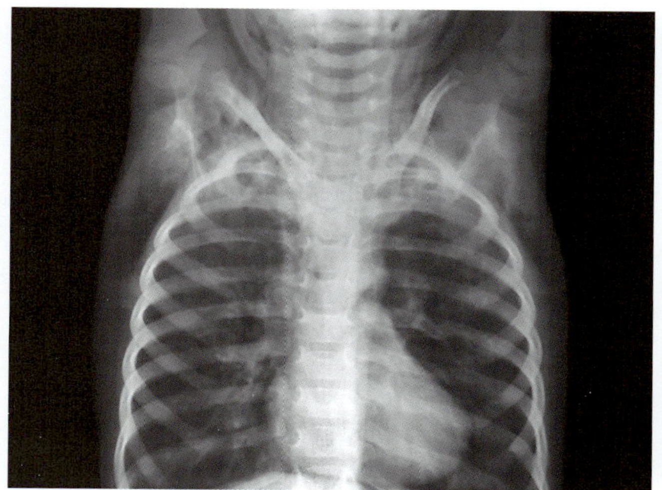

Fig. 12: X-ray chest PA view showing radiolucent shadows within the soft tissue: Surgical emphysema.

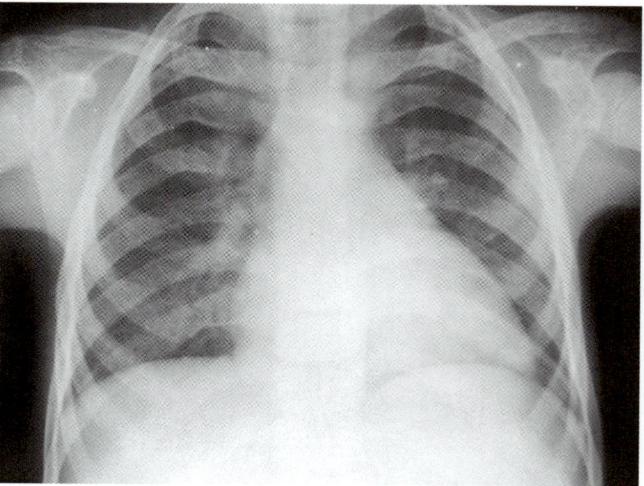

Fig. 13: X-ray PA view of the chest showing cardiomegaly and widening of the anterior ends of the ribs.

X-ray Number 13

Interpretation: This is an X-ray PA view of the chest showing cardiomegaly and widening of the anterior ends of the ribs with decreased mineralization **(Fig. 13)**.

Diagnosis: Chronic hemolytic anemia with cardiomegaly

X-ray Number 14

Interpretation: This is a segment of chest X-ray showing erosion of the inferior margin of the 3rd and 4th right ribs.

Diagnosis: Rib notching due to coarctation of aorta/ interrupted aortic arch **(Fig. 14)**

Must remember other causes of notching of ribs.

Causes of inferior rib notching:

- *Aortic obstruction:*
  - Takayasu arteritis
  - Coarctation of aorta
- *Subclavian artery obstruction:*
  - Classic BT shunt
  - Takayasu arteritis
- Chronic SVC obstruction
- Intercostal AV fistula
- Neurofibromatosis

Causes of superior rib notching:

- Poliomyelitis
- Osteogenesis imperfecta

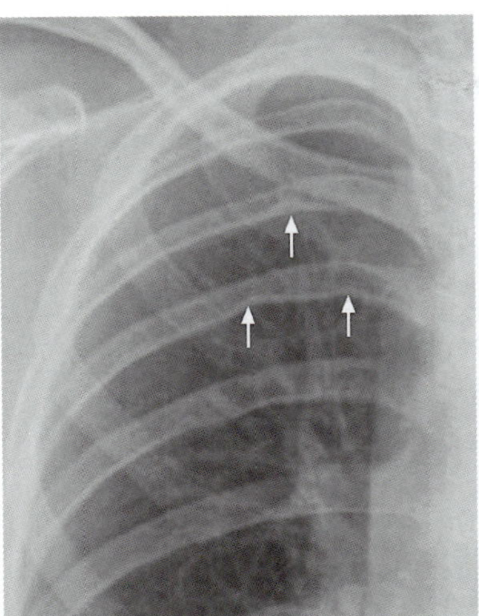

Fig. 14: Chest X-ray showing—rib notching due to coarctation of aorta/interrupted aortic arch.

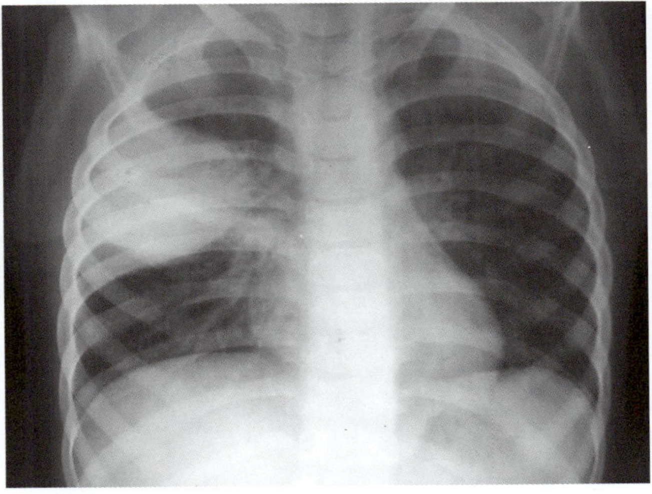

Fig. 16: Chest X-ray PA view of the thorax showing rounded homogeneous opacity in the right upper and mid zone.

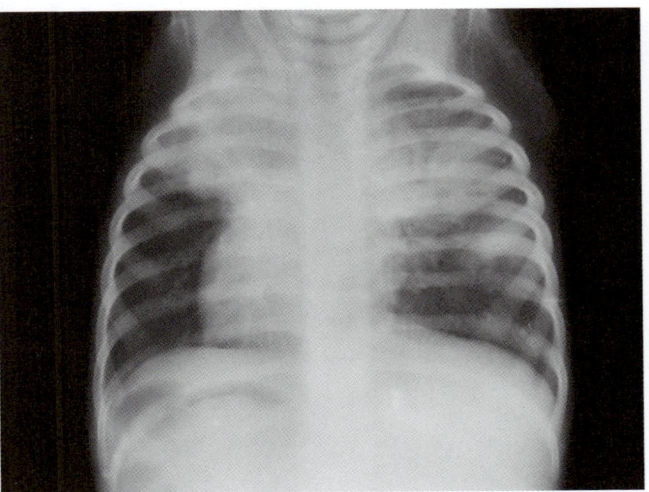

Fig. 15: Chest X-ray AP view showing homogeneous opacity: Lobar pneumonia.

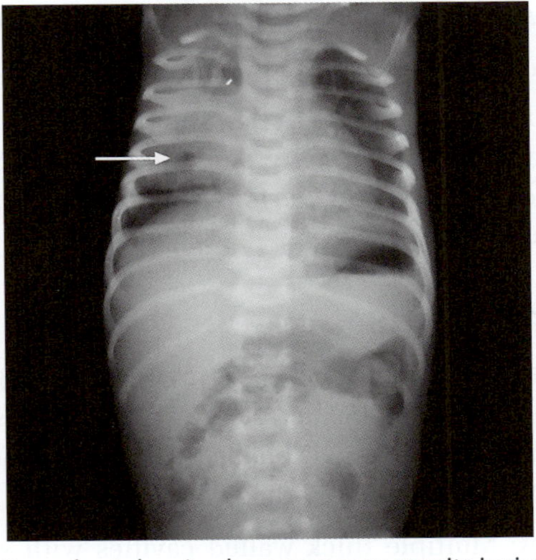

Fig. 17: X-ray chest showing homogeneous opacity in right upper zone and midzone.

- Neurofibromatosis
- Marfan's syndrome
- Collagen vascular disease
- Hyperparathyroidism

X-ray Number 15

Interpretation: This is chest X-ray AP view showing homogeneous opacity in the right upper zone and mid zone and left upper zone showing air bronchogram **(Fig. 15)**.

Diagnosis: Lobar pneumonia in right and left upper lobe (air space pneumonia).

X-ray Number 16

Interpretation: Chest X-ray PA view of the thorax **(Fig. 16)** showing rounded homogeneous opacity in the right upper and mid zone with air bronchogram.

Diagnosis: Round pneumonia

Usually seen in children below 7 years of age.

Differential diagnosis: Coin lesion in adults.

X-ray Number 17

Interpretation: X-ray chest PA view **(Fig. 17)** showing radiolucent pocket within homogeneous opacity in the right upper and mid zone.

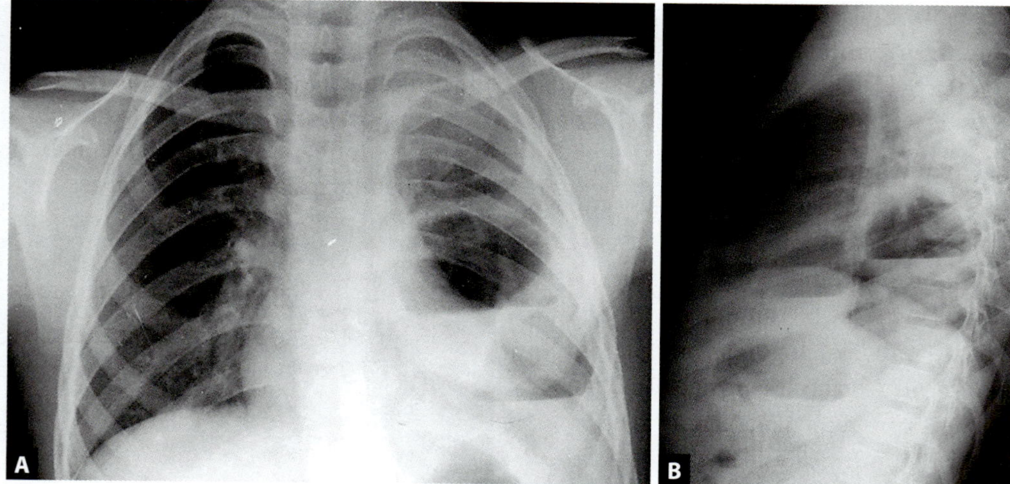

Figs. 18A and B: (A) X-ray chest showing obliteration of left costophrenic angle; (B) Lateral view of the thorax showing multiple lung abscesses.

Diagnosis: Pneumatocele with right upper lobe pneumonia

Causes of pneumatocele: Pneumonia due to *Staphylococcus*

Others: Streptococcus pneumoniae, Haemophilus influenzae, Escherichia coli, group A streptococci, *Serratia marcescens, Klebsiella pneumoniae,* adenovirus, and tuberculosis

X-ray Number 18A

Interpretation: This is a chest X-ray PA view **(Fig. 18A)** with normal soft tissue, normal clavicles, and ribs. Right costophrenic angles is visible, left costophrenic angle is obliterated with normal cardiac silhouette.

Findings: Multiple thick walled cavities with smooth margins containing air-fluid levels in the mid and lower zone of the left lung.

Diagnosis: Multiple lung abscesses with left sided pleural effusion (empyema).

X-ray Number 18B

Same child with left lateral view of chest **(Fig. 18B)**.

X-ray Number 19

This is a chest X-ray PA view **(Fig. 19)** with normal soft tissue, normal clavicles, and ribs.

Findings:

- Left costophrenic angle is visible.
- Right costophrenic angle is obliterated.

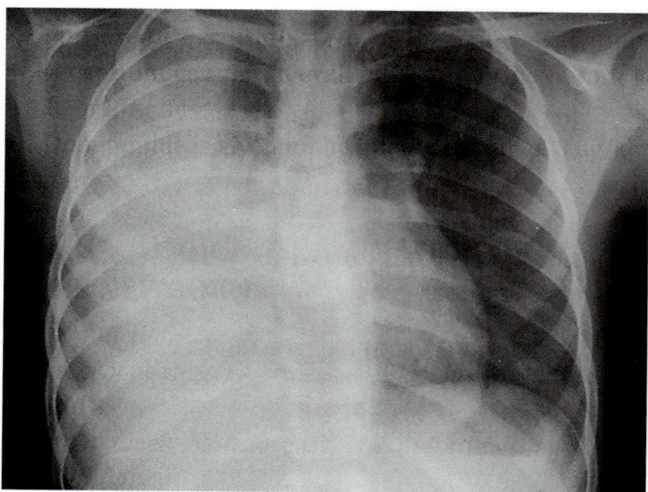

Fig. 19: X-ray showing right-sided homogeneous opacity with obliterated right costophrenic angle.

- Homogeneous opacity in the right hemithorax with air-bronchogram
- Ellis s-shaped curve
- Shift of the mediastinum to the left

Diagnosis: Consolidation in the right lung with right-sided pleural effusion.

X-ray Number 20

Interpretation: This is a chest X-ray PA view **(Fig. 20)** with normal soft tissue, normal clavicles and ribs, trachea is shifted to the right. Costophrenic angles are visible.

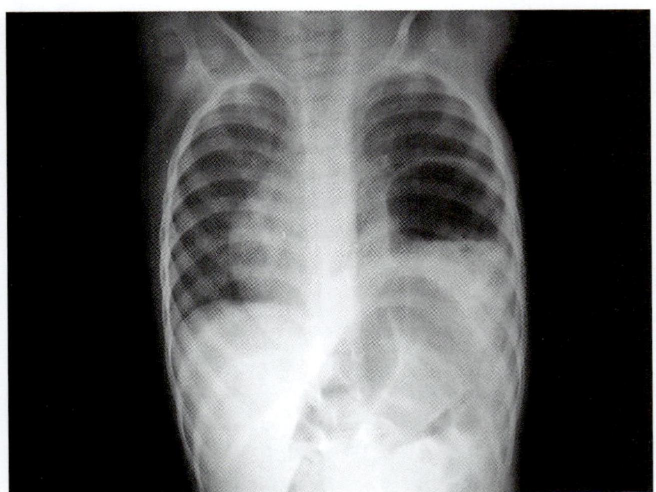

Fig. 20: X-ray chest showing left hemidiaphragm at a higher level than the right with mediastinal shift.

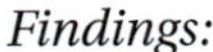

Findings:

- With normal cardiothoracic ratio
- Left hemidiaphragm at a higher level than the right
- Gas shadow present below the left hemidiaphragm
- Mediastinum shifted to the right

Diagnosis: Eventration/palsy of the left hemidiaphragm

The main difference between diaphragmatic eventration and diaphragmatic palsy is that eventration affects a portion of the diaphragm, while palsy affects the entire side.

X-ray Number 21

Interpretation: This is a chest X-ray AP view **(Fig. 21)** showing normal soft tissues and visualized bones with trachea shifted to the right.

Findings:

- Endotracheal tube present
- Mediastinal shift to the right
- Bowel loops in the left hemithorax

Diagnosis: Congenital diaphragmatic hernia (left sided—Bochdalek's hernia).

X-ray Number 22

Interpretation: This is chest X-ray PA view **(Fig. 22)** showing normal soft tissue, normal bony contours, normal cardiothoracic ratio, and visible costophrenic angles.

Multiple nodules 1–2 mm in size scattered throughout both the lung fields more prominent in the right lower zone.

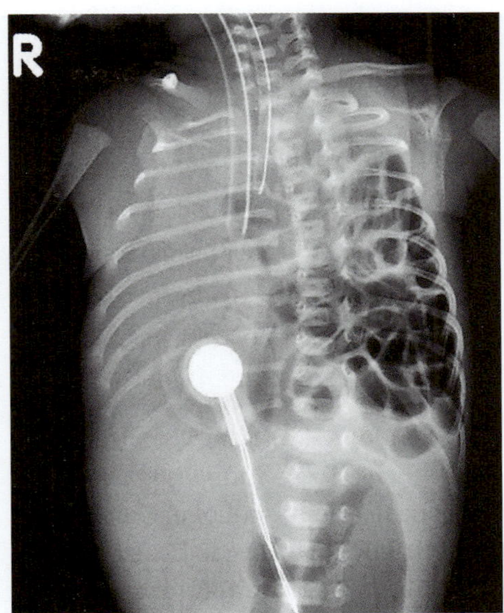

Fig. 21: X-ray AP view showing trachea shifted to the right with bowel loops in the left hemithorax.

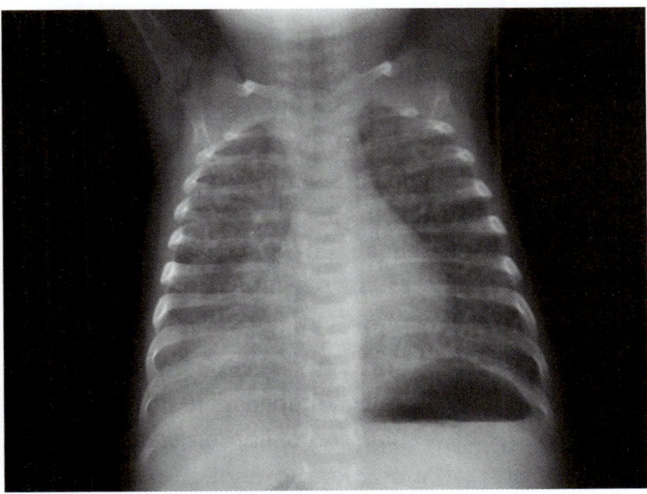

Fig. 22: Chest X-ray showing multiple nodules 1–2 mm in size scattered throughout both the lung fields.

Diagnosis: Miliary mottling

Causes:

- Miliary tuberculosis
- Varicella pneumonia
- Bronchopneumonia
- Pulmonary edema
- Tropical pulmonary eosinophilia

X-ray Number 23

Interpretation: This is chest X-ray PA view **(Fig. 23)** showing normal soft tissue, normal ribs and clavicles,

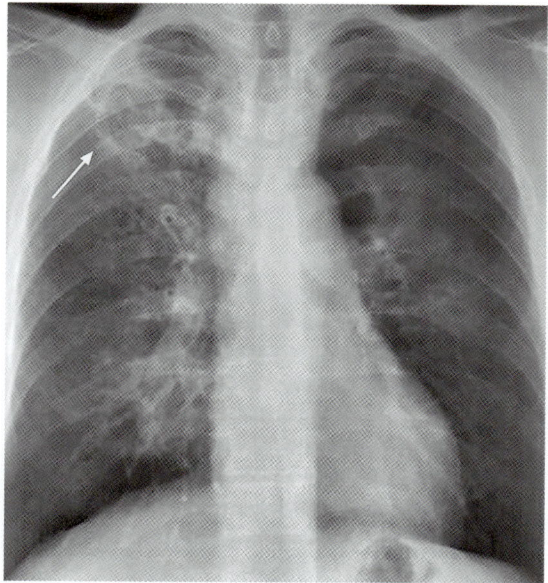

Fig. 23: X-ray chest showing cavitary lesion in the upper zone of the right lung with enlargement and calcification of the hilar lymph nodes.

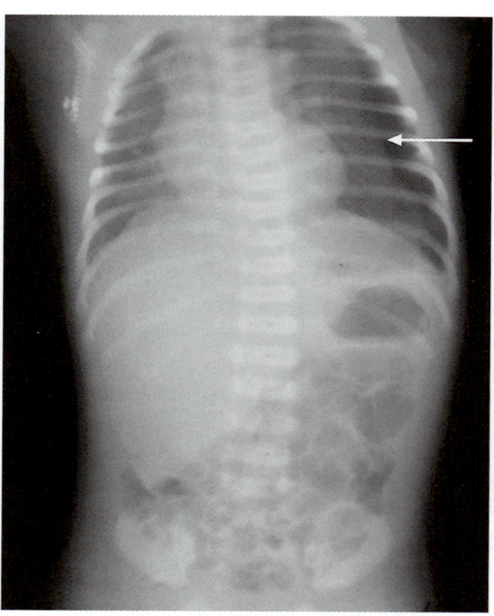

Fig. 24: CXR PA view showing mediastinal shift to right side with collapse left lung border. (CXR: chest X-ray)

normal cardiothoracic ratio, and centrally placed trachea.

Findings:

- Cavitary lesion in the upper zone of the right lung
- Enlargement and calcification of the hilar lymph nodes

Diagnosis: Tuberculosis with cavitation

X-ray Number 24

Interpretation: This is a chest X-ray PA view **(Fig. 24)** with normal soft tissue, visualized bones. Costophrenic angles are visible, normal cardiothoracic ratio.

Findings:

- Trachea shifted to the right side
- Mediastinal shift to the right side
- Collapsed lung border on the left side
- Absent bronchovascular markings on the left side
- Hyperlucency of left peripheral lung fields

Diagnosis: Left-sided pneumothorax

X-ray Number 25

See **Figure 25**.

X-ray Number 26 (Normal Chest X-ray)

Interpretation: Normal chest X-ray **(Fig. 26)**.

X-ray Number 27

Interpretation: Cardiomegaly can be ascertained if A + B >50% of C **(Fig. 27)** [in neonates, cardiomegaly is diagnosed radiologically if A+B >60% of C]

Draw a perpendicular line through the middle of the vertebral body (spinus processes) and then draw horizontal lines maximum to the right (A) and maximum to the left (B) of cardiac shadow.

A transverse line (C) is drawn to depict maximum thoracic diameter. Some authorities prefer a transverse line through the uppermost point of right dome of diaphragm.

X-ray Number 28

Interpretation: This is a chest X-ray PA view with normal soft tissue, normal bony structures with trachea at midline **(Fig. 28)**. Costophrenic angles are visible, with cardiac apex in the right hemithorax and increased cardiothoracic ratio with fundic gas below the right hemidiaphragm suggesting stomach on the right side.

Diagnosis: Situs inversus totalis (dextrocardia and rotation of gastrointestinal system so that the liver lies below the left hemidiaphragm and the fundus of the stomach lies below the right hemidiaphragm):

- *Situs inversus thoracalis*—only dextrocardia
- *Situs inversus abdominalis*—levocardia with the liver lying below the left hemidiaphragm and the fundus of the stomach lies below the right hemidiaphragm.

Cardiac silhouette

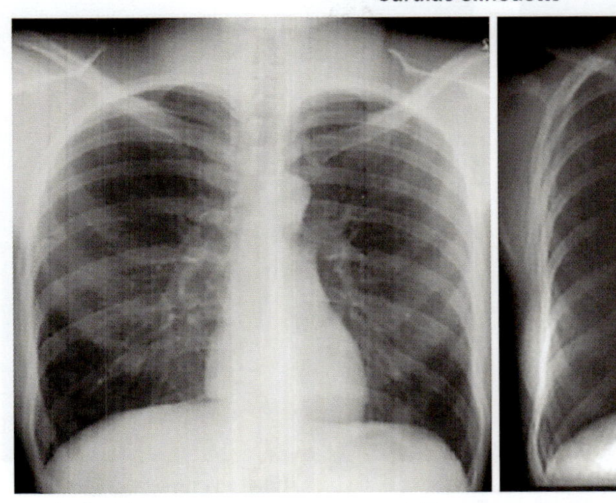

1. R atrium
2. R ventricle
3. Apex of L ventricle
4. Superior vena cava
5. Inferior vena cava
6. Tricuspid valve
7. Pulmonary valve
8. Pulmonary trunk
9. R PA 10. L PA

Fig. 25: CXR PA view showing cardiac borders and vascular system. (CXR: chest X-ray)

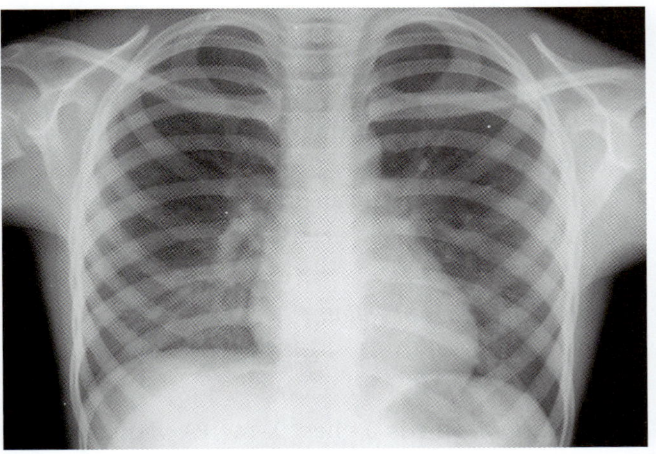

Fig. 26: Normal chest X-ray.

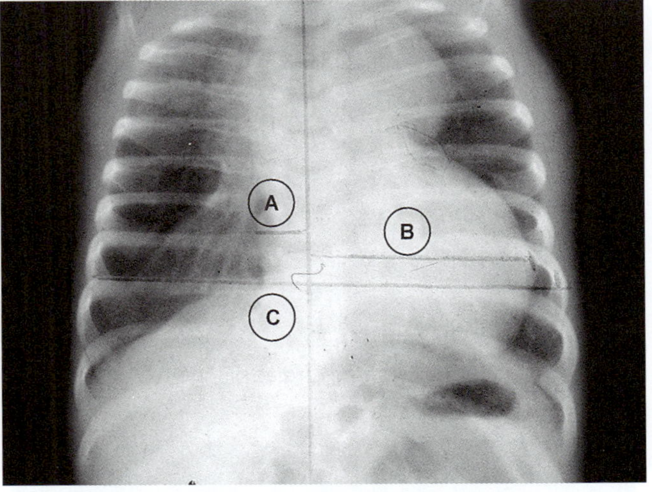

Fig. 27: Cardiomegaly interpretation.

X-ray Number 29

Interpretation: This is a chest X-ray PA view **(Fig. 29)** with normal soft tissue, visualized bones with normally positioned trachea. Costophrenic angles are visible, with enlarged cardiac silhouette (increased cardiothoracic ratio).

Findings:

- Enlarged cardiac silhouette
- Loss of normal contour with stencilled outline of the heart
- Pulmonary oligemia

Diagnosis: Pericardial effusion

Here the contour of cardiac silhouette is preserved. But in cardiomyopathy, this contour is distorted.

X-ray Number 30

Interpretation: This is a chest X-ray PA view **(Fig. 30)** showing meagre soft tissue shadows. Visualized bones and tracheal position normal. There is hugely enlarged cardiac shadow with loss of contour.

Diagnosis: Cardiomyopathy

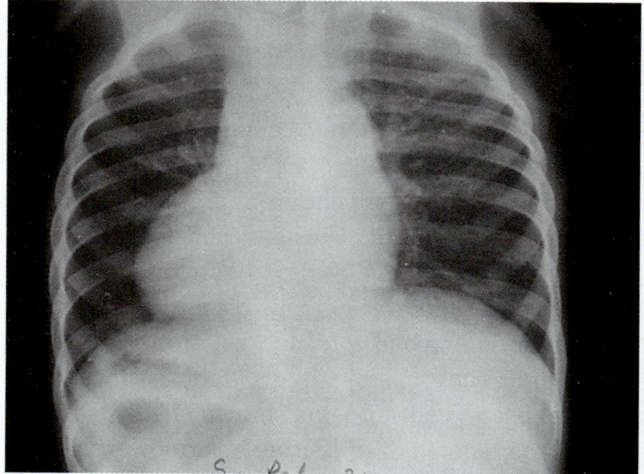

Fig. 28: CXR PA view showing dextrocardia with liver on left side. (CXR: chest X-ray)

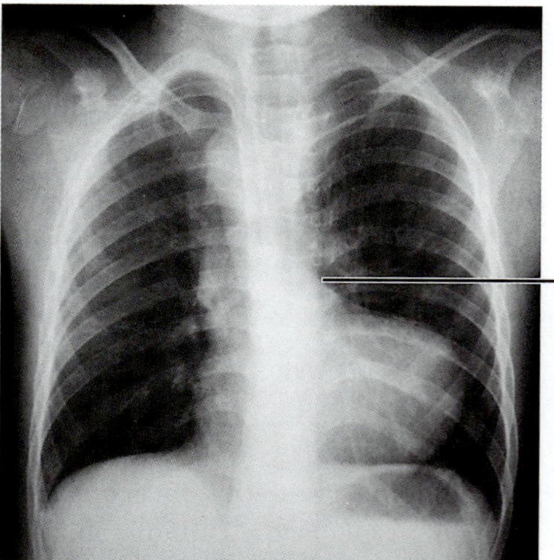

Fig. 31: Tetralogy of Fallot.

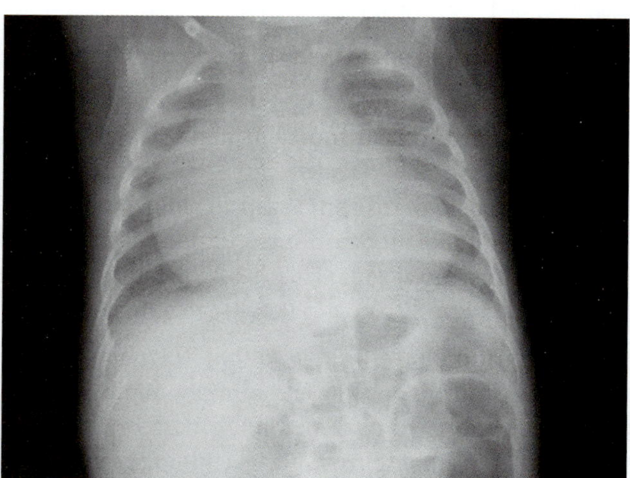

Fig. 29: Enlarged cardiac silhouette.

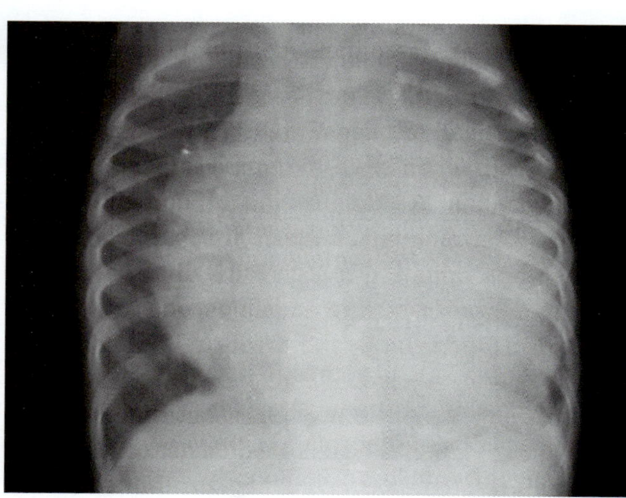

Fig. 30: Hugely enlarged cardiac shadow with loss of contour.

X-ray Number 31

Interpretation: This is a chest X-ray PA view **(Fig. 31)** with normal soft tissue, normal clavicles and ribs, and centrally positioned trachea.

Findings:

- Costophrenic angles are visible
- With enlarged cardiac silhouette (increased cardiothoracic ratio)
- *Boot-shaped heart* with an upturned cardiac apex
- Concave pulmonary arterial segment *(Coeur-En-Sabot-boot shaped)*

Diagnosis: Tetralogy of Fallot

X-ray Number 32

Interpretation: This is a chest X-ray PA view **(Fig. 32)** showing normal soft tissue, normal bony contours, normal cardiothoracic ratio, visible costophrenic angles with haziness both lower zones due to breast shadows (summation shadows).

Findings:

- Double aortic knuckle
- Posterior rib notching

Diagnosis: Coarctation of aorta

X-ray Number 33

Interpretation: X-ray AP view **(Fig. 33)** of the chest showing:

- Meagre soft tissue
- Hyperaeration on right lung field
- Patchy radiopacities both upper lung fields

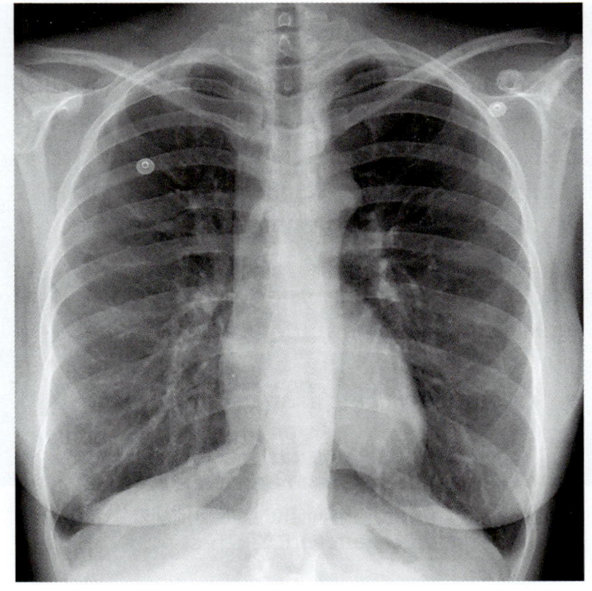

Fig. 32: CXR showing with haziness both lower zones due to breast shadows. (CXR: chest X-ray)

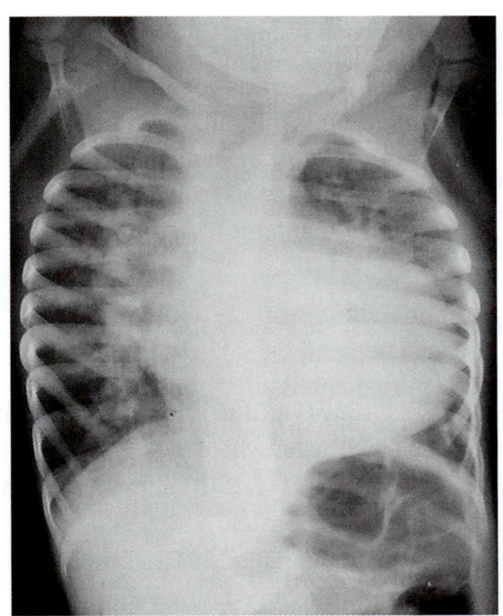

Fig. 33: CXR showing patchy radiopacities both upper lung fields with gross cardiomegaly.

- Gross cardiomegaly
- Biventricular hypertrophy
- Pulmonary plethora (pulmonary vessels are enlarged more than the adjacent bronchi)

Diagnosis: VSD with Eisenmenger syndrome along with right and left upper lobe pneumonia

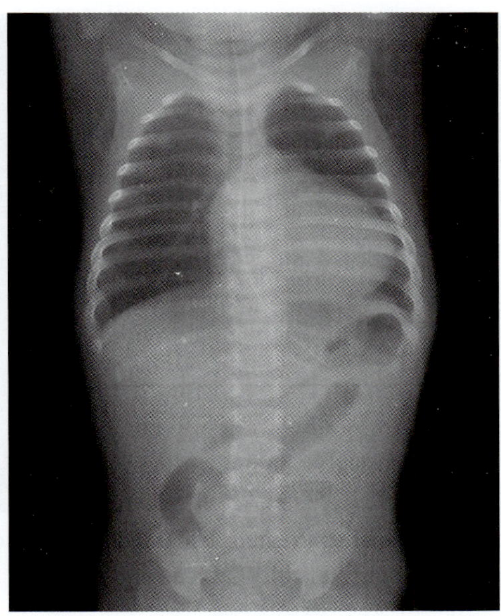

Fig. 34: CXR showing increased cardiothoracic ratio with oligemic lung fields.

X-ray Number 34

Interpretation: This is a chest X-ray PA view **(Fig. 34)** with normal soft tissue, normal clavicles and ribs, costophrenic angles are visible. Cardiac silhouette is enlarged (increased cardiothoracic ratio) with oligemic lung fields.

Findings:

- Enlarged cardiac silhouette with cardiac contour classically described as *"egg on a string"* appearance
- Narrowing of superior mediastinum

Diagnosis: Transposition of great arteries

X-ray Number 35

Interpretation: Chest X-ray PA view **(Fig. 35)** showing right ventricular preponderance showing boot-shaped heart with no pulmonary atresia.

Diagnosis: Cyanotic congenital heart disease with Fallot's physiology.

X-ray Number 36

Interpretation: Chest X-ray PA view **(Fig. 36)** showing smudgy opacities over the bases of both the lungs, simulating bat wing appearance.

Diagnosis: Pulmonary edema

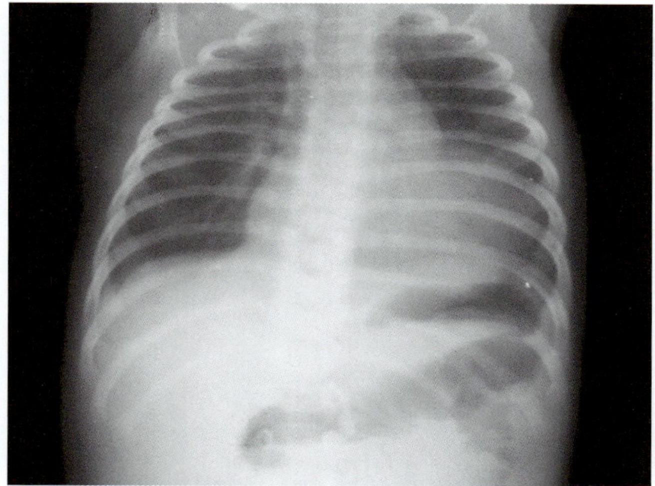

Fig. 35: CXR showing boot-shaped heart with no pulmonary atresia. (CXR: chest X-ray)

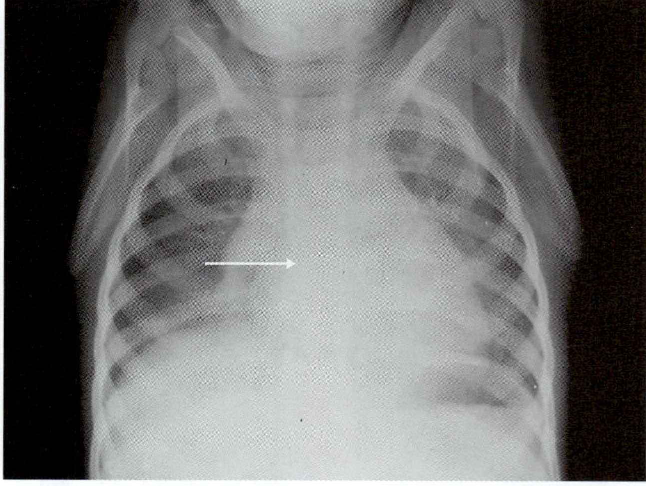

Fig. 37: CXR showing mediastinal widening with a sail like projection (arrow). (CXR: chest X-ray)

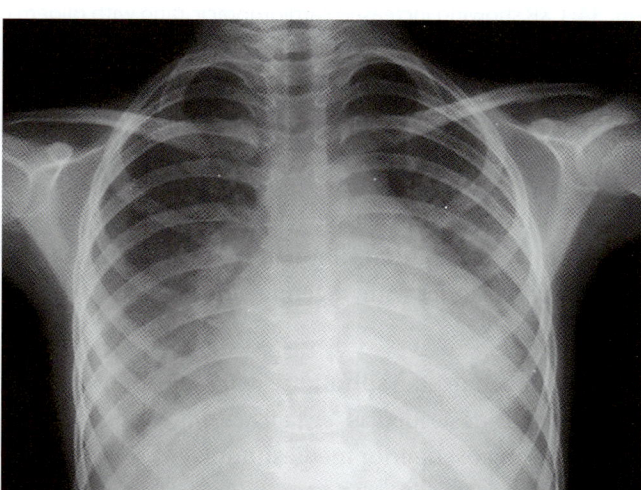

Fig. 36: Bat wing appearance in CXR.

X-ray Number 37

Interpretation: Chest X-ray PA view **(Fig. 37)** showing mediastinal widening with a sail like projection (brown arrow) from right border of heart (Sail sign)

Diagnosis: Most probable *thymic enlargement (right lobe).*

Chest X-ray Newborn

Characteristics of newborn chest X-rays: Anatomical and physiological differences:

Transitional changes:

- Anatomical landmarks
- Congenital defects
- False confidence in interpretation

Causes of respiratory distress in newborn:

- *Systemic diseases:* Metabolic, birth asphyxia, etc.
- *Extrathoracic causes:*
  - Central nervous system (CNS)
  - Neuromuscular
  - Skeletal abnormalities
  - Abdominal
- *Intrathoracic causes:*
  - Surgical causes
  - Medical causes

X-ray Number 38

Interpretation:

A. Chest X-ray AP view **(Fig. 38A)** showing reticulonodular opacities all over the lung field

B. Chest X-ray AP view **(Fig. 38B)** showing ground glass opacity all over the lung field

C. Chest X-ray AP view **(Fig. 38C)** showing complete whiteout lungs and reduced lung volumes

Diagnosis: Respiratory distress syndrome in neonate

X-ray Number 39

Chest X-ray PA views **(Figs. 39A and B)** show streaky linear opacities spreading from hila to peripheral lung fields (fanning), lung volumes are slightly enlarged.

Impression: Transient tachypnea of newborn

Typical radiological features are normal or slightly high lung volume, streaky linear shadows fanning from hila,

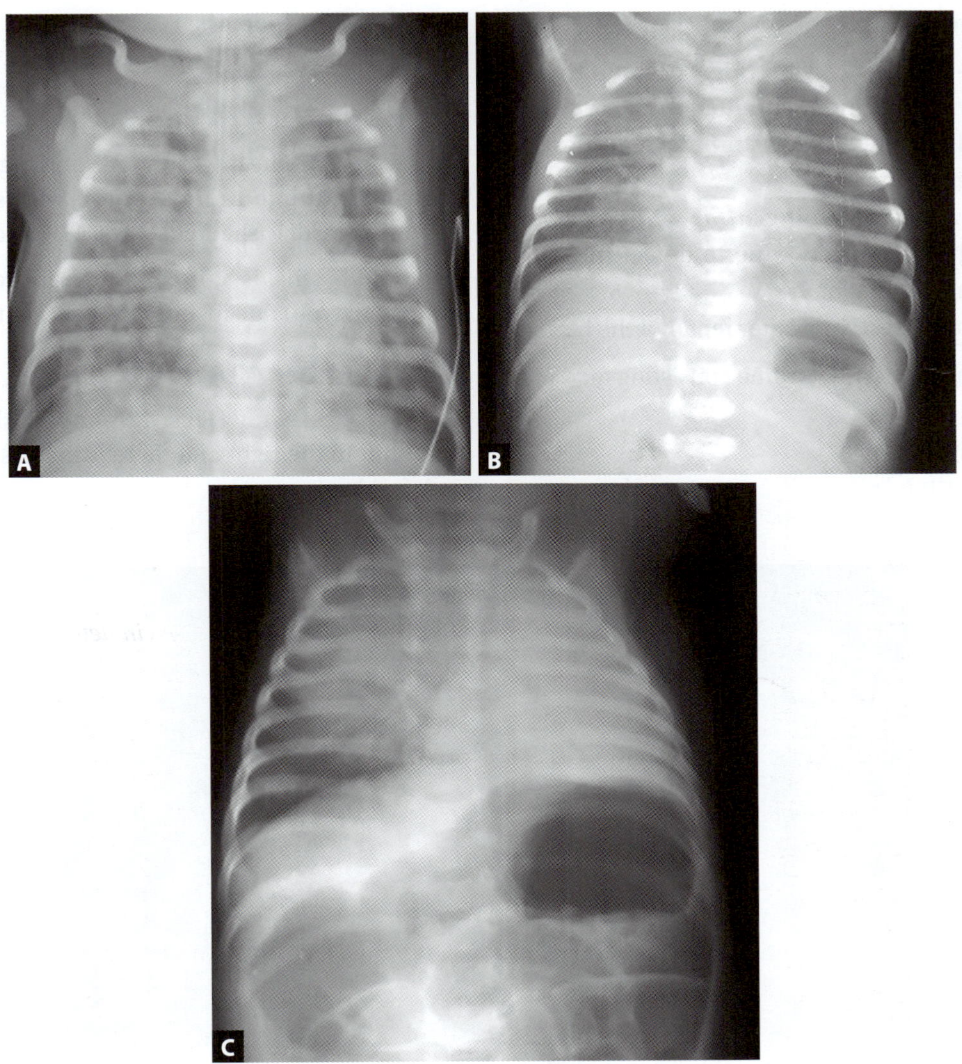

Figs. 38A to C: Chest X-ray AP view showing Respiratory distress syndrome in neonate

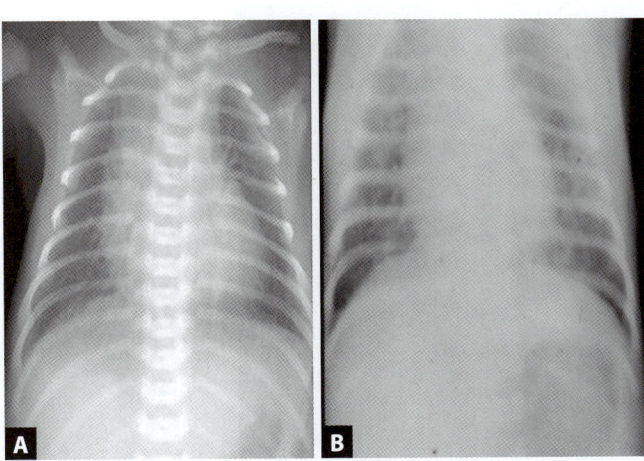

Figs. 39A and B: Streaky linear opacities spreading from hila to peripheral lung fields.

there may be visible transverse fissure on right lung and in rare cases pleural effusion as well.

Lung volume in neonatal pulmonary diseases:

Increased lung volume:

- TTN
- Meconium aspiration
- Congenital heart disease

Normal/decreased lung volume:

- HMD
- Immature lung

Variable lung volume:

- PPHN
- Pneumonia

X-ray Number 40

Interpretation X-ray chest PA view **(Figs. 40A and B)**:

1. (Left) shows mediastinum is shifted to the right with multiple radiolucent shadows mimicking intestines within left hemithorax.

   Comment: Left-sided congenital diaphragmatic hernia (Bochdalek variety) due to defect in the left posterolateral diaphragm.
2. Right, one is the chest X-ray after repair of the hernia.

Diaphragmatic hernia is a syndrome consisting of:

- Hernia
- Pulmonary hypoplasia
- Lung immaturity
- Left heart hypoplasia
- Persistent pulmonary hypertension

X-ray Number 41A and B

These are the chest X-rays (AP and right lateral views showing multiple radiolucent shadows in the thorax, obscuring cardiac shadow) **(Figs. 41A and B)**.

Comment: This is congenital diaphragmatic hernia (Morgagni type) due to anterior defect of the diaphragm.

X-ray Number 42A and B

This is a chest X-ray **(Figs. 42A and B)** showing mediastinal shift to the right and there is increased radiolucency on left side.

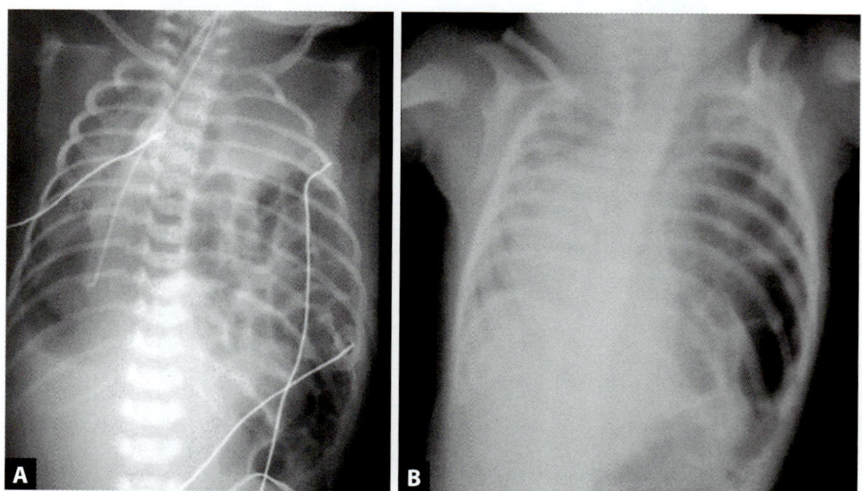

Figs. 40A and B: Mediastinum is shifted to the right with multiple radiolucent shadows.

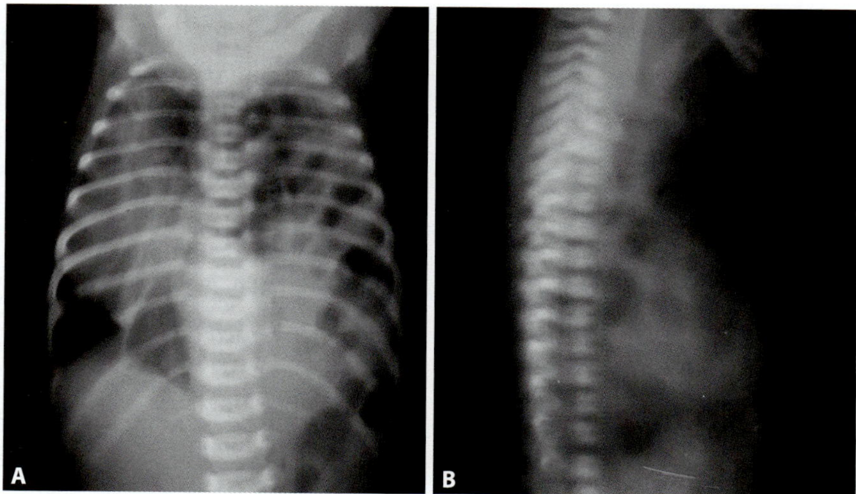

Figs. 41A and B: CXR showing multiple radiolucent shadows in the thorax.

CT chest axial view revealed multiple large cysts in left hemithorax.

Impression: Congenital pulmonary air way malformation left lung.

Radiologically 3 types of congenital pulmonary airway malformation (CPAM):

- *Type 1 (50%):* Single or multiple large cysts
- *Type 2 (30%):* Multiple small cysts
    - Congenital anomalies
    - Malignancy
- *Type 3 (10%):* Solid with microscopic cysts

X-ray Number 43A and B

These X-rays of chest PA views **(Figs. 43A and B)** show there is large radiolucency on left side almost encroaching superior mediastinum (most evident on right X-ray causing some shift of mediastinum to the right).

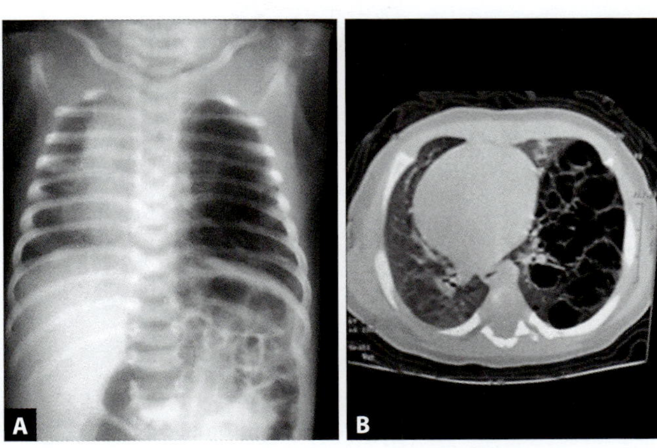

Figs. 42A and B: Chest X-ray showing mediastinal shift to the right and there is increased radiolucency on left side.

Comment: Congenital lobar overinflation (CLO)

X-ray Number 44A and B

Chest X-ray PA view (left) showing small areas of radiolucency right lower zone, which after coalescence turned into large pockets (right film) **(Figs. 44A and B)**.

Impression: Pulmonary interstitial emphysema (PIE)

PIE is the first sign of barotrauma in a baby when put in ventilator support which if not promptly acted may cause more damage to lung parenchyma.

X-ray Number 45A and B

These are the chest X-rays **(Figs. 45A and B)** of a newborn (4 Day baby) showing multiple small infiltrates throughout right lung field, possibly due to meconium aspiration syndrome (MAS).

The baby was on ventilator support for long. So, in right film at age of 24 days, there are patchy scattered opacities throughout lung fields on either side.

Impression: Bronchopulmonary dysplasia (BPD)

BPD develops in neonates due to prolong exposure to oxygen, causing injury to lung parenchyma.

X-RAY LIMBS

X-ray views commonly used are AP, lateral, oblique, and special views.

Step by step approach must be done:

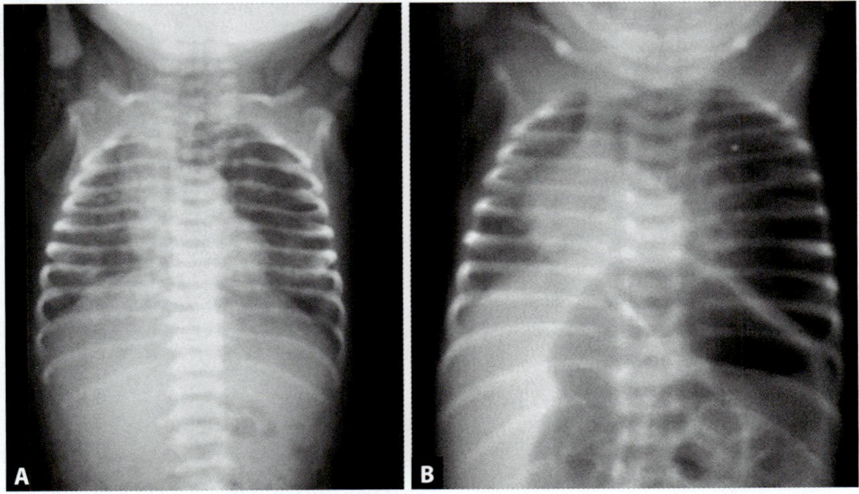

Figs. 43A and B: Large radiolucency on left side almost encroaching superior mediastinum.

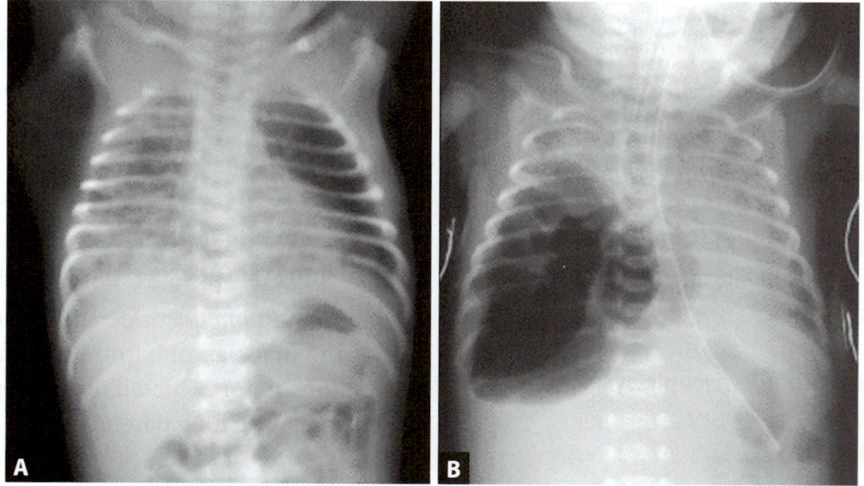

Figs. 44A and B: Small areas of radiolucency right lower zone.

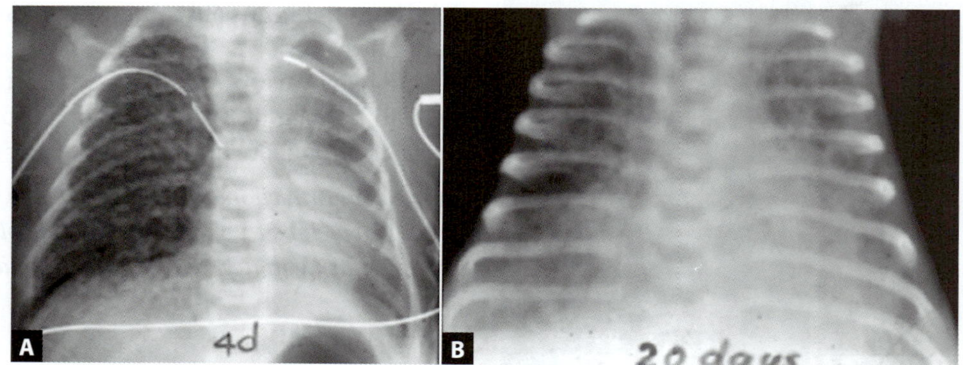

Figs. 45A and B: Multiple small infiltrates in right lung field due to meconium aspiration syndrome.

Soft tissues:

Bones:

- Size, shape, architecture, mineralization
- Diaphyses, metaphysis, epiphyses, and cortices

Joint space:

- Generalized/localized radiodensities or lucencies
- Within bones

X-ray Number 46A and B

This is X-ray knee AP and lateral view **(Figs. 46A and B)** showing soft tissue swelling around the knee joint with generalized under mineralization of visualized bones. Joint space is diminished. There is few dense transverse line at the diaphysis, called *Lines of Park.*

Impression: Rheumatoid arthritis

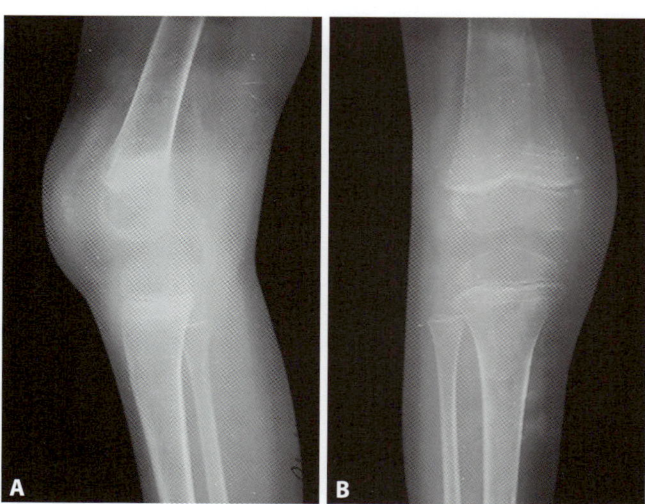

Figs. 46A and B: X-ray knee AP and lateral view showing soft tissue swelling around the knee joint with joint space diminished.

X-ray Number 47

These are the X-rays of knee and right wrist AP views **(Figs. 47A and B)** showing irregular discrete zones of calcification in the distal femoral and proximal tibial epiphyses, depicting epiphyseal dysgenesis.

X-ray wrists showing less number of carpal bones suggesting delayed bone age.

Impression: Hypothyroidism

X-ray Number 48

Interpretation: These are X-ray left wrist AP and lateral view **(Figs. 48A and B)** of the wrist joint (left side) showing widening at the wrist joint.

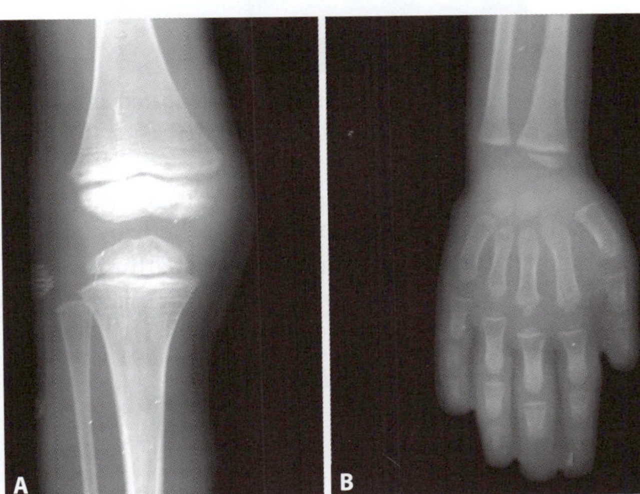

Figs. 47A and B: X-rays of knee and right wrist AP views showing irregular discrete zones of calcification in the distal femoral and proximal tibial epiphyses.

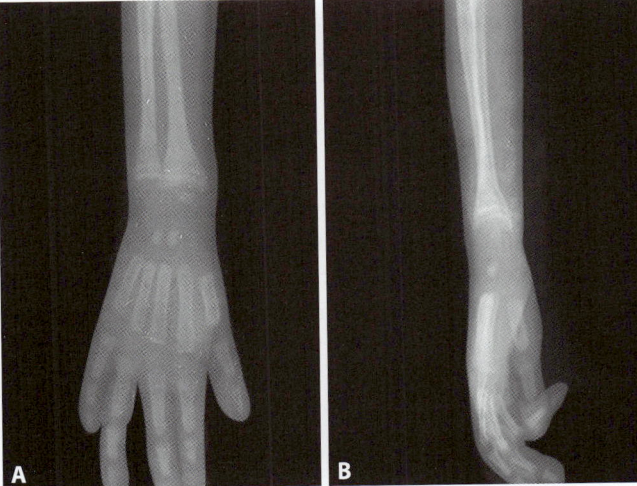

Figs. 48A and B: X-ray left wrist AP and lateral view showing widening at the wrist joint.

Findings:

- Loss of normal zone of provisional calcification
- Splaying (widening of distal end of the metaphysis)
- Fraying (edge of metaphysis loses its sharp border)
- Cupping (edge of the metaphysis changes from flat or convex surface to a more concave surface known as cupping)
- Coarse trabeculation of the diaphysis

Diagnosis: Rickets

X-ray Number 49

Interpretation: This is an AP view of the wrist joint **(Fig. 49)** showing trabeculations and thickening of the carpals and metacarpals.

Diagnosis: Chronic hemolytic anemia

X-ray Number 50

Interpretation: This is an X-ray of both lower limbs AP view **(Fig. 50)** showing:

- Pencil thin cortex
- Subperiosteal hemorrhage
- Osteoporosis (ground glass appearance)
- Scurvy line
- Trummerfeld zone (fragmentation above calcified cartilage)
- Marginal cleft (corner sign)
- Pelkan spur (lateral prolongation of white line under triangular area of rarefaction)
- Epiphyseal fracture

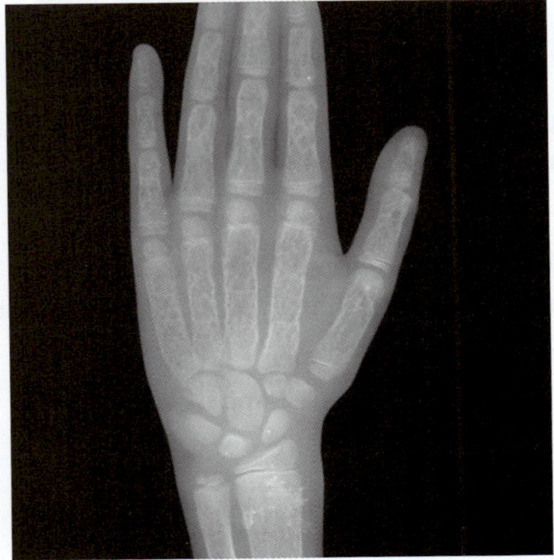

Fig. 49: Wrist joint showing trabeculations and thickening of the carpals and metacarpals.

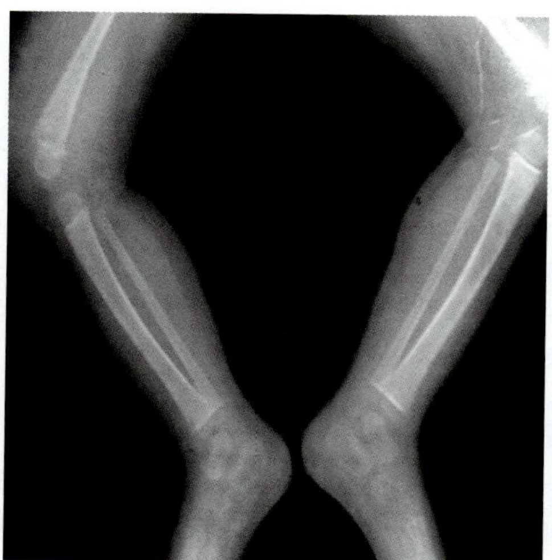

Fig. 50: X-ray of both lower limbs showing pencil thin cortex and subperiosteal hemorrhage.

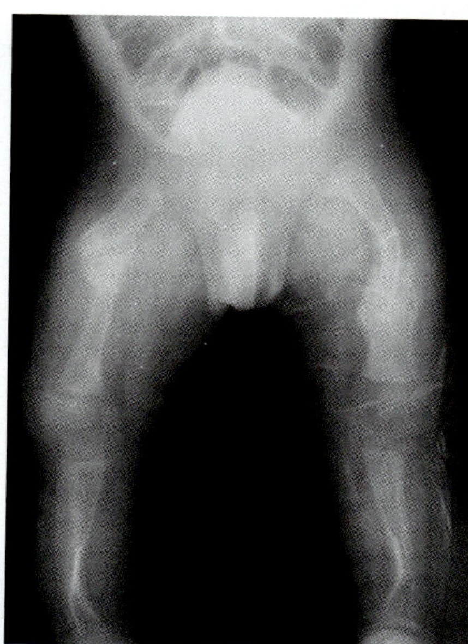

Fig. 51: X-ray of pelvis and both lower limbs showing multiple fractures and callous formation with pseudoarthrosis.

- Increased calcification (Wimberger line)
- Signet ring sign (sharply outlined epiphysis with central rarefaction)

Note: White line of Frankel is seen in some cases.

Diagnosis: Scurvy

X-ray Number 51

Interpretation: This is an X-ray AP view **(Fig. 51)** showing the pelvis and both lower limbs.

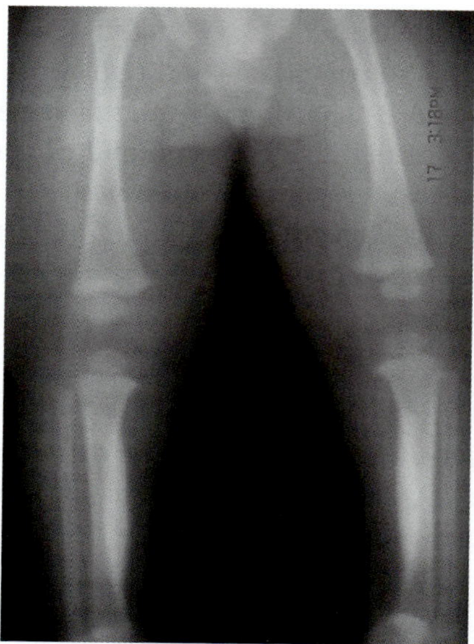

Fig. 52: X-ray both lower limbs showing elongated fusiform thickening at both tibial diaphyses.

Findings:

- Multiple fractures in the long bones of both lower limbs
- Multiple callous formation with pseudoarthrosis

Diagnosis:

- *Osteogenesis imperfecta*
- *Nonaccidental injury (child abuse)*

X-ray Number 52

X-ray both lower limb AP **(Fig. 52)** view showing elongated fusiform thickening (hyperostosis) at the both tibial diaphyses.

Comment: Diaphyseal dysplasia

There are several varieties of diaphyseal dysplasia namely Camurati–Engelmann disease, Ghosal's hemato-diaphyseal dysplasia, etc.

X-ray Number 53

X-ray both femur AP view shows hyperopaque visualized bones **(Fig. 53)**. There is a displaced fracture at the upper end of shaft of left femur. There is bone in bone appearance in all the bones with metaphyseal flaring mimicking rickets.

Impression: Osteopetrosis

X-ray Number 54

X-ray left humerus AP view **(Fig. 54)** shows a large lytic lesion at the proximal end of humerus.

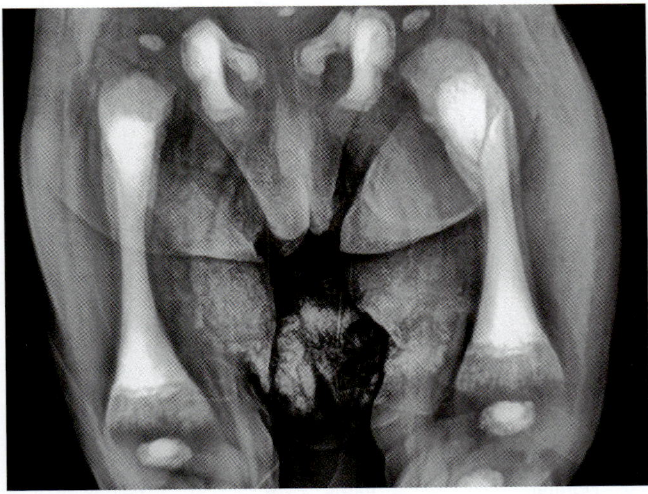

Fig. 53: X-ray both femur showing hyperopaque visualized bones and there is a displaced fracture at the upper end of shaft of left femur.

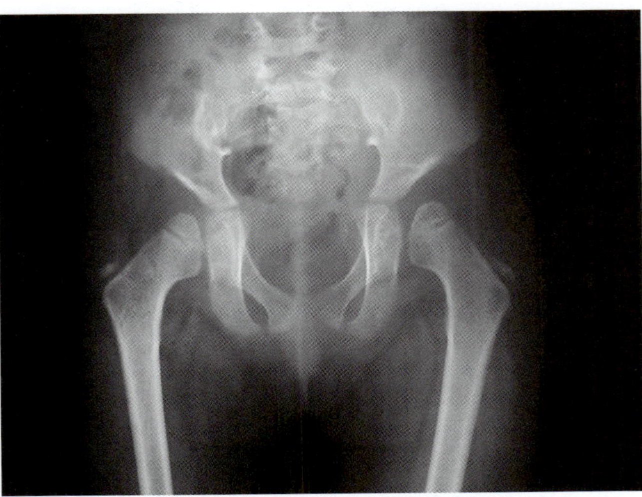

Fig. 55: X-ray pelvis showing flaring of ilial bones, shallow acetabular roof, coxa vara deformity of femur.

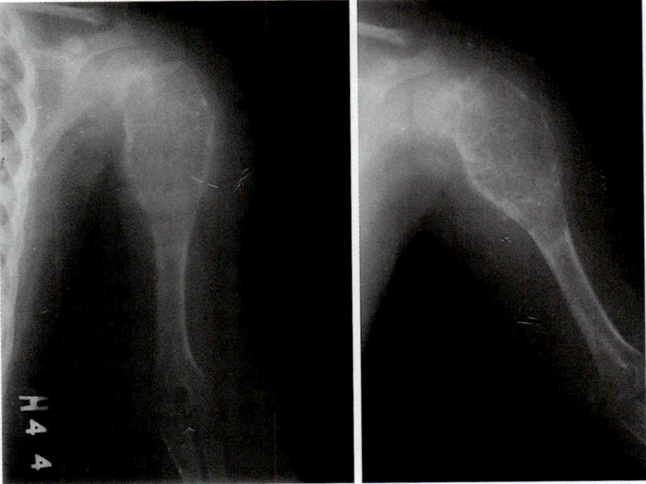

Fig. 54: Humerus showing a large lytic lesion at the proximal end of humerus.

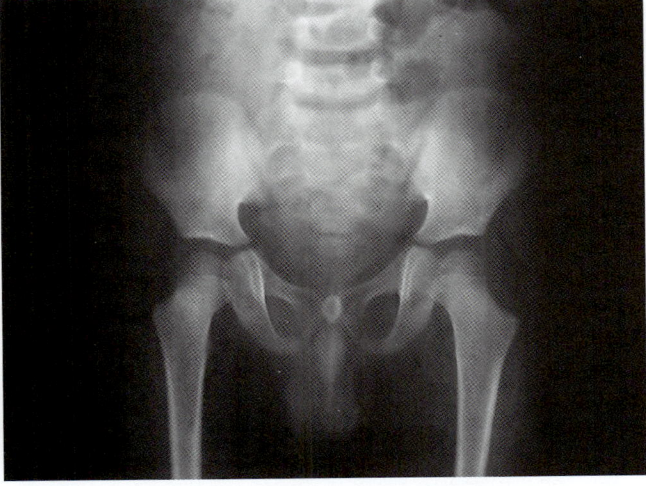

Fig. 56: X-ray pelvis showing a small round radiopaque shadow just over symphysis pubis.

Comment: Aneurysmal bone cyst proximal end of left humerus.

X-RAY PELVIS

Step-wise approach is needed:

- Soft tissues
- *Bones:*
  - Long and flat
  - Size and shape
  - Architecture, mineralization
  - Lumbar vertebrae, sacrum, ilial wings, acetabular roof, and sacrosciatic
  - Notch, ischium and symphysis pubis, femoral head
- Any other obvious finding (calculi, exostosis, etc.)

X-ray Number 55

This is a X-ray pelvis AP view **(Fig. 55)** showing flaring of ilial bones, shallow acetabular roof, and coxa vara deformity of femur.

Comment: Possibility of mucopolysaccharidoses.

X-ray Number 56

This is X-ray pelvis AP view **(Fig. 56)** showing a small round radiopaque shadow just over symphysis pubis.

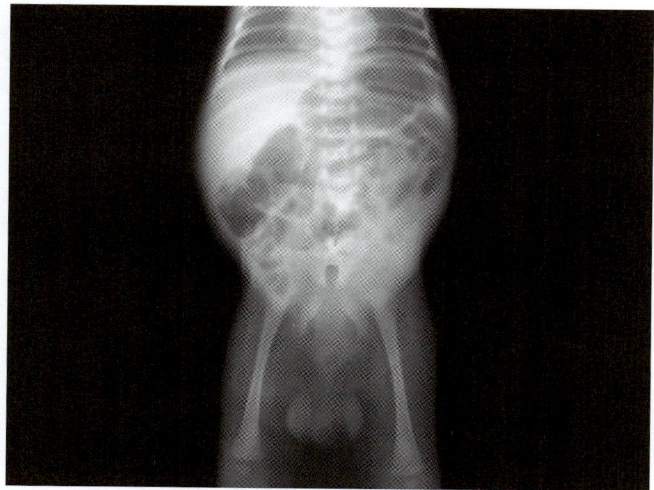

Fig. 57A: X-ray pelvis showing absence of sacrum.

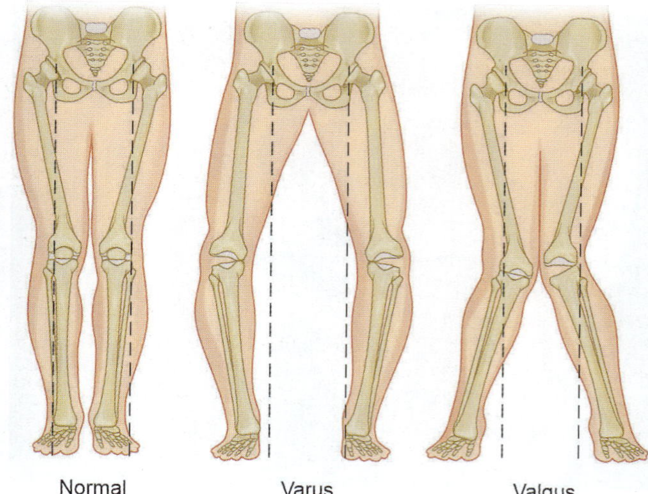

Fig. 57B2: Genu valgus and Genu Varus.

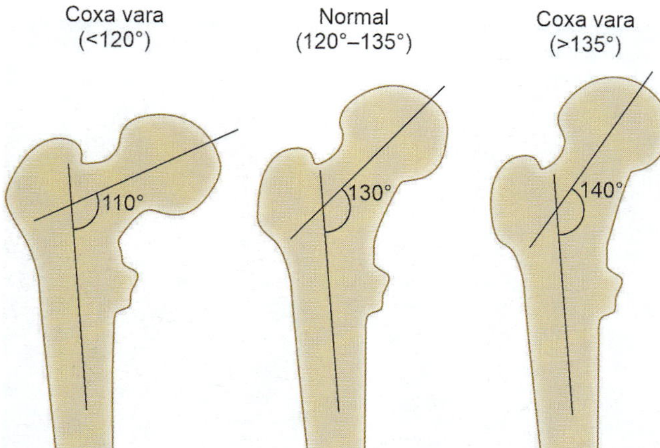

Fig. 57B1: Angle between femoral neck and shaft.

Comment: Stone at the neck of urinary bladder (vesical urolithiasis).

X-ray Number 57

X-ray pelvis AP view **(Fig. 57A)** showing absence of sacrum.

Comment: Caudal regression syndrome

X-RAY WRISTS

Again a systematic approach needed to interpret wrist X-rays.

- Soft tissues
- *Bones:*
  - Size and shape **(Fig. 57B1 and B2)**
  - Architecture
  - Mineralization, trabeculation
- Short bones (carpal, metacarpal, phalanges—number, any special character)
- Metaphyseal ends, epiphyses
- Bone age determination

X-ray Number 58

This is a X-ray left wrist AP view **(Fig. 58)** showing erosion of terminal phalanges, metacarpals are inverted bullet or bottle shaped, squaring of 1st metacarpal bone. Less number of carpal bones. The distal ends of ulna and radius are tipping toward each other.

Comment: Changes are suggestive of mucopolysaccharidoses.

X-ray Number 59A and B

X-rays of both wrists AP views **(Figs. 59A and B)** showing multiple cartilaginous projection from distal ends of long bones as well as phalanges.

Comment: Multiple enchondromatosis (Ollier disease)

X-RAY SPINE

A systematic approach should be adopted:

- Views: AP and lateral views
- Curvature of vertebral column
- Vertebral bodies—size, shape, architecture, and mineralization
- Intervertebral disk space
- Paravertebral space

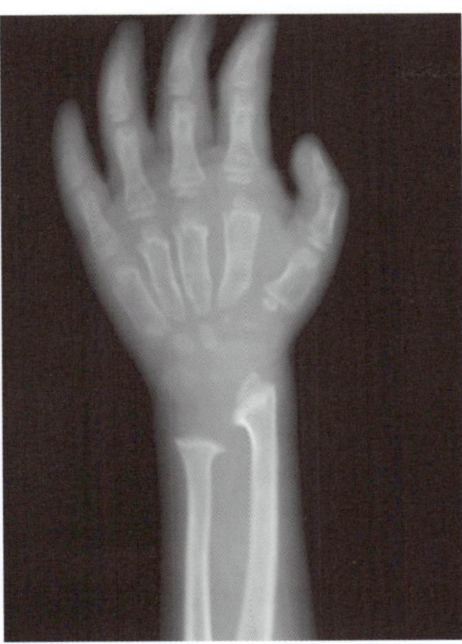

Fig. 58: X-ray left wrist showing erosion of terminal phalanges, metacarpals are inverted bullet or bottle shaped.

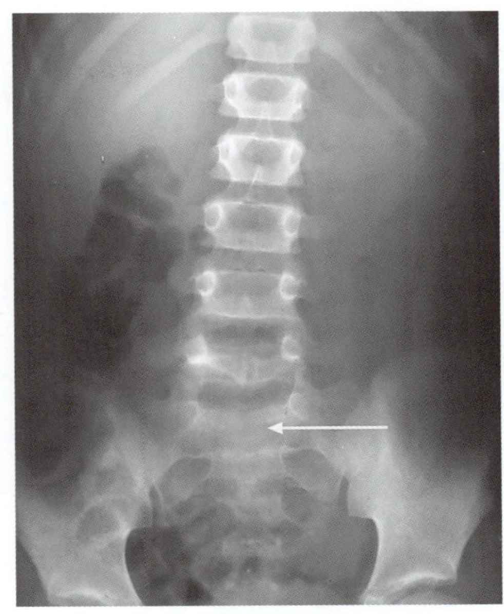

Fig. 60: X-ray lumbosacral spine showing a cleft at the middle of body of 5th lumbar vertebra.

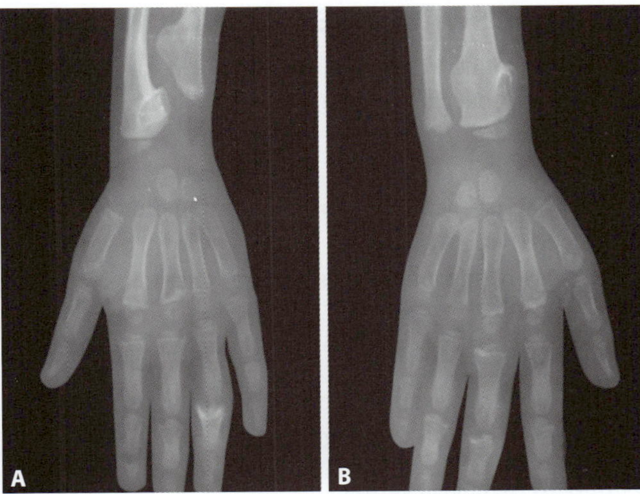

Figs. 59A and B: X-rays of both wrists showing multiple cartilaginous projection from distal ends of long bones as well as phalanges.

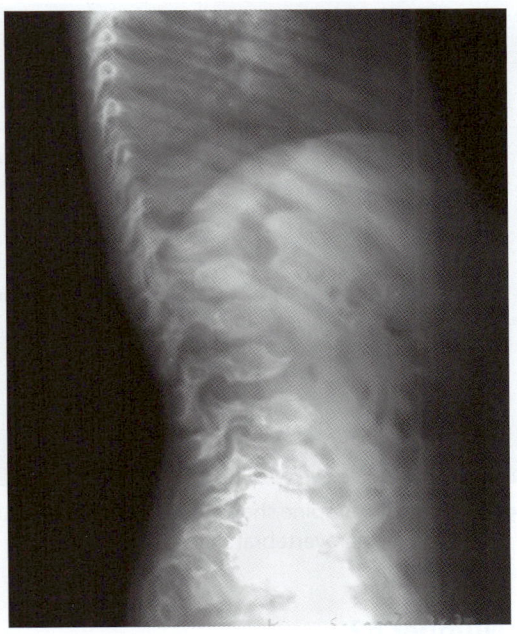

Fig. 61: X-ray dorsolumbar spine AP view shows beaking.

X-ray Number 60

X-ray lumbosacral spine AP view **(Fig. 60)** shows a cleft at the middle of body of 5th lumbar vertebra.

Comment: Spina bifida occulta

X-ray Number 61

X-ray dorsolumbar spine AP view **(Fig. 61)** shows beaking of:

Vertebral bodies mainly lumbar region

Comment: Changes are suggestive of mucopolysaccharidosis.

Other causes of beaking of vertebrae are achondroplasia, congenital hypothyroidism, pseudoachondroplasia, etc.

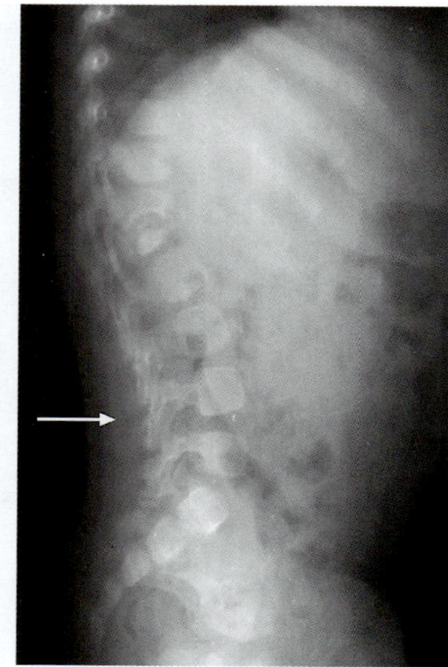

Fig. 62: X-ray lumbosacral spine lateral view shows compressed 1st lumbar vertebra.

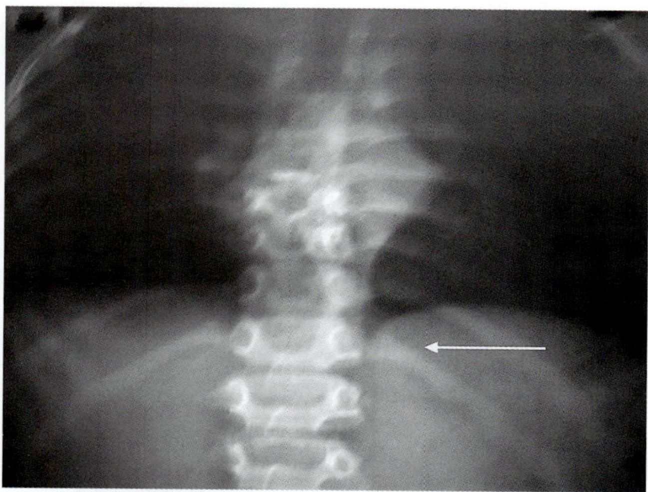

Fig. 63: X-ray dorsal spine showing fusiform radiopaque paravertebral shadow.

X-ray Number 62

X-ray lumbosacral spine lateral view **(Fig. 62)** shows necrosed and compressed 1st lumbar vertebra.

Comment: Caries spine

X-ray Number 63

X-ray dorsal spine AP view **(Fig. 63)** shows fusiform radiopaque paravertebral shadows lower thoracic vertebrae.

Comment: Cold abscess thoracic spine

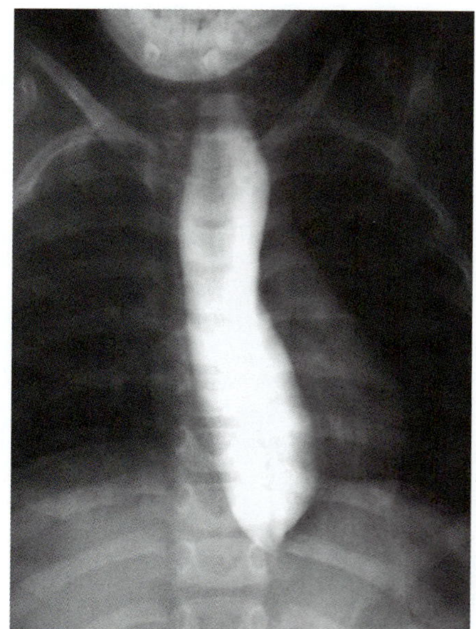

Fig. 64: Barium swallow examination showing abrupt narrowing of the esophagus.

BARIUM SWALLOW EXAMINATION

For interpretation of barium swallow examination, stepwise approach should be followed as below:

- Soft tissue
- Bones
- Esophagus—width, mucosal pattern, peristalsis, filling defects
- Passage of barium from esophagus to stomach

X-ray Number 64

Barium swallow examination abrupt narrowing of the esophagus at cardio-esophageal junction **(Fig. 64)**.

Comment: Achalasia cardia

X-ray Number 65

This is a barium swallow examination **(Fig. 65)** showing passage of barium from esophagus to stomach with multiple filling defect in esophagus.

Comment: Esophageal varices

X-ray Number 66

These are the barium swallow examination of esophagus AP and lateral views **(Fig. 66)** showing constriction at the mid part of esophagus with very little amount of barium passing into stomach.

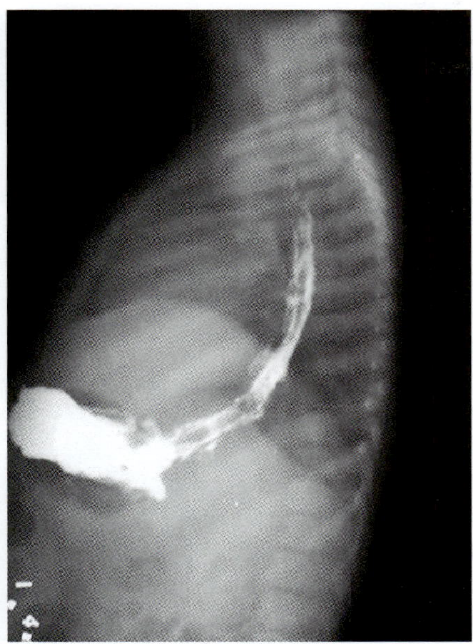

Fig. 65: Barium swallow examination showing multiple filling defect in esophagus.

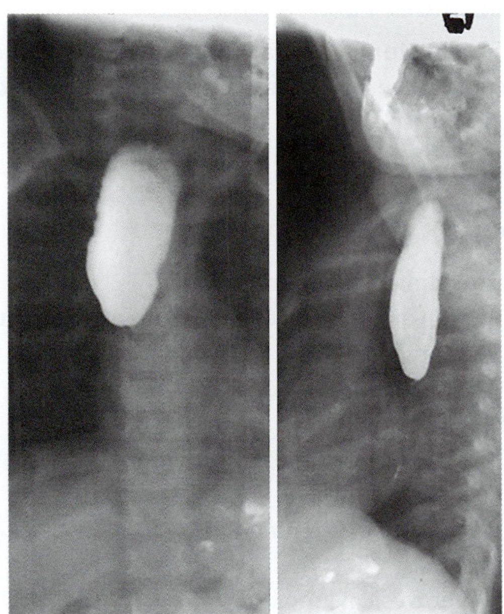

Fig. 66: Barium swallow examination of esophagus AP and lateral views showing constriction at the mid part of esophagus.

Comment: Stricture esophagus (may be due corrosive esophagitis due ingestion of corrosive agent).

BARIUM MEAL EXAMINATION

Again a systematic approach is mandatory to study a barium meal examination (and follow through).

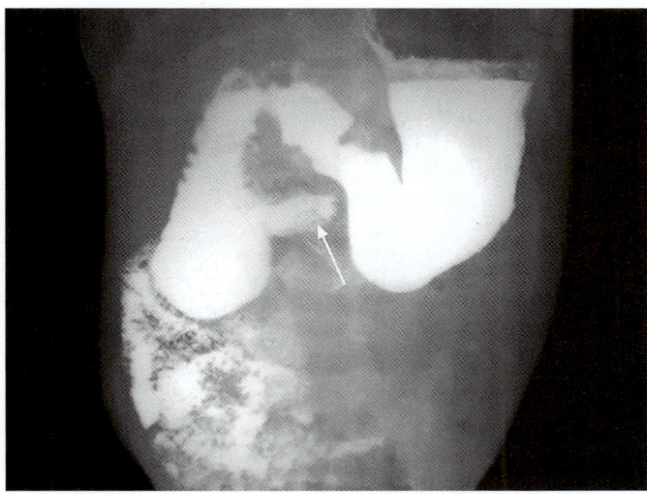

Fig. 67: Barium meal examination showing irregular margin of duodenum with an outpouching (arrow) from 2nd part, 3rd part is dilated.

Steps:

- *Stomach* (size, shape, *position, mucosal pattern, peristalsis, pylorus, and reflux of dye in esophagus)*
- *Duodenum* (cap, c-loop, and mucosal pattern)
- *Small intestines* (position, distribution, mucosal pattern, peristalsis, passage of dye, and ileocecal region)
- *Large intestines* (position, distribution, mucosal pattern, caliber, and cecal position)
- *Appendix*

X-ray Number 67

Barium meal examination **(Fig. 67)** showing normal position, size, and mucosal pattern of stomach, but irregular margin of duodenum with an outpouching (arrow) from 2nd part, 3rd part is dilated. Barium has passed to small intestines.

Comment: Duodenal diverticulum

X-ray Number 68

This is a barium meal examination **(Fig. 68)** showing distended stomach, increased rugosities of duodenal mucosa with proximal dilatation, and obstruction of passage of barium from duodenum to jejunum, producing a V-shaped deformity.

Comment: Duodenal web (Windsock sign)

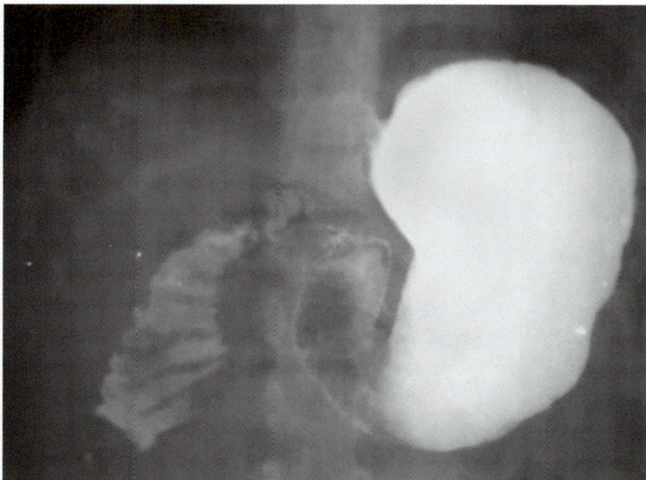

Fig. 68: Barium meal examination showing distended stomach, increased rugosities of duodenal mucosa with proximal dilatation and obstruction of passage of barium from duodenum to jejunum.

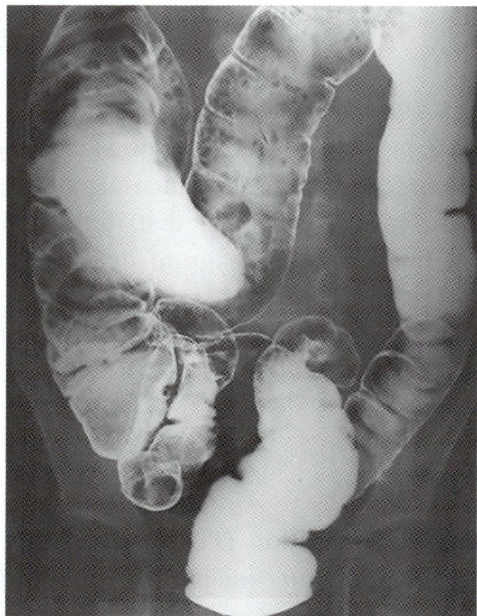

Fig. 69: Barium enema showing multiple filling defects throughout the colon.

BARIUM–ENEMA EXAMINATION

- Rectum and colon (position, haustration, dilation, mucosal pattern, and filling defects)
- Evacuation—complete or incomplete

X-ray Number 69

Barium-enema examination **(Fig. 69)** shows multiple filling defects throughout the colon.

Comment: Juvenile intestinal polyposis.

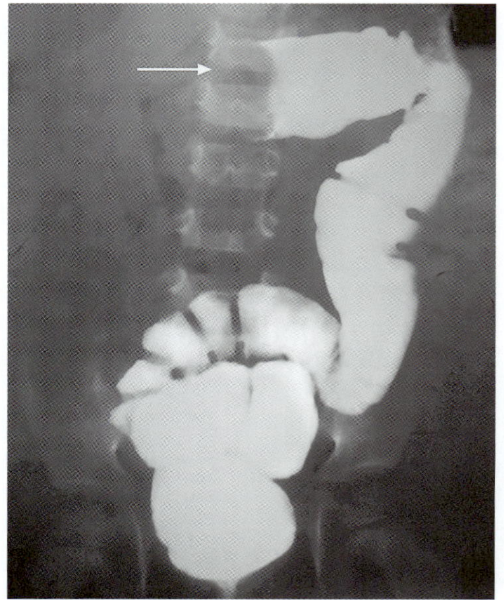

Fig. 70: Barium–enema study showing figure of 3 or claw sign.

X-ray Number 70

This is a barium-enema study **(Fig. 70)** showing obstruction in the level of transverse colon, Figure of 3, or claw sign is seen.

Diagnosis: Intussusception

IVP (IVU) EXAMINATION

- Control film of abdomen—a must
  - See the distribution of gas of stomach and intestine
  - Vertebral bodies
  - Any radiopaque shadow
- IVP at different times:
  - Kidneys (size, shape, and position)
  - Pelvicalyceal system
  - Pelviureteric (pu) junction
  - Ureters
  - Ureterovesical junction
  - Urinary bladder (position, shape, and mucosal pattern)
  - Urethra in MCU following IVP

X-ray Number 71

IVP at 15 minutes **(Fig. 71)** shows both kidneys are in normal position. Shapes and sizes with visible some pelvicalyceal system and PUJ. The dye has reached the urinary bladder, which is also normal in position, shape, and mucosal pattern.

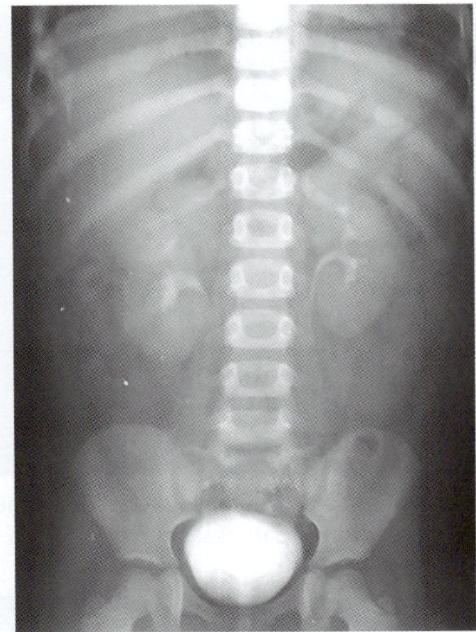

Fig. 71: Normal IVP.

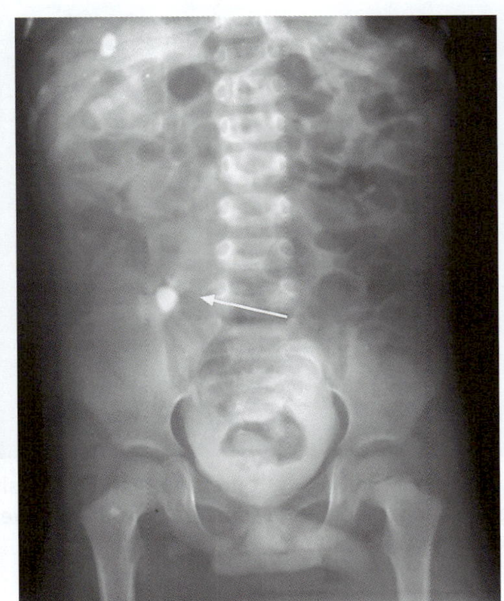

Fig. 72: IVP shows the right kidney in ectopic position.

Comment: Normal IVP though full study should be seen as well as post void film to ascertain the residual volume (best modality to measure the residual urine is USG though).

X-ray Number 72

IVP at 5 minutes shows **(Fig. 72)** the right kidney is in ectopic position at the level of pelvic brim.

Comment: Ectopic kidney right side (failure of accent of right kidney).

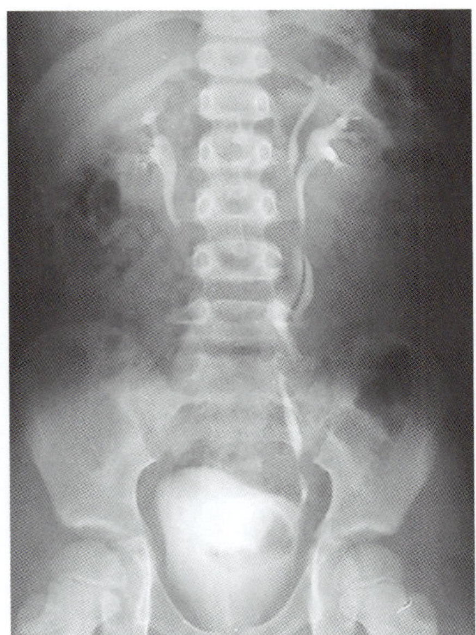

Fig. 73: IVP shows double ureters on left kidney.

X-ray Number 73

IVP at 15 minutes shows **(Fig. 73)** normal position of both kidneys but there are double ureters on left kidney. Urinary bladder appears normal.

Comment: Double ureters of left kidney

X-ray Number 74

IVP shows **(Fig. 74)** clubbing of pelvicalyceal system right kidney due to early hydronephrotic changes.

Comment: Right-sided hydronephrosis.

X-ray Number 75

This is the IVP control film **(Fig. 75)** showing radiopaque shadows both kidneys simulating pelvicalyceal systems.

Comment: Staghorn calculi.

X-ray Number 76

This is IVP showing **(Fig. 76)** a small radiopaque shadow on right side at the level of upper part of sacrum.

Comment: Ureteric stone in right ureter

MICTURATING CYSTOURETHROGRAM

- *Bladder (size, shape, position, mucosal pattern, diverticuli, and UV junction)*
- *Ureter—if visible in reflux grades?*
- *Urethra—mucosa and width*
- *Residual urine*

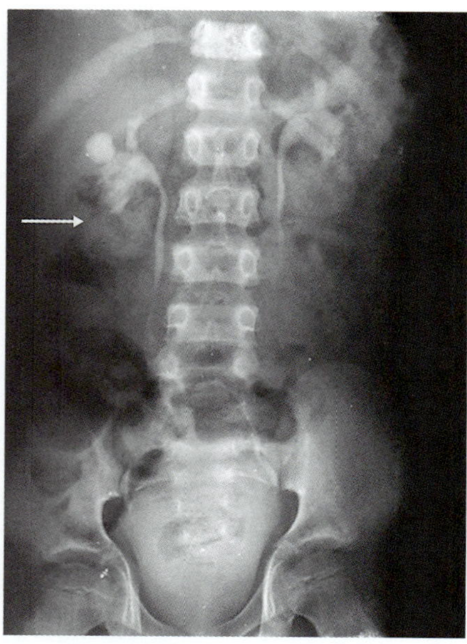

Fig. 74: IVP shows clubbing of pelvicalyceal system due to early hydronephrotic changes.

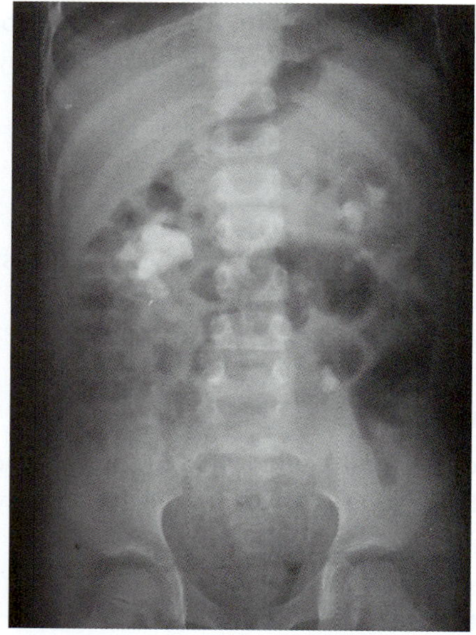

Fig. 75: IVP control film showing radiopaque shadows both kidneys

X-ray Number 77

This is micturating cystourethrogram (MCUG) showing **(Fig. 77)** distended urinary bladder with some out pouching (diverticula) with irregular mucosal pattern. The proximal part of urethra appears dilate, possibly due to obstruction distally.

Diagnosis: Posterior urethral valve with vesical diverticuli.

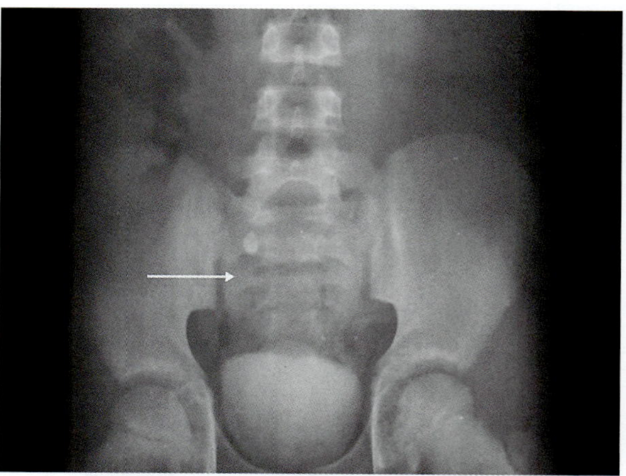

Fig. 76: IVP showing a small radiopaque shadow at the level of upper part of sacrum.

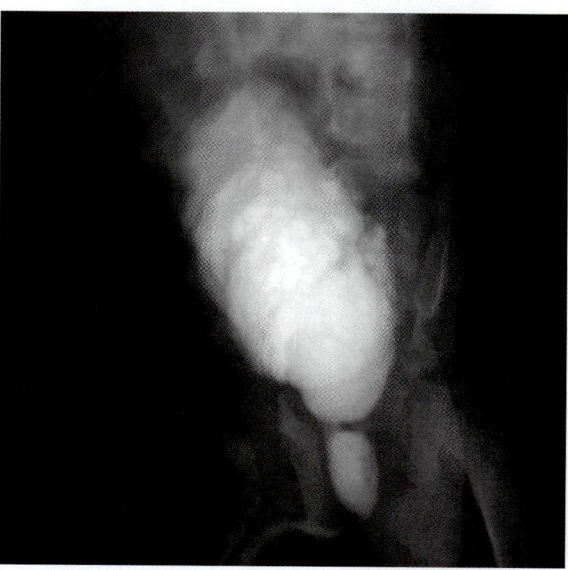

Fig. 77: This is micturating cystourethrogram (MCUG) showing distended urinary bladder with some out pouching (diverticula) with irregular mucosal pattern.

X-ray Number 78

This is MCU **(Figs. 78A and B)** showing dilated tortuous ureters on both sides with dilated pelvicalyceal systems also.

Comment: Grade V vesicoureteral reflux (VUR).

X-RAYS OF NEWBORN

X-ray Number 79

X-ray abdomen AP view **(Fig. 79)** in supine posture showing radiolucent shadows (Gas) within the walls of visualized intestines.

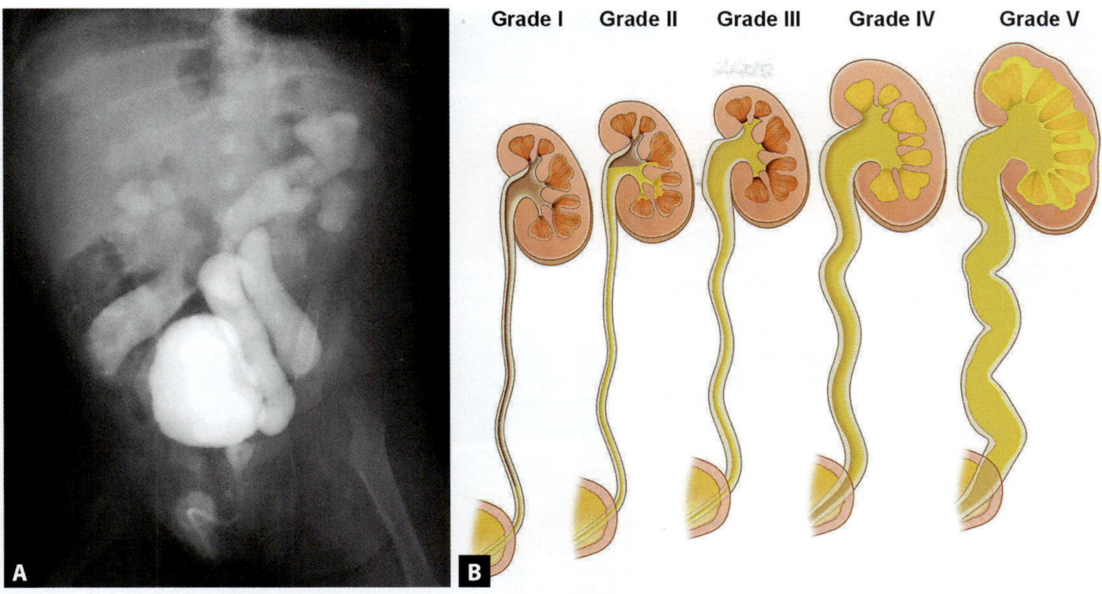

Figs. 78A and B: MCU showing dilated tortuous ureters with dilated pelvicalyceal systems.

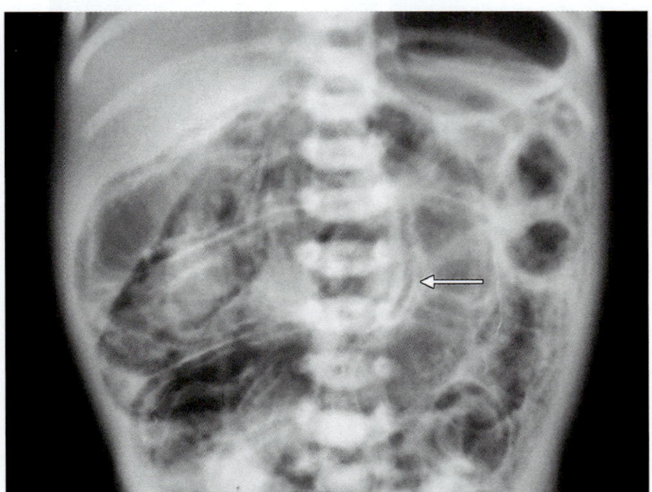

Fig. 79: X-ray abdomen showing gas within the walls of visualized intestines.

Comment: Pneumatosis intestinalis possibly due to necrotizing enterocolitis (NEC).

Cross-table lateral decubitus films yield better visualization of pneumatosis and free air within peritoneum.

X-ray Number 80

Different stages of NEC (free gas under the diaphragm, football sign) **(Fig. 80)**.

X-ray Number 81

Portal venous gas in stage 2 of NEC **(Fig. 81)**.

X-ray Number 82

Invertogram showing high anorectal anomaly **(Fig. 82)**.

But nowadays this view is obsolete A prone cross-table lateral view is newer as it is comfortable to the babies (X-ray 86).

X-ray Number 83

See **Figure 83**.

X-ray Number 84

This is X-ray of pelvis and upper part of lower limbs of a newborn **(Fig. 84)** showing alternate longitudinal bands of radiopacities and radiolucencies at the distal femoral metaphyseal ends, simulating Celery stalk appearance.

Diagnosis: Congenital rubella

X-ray Number 85

X-rays both upper and lower limbs AP views **(Fig. 85)** show panosteitis of long bones with looser zones (radiolucent bands at the metaphyses). There is periosteal elevation along with symmetrical erosion at the medial aspects of proximal ends of both tibia (Wimberger's sign).

Diagnosis: Congenital syphilis

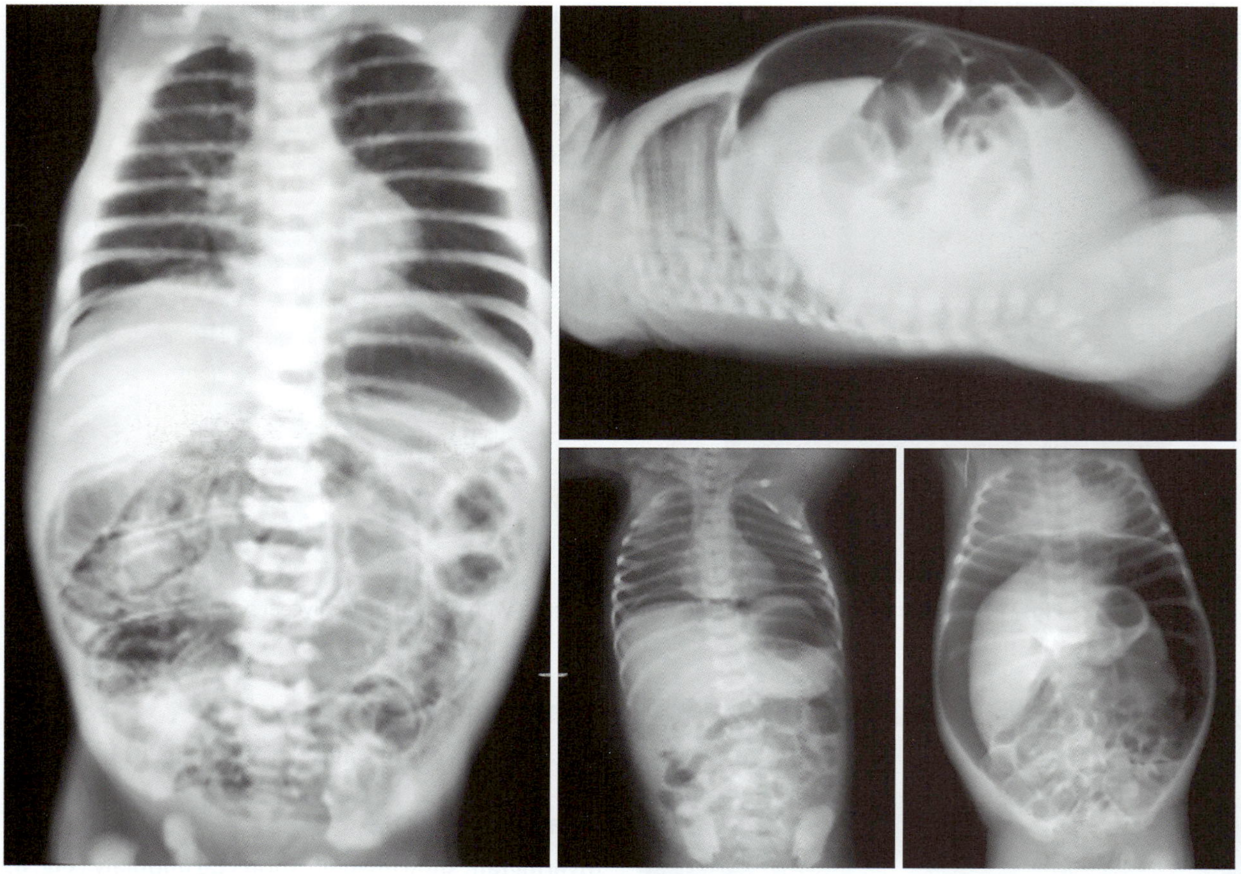

Fig. 80: Different stages of NEC.

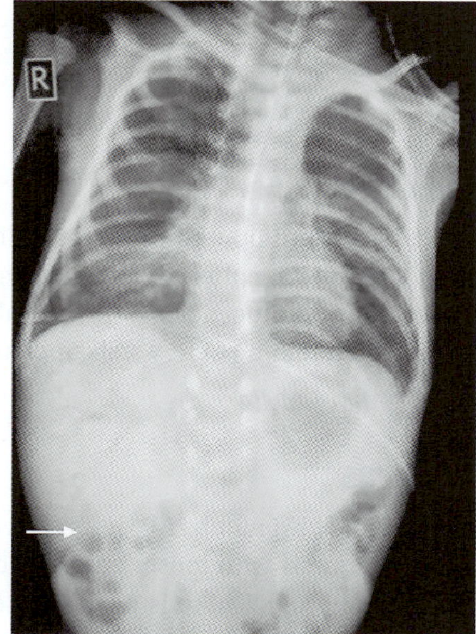

Fig. 81: Stage 2 NEC.

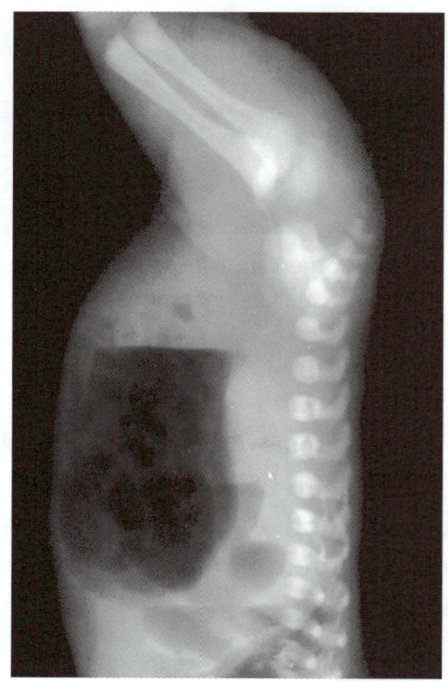

Fig. 82: Invertogram showing anorectal anomaly.

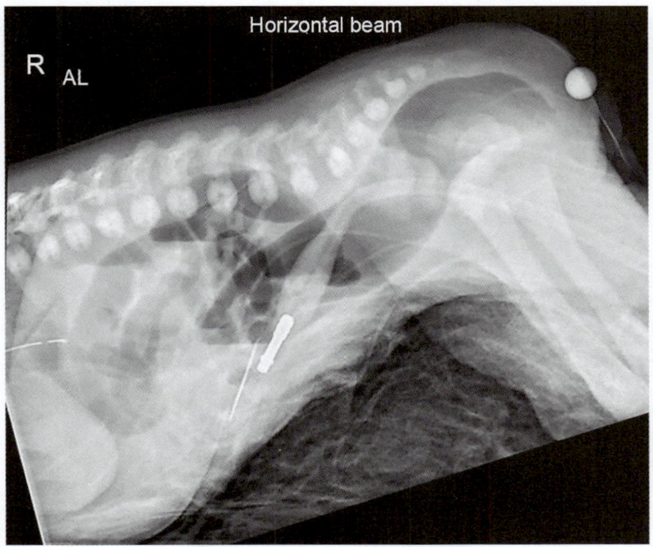

Fig. 83: High anorectal anomaly

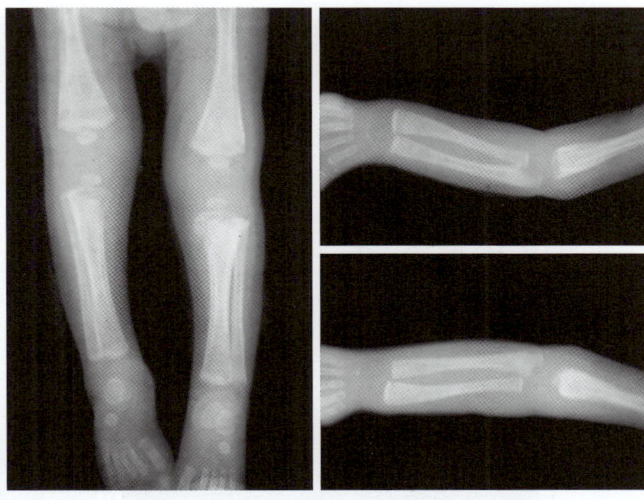

Fig. 85: X-rays both upper and lower limbs showing periosteal elevation along with symmetrical erosion at the medial aspects of proximal ends of both tibia (Wimberger's sign).

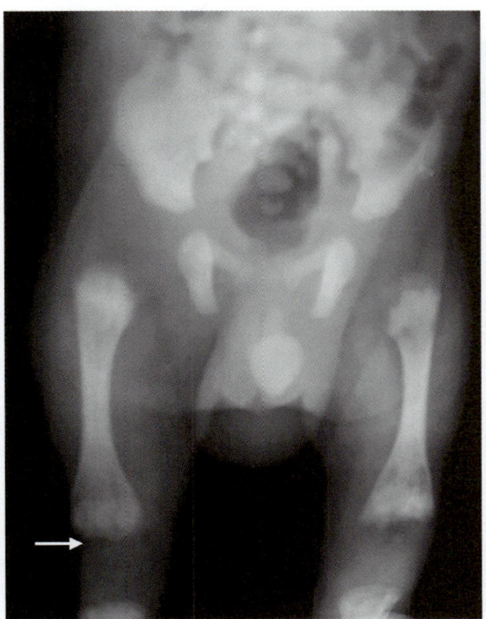

Fig. 84: Lower limbs of a newborn showing alternate longitudinal bands of radiopacities and radiolucencies at the distal femoral metaphyseal ends.

Initially just after birth of a newborn, all these changes may not be there, but within 8 weeks, florid pictures are visible if left untreated. On the contrary, the changes of congenital rubella are evident in early neonatal days and changes disappear with time.

X-ray Number 86

This is an AP view of neck and chest **(Fig. 86)** showing a huge soft tissue shadows on left side of neck slightly encroaching upper part of left side of chest.

Comment: Cystic hygroma left side of neck.

X-ray Number 87

X-ray neck and chest lateral view **(Fig. 87)** shows the radiopaque rubber tube not passing into distal part of esophagus, but gas shadows are visible in abdomen.

Diagnosis: Esophageal atresia with tracheoesophageal fistula.

X-ray Number 88

X-ray chest PA view **(Fig. 88)** shows multiple small radiopaque shadows scattered throughout the lung fields, simulating large military shadows.

Comment: Congenital tuberculosis

Miliary shadows, or miliary nodules, are usually 1–3 mm in diameter, but can be larger in some cases. In 10% of cases, the nodules may be greater than 3 mm in diameter.

X-ray Number 89

This is a barium enema examination **(Fig. 89)** showing very small caliber colon all through.

Comment: Microcolon (total colonic aganglionosis)

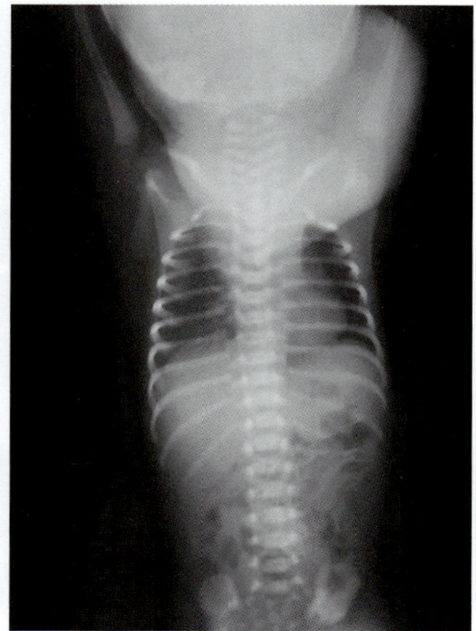

Fig. 86: AP view of neck and chest showing a huge soft tissue shadows on left side of neck.

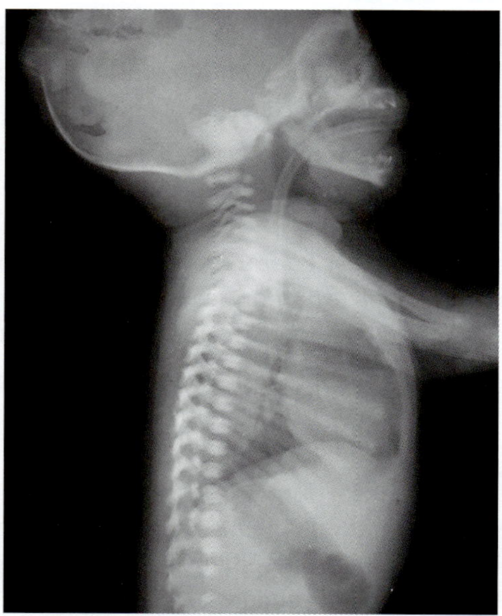

Fig. 87: X-ray neck and chest lateral view shows the radiopaque rubber tube not passing into distal part of esophagus.

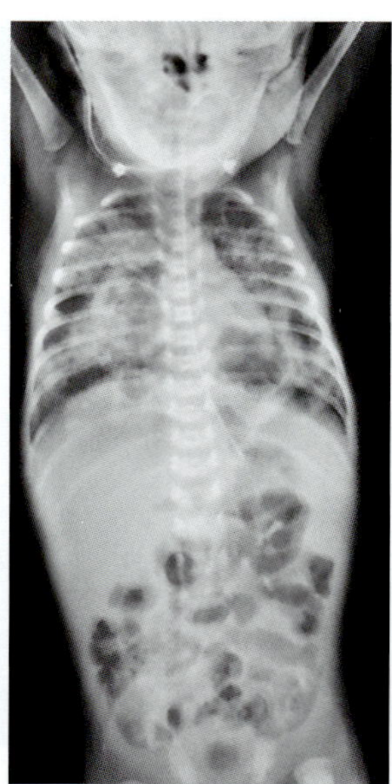

Fig. 88: X-ray chest PA view shows multiple small radiopaque shadows simulating large military shadows.

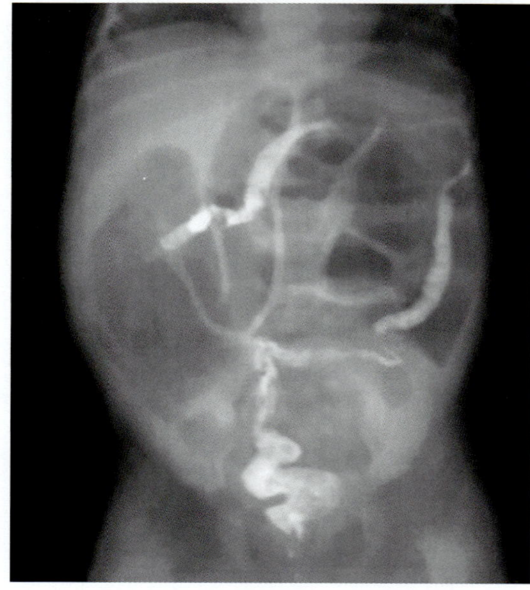

Fig. 89: Barium enema examination showing very small caliber colon.

If there is proximal atresia or obstruction, less amount of succus entericus enters the distal bowel loop, hence the distal segment gets atretic or hypoplastic.

MRI BRAIN

Introduction:

- MRI is a scan utilizing strong magnetic fields and radio waves to produce detailed images inside body.
- MRI scanner is a large tube that contains powerful magnets.
- MRI is perhaps the best application of superconductivity which directly helped people across the globe.
- MRI is increasingly being appreciated as an alternative to CT, not only for offering three-dimensional (3-D) imaging without radiation exposure at only slightly inferior spatial resolution, but also for its superior

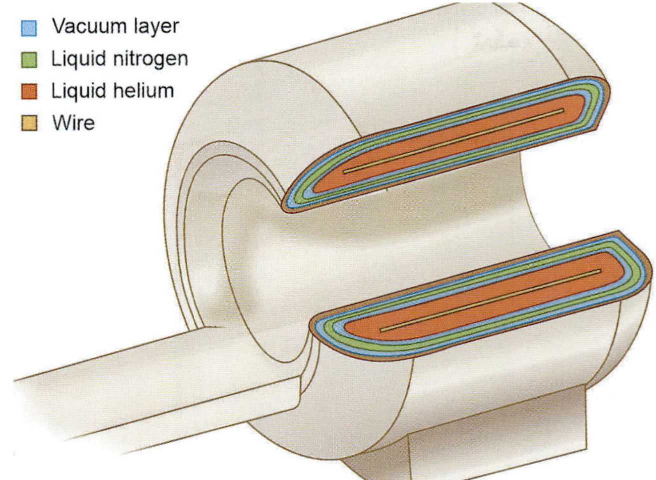

Fig. 90: MRI machine structure.

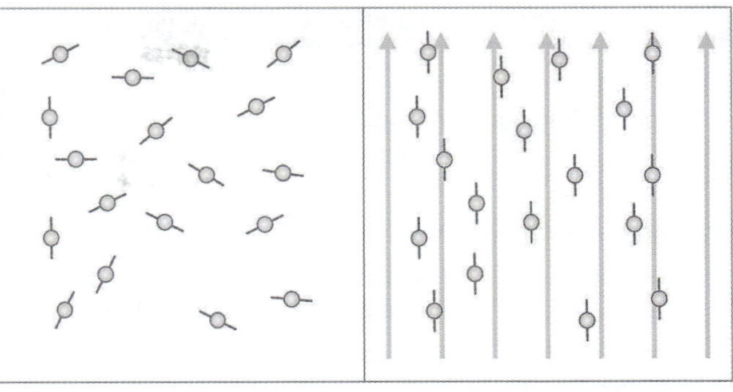

Fig. 91: Radio waves generated by electromagnetic fields > realign hydrogen atoms those naturally exist in our body.

soft-tissue contrast and exclusive morpho-functional imaging.

- Keeping an MRIs magnetic current superconductive requires extreme cold **(Fig. 90)**. That is where helium comes in: With a boiling point of minus 452°F, liquid helium is the coldest element on Earth. Pumped inside an MRI magnet, helium lets the current travel resistance-free.

History of MRI:

- In 1937–1938, Professor Isidor Isaac Rabi sent a beam of molecules through a magnetic field and found nuclei emit radio waves at specific frequencies. Professor Rabi was awarded Nobel Prize in Physics in 1944.
- Felix Bloch and Edward Mills Purcell subsequently extended this work to solids and liquids—they both were awarded Nobel Prize in 1952 (Physics)
- MR relaxation times could be used to distinguish cancer from healthy tissue (Damadian, 1971)
- Paul Lauterbur (1971) demonstrated image from the frequency signals
- First human image was produced in 1977 (Nobel Prize in 2003)
- Raymond Damadian is the inventor of the first magnetic resonance scanning machine. Damadian, a physician, performed the first full-body scan of a human being in 1977.
- As per the International System of Units (often abbreviated to SI*), one Tesla is equal to the one weber of magnetic induction per square meter of area.*
- The SI unit of magnetic induction is named in honor of the Serbian-American engineer and inventor Nikola Tesla, upon the Slovenian inventor and electrical engineer France Avcin.
- Now, MRI machines are available from 1.5 to 7.0 Tesla.

Working principles:

- No radiation
- Radio waves generated by electromagnetic fields > realign hydrogen atoms those naturally exist in our body **(Fig. 91)**.
- As these hydrogen atoms return to their usual alignment, they emit different amount of energy depending upon type of the tissue they are in.
- The scanner captures this energy and creates a picture using this information.
- In most of the MRI unit, the magnetic field is produced by passing an electric current through wire coils. The other coils are inside the machine surrounding the patient lying on table.
- A computer processes the signals and creates series of images, each of which shows a thin slice of the body.

Paramagnetic materials are attracted by external magnetic fields whereas diamagnetic materials are repelled. Air is paramagnetic.

Advantages of MRI brain **(Table 1)**:

- No radiation exposure risk
- Images easily acquired in multiple planes (axial, sagittal, coronal, or oblique) **(Figs. 92-95)**
- Superior soft tissue contrast in comparison to CT
- MRA may be done even without contrast material unlike CT
- Advance techniques of MRI like diffusion, spectroscopy, perfusion studies are added advantages in comparison to CT

TABLE 1: Comparison of CT and MRI.

	CT	*MRI*
Principle of imaging	Absorption of X-ray	Magnetic resonance phenomenon
Radiation exposure	Yes	No
Tissue resolution	Good (physical information)	Excellent (scientific information)
Dynamic diagnostic information	Difficult	Easy
Influence by bone, air	Yes	No
Image plane	Transverse plane	Arbitrary section plane
Examination noise	No	Yes
Examination time	Short (5–10 mins)	Long (15–30 mins)
Preferred area	Lung, abdomen, bones, etc.	Brain, spinal cord, lungs

- Functional MRI can pick up active part of brain during certain activities
- Tissue resolution is far superior except in bones (but marrow can be seen)
- Provides better differentiation than CT for water, fat, iron, and blood
- It can pick up tumors as small as 0.3 mm
- Provides high-resolution details of posterior fossa, base of skull, and orbit than CT

Disadvantages of MRI brain:

- More expensive than CT
- Takes longer time for acquisition
- High noise may cause discomfort to children
- More claustrophobic than CT as more enclosed bore (but not in open MRI)
- MRI images are subject to unique artifacts that must be recognized
- MRI scan may not be safe in patients with metal implants and foreign bodies.

Items to be avoided during MRI procedure:

- Metals and electronic items to be avoided in examination room, as it may cause burn, interfere magnetic field and malfunction of items carried.
- Jewelry, watches, credit cards, and hearing aids
- Pins, hairpins, metal zippers, and metallic items
- Removable dental work

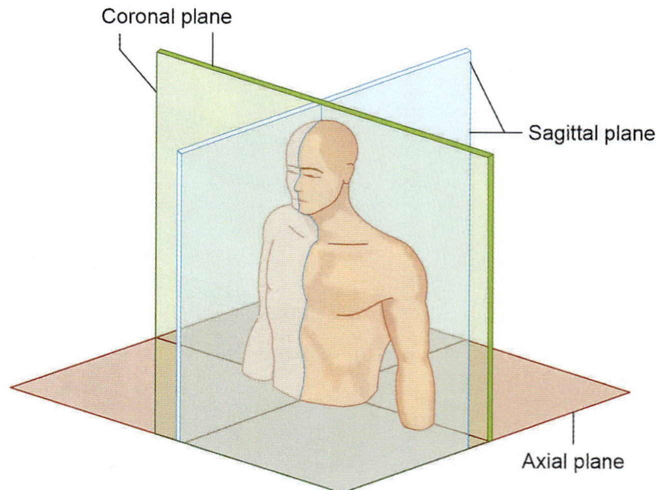

Fig. 92: Planes of MRI brain.

- Pens, pocket knives, and eyeglasses
- Body piercings
- Mobile phones, electronic watches, and tracking devices
- In majority of cases, MR examination is safe for patients with metal implants, except a very few.
- People with following implants should not be scanned until evaluated properly.
- Some cochlear implants
- Some types of clips used in brain aneurysm
- Some type of metal coils in vessels (PDA banding)
- Some older cardiac defibrillators and pacemakers
- Vagal nerve stimulators

Relative contraindications:

- Agitated/uncooperative patients or with uncontrolled movement disorder
- Hugely obese patients who cannot fit into MRI tube
- Claustrophobic patients
- Critically ill patients requiring ventilation support and IV pump (few ventilators are MRI compatible or may use pediatric MRI length dual-limb breathing circuit) but IV pumps cannot be used.
- MRI conditional Moduflex Bain-type circuit is used during MRI study.

Terminology in MRI:

- Images described by *intensity*
- Hyperintense means bright
- Hypointense means dark

MRI sequences:

- T1 and T2-weighted sequences **(Fig. 104)**

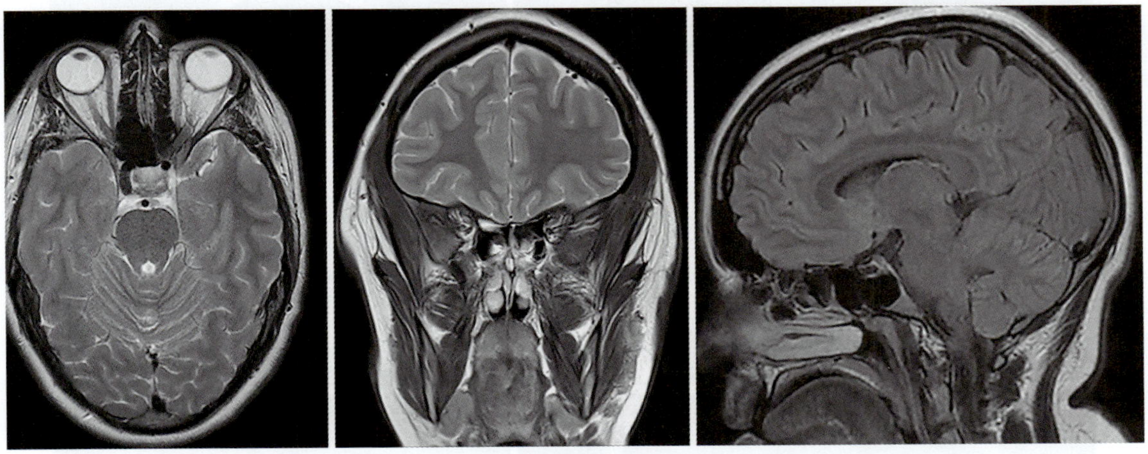

Axial

Coronal

Sagittal

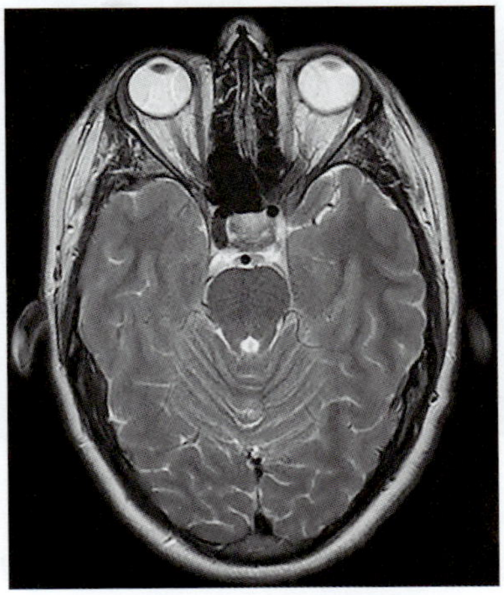

Axial

Right

Left

Fig. 93: Axial section for MRI brain.

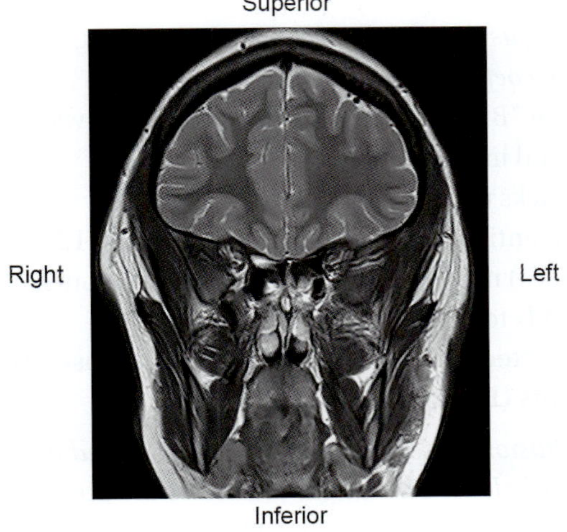

Fig. 94: Coronal view of MRI brain.

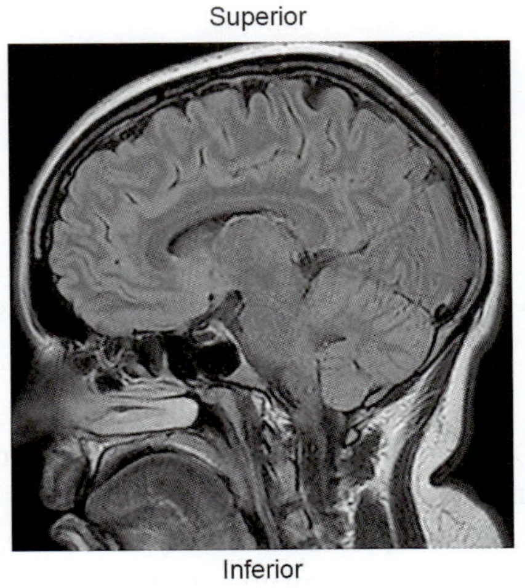

Fig. 95: Sagittal section of MRI brain.

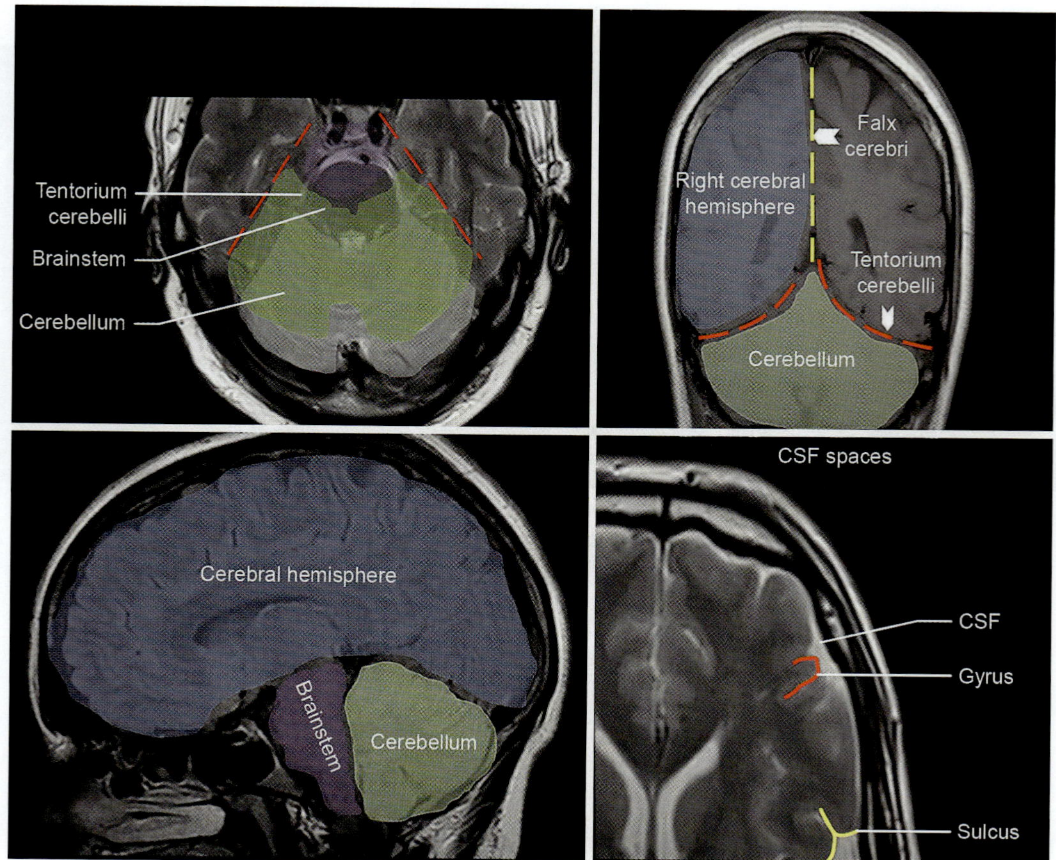

Fig. 96: Anatomy of brain.

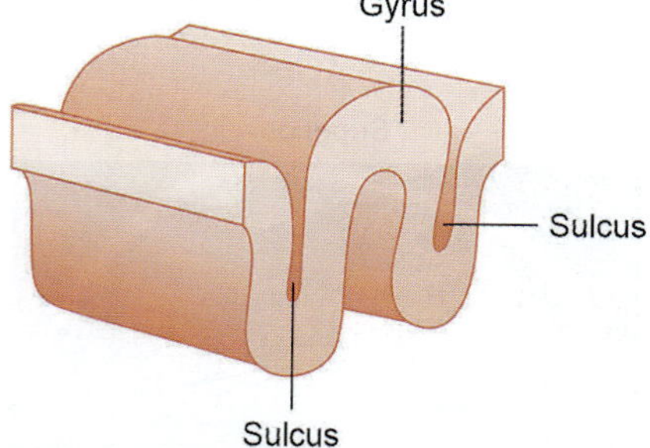

Fig. 97: Schematic representation of sulci and gyri.

- *On T1:* White matter appears white and gray matter appears grey and CSF is black
- *On T2:* It is the opposite. CSF is hyperintense, thalamus is darker than the corpus striatum (putamen and caudate) which are darker than cortical gray

- *FLAIR (fluid-attenuation inversion recovery)* **(Fig. 107)**:
  - Commonly used sequence
  - Similar to T2, but the fluid is darker or "suppressed"
  - Useful for areas of edema or inflammation
  - Used to identify plaques in multiple sclerosis (especially periventricular)

DWI (diffusion-weighted image) and ADC (apparent diffusion coefficient) **(Fig. 105)**:

- These "Blocky" images show how easily water moves around in the tissues.
- WI picks up very small and early infarcts.
- Conventional MRI sequences (T1 and T2 weighted images) may not detect infarct before 6 hours.
- CT fails to detect small infarct.
- Restricted diffusion occurs in strokes, abscesses, and tumors **(Fig. 106)**.

DTI (diffusion tensor imaging): (Figs. 107A and B)

Hydrocephalous: The lateral ventricles are grossly dilated along with 3rd ventricle **(Fig. 108)**. Changes are suggestive of hydrocephalous.

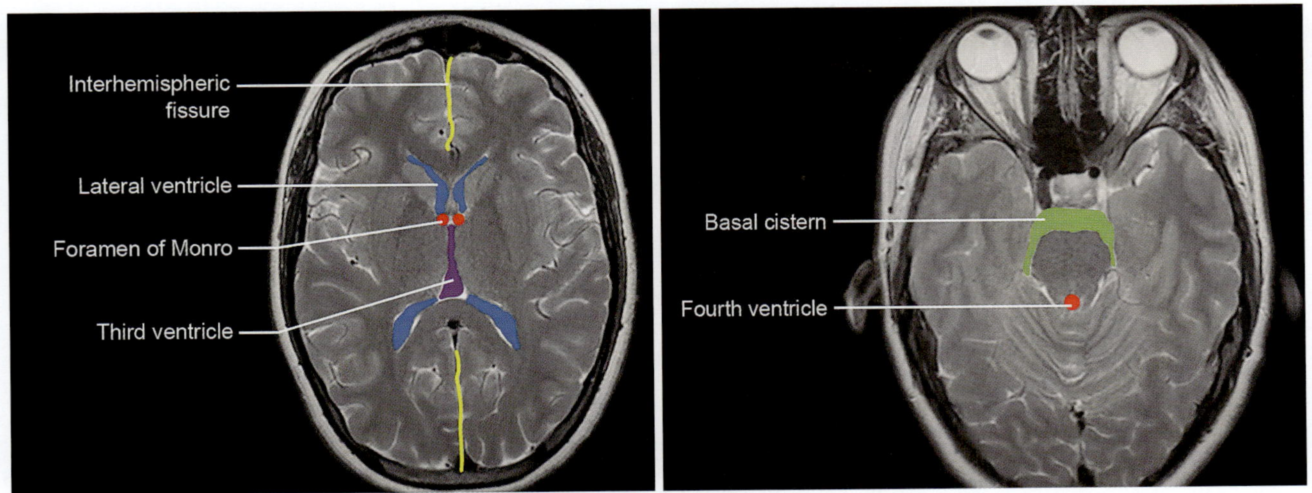

Fig. 98: Ventricles in brain.

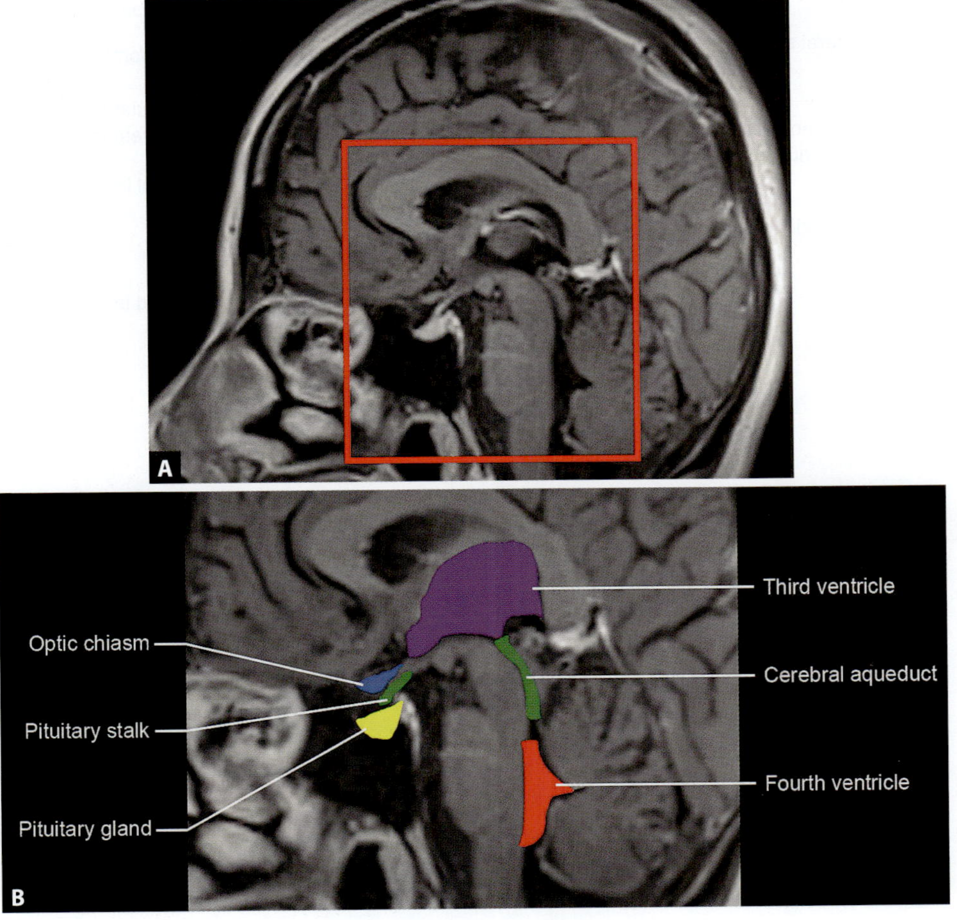

Figs. 99A and B: Sagittal view of brain.

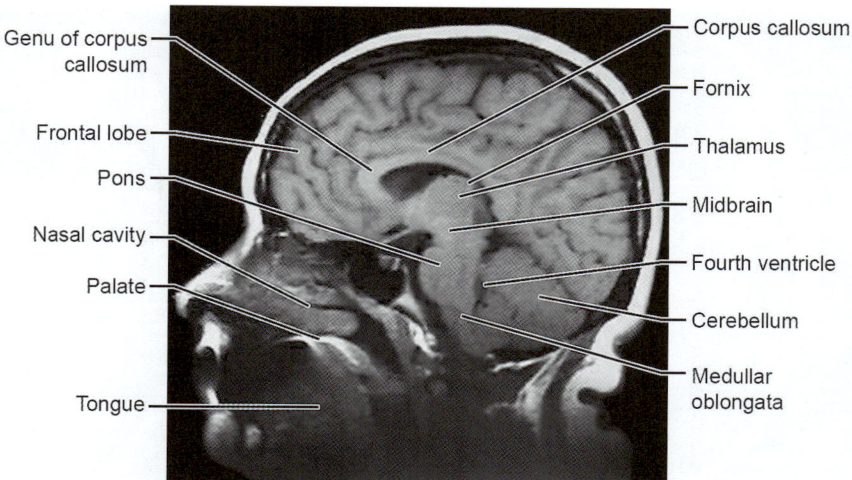

Fig. 100: Parts of brain in sagittal view.

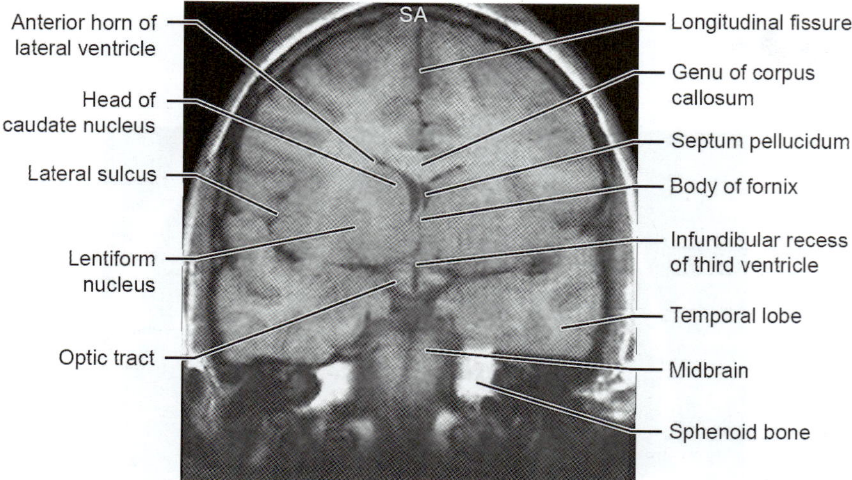

Fig. 101: Parts of brain in coronal view.

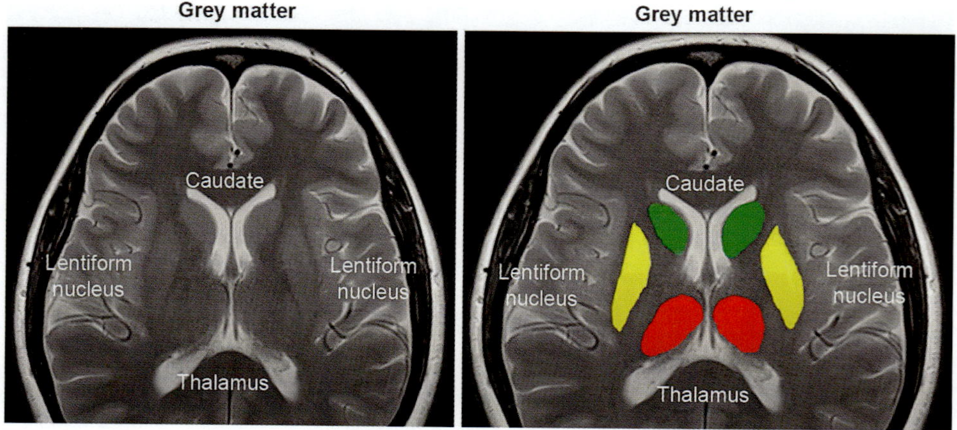

Fig. 102: Parts of midbrain.

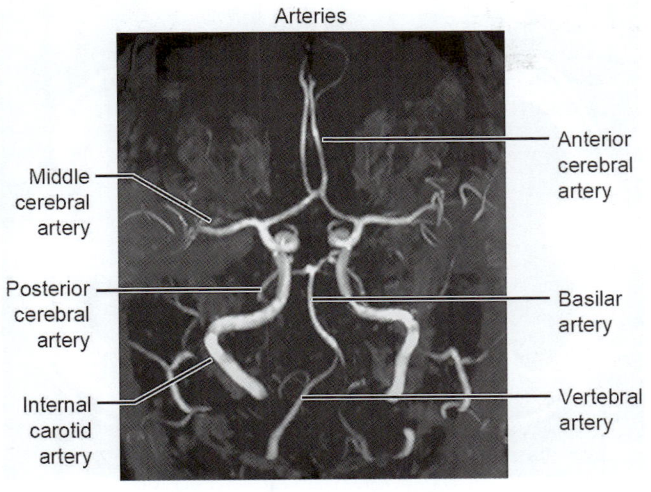

Fig. 103: Vascular system of brain.

Lissencephaly: Surface of brain parenchyma is very smooth with little number of sulci and gyri in comparison to normal brain surface **(Figs. 96, 97 and 109)**.

Open lip schizencephaly:

- *Open lip:* The cleft walls are separated and filled with CSF **(Fig. 110)**
- *Closed lip:* The cleft walls are in apposition **(Fig. 111)**

Closed lip schizencephaly:

Porencephalic cyst: The term porencephaly **(Fig. 112)** is taken to mean the following: a cystic lesion of the brain due to an encephaloclastic insult (e.g., intrauterine infections and ischemia), lined by white matter, which communicates with the ventricles and/or the subarachnoid space.

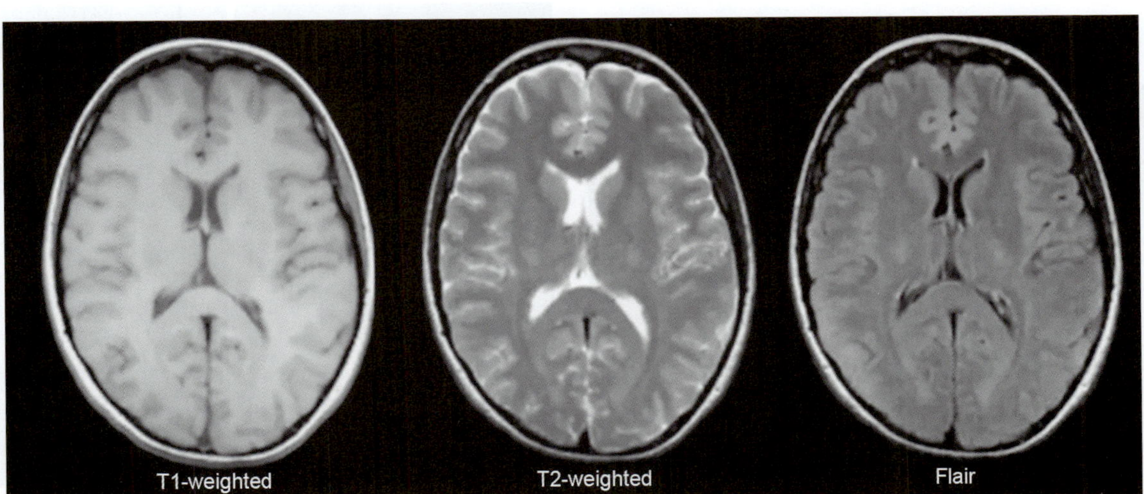

Fig. 104: MRI sequences.

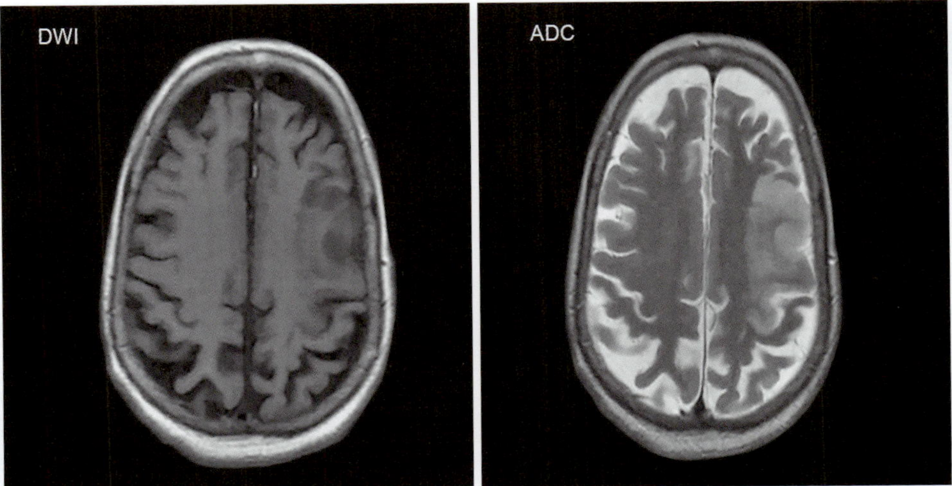

Fig. 105: DWI (diffusion-weighted image) and ADC (apparent diffusion coefficient).

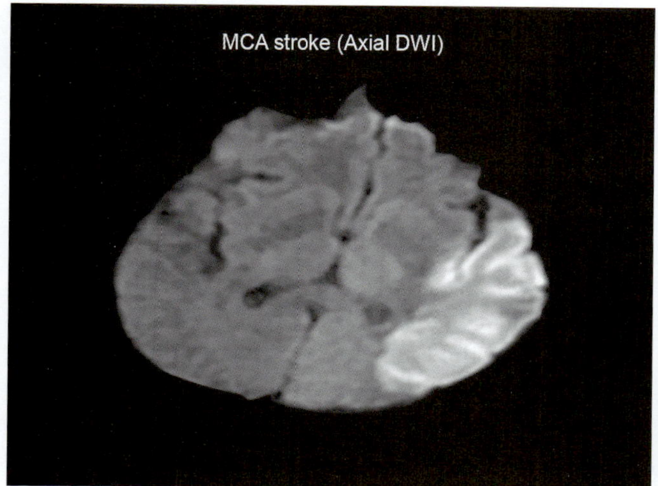

Fig. 106: Middle cerebral artery stroke.

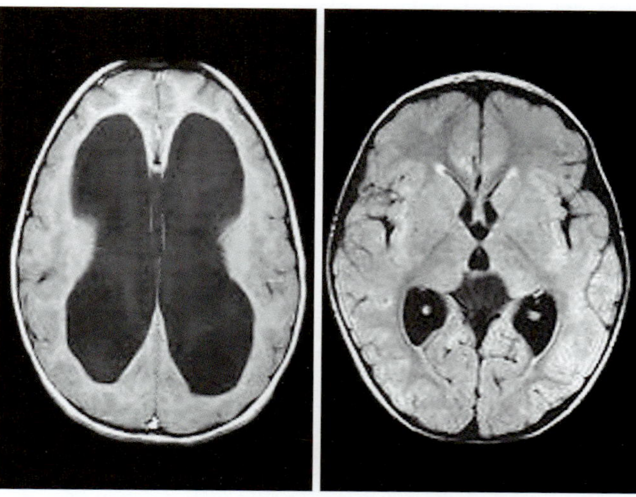

Fig. 108: Grossly dilated lateral and 3rd ventricle.

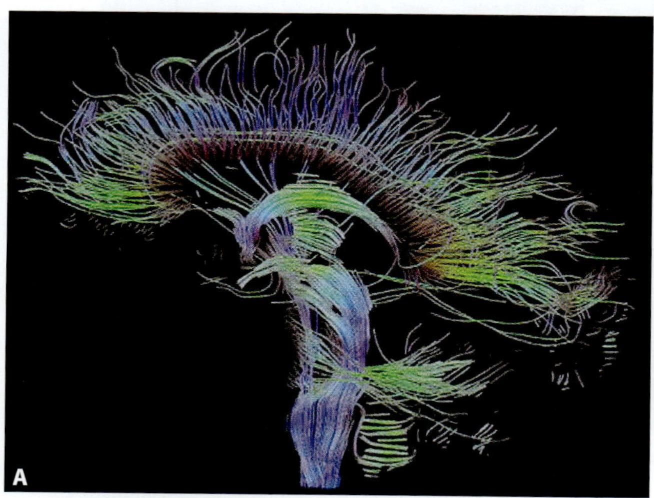

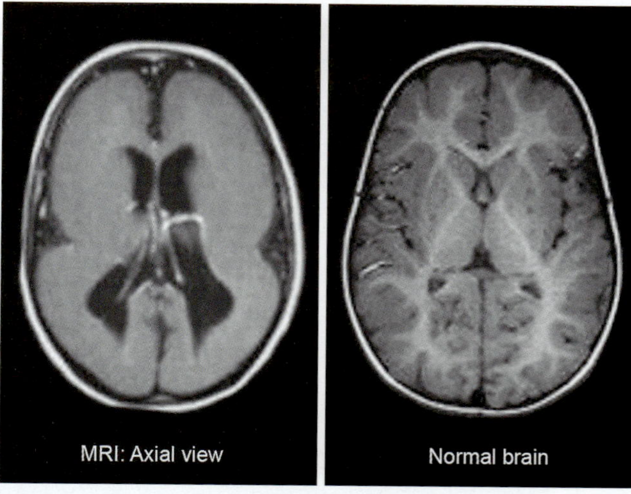

Fig. 109: With little number of sulci and gyri in comparison to normal brain surface.

Figs. 1107A and B: DTI (Diffusion tensor imaging)

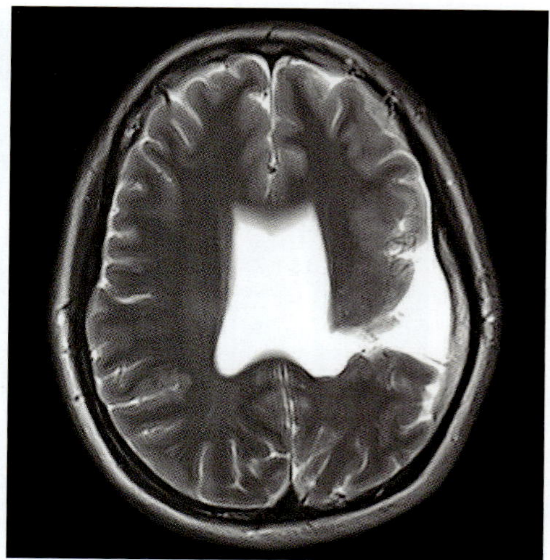

Fig. 110: Open lip schizencephaly.

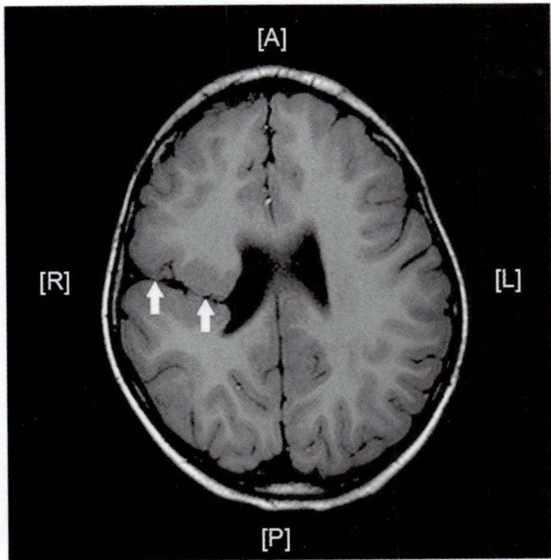

Fig. 111: Closed lip schizencephaly.

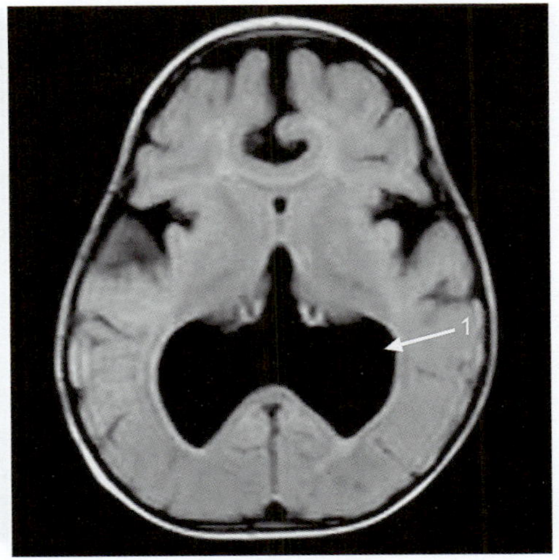

Fig. 113: Congenital brain malformation resulting from incomplete separation of the two hemispheres.

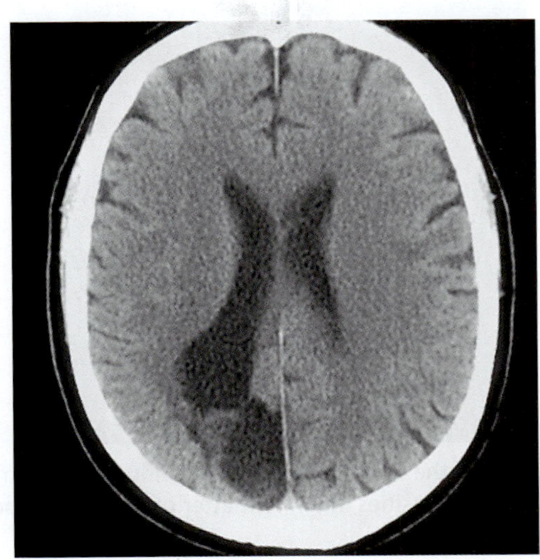

Fig. 112: A cystic lesion lined by white matter, which communicates with the ventricles.

Holoprosencephaly:

- Holoprosencephaly (HPE) **(Fig. 113)** is a rare congenital brain malformation resulting from incomplete separation of the two hemispheres.
- Classically three subtypes have been recognized, however additional entities are now included in the spectrum of the disease. The three main subtypes, in order of decreasing severity are:
  1. Alobar holoprosencephaly
  2. Semilobar holoprosencephaly
  3. Lobar holoprosencephaly

White matter disease:

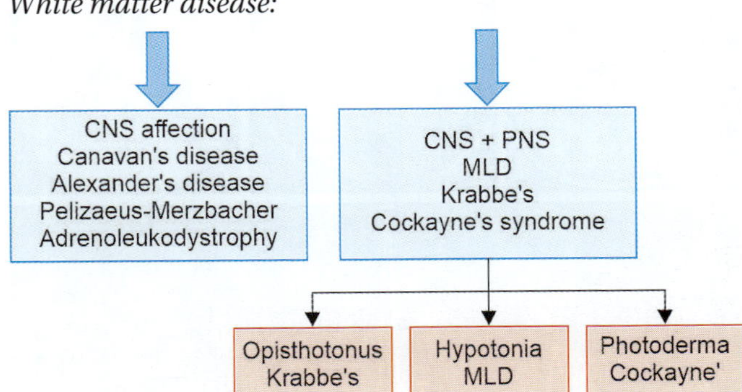

Alexandar disease: It is characterized by encephalopathy, failure to thrive, macrocephaly, motor delay, and seizures.

There are hyperintense signal from both frontal lobes.

Atrophy of medulla and upper cervical cord: *chipmunk sign* **(Fig. 114).**

Canavan disease: This is a leukodystrophy clinically characterized by megalencephaly, severe mental and neurological deficits, and blindness. There are hyperintense signals in white matter throughout the brain particularly occipital lobes **(Figs. 115A to D)**.

MR spectroscopy: Markedly elevated NAA and NAA: creatine ratio are pathognomonic for the condition.

This can be remembered using the mnemonic *CaNAAvan.*

Adrenoleukodystrophy: MRI of the brain **(Fig. 116)** demonstrates confluent and symmetric bilateral hyper-intensities in white matter of the parieto-occipital regions,

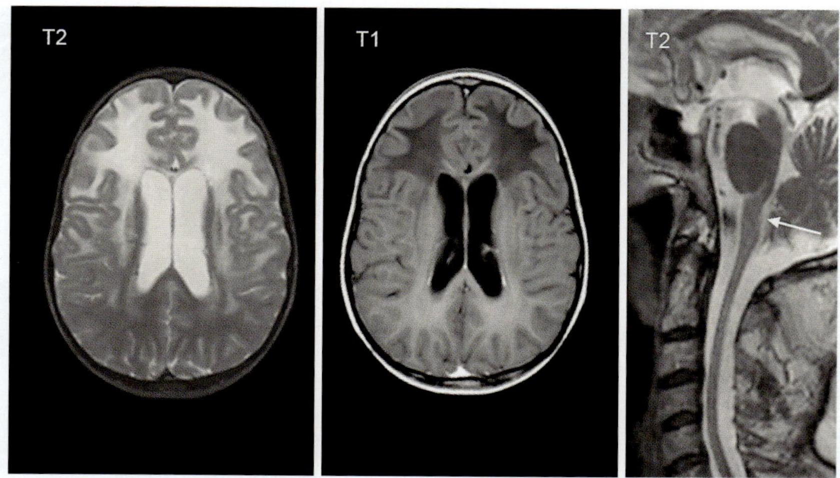

Fig. 114: Atrophy of medulla and upper cervical cord: Chipmunk sign.

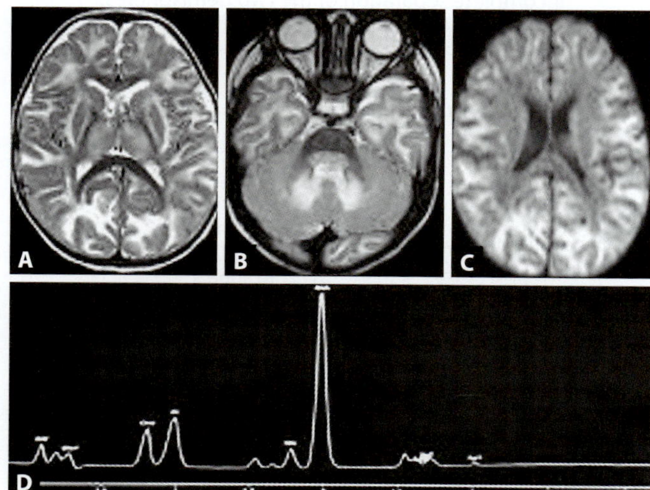

Figs. 115A to D: MRI shows hyperintense signals in white matter throughout the brain particularly occipital lobes.

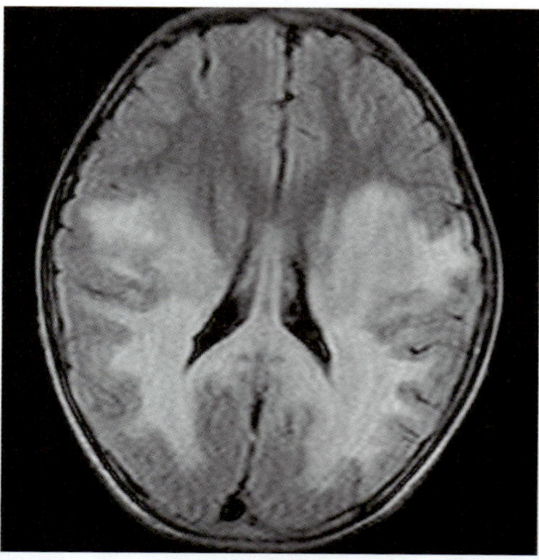

Fig. 116: MRI of the brain demonstrates confluent and symmetric bilateral hyperintensities in white matter of the parieto-occipital regions.

corpus callosum, acoustic radiation, inferior colliculus, lateral lemniscus, pons, cerebellar peduncle, etc. These dysfunctions are related to excessive accumulation of very long chain fatty acid (VLCFA) in tissues and plasma.

Clinically the child presents with fever, gait disturbance, and visual loss.

Metachromatic leukodystrophy: This is peri-atrial and to a lesser extent frontal horns leukodystrophy as well as periventricular perivenular sparing results in "*tigroid pattern*" **(Fig. 117)**.

Serum/urine arylsulfatase A levels: Reduced

Metachromatic leukodystrophy (MLD) is the most common hereditary (autosomal recessive) leukodystrophy and is one of the lysosomal storage disorders.

Dysmyelination refers to malformed and defective myelin sheath as opposed to the destruction of previously normal myelin that is seen in demyelination.

Pelizaeus-Merzbacher disease: Pelizaeus–Merzbacher disease (PMD) is an X-linked *leukodystrophy* which is characterized by **(Figs. 118A and B)** an arrest in myelin development.

Clinical presentation:

Patients may present with:

- Pendular eye movements (nystagmus)
- Hypotonia
- Pyramidal disease
- Ataxia

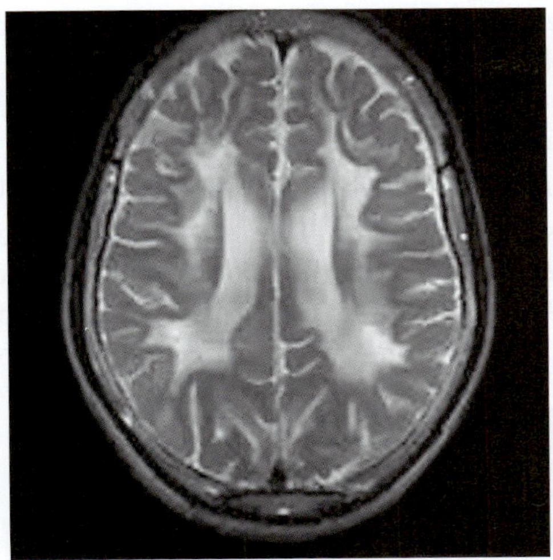

Fig. 117: MRI brain showing peri-atrial as periventricular perivenular sparing results in *"tigroid pattern"*.

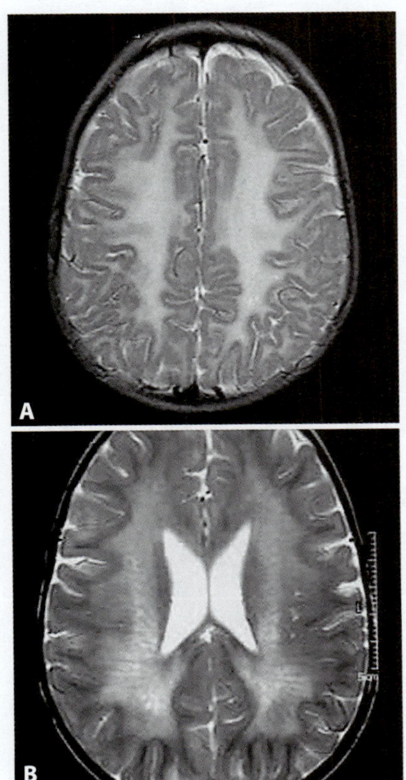

Fig. 118A and B: MRI brain showing arrest in myelin development.

Band heterotopia: Subcortical band heterotopia is a condition in which nerve cells (neurons) do not move (migrate) to their proper locations in the fetal brain during early development (heterotopia means "out of place") **(Fig. 119)**.

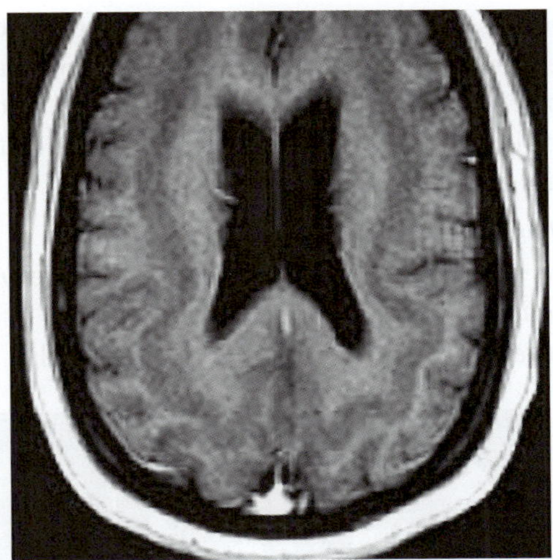

Fig. 119: MRI brain showing cerebral cortex is distributed in a well-organized and multilayered way.

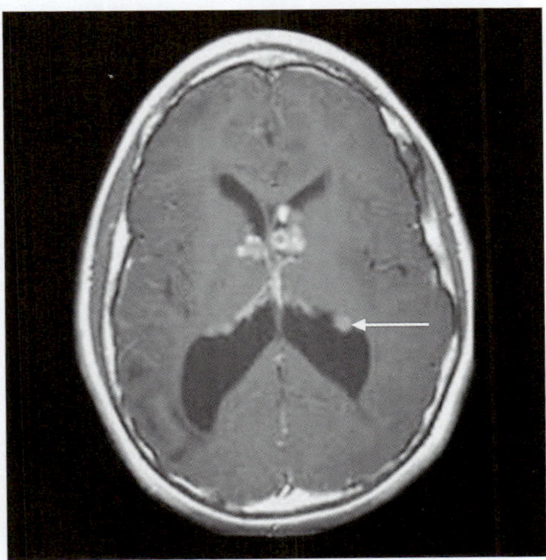

Fig. 120: MRI shows cortical or subependymal tubers.

Normally, the neurons that make up the outer surface of the brain (cerebral cortex) are distributed in a well-organized and multilayered way.

Brain develops from the core outward. Each migrating neuron, before arriving at its own predetermined site in the cortex, must travel outward through all the neurons that *have migrated and settled.*

Band heterotopia, also known as double cortex syndrome, is a form of diffuse *gray matter heterotopia* affecting *almost only women.*

Refractory epilepsy is present in nearly all affected patients, with partial complex and atypical absence epilepsy being the most common syndromes.

Tuberous sclerosis: Cortical or subependymal *tubers* and white matter abnormalities **(Fig. 120)**.

Tuberous sclerosis, also known as tuberous sclerosis complex or Bourneville disease, is a neurocutaneous disorder (*phakomatosis*) characterized by the development of multiple benign tumors of the embryonic ectoderm (e.g., skin, eyes, and nervous system).

Clinical presentation:

Tuberous sclerosis was classically described as presenting in childhood with a triad (Vogt triad) of:

1. *Seizures*: Absent in one-quarter of individuals
2. *Intellectual disability*: Up to half have normal intelligence
3. *Adenoma sebaceum*: Only present in about three-quarters of patients

   The full triad is only seen in a minority of patients (~30%).

Rasmussen encephalitis: There are T2 hyperintensities **(Fig. 121)** in subcortical and deep white matter of right cerebral hemisphere with right-sided cerebral atrophy and ventricular dilatation.

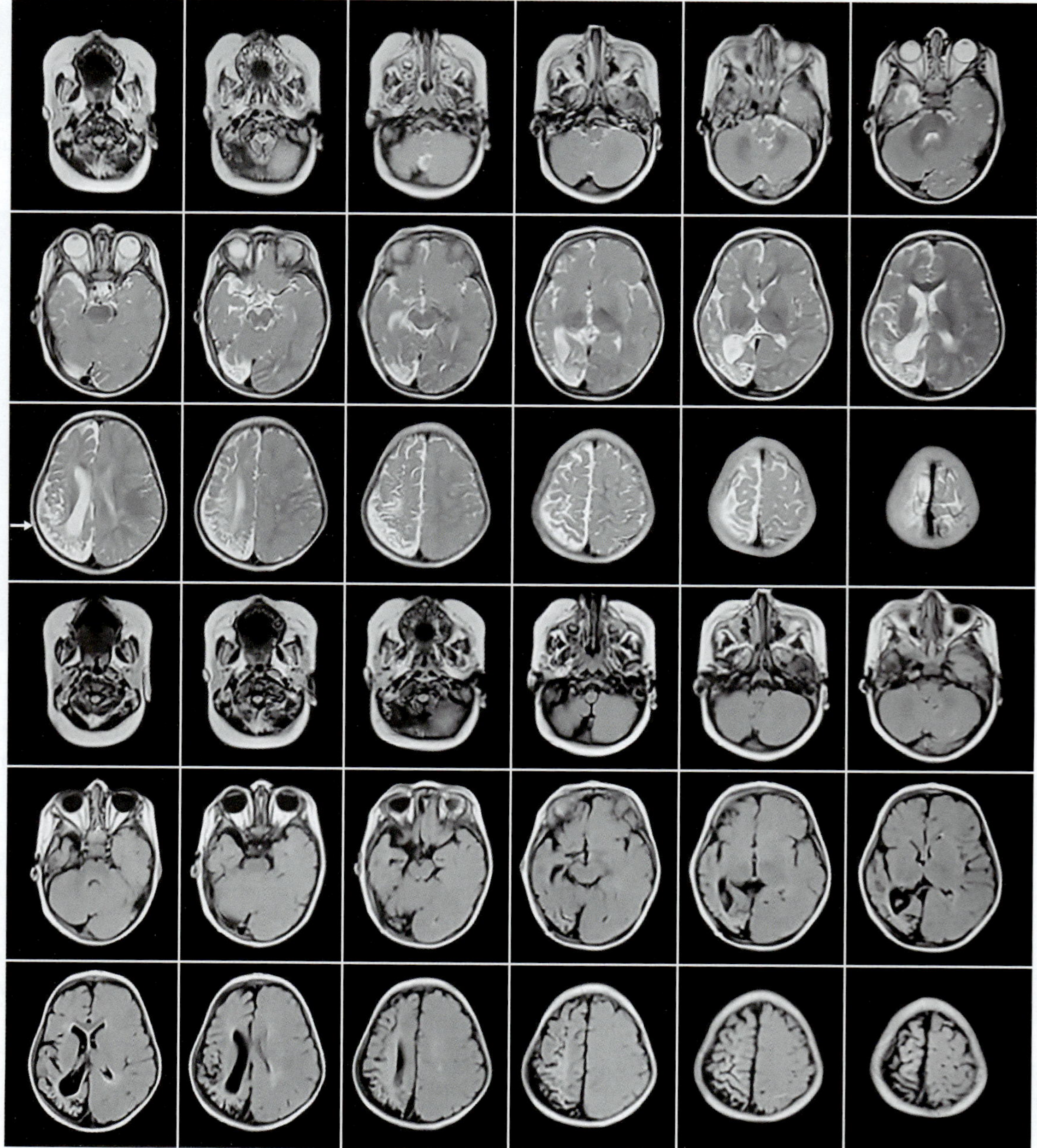

Fig. 121: MRI T2 showing hyperintensities in subcortical and deep white matter of right cerebral hemisphere with right-sided cerebral atrophy and ventricular dilatation.

Hypoxic-ischemic encephalopathy (HIE): Injury of basal ganglia and thalamus **(Figs. 122A and B)** in a term newborn—features of acute asphyxia. The lesions are hyperintense in all types of sequences (T1, T2, and FLAIR); they show diffusion restriction. (A) SE/T1, ax; (B) DWI

Bilateral, symmetrical paraventricular gliosis **(Figs. 123A and B)**, uneven external outlines of the lateral ventricles, thinning of the white matter layer—classic pattern of hypoxic-ischemic lesions in a baby born between 32 and 36 week of gestation. (A) FLAIR,ax; (B) FSE/T2, ax.

Ulegyria: A mushroom-shaped morphology of gyri is the characteristic appearance of ulegyria **(Figs. 124A and B)**.

Ulegyria refers to a shrunken and flattened cortex usually due to global *hypoxic-ischemic injury* in term infants, centering on the deepest portion of gyri, usually in the parasagittal region. It is here that perfusion is most tenuous and, therefore, most susceptible to ischemic damage.

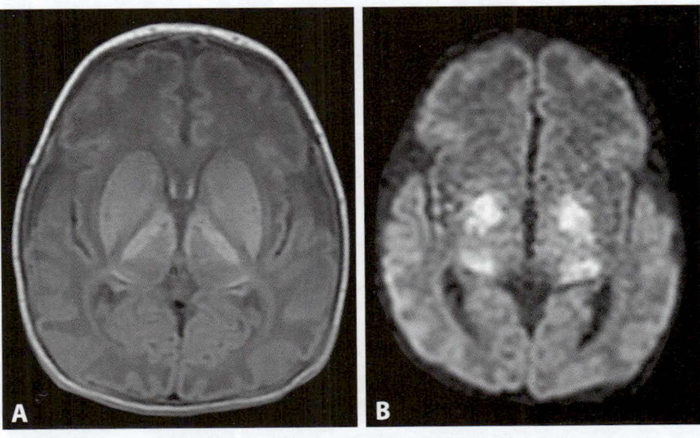

Figs. 122A and B: MRI shows hyperintense injury of basal ganglia and thalamus.

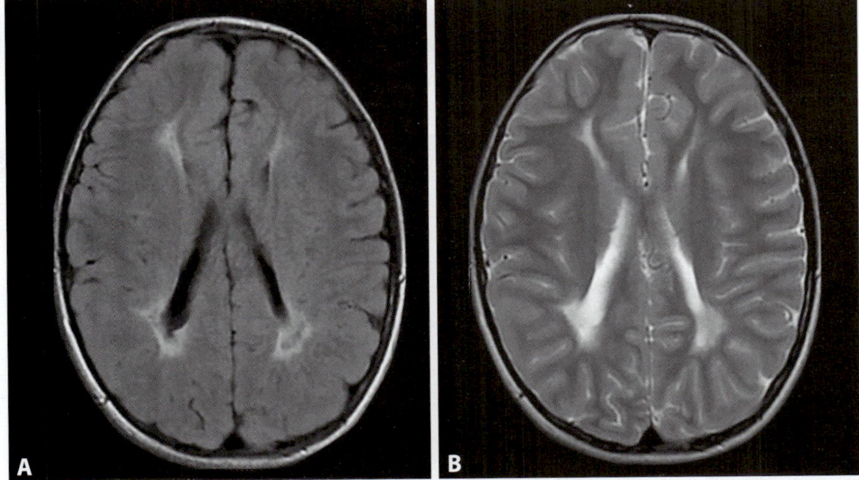

Figs. 123A and B: MRI showing bilateral, symmetrical paraventricular gliosis with thinning of the white matter layer.

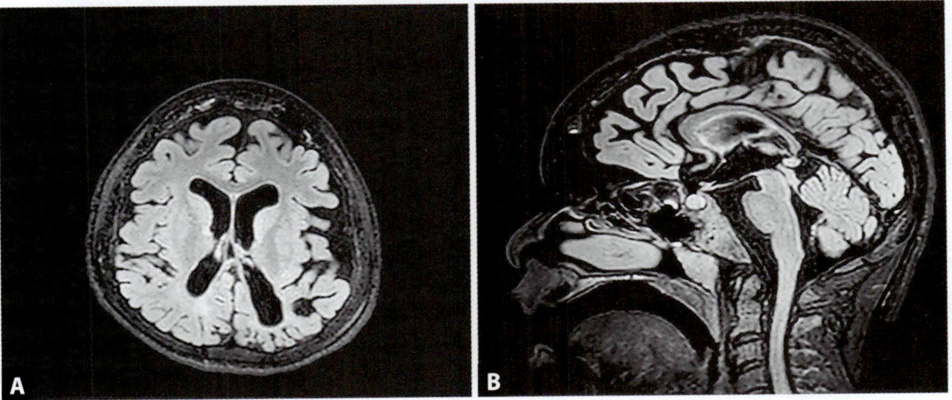

Figs. 124A and B: MRI brain shows mushroom-shaped morphology of gyri.

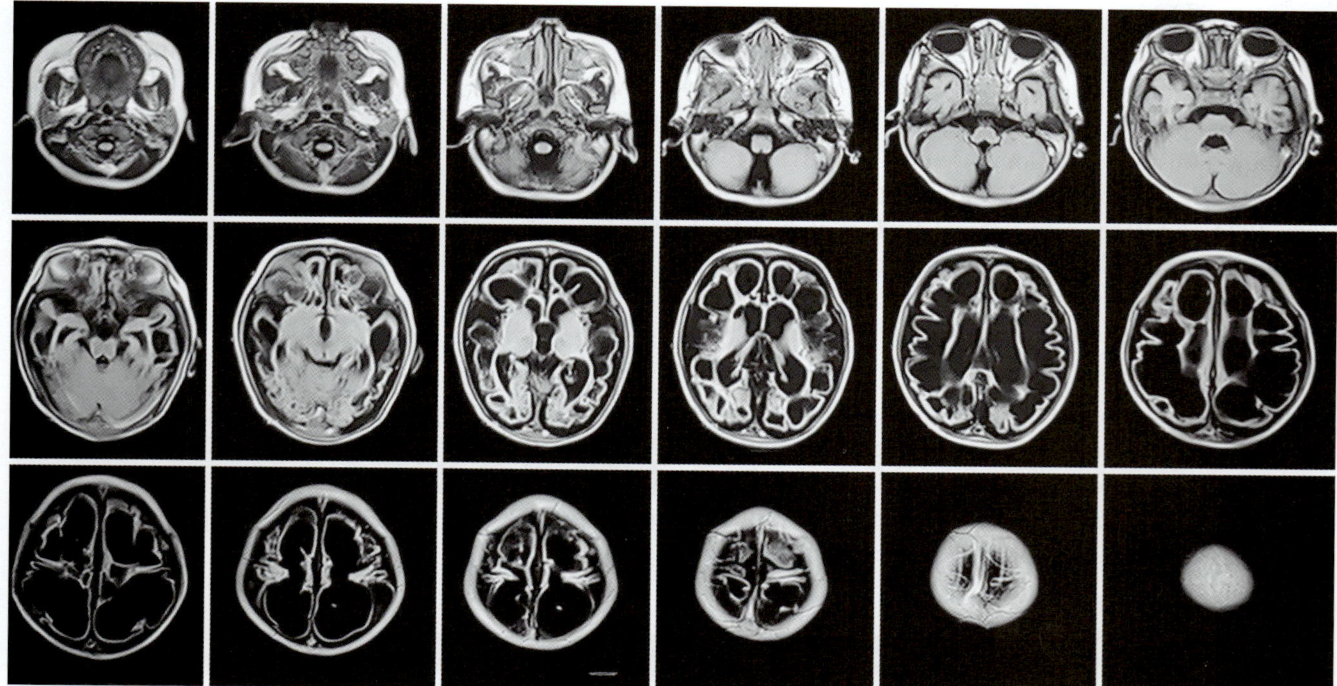

Fig. 125: MRI brain shows multicystic lesions post HIE.

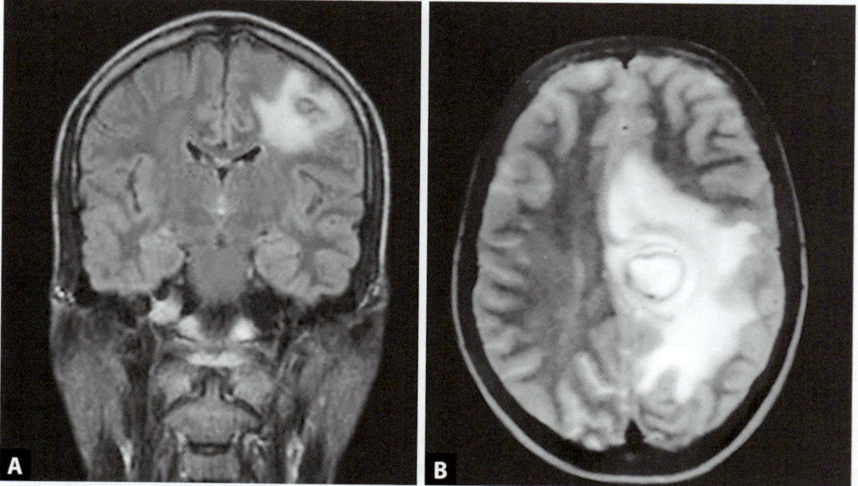

Figs. 126A and B: MRI brain showing single solitary ring enhancing lesion with surrounding edema.

Multicystic encephalopathy in HIE (Fig. 125):

Neurocysticercosis:

Tuberculoma:

Tuberculoma versus NCC:

Tuberculoma **(Figs. 126A and B)***:*

- *Size:* >20 mm
- *Shape:* Lobulated, irregular
- Marked edema with midline shift
- Seen mostly in post fossa

NCC **(Figs. 127A to C)***:*

- Size <20 mm
- Shape: Round or oval
- Edema present but no midline shift
- Seen over gray and white matter junction of cerebral cortex

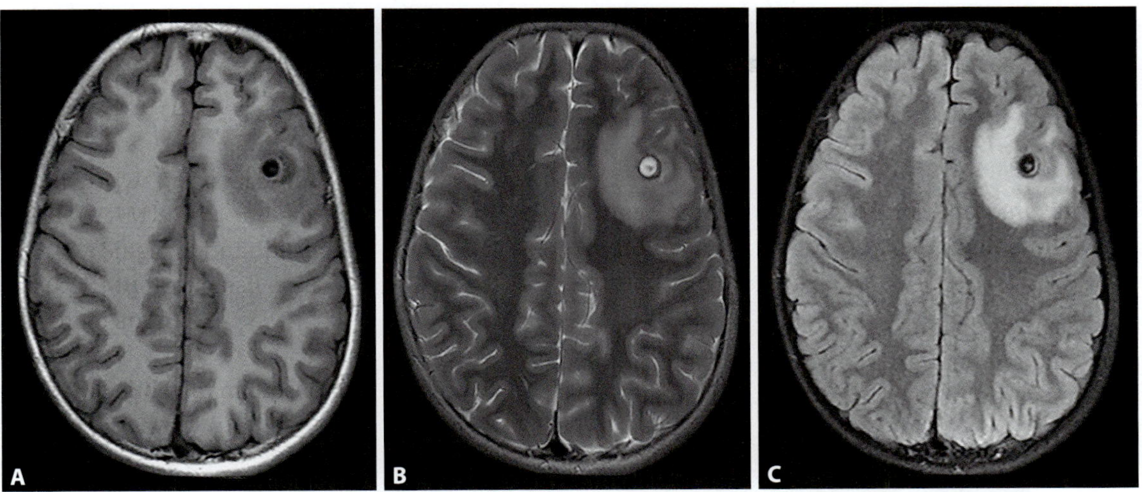

Figs. 127A to C: MRI shows single solitary ring enhancing lesion.

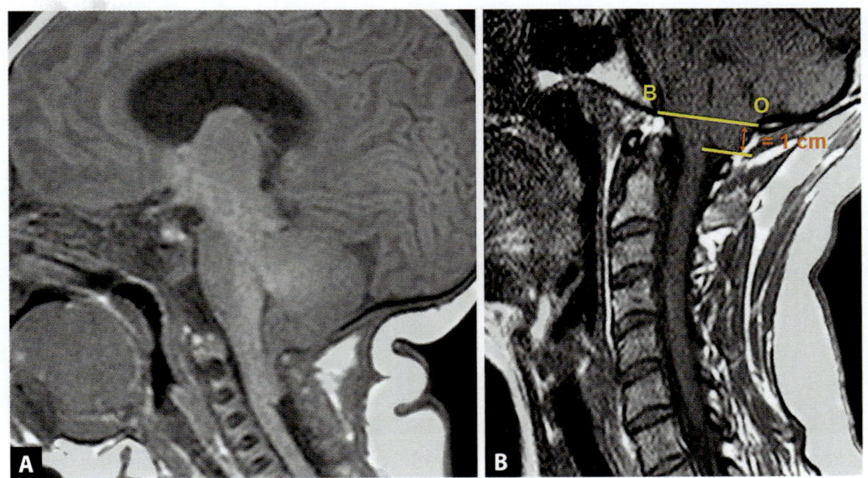

Figs. 128A and B: MRI showing Chiari II malformation.

Chiari II malformation: Drawing a line at the foramen magnum **(Figs. 128A and B)** from the inner margin of the opisthion to the basion, and then measuring the distance from that line to the inferior most margin of the cerebellar tonsils.

Herniation more than 3–5 mm varies according to age.

Classic features are >5 mm descent of the caudal tip of cerebellar tonsils past the foramen magnum **(Fig. 129)**; however, as little as <3 mm caudal cerebellar descent may be seen in a child presenting early with Chiari 1.

Near total callosal agenesis **(Fig. 130)***:*

Glutaric aciduria type 1: The MRI brain shows frontal hygroma (excessive extra-axial CSF collection) and wide open sylvian fissure **(Fig. 131)**.

The child presents with GDD and microcephaly sometimes mimicking cerebral palsy.

ADEM: MRI brain showing multiple hyperintense signals involving multiple areas of white matter in one of our child with MIS-C **(Fig. 132)**.

Dandy-Walker malformation **(Figs. 133 and 134)***:*

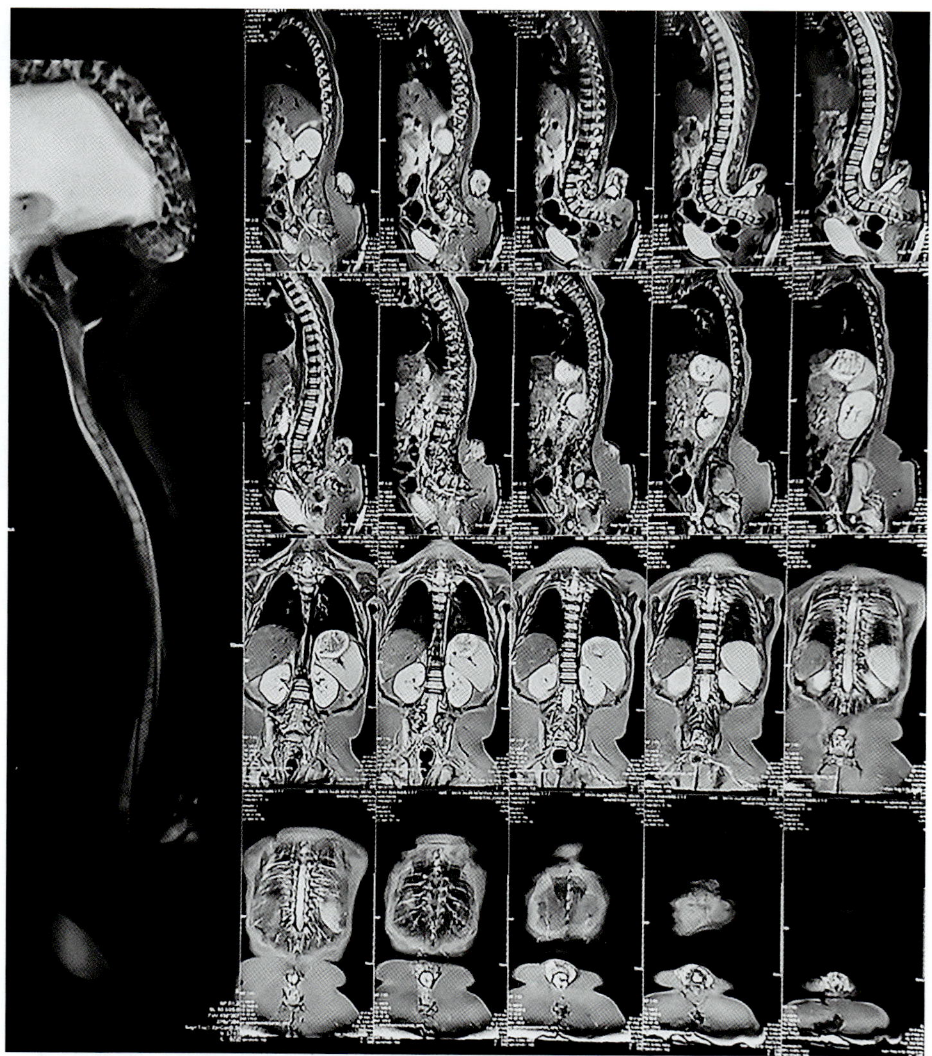

Fig. 129: Classic features are a >5 mm descent of the caudal tip of cerebellar tonsils past the foramen magnum.

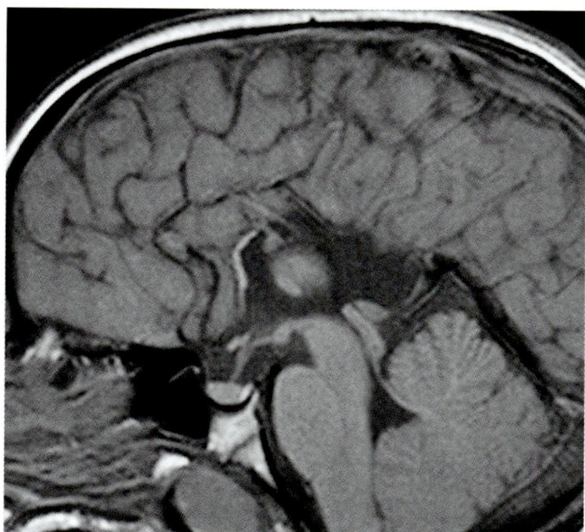

Fig. 130: MRI brain shows near total callosal agenesis.

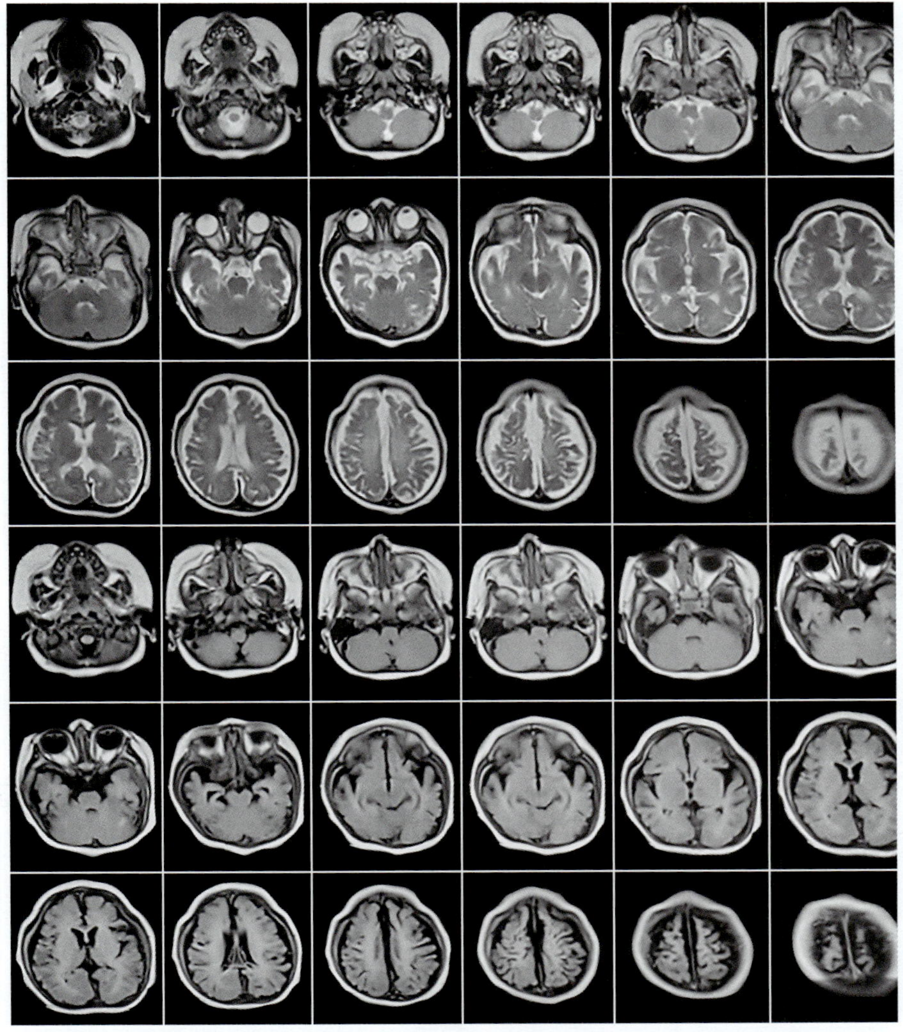

Fig. 131: MRI brain shows frontal hygroma (excessive extra-axial CSF collection) and wide open sylvian fissure.

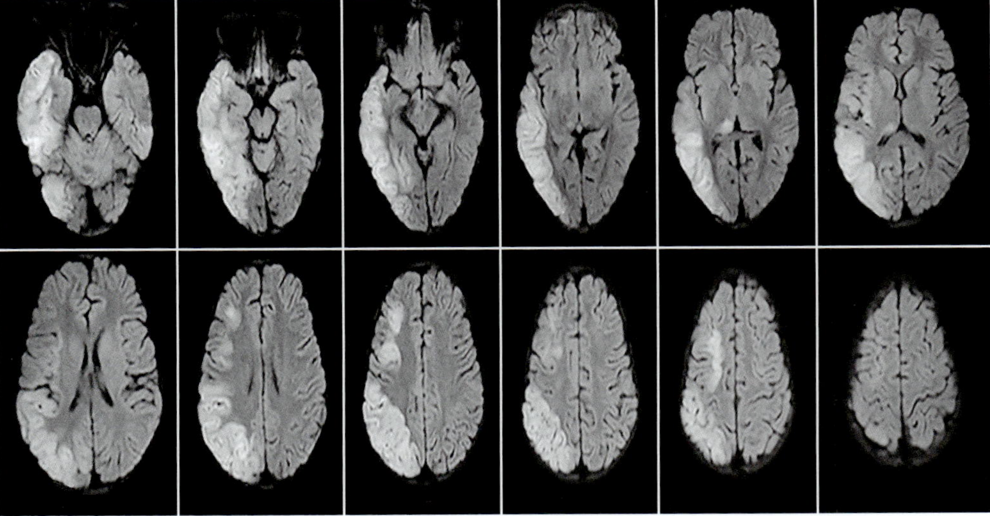

Fig. 132: MRI brain showing multiple hyperintense signals involving multiple areas of white matter.

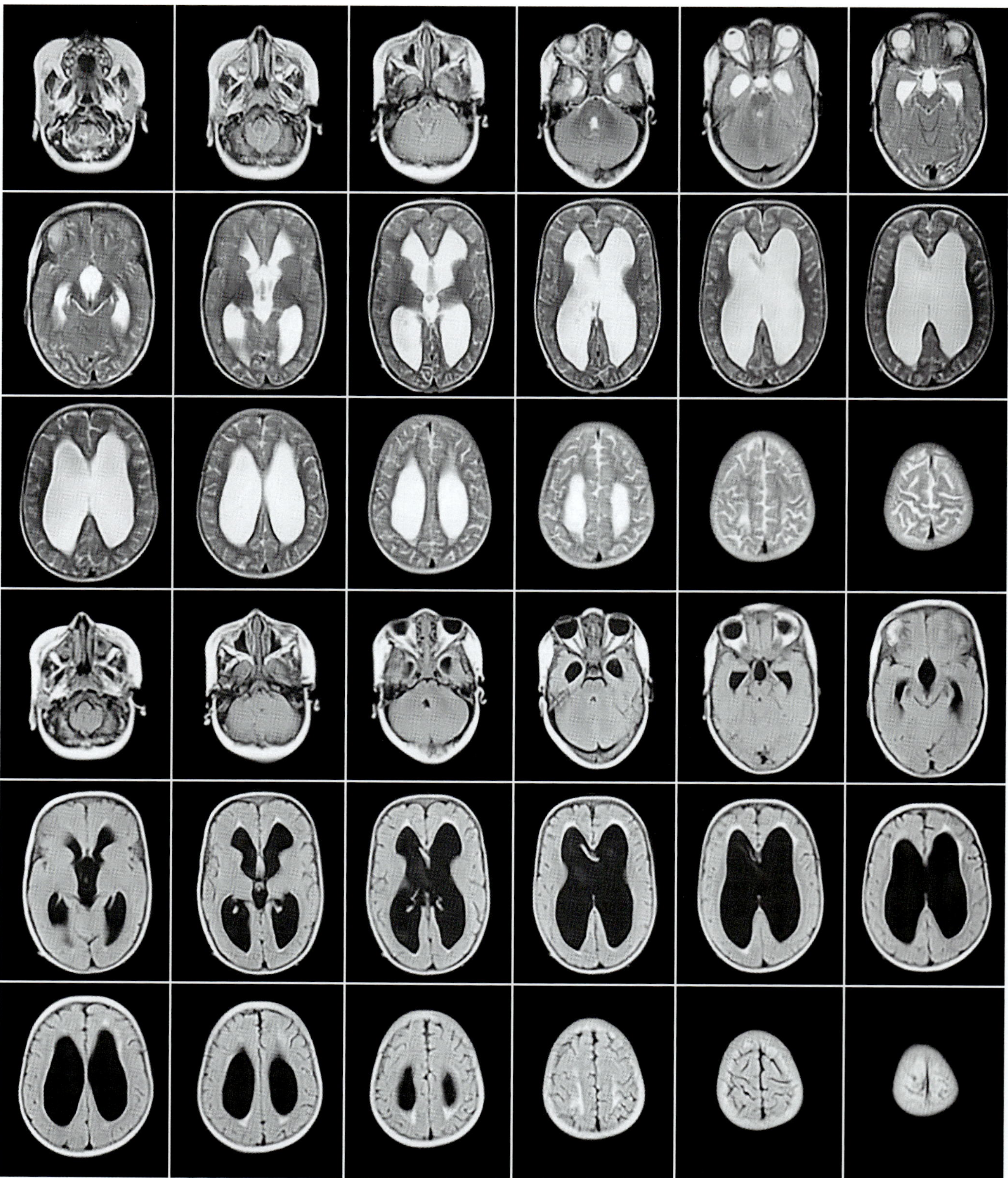

Fig. 133: MRI brain showing Dandy–Walker malformation.

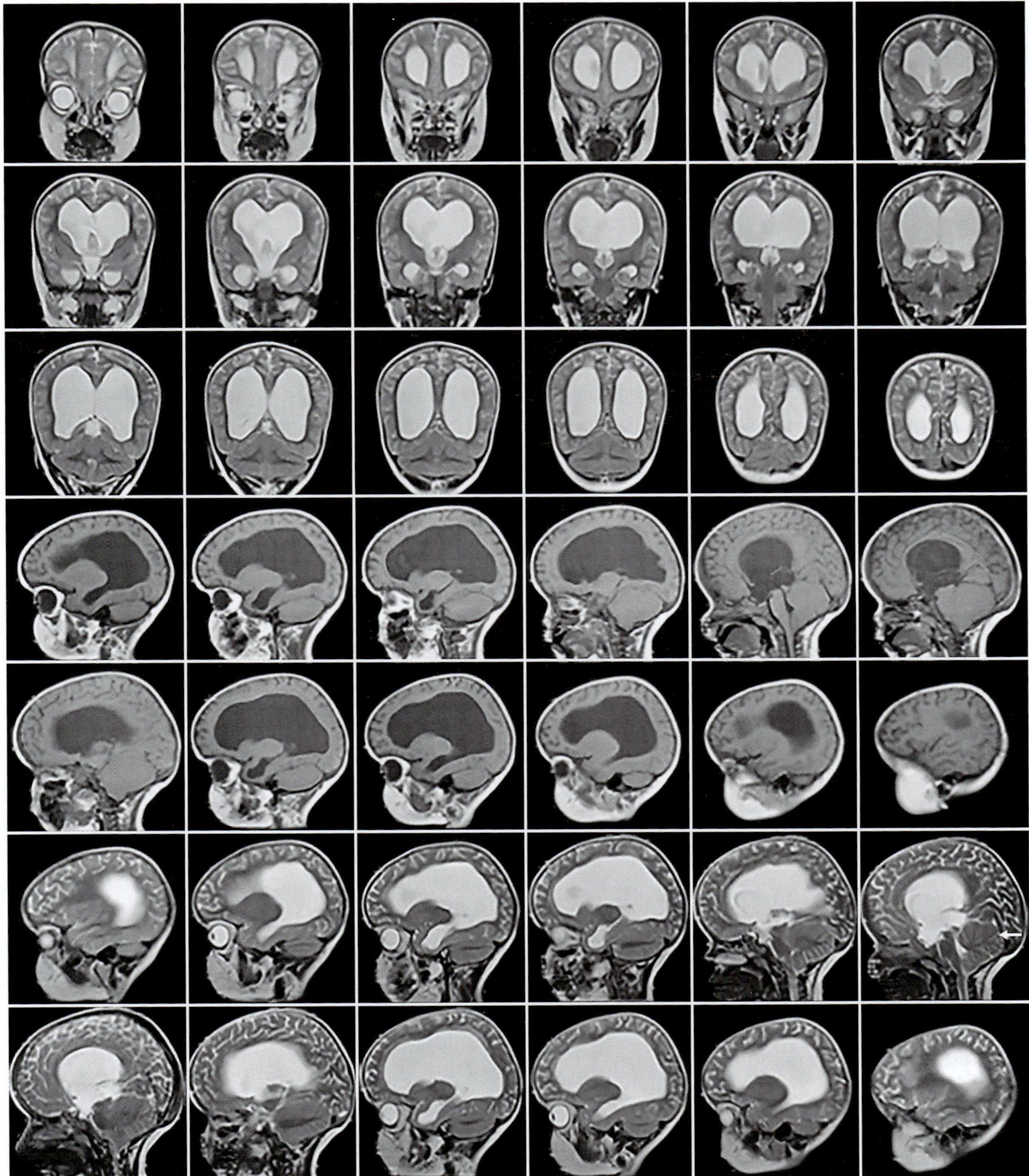

Fig. 134: Sagittal view MRI of Dandy–Walker syndrome.

Dandy–Walker malformation is characterized by:

- Agenesis or hypoplasia of the cerebellar vermis
- Dilatation of the fourth ventricle
- Enlargement of the posterior fossa

Day-by-day scope of MRI brain is getting unveiled to detect several diseases in children. In future, this modality without radiation hazards would more popularity and utility in treatment of ailing children as well as adults.

CHAPTER 15

Vaccines

Subhasish Bhattacharyya, Mousumi Das

Q1. What are humoral and cell-mediated immunity?

Ans. Understanding humoral and cell-mediated immunity:

The immune system is crucial for protecting the body against pathogens. It comprises two main types of immunity: humoral and cell-mediated.

Humoral immunity:

Definition: A type of immune response that involves antibodies produced by B cells.

Mechanism of action:

- B cells recognize specific antigens.
- Upon activation, B cells differentiate into plasma cells that secrete antibodies.
- Antibodies bind to pathogens, neutralizing them or marking them for destruction.

Key components:

- *B cells:* Specialized lymphocytes that mediate humoral immunity
- *Antibodies (immunoglobulins):* Proteins that specifically target antigens
- *Memory cells:* B cells that remember past infections for quicker responses in future encounters

Cell-mediated immunity:

Definition: A type of immune response involving T cells that help eliminate infected or cancerous cells.

Mechanism of action:

T cells recognize infected cells through specific antigen presentation on MHC molecules. Activation of T cells leads to the proliferation of cytotoxic T cells that destroy infected cells and support other immune cells.

Key components:

- *T cells:* Including helper T cells (CD4+) and cytotoxic T cells (CD8+)
- *Cytokines:* Signaling molecules that facilitate communication between immune cells
- *MHC (major histocompatibility complex):* Molecules that present antigens to T cells

Both humoral and cell-mediated immunity play essential roles in the immune response.

Humoral immunity is primarily effective against extracellular pathogens, while cell-mediated immunity targets intracellular infections and tumors.

Q2. What are T and B cells? What role do they play in immunology of vaccines?

Ans. Introduction to immunology of vaccines:

Vaccines stimulate the immune system to develop immunity against specific pathogens without causing disease. B and T cells are essential components of this adaptive immune response.

Key roles of B cells:

- *Antibody production:* B cells are responsible for producing antibodies that bind to antigens, neutralizing pathogens, and marking them for destruction by other immune cells.
- *Memory formation:* After exposure to a vaccine, some B cells develop into memory B cells, which remain long-term in the body and can quickly produce antibodies upon re-exposure to the same pathogen.
- *Class switching:* B cells can undergo class switching, allowing them to produce different types of antibodies (IgM, IgG, IgA, etc.) tailored to the specific type of infection.

Key roles of T cells:

- *Helper T cells (CD4+ T cells):* These cells assist in activating B cells and cytotoxic T cells through the release of cytokines, enhancing the immune response.
- *Cytotoxic T cells (CD8+ T cells):* These cells can directly kill infected cells, playing a crucial role in controlling viral infections and tumor cells.
- *Memory T cells:* Similar to memory B cells, memory T cells persist after vaccination to provide a faster and more effective response during subsequent exposures.

The interaction between B and T cells is critical for generating a robust immune response to vaccines.

Together, they ensure both immediate and long-lasting immunity against diseases.

Q3. What are adjuvants? How do they affect performance of vaccines?

Ans.

Definition of adjuvants: Adjuvants are substances that enhance the body's immune response to an antigen.

Purpose of adjuvants: To improve the effectiveness of vaccines. To reduce the required dose of antigen needed in a vaccine.

Mechanisms of action: Adjuvants can stimulate the innate immune system. They can also enhance the immunogenicity of the antigen through various pathways.

Types of adjuvants:

- *Alum:* One of the most commonly used adjuvants in human vaccines
- *Oil-in-water emulsions:* Such as MF59 that boosts immune response
- *TLR agonists:* Target toll-like receptors to enhance the immune response

Applications in vaccines:

- Used in various vaccine formulations to improve efficacy against infectious diseases
- Essential in pandemic vaccine strategies to respond effectively to outbreaks

Safety and efficacy:

- Overall considered safe, though some adjuvants may cause side effects.
- Continuous research is needed to develop new adjuvants that are both effective and safe.

Q4. What are the differences between live attenuated and inactivated vaccines?

Ans. This note outlines the key differences between live attenuated and inactivated vaccines, which are two primary types used in immunization. Both types serve to train the immune system but operate through different mechanisms.

Live attenuated vaccines:

Definition: Contain a weakened form of the virus or bacterium that causes the disease

Mechanism of action: Stimulate a strong and long-lasting immune response by mimicking a natural infection. *Examples:* Measles, mumps, rubella (MMR), and rotavirus vaccines.

Advantages: Strong and prolonged immunity. Often provide lifelong protection with fewer doses.

Disadvantages: Not suitable for immunocompromised individuals. Potential risk of reversion to virulence in rare cases.

Inactivated vaccines:

Definition: Contain killed or inactivated pathogens that cannot replicate or cause disease.

Mechanism of action: Induce immune response without the risk of causing disease, usually requiring multiple doses. *Examples*: Polio (inactivated polio vaccine), hepatitis A, and some influenza vaccines.

Advantages: Safe for immunocompromised individuals. No risk of causing the disease.

Disadvantages: Weaker immune response often requiring booster doses. May not confer long-lasting immunity compared to live vaccines.

Summary—immune response: Live attenuated vaccines generally produce a stronger and longer-lasting immune response compared to inactivated vaccines.

Safety and suitability: Inactivated vaccines are safer for at-risk populations but often require additional doses to maintain immunity.

Usage: Choice of vaccine type depends on individual health, age, exposure risk, and specific disease considerations.

Q5. What are the differences between T-dependent and T-independent immune response?

Ans. The immune response can be classified into T-dependent and T-independent responses based on how B cells are activated. Understanding these two types of responses is crucial for comprehending the adaptive immune system's functionality.

T-dependent response:

Definition: This type of immune response requires T cell help for B cell activation.

Activation process: Antigen presentation by antigen-presenting cells (APCs) to T helper cells. Activation of T cells leads to the secretion of cytokines that support B cell activation. Differentiation of B cells into memory and plasma cells that produce antibodies.

Characteristics: Generates a robust response with high-affinity antibodies. Leads to the formation of memory B cells, providing long-lasting immunity. Involves isotype switching of antibodies, allowing for different antibody classes (IgG, IgA, etc.).

T-independent response:
Definition: This immune response does not require T cell help for B cell activation.

Activation process: B cells can directly recognize and respond to antigens, commonly polysaccharides and lipids. Cross-linking of B cell receptors by repeated epitope structures on antigens leads to activation.

Characteristics: Generates a weaker response compared to T-dependent responses. Produces primarily IgM antibodies without isotype switching. Limited generation of memory B cells, resulting in a short-lived response.

Key differences—requirement for T cell help: T-dependent responses need help, T-independent do not.

Antibody class produced: T-dependent responses involve various isotypes, T-independent primarily produces IgM.

Memory formation: T-dependent can lead to memory B cells, T-independent generally does not.

Response strength: T-dependent responses are more robust and durable compared to T-independent responses.

Q6. What are the conjugated vaccines?
Ans. Conjugated vaccines play an essential role in immunization, particularly against certain types of bacteria. These vaccines improve the body's immune response by linking a weak antigen to a strong antigen, enhancing the recognition and elimination of pathogens.

Key aspects of conjugated vaccines:
Definition: Conjugated vaccines are made by linking bacterial polysaccharides to a protein carrier.

Mechanism of action: polysaccharide component stimulates a T-cell-dependent immune response. This results in memory cell formation, leading to long-lasting immunity.

Examples:
- *Haemophilus influenzae type b (Hib) vaccine:* Protects against bacterial infections that can cause pneumonia and meningitis.
- *Pneumococcal conjugate vaccine (PCV):* Targets *Streptococcus pneumoniae*, reducing instances of pneumonia, meningitis, and sepsis.
- *Meningococcal conjugate vaccines:* Protect against *Neisseria meningitidis*, lowering the risk of meningococcal disease.

Advantages of conjugated vaccines:
- *Enhanced immune response:* Increased effectiveness in young children, who typically have weaker immune systems.
- *Long-term protection:* Often leads to longer-lasting immunity compared to polysaccharide vaccines alone.
- *Reduction in carriage:* Decreases the number of vaccinated children who carry bacteria, contributing to herd immunity.

Conclusion: Conjugated vaccines are crucial in preventing serious bacterial infections, especially in children, and play a significant role in public health.

The immune response to live vaccines exhibits several notable characteristics:
Strong immune response: Live vaccines stimulate both B-cell and T-cell responses effectively. Induction of long-lasting immunity. Live vaccines closely replicate natural infections, providing a robust immune reaction similar to the actual disease.

Types of immunity-induced: Primarily induces cell-mediated immunity (CMI) alongside humoral immunity. The response includes the activation of cytotoxic T lymphocytes (CTLs).

Single dose efficacy: Often, a single dose can provide sufficient immunity, reducing the need for booster shots.

Rapid onset of immunity: Immunity typically develops within days to weeks after vaccination.

Potential for reactogenicity: Live vaccines can cause mild, temporary side effects similar to the disease, due to the active viral/bacterial replication.

Possible shedding: In certain vaccines, there may be a risk of shedding the live vaccine virus/bacteria, with the potential for transmission to nonimmune individuals.

Q7. What determines the intensity and duration of immune response?
Ans. The intensity and duration of the immune response are influenced by various factors including:
- Type of pathogen, virulence of the pathogen
- Whether the pathogen is a virus, bacterium, or allergen.
- Nature of antigen
- Size, complexity, and stability of the antigen
- Presence of adjuvants that can enhance the immune response

Route of entry: How the pathogen enters the body (e.g., inhalation, ingestion, skin). Different routes may elicit different immune pathways.

Host factors:
- Genetic factors of the host, including variations in immune genes
- Age and overall health of the individual

- The presence of pre-existing immunity (from past infections or vaccinations)

Immune system components:

- Responses from innate versus adaptive immunity. Activation of various immune cells like T-cells, B-cells, macrophages, etc.
- Local cytokine levels and the presence of other immune cells
- Tissue repair and inflammation status

Q8. What is primary and secondary immune response?

Ans. Understanding these factors can help in predicting how effective and lasting the body's immune response will be against specific pathogens.

Primary immune response: The primary immune response occurs when the immune system is first exposed to a specific pathogen or antigen. This response typically takes time to develop as the body needs to recognize the pathogen and generate the necessary antibodies.

Key stages include:

- Recognition of the pathogen
- Activation of B-cells and T-cells
- Production of antibodies by B-cells

The response may take several days to weeks to become fully effective.

Secondary immune response: The secondary immune response, also known as the anamnestic response, occurs upon subsequent exposure to the same pathogen. This response is faster and more robust due to the memory cells (B- and T-cells) developed during the primary immune response.

Key features include:

- Quick recognition of the pathogen by memory cells
- Rapid proliferation of specific B-cells and T-cells
- Immediate antibody production, often of a higher affinity and concentration than during the primary response

The primary response is slower and initially produces fewer antibodies due to first-time exposure. In contrast, the secondary response is quicker, stronger, and ideally suited for fighting previously encountered pathogens.

Q9. Why is number of dose of each vaccine different?

Ans.

Main reasons for different vaccine doses:

Vaccine type: Different vaccines are designed using different technologies which impacts dosage requirements, e.g. mRNA vaccines, viral vector vaccines, protein subunit vaccines.

Immune response: Each vaccine elicits varied immune responses depending on its formulation and target pathogens.

Some vaccines stimulate a stronger immune response with fewer doses. Others require more doses for adequate protection.

Duration of immunity: Different vaccines provide varying lengths of immunity, influencing how often booster shots are necessary.

Some vaccines may require multiple doses to maintain immunity over time.

Population differences: Vaccination schedules may vary based on age groups, populations, and health conditions.

Higher-risk groups may necessitate extra doses.

Regulatory guidelines: Clinical trial outcomes and regulatory reviews can lead to different recommended dosage schedules.

Regulatory agencies (e.g., FDA, WHO) determine approved dosing regimens based on safety and efficacy data.

Additional considerations booster shots: Depending on the vaccine and emerging variants, booster doses may become necessary to enhance protection.

Public health recommendations: Changes in public health policy based on new research can affect recommended doses.

Q10. Why do we need booster vaccine? Discussion on the necessity of booster vaccines.

Ans.

Reasons for booster vaccines:

Enhanced immunity: Booster vaccines help in reinforcing the immune response to ensure continued effectiveness against diseases.

Waning immunity: Over time, immunity can diminish; booster shots help maintain sufficient antibodies in the system.

Adaptation to variants: New variants of viruses may emerge; boosters can be updated to tackle these changes effectively, and contribute to herd immunity, protecting the community at large.

Conclusion: Booster vaccines play a crucial role in maintaining health and safety against infectious diseases.

Q11. What are the safe injection practices?

Ans. Safe injection practices are essential protocols designed to prevent infections and ensure patient safety during injections. These practices are crucial for healthcare providers, especially in settings such as hospitals, clinics, and home care environments. Below are the main headings and details regarding safe injection practices:

General principles: Follow standard precautions to minimize the risk of infection. Always perform hand hygiene before and after each injection.

Preparation of injections: Use aseptic technique throughout the injection process. Check the medication vial for integrity and expiration date. Clean the vial septum with an alcohol swab before inserting a needle.

Equipment handling: Use sterile, single-use needles and syringes for every injection. Never share needles, syringes, or any other injection equipment.

Injection technique: Properly select the injection site based on the type of injection (intradermal, subcutaneous, and intramuscular). Rotate injection sites for repeated injections to prevent tissue damage.

Postinjection practices: Dispose of needles and syringes immediately in a designated sharps container. Monitor the injection site for adverse reactions or complications.

Education and training: Regularly train healthcare staff on safe injection practices. Provide resources for patients about the importance of safe injections. These measures collectively ensure that injections are administered safely, protecting both healthcare providers and patients from potential health risks.

Q12. What are the general instructions on administration of parenteral vaccines?

Ans.

Preparation for administration:

- Verify vaccine type and expiration date
- Ensure proper storage conditions prior to use
- Gather necessary equipment (syringes, needles, and alcohol swabs)

Site selection: Identify appropriate injection sites based on age and muscle development:

- Infants and smaller children: anterolateral thigh (vastus lateralis)
- *Bigger children and adults*: upper arm (deltoid muscle)

Injection technique:

- Wash hands
- Clean injection site with an alcohol swab
- Use a new, sterile needle and syringe for each vaccine
- Insert needle at the correct angle:
  - 90° for intramuscular
  - 45° for subcutaneous
- Aspirate (if recommended) to check for blood return
- Inject the vaccine slowly and steadily
- Withdraw the needle quickly and apply gentle pressure with a cotton ball

Postadministration care:

- Observe the patient for 15–30 minutes for any immediate allergic reactions
- Provide information on potential side effects and care
- Document the administration details (date, time, site, and vaccine type)

Special considerations:

- Adjust technique based on patient age and specific vaccine guidelines
- Be aware of contraindications and precautions for certain vaccines

Q13. What should be the ideal spacing between multiple doses of same vaccines?

Ans. The minimum interval between two doses of inactivated vaccines is usually 4 weeks (exception rabies).

- Vaccine doses administered up to 4 days before the minimum interval or age can be counted as valid (exception rabies). If the vaccine is administered >5 days before minimum period, it is counted as invalid dose and has to be repeated. This rule does not apply to live, parenteral vaccines.

Q14. What should be the spacing of different vaccines?

Ans. Whenever multiple vaccinations (including two live parenteral vaccines) are to be given simultaneously, they should be administered in the same sitting or they should be administered on the same clinic day (conventionally a clinic day consists of 6 hours). When two or more live parenteral/intranasal vaccines are not administered on the same day, they should be given at least 28 days (4 weeks) apart; this rule does not apply to live oral vaccines.

Q15. How many different vaccines can be administered simultaneously?

Ans. Any number of antigens can be given on the same day. Two or more inactivated or inactivated and live vaccines can be administered at any interval between them. Two or more live, parenteral vaccines should be administered on the same day or 4 weeks apart.

Q16. Why intramuscular route is preferred for certain vaccines and subcutaneous or intradermal for some other vaccines?

Ans. Vaccination can be administered using different routes, primarily intramuscular (IM), subcutaneous (SC), and intradermal (ID). The choice of route depends on several factors pertaining to the vaccine's properties, efficacy, and target group.

Main reasons for route preference:

Intramuscular:

- Allows for larger volumes of the vaccine to be administered, which is beneficial for certain formulations
- Suitable for vaccines that require deep muscle penetration for optimal vaccine delivery and absorption

Subcutaneous (SC):

- Preferred for vaccines that do not require a high volume or deep penetration. Suitable for vaccines that can induce a good immune response even at lower volumes
- Commonly used in easily absorbable products or live vaccines

Intradermal (ID): This route is less common but may be used for specific vaccines that necessitate a targeted immune response at the skin level. May require less vaccine volume and is often associated with higher local immune response and fewer systemic side effects.

Safety and tolerability:

Side effects: IM injections tend to be associated with muscle soreness but are usually well tolerated. SC injections may have a lower risk of pain and local reactions than IM injections. ID routes generally show minimal systemic reactions but require proper training for administration.

Vaccine characteristics:

Formulation: Some vaccines need specific adjuvants or formulations that work best when delivered via the IM route. Others, particularly live attenuated vaccines, might be better suited for SC or ID routes due to their design.

Conclusion: Key considerations for vaccine route selection include the desired immune response and safety profile, along with practical factors like volume and ease of administration.

Q17. How should a serious anaphylaxis reaction, to a vaccine be managed?

Ans. Overview of anaphylaxis: Anaphylaxis is a severe, potentially life-threatening allergic reaction. It can occur in response to various triggers, including vaccines.

Immediate steps for management:

Recognition of symptoms:

- Difficulty breathing or shortness of breath
- Swelling of the face, throat, or tongue
- Rapid or weak pulse
- Skin reactions (hives, redness)
- Dizziness or fainting

Administer epinephrine: Administer intramuscular epinephrine immediately (usually in the thigh) when anaphylaxis is suspected. Dosage: 0.3–0.5 mg for adults; 0.01 mg/kg for children (maximum 0.3 mg).

Emergency response:

- Call emergency services
- Seek immediate medical assistance after administering epinephrine

Monitor patient: Continuously monitor the patient's vital signs and symptoms.

Secondary treatments:

- *Antihistamines:* Consider administering antihistamines postepinephrine for symptom relief (not a substitute for epinephrine).
- *Oxygen therapy:* Provide supplemental oxygen if the patient has difficulty breathing.

Follow-up care:

- *Observation period:* Patients should be observed for at least 2–3 hours postreaction in a healthcare setting as symptoms may recur.
- *Documentation:* Document the reaction, treatment provided, and any follow-up actions needed.

Prevention:

Emergency plans: Ensure that vaccination sites have protocols in place for handling allergic reactions, including having epinephrine readily available.

Patient education: Inform patients about the signs of anaphylaxis and the importance of seeking immediate help.

Q18. What precautions should be observed for proper storage and handling of vaccines?

Ans. Maintain appropriate temperature ranges: Cold chain requirements must be met to ensure vaccine efficacy.

Store vaccines in designated refrigeration: Use calibrated refrigerators to avoid temperature fluctuations.

Handling protocols:

Follow strict hygiene practices: Use gloves when handling vaccines. Disinfect surfaces and equipment before and after use.

Check expiry dates: Regularly inspect vaccine stocks to avoid using expired vaccines.

Transportation guidelines: Ensure temperature monitoring during transport:

- Use temperature loggers to track conditions
- Limit the duration outside of recommended storage conditions
- Minimize exposure to heat during transportation

Q19. What are the special situations for vaccination?

Ans. Vaccination plays a crucial role in public health, but there are specific circumstances where the approach to vaccination may vary.

The following outlines key special situations regarding vaccination:

- *Pregnancy:* Safety of vaccines during pregnancy: Recommended vaccines (e.g., Tdap, Influenza)
- *Timing for administration in immunocompromised individuals:* Types of immunocompromised status (e.g., HIV, cancer treatment)—some live attenuated vaccines contraindicated, inactivated vaccines recommended.
- *Travel vaccination:* Required vaccines for international travel (e.g., Yellow fever, hepatitis A)
- Timing and planning for vaccination prior to travel
- *Postexposure prophylaxis:* Vaccination following potential exposure (e.g., rabies, measles)—importance of timely intervention

Q20. What are the issues faced by the clinicians in vaccinating an immunocompromised individual?

Ans. When vaccinating immunocompromised individuals, clinicians encounter several key challenges:

- *Understanding the immune status:* Variability in immune response due to different types of immunocompromised states (e.g., due to therapies, diseases). Need for tailored vaccination strategies based on individual assessment
- *Vaccine selection:* Deciding which vaccines are appropriate and safe for the individual
- Awareness of live attenuated vaccines that may pose risks.
- *Timing of vaccination:* Determining the ideal timing for vaccinations, especially in relation to immunosuppressive treatments.
- Need to catch up on missed vaccinations while balancing safety.
- *Monitoring adverse reactions:* Increased vigilance required for monitoring vaccine responses and adverse effects
- Awareness of altered reaction profiles in immunocompromised patients

Patient education and communication: Importance of educating patients about the necessity and potential risks of vaccination

Q21. What is the definition of adverse events following immunization?

Ans. Adverse events following immunization (AEFI) refer to any untoward medical occurrence that follows immunization and does not necessarily have a causal relationship with the vaccine. It is essential to monitor and assess these events to ensure vaccine safety and effectiveness.

Key points about AEFI include:

Definition: An adverse event is any negative health outcome that occurs after vaccination.

Types of AEFI:

- *Mild reactions:* Common, self-limiting reactions such as fever, soreness at the injection site, or mild rashes
- *Severe reactions:* Rare but serious events such as anaphylaxis or Guillain–Barré syndrome that require immediate medical attention

Importance of reporting: Health professionals and vaccine recipients are encouraged to report any AEFI to assess the vaccine's safety profile and identify potential risks.

Monitoring: Continuous surveillance systems exist to monitor the safety of vaccines, including postmarketing studies and clinical trials.

Causality assessment: Investigating whether there is a causal relationship between the immunization and the adverse event for proper risk management and communication.

Q22. What are the serious vaccine reactions?

Ans. Common serious vaccine reactions:

Anaphylaxis: A severe allergic reaction that can occur within minutes to hours after vaccination.

Symptoms include: Difficulty breathing, swelling of the face and throat, rapid heartbeat, rash, or hives.

Thrombosis with thrombocytopenia syndrome (TTS): Rare blood clotting condition associated with certain vaccines.

Symptoms may include: Severe headache, abdominal pain, leg swelling, and skin rash.

Myocarditis and pericarditis: Inflammation of the heart or its surrounding tissue, commonly reported with mRNA vaccines. Symptoms include: Chest pain, shortness of breath, feelings of having a fast-beating or fluttering heart.

Guillain-Barré syndrome (GBS): A rare neurological disorder that may occur following vaccination, characterized by—weakness and tingling in extremities, rapid muscle weakness leading to paralysis.

Monitoring and reporting: VAERS (vaccine adverse event reporting system): A system established to monitor vaccine safety and allows anyone to report adverse reactions. It is essential to report any serious reactions to ensure vaccine safety.

Conclusion: While serious reactions to vaccines are rare, awareness and prompt treatment are critical. Healthcare providers should be prepared to manage these reactions and empower patients with knowledge about potential risks.

Q23. What precautions should be taken while reconstituting a vaccine, with diluents?

Ans. When reconstituting a vaccine with a dry element, several precautions should be taken to ensure safety and efficacy:

Aseptic technique: Always maintain strict hygiene and sterile conditions to prevent contamination.

Check expiration dates: Ensure that the vaccine and diluent are within their expiration dates before use.

Proper mixing: Follow the proper methods for mixing the dry element with the diluent to achieve a homogeneous solution.

Volume accuracy: Measure the correct volume of diluent as per the vaccine manufacturer's guidelines.

Observe for particulates: Inspect the reconstituted solution carefully for any particulates or discoloration before administration.

Storage conditions: After reconstitution, store the vaccine as instructed, usually under refrigeration, and use it within the recommended time frame.

Q24. What is cold chain? What is the importance of cold chain?

Ans. Cold chain refers to the temperature-controlled supply chain used to preserve and maintain the quality of perishable goods such as pharmaceuticals, food products, and biological samples.

The importance of cold chain includes:

- *Preservation of quality:* Maintains the efficacy and longevity of sensitive products, preventing spoilage and degradation.
- *Regulatory compliance:* Adherence to strict regulations and standards for storage and transportation of temperature-sensitive goods
- *Market expansion:* Facilitates access to global markets by enabling the transport of perishable goods over long distances without compromise.
- *Cost efficiency:* Reduces waste and losses by ensuring products reach consumers in optimal condition.

Q25. Which are cold-sensitive vaccines?

Ans. Freeze-sensitive vaccines are vaccines that lose potency and are irreversibly damaged when exposed to freezing temperatures. This is because freezing can cause adjuvants in the vaccine, particularly those containing aluminum salts, to clump together, compromising the vaccine's immunological properties.

Examples of freeze-sensitive vaccines include:

- *Inactivated vaccines:* Many inactivated vaccines, such as diphtheria, tetanus, pertussis (DTP/DTaP), hepatitis B (HepB), and inactivated poliovirus (IPV), are freeze-sensitive.
- *Other freeze-sensitive vaccines:* Hepatitis A, human papillomavirus (HPV), meningitis C, pneumococcal (PCV), influenza, and typhoid vaccines are also freeze-sensitive.

Important considerations:

- *Storage and transportation:* Freeze-sensitive vaccines must be stored and transported at temperatures between 0°C and 10°C (32°F and 40°F) to prevent freezing.
- *Damage from freezing:* Even brief exposure to freezing temperatures can damage freeze-sensitive vaccines, rendering them ineffective.
- *Cold chain management:* Proper cold chain management, including monitoring temperatures and using freeze-preventive measures, is crucial for ensuring the integrity of freeze-sensitive vaccines.
- *Visual freeze indicators:* Freeze indicators, such as freeze-tags, can help detect if a vaccine has been exposed to freezing temperatures, although they do not detect the specific temperature.

Q26. Which vaccines are light sensitive?

Ans. Several vaccines are sensitive to light and require specific storage conditions to maintain their potency. These include BCG, measles, and some influenza vaccines. Exposure to light can degrade the vaccine, making it less effective or potentially harmful. Reconstituted BCG, measles, and JE vaccines are particularly light-sensitive.

Here is a more detailed look at light-sensitive vaccines:

- *BCG (Bacillus Calmette-Guérin):* This vaccine, used to prevent tuberculosis, is highly sensitive to both heat and light. It is typically supplied in an amber-colored bottle to protect it from light.
- *Measles:* Measles vaccine, especially when reconstituted, is susceptible to damage from light and heat.
- *Japanese encephalitis (JE):* Similar to measles, JE vaccine is sensitive to light and heat, especially after reconstitution.
- *Other light-sensitive vaccines: Immunize.org* and the *Centers for Disease Control and Prevention (CDC)* mention that some influenza vaccines, certain meningococcal vaccines, and HPV vaccines should also be protected from light.
- *Storage:* Vaccines should always be stored in their original packaging, away from direct sunlight and fluorescent lights. Doors of storage units should be kept closed to avoid unnecessary exposure to light.

Q27. If the baby does not develop a scar after BCG vaccination, what to do?

Ans. Scar failure rate following BCG neonatal vaccination of 8.6% and 10% has been reported in Indian studies. Failure of formation of BCG scar at the site of BCG vaccination may not necessarily imply failure of immunization because majority of them elicit positive in vitro lymphocyte migration inhibition (LMI) response. The presence of BCG scar is the only simple way of determining previous vaccination in clinical settings as well as in health surveys to assess vaccine uptake in spite of studies indicating that scar development is not a reliable indicator of the immunological response to BCG. Hence, a single repeat dose of BCG may be administered to infants who fail to demonstrate a scar beyond 6 months of vaccination. If there is a failure of scar formation after the second vaccination, no further doses are warranted. Pre-BCG Mantoux test is not necessary.

Q28. What are the different vaccines available for polio?

Ans. Inactivated polio vaccine (IPV), first developed and licensed in 1955, is given by injection and is available only in trivalent form containing the three virus serotypes PV1, PV2, and PV3. OPV as a monovalent (mOPV) vaccine was initially licensed in 1961 followed by a trivalent version (tOPV) in 1963. Bivalent OPV (bOPV containing types 1 and 3 Sabin viruses) has been licensed and used in some settings since December 2009. Following the planned global switch from tOPV to bOPV in April 2016, tOPV is now not available. mOPV will be stockpiled for future outbreaks.

Q29. What is VDPV?

Ans. The attenuated viruses in live OPV vaccines may reacquire neurovirulence and transmission capacity through replication and genetic divergence effect. Such mutated viruses can circulate in a community for an extended period of time and cause paralysis, which is known as cVDPV. 90% of reported cVDPV are due to type 2 polio virus.

Key risk factors for cVDPV emergence and spread are: (1) development of immunity gaps arising from low-OPV coverage, (2) prior elimination of the corresponding WPV serotype, (3) emphasis on use of mOPV and bOPV in national immunization days (NIDs) and subnational immunization days, leading to increasing susceptibility to type 2 in the population, and (4) insensitive AFP surveillance. These viruses are further subdivided into three categories:

1. Circulating VDPVs, when evidence of person-to-person transmission in the community exists
2. Immunodeficiency-associated VDPVs (iVDPVs), which are isolated from people with primary B-cell or combined immunodeficiency disorders
3. Ambiguous VDPVs(aVDPVs), which are either clinical isolates from a person with no known immunodeficiency or sewage isolates of unknown origin.

Q30. What are the merits and demerits of OPV and IPV?

Ans.

Merits of OPV:

- *Effective in stopping transmission:* OPV induces strong immunity in the gut, preventing the virus from replicating and spreading through the fecal-oral route.
- *Long-lasting protection:* OPV provides long-lasting immunity against all three types of polioviruses.
- *Cost-effective:* OPV is relatively inexpensive to produce and administer, making it a cost-effective option for widespread vaccination campaigns.

Demerits of OPV:

- *Risk of vaccine-associated paralytic poliomyelitis (VAPP):* In rare cases, OPV can cause paralysis in individuals vaccinated, though this is a very low risk.
- *Potential for circulating vaccine-derived poliovirus (cVDPV) emergence:* OPV can revert to a wild form, causing outbreaks of cVDPV in areas with poor sanitation and inadequate vaccination coverage.

- *Not ideal for individuals with weakened immune systems:* OPV is not recommended for individuals with certain weakened immune systems due to the risk of VAPP and the potential for the vaccine virus to cause illness.

Merits of IPV:

- *Eliminates the risk of VAPP*: IPV does not contain a live virus, so it cannot cause VAPP.
- *High efficacy*: IPV is highly effective in preventing paralytic disease caused by all three types of polioviruses.
- *Safe*: IPV is one of the safest vaccines in use, with minimal side effects.
- *Suitable for individuals with weakened immune systems*: IPV is safe to administer to individuals with weakened immune systems.

Demerits of IPV:

- *Does not stop transmission:* IPV does not induce gut immunity and, therefore, does not stop the spread of the virus through the fecal-oral route.
- *More expensive than OPV:* IPV is more expensive to produce and administer than OPV, making it less cost-effective for widespread vaccination campaigns.
- *Not as effective in areas with high fecal-oral transmission:* In areas where fecal-oral transmission is common, IPV may not be as effective as OPV in preventing outbreaks.

Q31. What are cellular and acellular DTP vaccines?

Ans. Popularly known as triple antigen, DTwP is composed of tetanus and diphtheria toxoids as well as killed whole-cell pertussis (wP) bacilli adsorbed on insoluble aluminum salts which act as adjuvants.

The content of diphtheria toxoid varies from 20 to 30 Lf that of tetanus toxoid (TT) varies from 5 to 25 Lf per dose and whole cell pertussis >4 IU per dose.

Once disease rates declined, concerns about frequent local side effects, as well as public anxiety about the safety of wP vaccines, led to the development of acellular pertussis (aP) vaccines in Japan in 1981.

These were licensed in the US in 1996 and have now replaced the whole-cell vaccines in most developed countries. All aP vaccines are associated with significantly lesser side effects, and thus the replacement of the wP vaccines was mainly driven by the safety profile of these vaccines. The other important advantage of the aP vaccines is the reproducible production process with its use of purified antigens and the removal of lipopolysaccharides (LPS) and other parts of the bacterial cell wall during the purification of soluble antigenic material. These vaccines contain ≥1 of the separately purified antigens pertussis toxin (PT), filamentous hemagglutinin (FHA), pertactin (PRN), and fimbrial hemagglutinins 1, 2, and 3 (FIM type 2 and type 3).

Q32. What are contraindications to whole cell DPT vaccine?

Ans. Moderate to severe hypersensitivity reaction occurring after the previous administration of any dose of DPT-containing vaccines. It is also contraindicated in those with known hypersensitivity to any of the vaccine constituents. It is also contraindicated in infants who developed an acute encephalopathy of unknown etiology, within 7 days of previous administration of DPT-containing vaccine. Infants with a progressive neurological illness should not receive this vaccine. Acute moderate to severe illnesses are a precaution for administration of this vaccine.

Q33. What are the contraindications of MMR vaccine?

Ans.

Contraindications: Subjects with moderate to severe allergic reaction to previous dose of the vaccine or known hypersensitivity to any other component of the vaccine, pregnancy. Pregnancy should be avoided for 1 month following vaccination.

Other contraindications: Moderate to severe immuno-suppression due to drugs, radiation, advance lymphoma, serious malignant disease, or some congenital disorders of immunity.

Q34. How many types of hepatitis A vaccines are available in India? What are the dose, route, and age for hepatitis A vaccine?

Ans. Two types—inactivated and live attenuated

Inactivated vaccines available in India: Most of the currently available vaccines are derived from HM 175/ GBM strains and grown on MRC-5 human diploid cell lines.

Another type—live attenuated

IAP recommendations: Hepatitis A vaccine schedule

Routine vaccination:

- *Inactivated vaccines:* >12 months: Two doses administered intramuscular (IM) at 0 and 6–18 months
- *Live vaccines:* >12 months: Single dose administered subcutaneous (SC)

Catch-up vaccination:
- *Inactivated vaccines:* Two doses administered IM at 0 and 6–18 months
- *Live vaccines:* single dose administered SC
- For catch-up vaccination, prevaccination screening for hepatitis A antibody is recommended in children >10 years, as at this age, the estimated seropositive rates exceed 50%.

Q35. What are the types of typhoid vaccine available in India? What is the age for giving different types of typhoid vaccine?

Ans. Clinical trials, some conducted decades ago, have demonstrated efficacy of a range of typhoid vaccines which include:
- Whole cell inactivated vaccines
- Virulence capsular polysaccharide vaccines
- Live-attenuated vaccines; and more recently
- Virulence conjugate vaccines

The new generation current typhoid fever vaccines include oral live-attenuated Ty21a vaccine, parenteral Vi polysaccharide, and Vi-polysaccharide (Vi-PS) capsular conjugate vaccines. Oral live-attenuated Ty21a vaccine is not available in the country.

IAP recommendations:

Typhoid vaccines:
- Both Vi-PS (polysaccharide) and Vi-PS conjugate vaccines
- *Minimum ages:*
  - Vi-PS conjugate (Typbar-TCV®): 6 months
  - Vi-PS (polysaccharide) vaccines: 2 years
- *Vaccination schedule:*
  - *Vi-PS (polysaccharide) vaccines*: Single dose at 2 years; revaccination every 3 years (no evidence of hyporesponsiveness on repeated revaccination so far)
  - *Vi-PS conjugate (Typbar-TCV®)*: Single dose at 9–12 months
- *Catch-up vaccination:*
  - Recommended throughout the adolescent period, i.e., till 18 years
  - IAP prefers the use of Vi-PS conjugate vaccine.

Q36. What are the types of JE vaccine available in India? What are the age and schedule of JE vaccination?

Ans. World over, following vaccines were available for use against JE:
- *Mouse brain-derived inactivated JE vaccine (JE-VAX):* This vaccine is no longer in clinical usage
- Inactivated primary hamster kidney cells with P3—China
- Live attenuated, cell culture-derived SA 14-14-2

Newer JE vaccines:
- Inactivated SA 14-14-2 vaccine
- Inactivated Vero cell culture-derived Kolar strain, JE vaccine
- Live-attenuated recombinant SA 14-14-2 chimeric vaccine
- Inactivated Vero cell-derived JE vaccine (Beijing-1 JE strain by Biken and Kaketsuken, Japan) not available in India.

Owing to many drawbacks (high cost, complicated dosing schedule, requirement of numerous doses and boosters, concerns about side effects, and reliance neurological tissue for production) and availability of better vaccines, the first two vaccines, i.e., mouse brain-derived and primary hamster kidney cells with P3 are no longer being produced.

Japanese encephalitis (JE) vaccines: IAP recommendations:

Routine vaccination:
- Recommended only for individuals living in endemic districts. Both rural and urban children in a district should be vaccinated.
- Three types of new generation JE vaccines are licensed in India:
  1. Live-attenuated, cell culture-derived SA 14-14-2
  2. Inactivated JE vaccines, namely "Vero cell culture-derived SA 14-14-2 JE vaccine"
  3. "Vero cell culture-derived, 821564XY, JE vaccine"
- Live-attenuated, cell culture-derived SA-14-14-2:
  - Minimum age: 8 months
  - Two-dose schedule, first dose at 9 months along with MR vaccine
  - Second dose at 16–18 months along with DTP booster
- Inactivated cell culture-derived SA 14-14-2:
  - *Minimum age*: 1 year (US-FDA: 2 months)
  - *Primary immunization schedule*: Two doses of 3 microgram/0.5 mL administered intramuscularly on days 0 and 28 for children aged ≥1 to ≤3 years
  - Two doses of 6 microgram/0.5 mL for children >3 years and adults
  - Need of boosters still undetermined
- Inactivated Vero cell culture-derived Kolar strain, 821564XY, JE vaccine:
  - Minimum age: 1 year

- *Primary immunization schedule:* Two doses of 0.5 mL each administered intramuscularly at 4 weeks interval
- Need of boosters still undetermined

Catch-up vaccination: All susceptible children up to 15 years should be administered during disease outbreak or ahead of anticipated outbreak in campaigns.

Q37. What kind of vaccine varicella is? What are the age, route, and dosage of varicella vaccine?

Ans. Monovalent varicella vaccines available in India currently are approved by Central Drugs Standard Control Organization (CDSCO) after phase II and III immunogenicity and safety studies.

They are licensed for use in persons aged >12 months.

All of them employ live-attenuated VZV (Oka strain). They do differ in the number of plaque-forming units (PFUs) from 1,300 to 2,500 PFUs—though a dose of 200 PFU is immunogenic. WHO does not specify a minimum number of PFUs per vaccine dose, but is important for national regulatory authority, which licenses the vaccine. The ACVIP now recommends two doses of varicella vaccine for children of all age groups.

For primary immunization, the first dose is best administered at 15 months and the second dose should be given 3–6 months after the first dose. However, during an outbreak, the first dose may be administered at 12 months of age if it is ensured that the two-dose schedule will be completed by the individual child.

Q38. What are the types of pneumococcal vaccine available in India? what is the earliest age for pneumococcal vaccination?

Ans. Currently, two types of vaccines are licensed for use: (1) Pneumococcal polysaccharide vaccine (PPSV) and (2) Pneumococcal conjugate vaccines.

The unconjugated PPSV is a 23-valent vaccine (PPSV23) containing 25 µg per dose of the purified polysaccharide of the following 23 serotypes of pneumococcus.

The earliest age for pneumococcal vaccination—6 weeks for conjugated, 2 years—for polysaccharides

Q39. Whom to give Influenza vaccine and at what schedule?

Ans. Influenza vaccine recommended for

1. Children 6 months to 5 years age
2. The high risk children aged >5 years which includes following:
    a. Chronic cardiac, pulmonary (excluding asthma), haematologic and renal (including nephritic syndrome), condition, chronic liver disease and diabetes mellitus.
    b. Congenital or acquired immunodeficiency (including HIV infection).
    c. Children on long term salicylate therapy.
    d. Laboratory personnel and health care workers.

Dosage and schedule:

- 0.5 mL (15 µg) >6 months of age
- From 6 months to 8 years for the first time, two doses of inactivated influenza vaccine (IIV) to be given 4 weeks apart
- *>8 years:* Single dose
- Revaccination is recommended with a single annual dose, till the age of 5 years.

In those at high risk of influenza complications, annual revaccination may be continued beyond the age of 5 years.

Q40. What are HPV vaccines? What are the dose, route, and age of vaccination of HPV vaccine?

Ans. The quadrivalent and nonvalent vaccines have been licensed globally. The bivalent vaccine has been withdrawn from the Indian market. Both vaccines are manufactured by recombinant DNA technology that produces noninfectious virus-like particles (VLPs) comprising the HPV-L1 protein.

4vHPV: Cervavac

Schedule for Cervavac:

- *9–14 years of age (boys and girls):* Two-dose schedule (0.5 mL at 0 and 6 months). The interval between the 1st and 2nd dose should not be <5 months.
- *15–26 years of age (females and males) and immunocompromised:* 3-dose (0.5 mL at 0, 2, and 6 months) schedule. The second dose should be administered at least 1 month after the first dose and the third dose should be administered at least 3 months after the second dose.

Age recommendations:

- Gardasil 4—Females: 9–45 years
- Gardasil 9—Females: 9–26 years
- Males: 9–14 years
- Cervavac—Males and females: 9–26 years

Q41. What are the vaccines important for the adolescent?

Ans. Indian Academy of Pediatrics, Advisory Committee on Vaccines and Immunization Practices recommended vaccines in adolescents (11–18 years).

Vaccine schedule:

- Tdap/Td—10 years

- HPV—9 years
- COVID vaccines—12 years onwards

Indian Academy of Pediatrics, Advisory Committee on Vaccines and Immunization Practices recommended vaccines in adolescents for catch-up.

Vaccine schedule:

- *MMR:* Two doses at 4–8 weeks' interval
- *Hepatitis B:* Three doses at 0, 1, and 6 months
- *Hepatitis A:* Two doses at 0 and 6 months (prior check for anti-HAV IgG may be cost-effective in children of age >10 years)
- *Typhoid TCV:* Single dose
- *Varicella:* Two doses at 4–8 weeks of interval
- *HPV:* 9–14 years (boys and girls): Two dose 6 months apart
- *15 years or older (girls and women):* 4vHPV: 0–2–6 months
- *9vHPV (females):* 15–26 years: 0–2–6 months

Indian Academy of Pediatrics, Advisory Committee on Vaccines and Immunization Practices recommended vaccines in adolescents in special circumstances:

Vaccine schedule:

- *Influenza:* One dose every year
- *Japanese encephalitis vaccine catch-up:* Up to 15 years*
- *PPSV23 (pneumococcal):* Maximum two doses 5 years apart
- *Rabies vaccine:* 0, 3, 7, 14, and 28 days

Q42. What are the vaccines contraindicated in AIDS patients?

Ans. Indian Academy of Pediatrics (IAP), World Health Organization (WHO), American Academy of Pediatrics (AAP), Advisory Committee on Immunization Practices (ACIP), and Centers for Disease Control and Prevention (CDC) recommend all the live vaccines in asymptomatic HIV-1 infected children except OPV. However, in a symptomatic child, all live vaccines are forbidden, but at times measles/MMR/varicella vaccines may be considered on individual merit. Yellow fever vaccine is contraindicated in symptomatic but can be given in asymptomatic and those at risk of exposure. For killed vaccines in an HIV-infected child, ideally postvaccination monitoring of seroconversion is desirable. In an HIV-infected child, there is a multifold enhanced risk of diseases such as tuberculosis, hepatitis (A and B), measles, influenza, varicella, pneumococcal, and meningococcal disease. Hence, in such situations, a judicious and intelligent decision of the physician is warranted.

*Only in endemic area as catch up

Q43. How will you modify vaccination following steroid therapy?

Ans. Children receiving oral corticosteroids in high doses (prednisolone 2 mg/kg/day for those weighing <10 kg or for those weighing >10 kg, 20 mg/day or its equivalent) for >2 weeks should not receive live-virus vaccines until the steroids have been discontinued for at least 1 month. Killed vaccines are safe but may be less efficacious. Children receiving oral corticosteroids in high doses (prednisolone 2 mg/kg/day for those weighing <10 kg or for those weighing >10 kg, 20 mg/day or its equivalent) for <2 weeks can receive live-virus vaccines after discontinuation of treatment. Children receiving oral corticosteroids in lower doses (prednisolone <2 mg/kg/day for those weighing <10 kg or for those weighing >10 kg, <20 mg/day or its equivalent) can receive live vaccines, while on therapy. These doses are not immunosuppressive. Children who are receiving only maintenance physiologic doses of corticosteroids can receive live-virus vaccines. Children on alternate day therapy, inhaled or topical therapy may be safely and effectively given their age-appropriate vaccines. Low or moderate doses of systemic corticosteroids or locally administered corticosteroids in children who have a disease (e.g., systemic lupus erythematosus) that in itself is considered to suppress the immune response should not receive live-virus vaccines during therapy, except in special circumstances during which the potential benefit of protection and the risk of adverse reaction are weighed.

Q44. What are the types of rabies vaccine availability in India?

Ans. The currently available vaccines are:

- The cell culture vaccines (CCVs) include purified chick embryo cell vaccine (PCECV), human diploid cell vaccine (HDCV), purified vero cell rabies vaccine (PVRV)
- *Purified duck embryo vaccine (PDEV)*

  It is to be noted that all CCVs and PDEV should have potency (antigen content) >2.5 IU per intramuscular dose irrespective of whether it is 0.5 mL or 1.0 mL vaccine by volume.

Q45. What are the vaccines that should be given to traveler?

Ans. Travellers need to be up to date in age recommended vaccinations Apart from routine vaccinations travellers also need some selective vaccines and country specific vaccines.

Selective use for travelers:

- Hepatitis A
- Typhoid fever
- Rabies
- Cholera
- Japanese encephalitis
- Tick-borne encephalitis

Country-specific mandatory vaccines for travelers:

- Yellow fever
- Meningococcal conjugate
- Oral poliovirus vaccines

Q46. What is current scenario of dengue and malaria vaccine?

Ans.

Dengue virus vaccine: Dengvaxia™ (also referred to as CYD-TDV) is a live recombinant tetravalent dengue vaccine developed by Sanofi Pasteur and administered in a three-dose schedule (0/6/12 months). Dengvaxia was first licensed in December 2015. Due to the occurrence of vaccine-induced antibody-dependent enhancement, in 2018, the World Health Organization (WHO) issued fresh recommendations for its use. The WHO recommended that only those persons with evidence of a past dengue infection should be vaccinated (based on an antibody test, or on a documented laboratory confirmed dengue infection in the past). Where prevaccination screening is not feasible, the vaccine should be administered only in those areas vaccination wherein recent serosurveys have documented seroprevalence rates of at least 80% by age 9 years.

Vaccines in phase III trials:

- The Takeda vaccine (TAK-003) is a tetravalent vaccine in which wild DEN2 is attenuated and the *Env* and *PrM* genes of DEN 1, 3, and 4 are inserted into the genome of the attenuated DENV2 backbone.
  In August 2022, Takeda's Qdenga® [Dengue Tetravalent Vaccine (live, attenuated)] received approval in Indonesia, for use regardless of prior dengue exposure.
- TetraVax-DV (NIH) is a combination of four monovalent attenuated DENVs—in phase 2 trial.

Other vaccines in phase II trials:

- *TDENV-PIV:* This is a purified inactivated vaccine which consists of all four dengue serotypes.

Vaccines in phase I trials:

- Merck's V180, a recombinant subunit dengue vaccine, adjuvanted with ISCOMATRIX, is in phase 1 study.

The Serum Institute of India is currently recruiting in Australia for its phase I trial of its Dengusiil™ dengue vaccine candidate.

Malarial vaccines: The RTS,S/AS01 vaccine is the only malaria vaccine to be recommended for use by the WHO. The WHO has recommended this vaccine for the prevention of *P. falciparum* malaria in children living in regions with moderate-to-high malaria transmission, as defined by WHO.

Schedule: Three primary doses at a minimum interval of 4 weeks between doses, beginning at 5 months of age, with a fourth dose provided approximately 12–18 months after the third dose.

Plasmodium falciparum Sporozoite (PfSPZ), an attenuated whole sporozoite vaccine, which is given intravenously, has shown a vaccine efficacy of 100% against Controlled Human Malarial Infection model up to 79 days of follow-up. It is now being under study.

The R21/Matrix-M vaccine has shown an efficacy of 71–76% against at least one malaria episode over 12 months (depending on adjuvant dosage).

RH5.1, which is a vaccine targeting blood stages, has completed phase 2 trials and Pfs230D1M, which is a transmission blocking agent, has completed phase 2 trials.

SUGGESTED READING

1. Bonanni P, Boccalini S, Bechini A. Efficacy, duration of immunity and effectiveness of vaccines. Vaccine. 2015; 33(4):552–60.
2. Centers for Disease Control and Prevention. Epidemiology and prevention of vaccine-preventable diseases (The Pink Book). 14th ed. Washington DC: CDC; 2021.
3. Indian Academy of Pediatrics Advisory Committee on Vaccines and Immunization Practices (ACVIP). IAP immunization timetable 2024. Indian Pediatr. 2024; 61(3):256–64.
4. Kliegman RM, St Geme JW, Blum NJ, Shah SS, Tasker RC, Wilson KM, editors. Nelson textbook of pediatrics. 22nd ed. Philadelphia: Elsevier; 2023.
5. Plotkin SA, Orenstein WA, Offit PA, Edwards KM. Plotkin's vaccines. 8th ed. Philadelphia: Elsevier; 2024.
6. Siegrist CA. Vaccine immunology. In: Plotkin SA, Orenstein WA, Offit PA, editors. Vaccines. 7th ed. Philadelphia: Elsevier; 2018. p. 16–34.
7. World Health Organization. Immunization in practice: a practical guide for health staff. 2015 update. Geneva: World Health Organization; 2015.

CHAPTER 16

Instruments

Ira Das, Sayan Chatterjee

ASTHMA DEVICES

Q1. What are the most common types of aerosol delivery devices used for children?

Ans.

- *pMDI*: Pressurized metered dose inhalers with spacer (with or without mask)
- *DPI* (dry powder inhalers)
- Nebulizers
- Soft mist inhalers

Metered Dose Inhalers

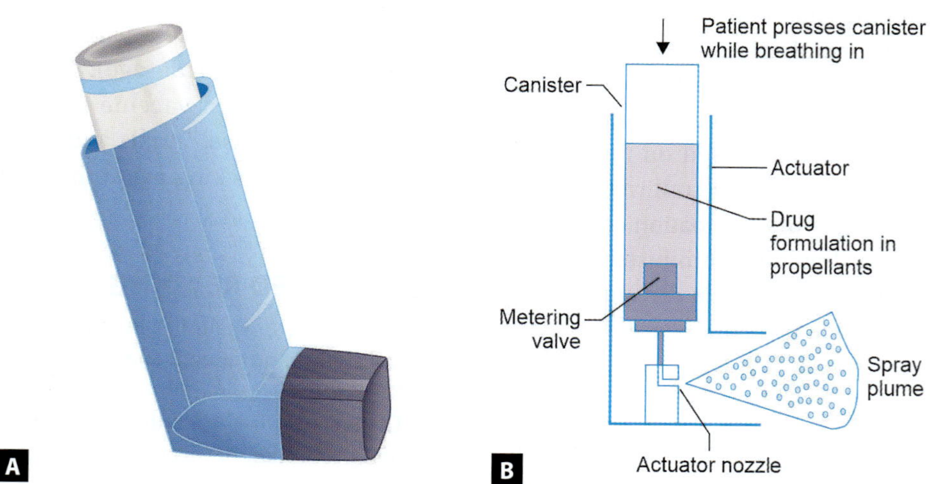

Figs. 1A and B: (A) Metered dose inhalers; (B) Parts of metered dose inhalers.

Q2. What are the different parts of pMDI?

Ans. The main parts of a pMDI **(Fig. 1B)** are:

- The canister
- The actuator
- The mouthpiece
- Dust cap

Q3. What is canister?

Ans. The canister is usually made of aluminum or stainless steel. It contains medicine along with a liquefied gas propellant (*HFA—hydrofluoroalkane*).

Q4. Why it is called metered dose inhaler?

Ans. MDI (*metered dose inhaler*) is a device that delivers a specific amount of medication in an aerosol form to the lungs. The metering valve present within the actuator delivers the metered quantity of the drug in the aerosol form **(Fig. 1A)**.

Q5. What is the function of propellant in MDI?

Ans. The propellant provides the force to generate the aerosol cloud and is also the medium where the active component must be suspended or dissolved.

Q6. What are the drugs delivered through MDI?

Ans.

- Beta$_2$ agonist
- Anticholinergics
- Corticosteroids
- Mast cell stabilizer

Q7. What are the uses of MDI?

Ans.

- Bronchial asthma (both reliver and controller therapy)
- Hyperkalemia
- Obstructive airway disease

Q8. How to use MDI?

Ans.

- Shake inhaler smoothly for 4–5 seconds by placing index finger on top of the canister and thumb on the bottom of the mouthpiece.
- Sit straight and extend the neck slightly.
- Remove the cap.
- Open mouth such that tongue cannot obstruct mouthpiece.
- Breath out normally.
- Put the inhaler between lips in mouth. Press the inhaler and start breathing (slow and deep breath).
- Hold breath for 4–10 seconds. Breath out slowly.
- Repeat after 30 seconds, if another dose is required.
- Rinse mouth after corticosteroid inhalation.
- Close the cap over mouthpiece.

Q9. Why hold breath for 4–10 seconds?

Ans. Gravitational deposition is the principal mechanism for drug deposition in lung, others are inertial impaction and diffusion, for which breath holding is needed.

Q10. What are the advantages of MDI?

Ans.

- Easily portable
- Multidose delivery system
- Lower risk of bacterial contamination
- No drug preparation
- Quick delivery
- Effective in acute management

Q11. What are the disadvantages of MDI?

Ans.

- Need for correct coordination of inhalation and actuation
- Oropharyngeal drug deposition
- Used with spacer (increases cost)
- Cold freon effect

Q12. What do you mean by the cold Freon effect?

Ans. During pMDI inhalation without spacer, pressurized propellants rapidly expand and evaporated causing feeling of cold in oropharynx which leads to *bronchospasm*.

Q13. How to use metered dose inhaler with spacer device and a mask?

Ans.

- Shake the MDI 4–5 times and remove the cap.
- Insert the mouthpiece of the MDI into the soft rubber ring at the open end of the spacer.
- Place the mask gently over child's face covering mouth and nose with good seal. Child can breathe in and out normally.
- Press down on the MDI canister at starting of inspiration to deliver drugs into the spacer and encourage the child to take tidal breathing with open mouth (if possible) for 5–6 breaths.
- Wait 30 seconds before repeating second puff.

Q14. How to use metered dose inhaler with spacer device?

Ans.

- Shake the MDI 4–5 times and remove the cap.
- Insert the mouthpiece of the MDI into the soft rubber ring at the open end of the spacer.
- Start breathing in and out slowly and notice the movement of valve.
- Once breathing pattern is established, press MDI canister once at starting of inspiration and take slow and deep breath, take 5–6 breaths after single actuation.
- Remove the device from the mouth and wait for 30 seconds, then repeat 2nd dose.
- Rinse mouth after corticosteroid inhalation.

Q15. Why must you shake the MDI?

Ans. For correct mixing of propellant and active drugs, because one is heavier than other.

Q16. How to prime MDI?

Ans. For a new metered dose inhaler (MDI), or if it has not been used for 1 week or longer, two actuations should be released into the air prior to use to ensure adequate mixing and proper device function.

Selection of device:

- MDI + spacer and mask <3–4 years
- MDI + spacer for 4–6 years
- MDI + spacer or DPI >6 years

Nebulizer—regardless of age:

- Describe the different particle size deposited in lung

MMAD—mass median aerodynamic diameter **(Table 1)**:

TABLE 1: MMAD and corresponding deposition in the respiratory tract.

MMAD 0.2–0.5 µm	Exhaled out with no deposition
MMAD 0.5–5 µm	Deposited in periphery of lung
MMAD >5 µm	Deposited in the oropharynx

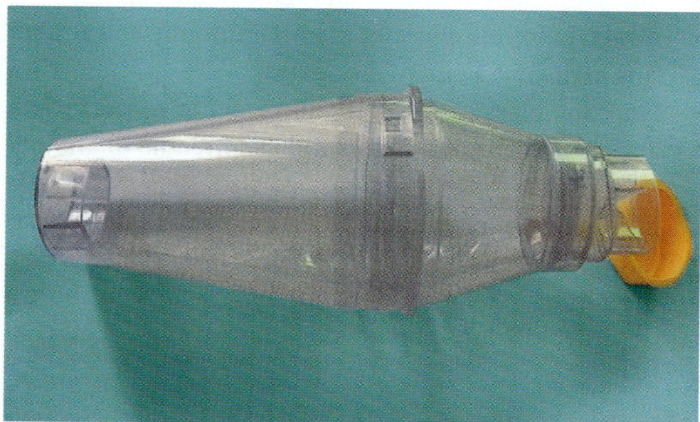

Fig. 2: Spacer (valved holding chamber/reservoir).

- Spacer devices can be used by children of any age.
- With/without valve
- Made of polyamide/polycarbonate electrostatic resistant plastics.
- Capacity 140–750 mL **(Fig. 2)**

Q17. What benefits does spacer offer?

Ans.

- Patient coordination is not necessary.
- More medication buildup in the lungs.
- 90% less deposition occurred in the oropharynx.
- Just as good as a nebulizer

Q18. What are the disadvantages of spacer?

Ans.

- Initiation can be more complex.
- More expensive
- Less portable than MDI alone

Q19. What are the methods for care and cleaning of spacer?

Ans.

- Clean hands first
- Separate different parts
- Soak all the parts in clean warm water with mild liquid dishwashing detergent
- Rotate the spacer and mask in a bowl of clean water using a gentle motion
- Do not use running water. Water pressure alters static nature of spacer.
- Allow the parts to air dry
- Do not use cloth or paper which alter static nature inside the spacer and drugs will stick to the sides.
- When completely dry, reuse spacer

Q20. How often should one wash spacer?

Ans. Spacers should be cleaned once a week.

Q21. How often do you need to replace spacers?

Ans. At least once a year

Q22. What are the advantages of zero stat spacer?

Ans.

- The static free polyamide material enables more drug available for inhalation due to lack of attraction of drug particles to spacer wall.
- The zero stat has an aerosol half-life of 45 seconds as compared to just 10 seconds in polycarbonate spacer.

Dry Powder Inhalers

Q23. In which age group, DPI can be used?

Ans. Children >6 years of age can use DPI.

Q24. What is the carrier of drugs in DPI?

Ans. Lactose.

Q25. How DPI work?

Ans. Gelatine capsules contain drugs, carrier substances (lactose). After piercing with inbuild needle drugs disaggregate and formed aerosol with patient's inspiratory flow.

Q26. What is the inspiratory flow required for DPI?

Ans. 30–60 L/min according to different devices.

Q27. How to use DPI (Rotahaler)?

Ans.

- Hold the rotahaler vertically
- Insert the rota cap, transparent end first, into the raised square hole **(Fig. 3)**
- Press the rota cap firmly such that the top end of rota cap is in the level with the top of hole.
- Rotate the base, the fin separates the two halves of the rota cap.
- After breath out fully, grip the mouthpiece between lips. Breath in through your mouth as deeply as you can.
- Remove the rotahaler and hold your breath as long as it is comfortable.
- After use, discard the empty rota cap shell.

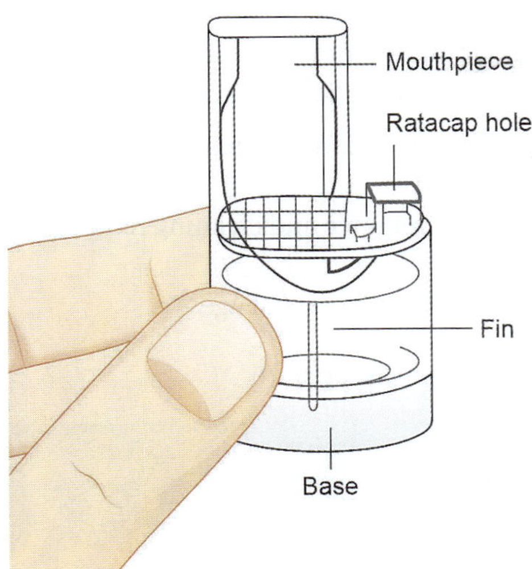

Fig. 3: Parts of Rotahaler.

Q28. What are the differences between MDI and DPI?

Ans. MDI:

- High velocity aerosols
- Requires hand breath coordination for delivery of medicine
- Use of a spacer improves medication delivery.
- Require propellants
- Time consuming to teach
- Can be used in any age group

DPI:

- More costly
- Aerosol velocity depends on inspiratory flow rate.
- No hand breath coordination requires
- Easy to teach
- Ambient humidity and heat may affect emitted dose.
- Can only be used from 6 years of age

Nebulizers (Fig. 4)

Q29. What are the different types of nebulizers?

Ans.

- Jet nebulizer
- Ultrasonic nebulizer
- Vibrating mesh nebulizer
- Small volume nebulizer
- Breath actuated nebulizer
- Handheld multidose nebulizer
- Large volume nebulizer

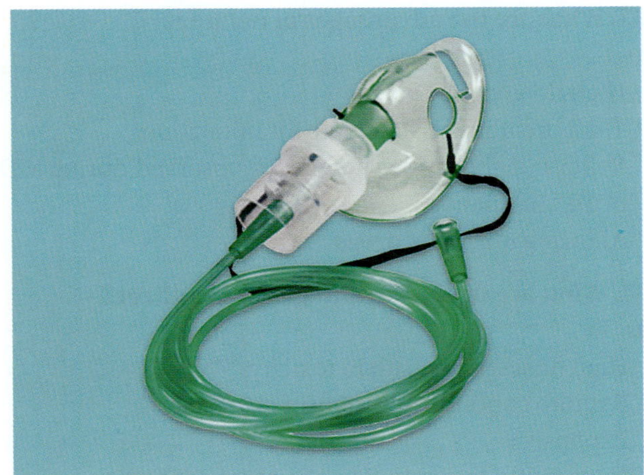

Fig. 4: Nebulizer mask.

Q30. What are the components of nebulizer?

Ans.

- Compressor
- Tubing
- nebulizer chamber
- Mouthpiece or face mask
- Nebulizer filter

Q31. What is the principle of jet nebulizer?

Ans. Aerosol generated by Venturi effect of Bernoulli's principle of gases.

Q32. What is the principle of ultrasonic nebulizer?

Ans. Aerosol is formed by ultrasonic wave (vibration of piezoelectric crystal).

Steps to use nebulizer:

- Wash your hands
- Connect to air compressor
- Fill the medicine cup with medicine
- Attach the other end to the mouthpiece and medicine cup
- Turn on the nebulizer machine
- Place the mouthpiece in mouth. If using a facemask, place it over the mouth and nose. Small children usually do better if they wear a mask.
- Breathe through mouth until all the medicine is used. This takes 5–20 minutes, depending on the device and medicine used.
- Turn off the machine when aerosol formation ends.
- As many patients are hypoxic, oxygen from central supply or an oxygen cylinder should be given, at a flow rate of 6–8 L/min in place of compressed air.

Q33. What are the advantages of nebulizer?

Ans.

- High dose can be given.
- Tidal breathing is adequate for inhalation.
- Reflex coughing does not occur (observed during MDI or DPI inhalation).
- Allowing mixing of drugs

Q34. What are the disadvantages of nebulizer?

Ans.

- High doses may result in toxicity.
- Require continuous supply of electricity
- Expensive
- Have risk of transmission of airborne infection
- All medicines not available in liquid forms
- Require more times

Q35. Which is more effective, MDI or nebulizer?

Ans. The use of MDI with spacer is more effective than nebulizer in young children because in MDI inhalation:

- Less time to stay in the emergency department
- Lower cost
- Easier to use
- Drug deposition in lungs 10–20% in case of MDI with spacer whereas <10% in case of nebulizer

Q36. Describe drug deposition in airway and oropharynx by different inhalational devices?

Ans. **Table 2** describe the drug deposition in airway and oropharynx by inhalational devices.

TABLE 2: Drug deposition in airway and oropharynx by inhalational devices.

Inhalational device	*Drug deposition airway*	*Drug deposition oropharynx*
MDI + spacer	10–20%	80%
MDI only	10%	80–90%
DPI	5–10%	40–50%
Nebulizer	<10%	50%++

(DPI: dry powder inhaler; MDI: metered dose inhaler)

Q37. What is soft mist inhaler?

Ans. Soft mist inhaler is a propellent free handheld multidose inhaler.

Q38. What are the advantages of soft mist inhaler?

Ans.

- Soft mist inhalers generate a fine mist of medication that is small and easily absorbed by the respiratory system, which increases the effectiveness of medication.
- Portable and compact, no need of spacer
- Breath actuated device that means they release medication automatically when user take a breath

Q39. What are the disadvantages of soft mist inhaler?

- More expensive
- Regular maintenance and cleaning required for proper functioning
- Useful more than 6 years of age

PEAK FLOW METER

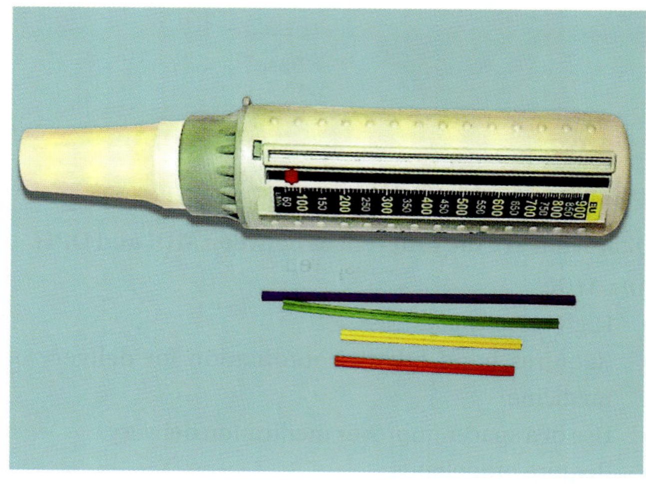

Fig. 5: Peak flow meter.

Q40. What is PEFR?

Ans. PEFR (peak expiratory flow rate) is the volume of air forcefully expelled from lungs in one exhalation.

Q41. What is the use of peak flow meter in children?

Ans. Peak flow meter (PFM) is used for asthma self-assessment plan. For diagnosis of asthma, diurnal PEF variability >20% if spirometry not available **(Fig. 5)**.

Q42. What is the normal PEFR in children?

Ans. Peak flow rate depends on age, height, and sex. Normal PEFR for children is between 150 and 450 L/min. The regression equation in both sexes based on height is: PEFR = 4.41 × HT (cm) – 328.26 L/min.

Q43. How to measure peak expiratory flow rate in children?

Ans. **Table 3** describes the PEFR-based asthma action plan zones indicating level of control and recommended interventions.

- Sliding marker should be at zero of scale
- Stand up and take a deep breath
- Blow out forcibly in a single breath
- Note the number where the sliding pointer stops

- Repeat the steps another two times
- Record highest of the three numbers

TABLE 3: PEFR-based asthma action plan zones indicating level of control and recommended interventions.

PEFR 80–100% of their personal best	Green zone, good control, need step down therapy
PEFR 50–80% of personal best	Yellow zone or caution zone, need rescue drugs and to increase controller medication
PEFR <50% of personal best	Red zone or stop zone, need immediate rescue drugs and emergency care

(PEFR: peak expiratory flow rate)

OXYGEN DELIVERY DEVICES

Q44. What are the different oxygen delivery devices?

Ans. Low-flow system [lower than patient's inspiration flow, variable fraction of inspired O_2 (FiO_2)]:

- Nasal cannula
- Simple face mask or Hudson mask
- Partial rebreathing mask
- Nonrebreathing mask

High-flow system (higher than patient's inspiration flow, consistent FiO_2):

- High-flow nasal cannula
- Venturi mask
- Continuous positive airway pressure mask

NASAL CANNULA

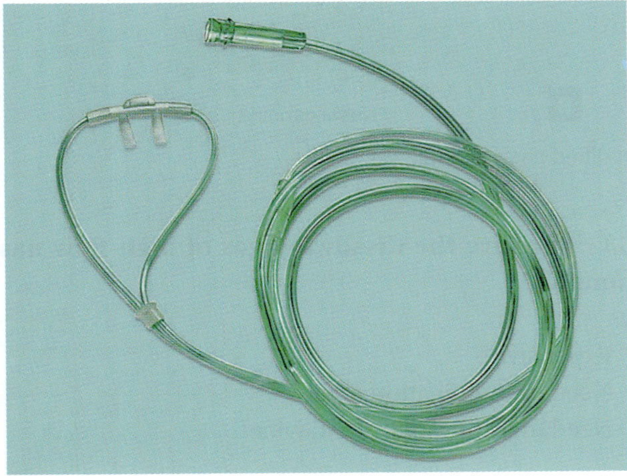

Fig. 6: Nasal cannula.

Q45. What is the indication of using nasal cannula?

Ans. Administration of oxygen where minimal O_2 requirement and recovery phase from acute episode (with gas flow rate of 2–4 L/min, it provides 30–40% of oxygen) **(Fig. 6)**.

Q46. What are the advantages of nasal cannula?

Ans.

- Leaves mouth free for nutritional purpose and talk
- Low cost

Q47. What are the disadvantages of nasal cannula?

Ans.

- Nasal dryness or irritation from nasal cannula
- Frequent displacement of nasal prongs
- Contraindicated in choanal atresia, deviated nasal septum

Q48. What is the difference between a nasal cannula and a high-flow nasal cannula?

Ans. HFNC means high flow nasal cannula. These devices blow humidified, heated oxygen into the nostrils. They can deliver up to 60 liters of oxygen per minute. Low-flow nasal cannula can only deliver a nasal cannula flow rate of 4–6 liters of oxygen per minute.

OXYGEN MASK

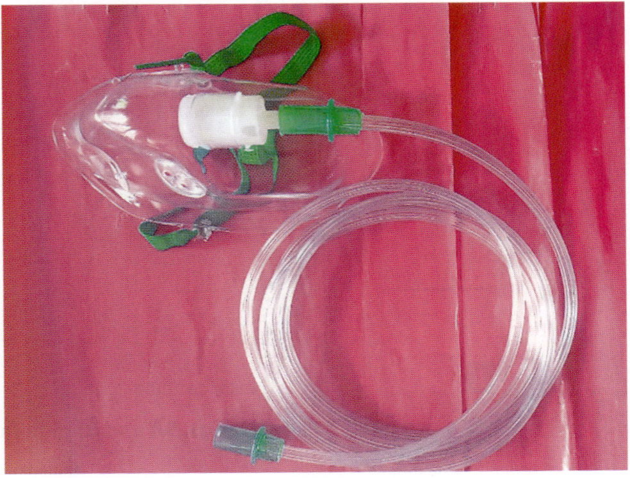

Fig. 7: Oxygen mask.

Uses of oxygen mask **(Fig. 7)**:

- Administration of oxygen (with gas flow rate of 5–10 L/min), it provides 30–60% of oxygen
- Nebulization

Q49. What are the disadvantages of oxygen mask?

Ans.

- If O_2 flow less than 6 L/min rebreathing of expired CO_2
- Difficulties during feeding and suctioning
- Tight mask not accepted by child
- Variable FiO_2 delivery

NONREBREATHER MASK

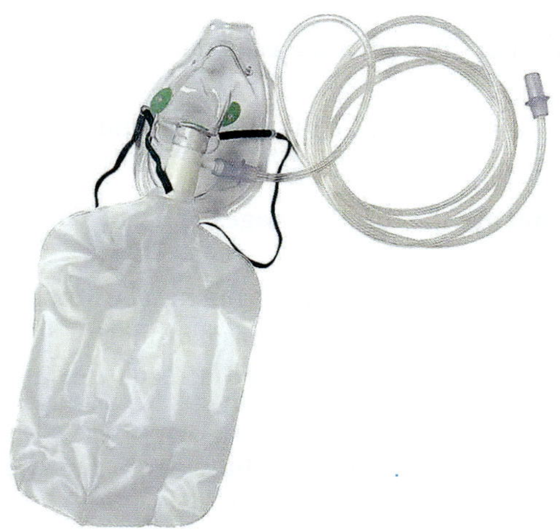

Fig. 8: Nonrebreather mask.

Indication of uses of nonrebreather mask **(Fig. 8)**: Used for the patient who are the hypoxic that require high FiO_2 (gas flow rate 10–15 L/min, FiO_2 60–100%)

Q50. What are the advantages of nonrebreather mask?

Ans. Can deliver close to 100% O_2

Q51. What are the disadvantages of nonrebreather mask?

Ans. Require tight seal on the face which often causes discomfort

HIGH-FLOW OXYGEN DELIVERY SYSTEM

High-flow Humidified Nasal Cannula (Figs. 9A and B)

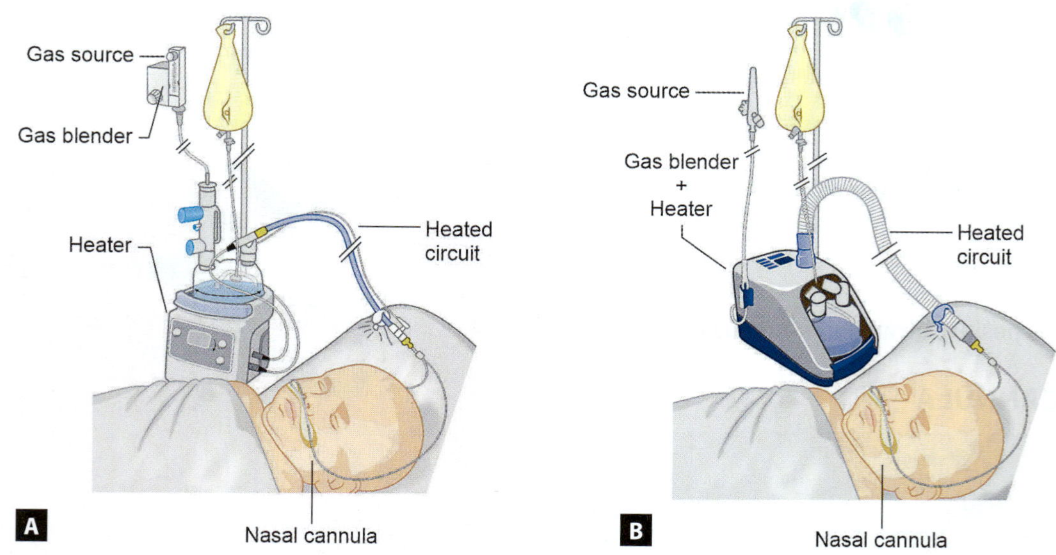

Figs. 9A and B: High-flow humidified nasal cannula.

Q52. What are the advantages of high-flow nasal cannula?

Ans.

- Comfortable and well tolerated
- Accurately titrate concentration of oxygen
- Can feed through mouth

Q53. What are the disadvantages of high-flow nasal cannula?

Ans.

- Expensive
- Need humidification device
- Need high-flow delivery device

Venturi Mask

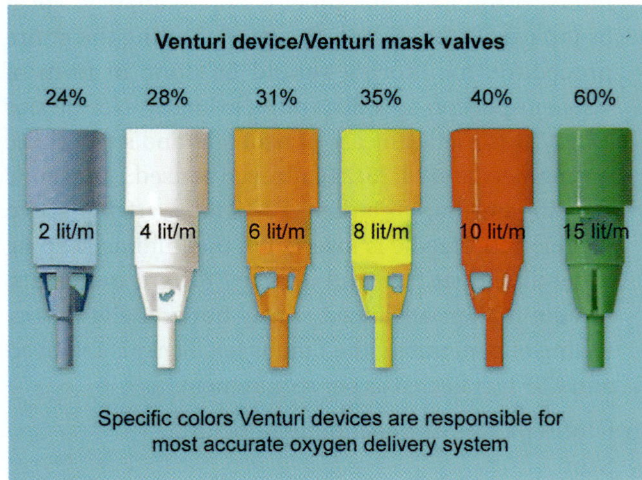

Fig. 10A: Venturi mask valves.

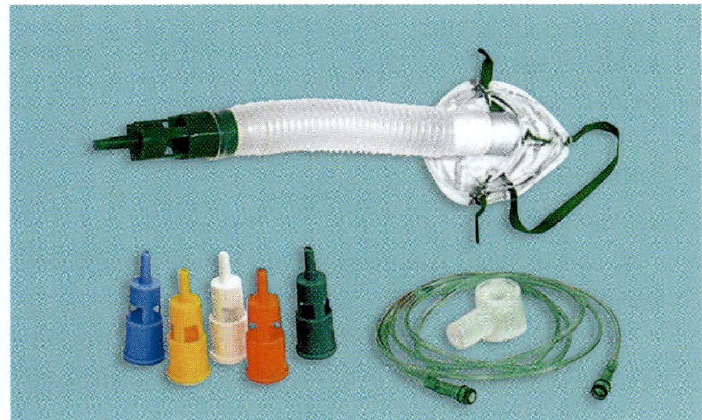

Fig. 10B: Parts of Venturi mask.

- It can deliver high-flow oxygen to children at a controlled rate. They can provide a constant oxygen concentration, even if the patient's breathing changes.
- The device uses different sizes of adaptors (of different color) to deliver a fixed or predicted FiO_2. The FiO_2 delivered depends on the flow rate and/or entrainment port size **(Table 4)**.

Q54. How does it work?

Ans. A venturi mask **(Fig. 10A)** uses a small jet to force oxygen through a mask, creating a high-velocity stream that pulls in room air. This process is based on Bernoulli's principle, which states that gas' velocity increases as it passes through a narrow tube, causing a drop in pressure.

Features: Venturi masks for children may include:

- Different sized ports to change the oxygen concentration **(Fig. 10B)**
- An adjustable nose clip
- A humidity cup
- Color-coded valves

TABLE 4: Estimated effective fractional concentration of oxygen in inspired gas (FiO_2) of low flow and reservoir oxygen delivery device.

Device	*Flow (L/min)*	*FiO_2 (%)*
Simple nasal cannula	2	28
	4	35
	6	40–45
Simple face mask	5	35–40
	10	50–60
Partial rebreathing mask	10–15	50–75
Nonrebreathing mask	15	95

LUMBAR PUNCTURE NEEDLE

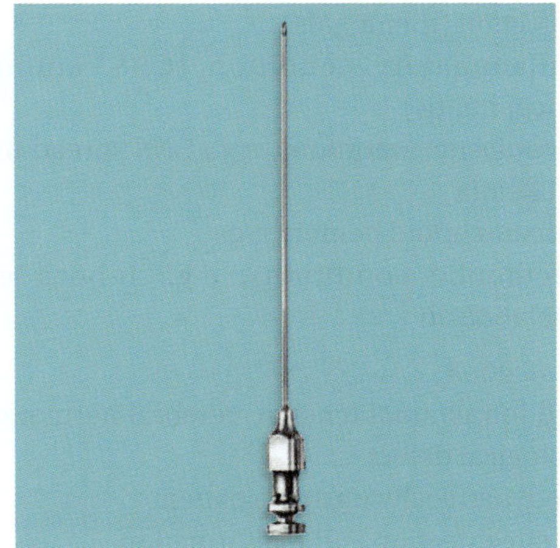

Fig. 11: Lumbar puncture needle (metallic).

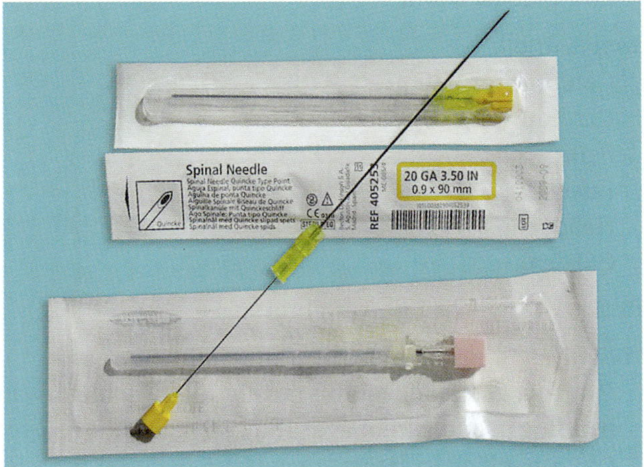

Fig. 12: Spinal needle, used for lumbar puncture.

Parts: Inner stellate and outer needle

General description: It is 10–12 cm long. Stellate of the needle has pin on one end which fits into the slot of the head of the needle. Previously, rigid metallic lumbar puncture **(Fig. 11)** needle was used, whereas nowadays spinal needle **(Fig. 12)** used for spinal anesthesia is used for doing lumbar puncture. This needle is a little bit malleable compared to conventional one.

Role of stellate: It helps to keep the lumen of the needle patent during puncturing through the structures.

Indications of lumbar puncture:

- *Therapeutics:*
  - Analgesia and anesthesia
  - *Administration of drugs:* Antibiotics, antifungal, and antineoplastic
  - Administration of dye in CSF rhinorrhea
- *Diagnostics:*
  - Infection (meningitis)
  - Inflammatory condition (GBS, autoimmune encephalitis)
  - Neoplastic conditions, e.g., CNS spread in case of leukemia
  - Subarachnoid hemorrhage
  - Metabolic conditions, e.g., inborn error of metabolism

Contraindication:

- Raised intracranial tension, cerebral herniation, focal neurological defect
- Hemodynamically unstable patient
- Local site infection and malformation
- Coagulopathy
- Low platelet count

Complication:

- Cerebral herniation
- Cardiorespiratory compromise
- Pain
- Infection
- Headache
- CSF leak

Site: L3-L4 or L4-L5 intervertebral space

Procedure:

- *Position:* Lateral decubitus mostly. Sitting with forward bending in adolescent age group
- Child is place in lateral decubitus position with hip flexed as much as possible over chest. This will increase the intervertebral space between the spinal processes. A line joining the top most point of both iliac crest with intersect the L4 spinal process approximately. Local or topical anesthesia may be given. During the entire procedure, monitoring should be done in form of visual inspection as well as pulse oximetry. Needle size 23/22/21 is used. (In case of neonates and small child, normal needle of 26/25/24 gauze can be used.) Antiseptic dressing and draping is done. L3-L4 intervertebral space is preferred. Needle is inserted in the midline keeping it parallel to surface and directed toward umbilicus. Needle is then advanced slowly horizontally till the feeling of penetrating the dura is felt. Stylet is removed and CSF is collected as per requirement.

Structures pierces during lumber puncture:

- Skin
- Subcutaneous tissue
- Back muscles
- Ligamentum flavum
- Epidural space
- Dura matter
- Arachnoid matter
- Subarachnoid space

Things seen in CSF:

- *Cell count:* WBC (neutrophil and lymphocyte), RBC, neoplastic cell
  - *Note:* Cells should be seen as early as possible because WBC and RBC are started to disintegrate within 1–2 hours
- *Biochemistry:* Sugar, protein, chloride, osmolality, etc.
- Culture
- Antigen detection
- Grams stain and Z-N stain

BONE MARROW ASPIRATION NEEDLE

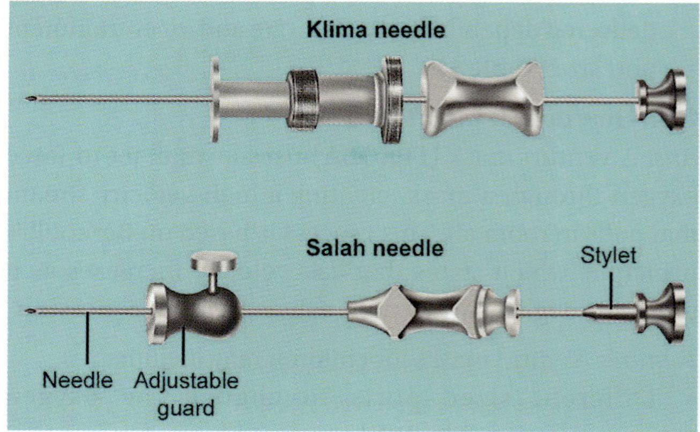

Fig. 13A

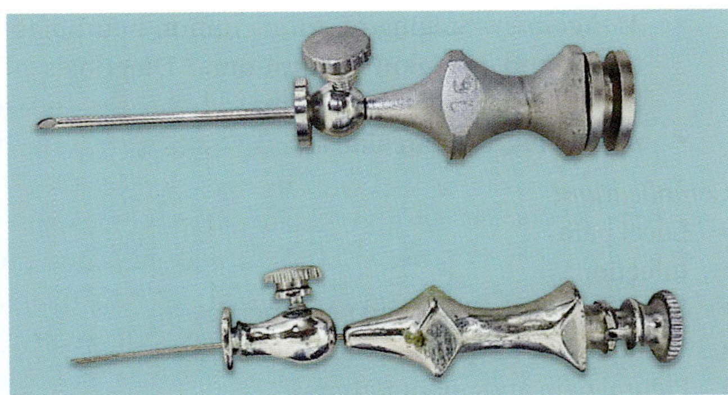

Fig. 13B

Figs. 13A and B: Bone marrow aspiration needle.

Types: Salah (with adjustable guard and screw) and Klima (guard is fixed at a particular distance) **(Figs. 13A and B)**

Parts: Stellate, thick body with nail and guard around 2 cm from the tip

- *Note:* Role of guard: It prevents excess or through and through penetration of the bone

Indication:

- *Diagnostic:*
  - Blood disorders like megaloblastic anemia, aplastic anemia, ITP, and myelofibrosis
  - Malignancy like leukemia, lymphoma, bone marrow involvement of other malignancy
  - Infection like Kala-azar
  - Storage disorder like Gaucher's disease
  - PUO
- *Therapeutic:*
  - Bone marrow transplantation,
  - Intraosseous drug administration

Contraindication:

- Coagulation disorders like hemophilia, DIC
- Local site skin infection
- Bone disorders like osteomyelitis, osteogenesis imperfecta

Site:

- *In pediatric age group:* Posterior superior iliac spine and iliac crest
- In newborn and small child—proximal tibia medial to tibial tuberosity
- In adult, sternum

Complication:

- Pain
- Bleeding
- Infection
- Fracture of bones

Procedure: Site is selected. Antiseptic dressing and draping is done. Anesthetize the area, skin, subcutaneous tissue, and periosteum with 1% Xylocaine. Introduce the needle by screwing (boring) motion, directing the needle perpendicular to bone. A loss of resistance is felt and needle gets fixed (does not sway side to side) when needle enters the bone marrow. Stellate is removed. A 10-mL or 20-mL syringe is attached and marrow is aspirated very slowly by negative suction. Entire needle and syringe is removed and marrow is smeared over glass slides.

BONE MARROW BIOPSY NEEDLE

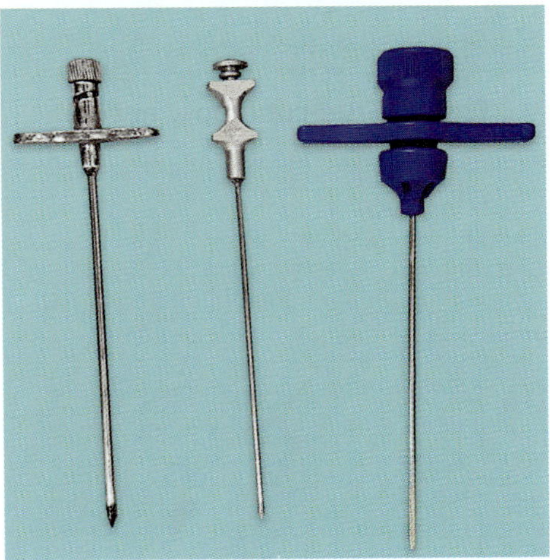

Fig. 14: Bone marrow biopsy needle. Blue one is Jamshidi needle.

Jamshidi needle is most commonly used. Currently disposable needles are also used **(Fig. 14)**.

Indications—are same as bone marrow aspiration needle.

But commonly done when there is dry tap (seen commonly in myelofibrosis, myelosclerosis, and aplastic anemia) during bone marrow aspiration and when diagnosis is inconclusive by bone marrow aspiration study.

Procedure: Selection of site, anesthesia, antiseptic dressing-draping same as bone marrow aspiration. Small skin incision is made. Needle is advanced through cortex of the bone into bone marrow by firm screwing movement. Stellate is removed. Needle is advanced a little further. Now move the needle sideways to about 20° for few times. Again move the needle same way but perpendicular to the last direction. In this way, a small piece of marrow material will be broken inside the needle. Now remove the needle, make imprint smear with the marrow chip and send the marrow chip for histopathological examination.

TRUE-CUT BIOPSY NEEDLE AND SEMIAUTOMATED BIOPSY GUN

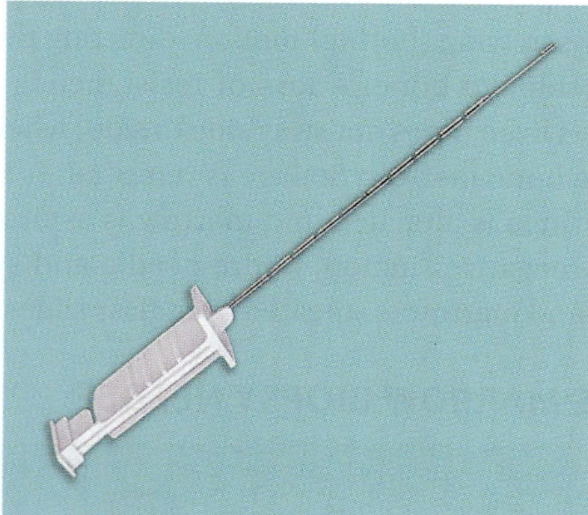

Fig. 15: True-cut biopsy needle.

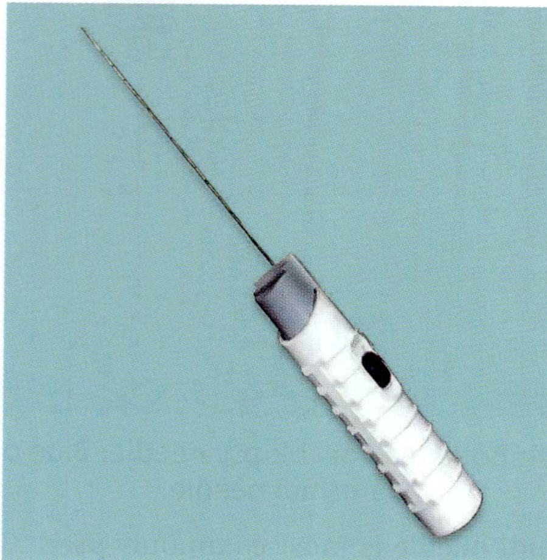

Fig. 16: Semiautomated biopsy gun.

These are biopsy needles **(Figs. 15 and 16)** used for:

- Liver biopsy
- Kidney biopsy
- Biopsy from any solid tumor with or without CT/USG guidance
- Rarely lung biopsy

Indication of liver biopsy:

- *Neonate:*
  - Neonatal hepatitis
  - Biliary atresia
  - Galactosemia
- *Children:*
  - Cirrhosis
  - Chronic hepatitis
  - *Metabolic:* Wilsons disease, tyrosinosis, and hemochromatosis
  - *Malignancy:* Staging of Wilms tumor, neuroblastoma, and Hodgkin's lymphoma. Diagnosis of hepatoma and hepatoblastoma
  - *Infiltration:* TB, sarcoidosis

Complication:

- Local pain
- Infection
- Bleeding—in the liver and peritoneum
- Intrathoracic and intraperitoneal bile leak
- Pleural pain and pneumothorax
- Penetration of other abdominal organs

Contraindication:

- Bleeding disorders
- Extreme dyspnea
- Pyogenic abscess of right lobe
- Biliary tract infection
- Peritoneal infection
- Hydatid disease

Site:

- If liver is larger than normal and extends well below subcostal margin, then it may be done by subcostal approach.
- If liver is shrunken, then right lateral approach, through 10th intercostal space in mid-axillary line
- Nowadays site is selected with help of USG/CT (USG guided or CT guided biopsy)

INFANT FEEDING TUBE/OROGASTRIC TUBE/NASOGASTRIC TUBE

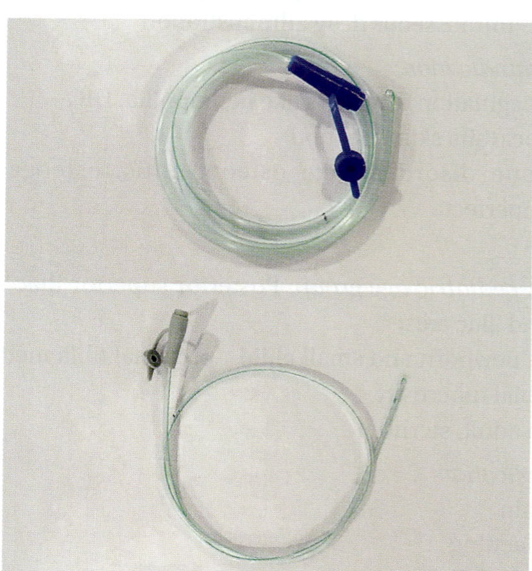

Fig. 17: Infant feeding tube. Blue one (8 Fr) and gray one (5 Fr).

- Plastic tube (polyethylene) with a blunt tip to prevent trauma to structures while introducing it **(Fig. 17)**.
- Opening on the lateral side close to the tip, to allow entry and exit of materials if tip is blocked
- Also had radiopaque maker throughout the length for better visualization on X-ray
- Sterilized by gamma irradiation

Indication:

- *Diagnostic:*
  - Bleeding in stomach and upper GI tract
  - Tuberculosis (gastric aspirate)
  - Tracheoesophageal fistula
  - Poisoning
  - Localization of esophageal strictures
  - Gastric analysis
- *Therapeutic:*
  - Nasogastric/orogastric feeding
  - Administration of drugs
  - Remove gastric contents in poisoning, persistent GI bleed, abdominal distension with bilious emesis, hepatic encephalopathy
  - Decompression of stomach in a child in ventilator/ CPAP

Contraindication:

- Head trauma
- Coagulopathy

Complication:

- Trauma to nose and nasopharynx
- Accidental placement in trachea
- Vomiting with aspiration
- Ulceration/infection of nasal mucosa

How much length to introduce?

Length from bridge of the nose to tragus + tragus to xiphisternum

What sizes are available?

6 Fr (green), 8 Fr (blue), 10 Fr (black). A smaller size of 5 Fr is also available. 5 Fr and 6 Fr used in neonates **(Fig. 17)**.

Other uses?

- As suction catheter
- As urinary catheter in newborn
- For giving oxygen as nasal and nasopharyngeal cannula
- As umbilical catheter

SUCTION CATHETER

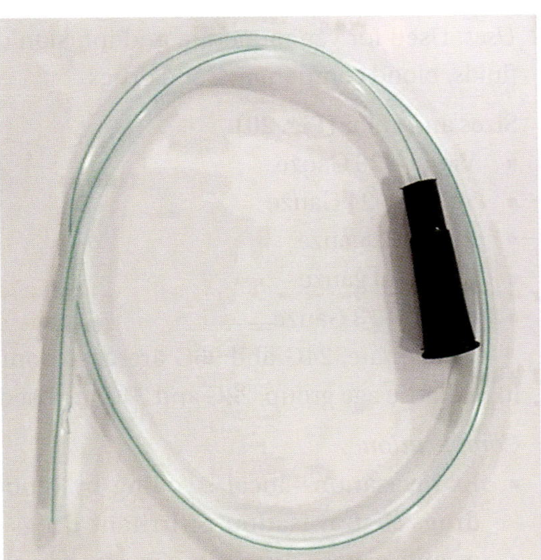

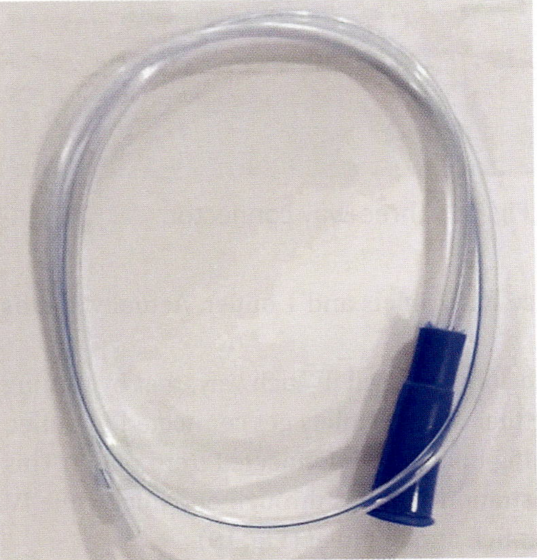

Fig. 18: Suction catheter. Black one (10 Fr) and blue one (6 Fr).

Used for suction from oral cavity, nose, pharynx, and endotracheal tube **(Fig. 18)**

Suction pressure: 80–100 mm Hg

Length of insertion: 3 cm for nose and 5 cm for mouth

Contraindication:

- Nasal bleeding
- Laryngospasm
- Severe bronchospasm
- Basal skull fracture

Complication:

- Trauma, bleeding
- Introduction of infection
- Vasovagal attack
- Laryngospasm and bronchospasm
- Vomiting

What sizes are available?

- 6 Fr (green), 8 Fr (blue), 10 Fr (black) **(Fig. 18)**

Sterilization:

- Gamma irradiation

THREE-WAY CONNECTOR

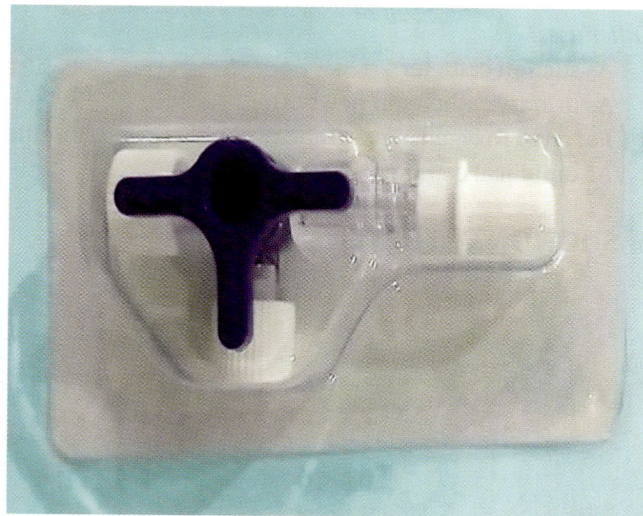

Fig. 19: Three-way connector.

This device has 2 inlets and 1 outlet. Actually 3 ends are open.

The connector is devised in such way, that by turning the handle, either of the 2 inlets get connected to outlet, while remaining inlet got disconnected from outlet. This helps administration of drugs through one inlet while IV fluids pass through another inlet **(Fig. 19)**.

Uses:

- Simultaneous administration of IVF and antibiotic
- Exchange transfusion
- Hemodialysis
- Pleural/ascitic tap
- CVP monitoring

INTRAVENOUS CANNULA

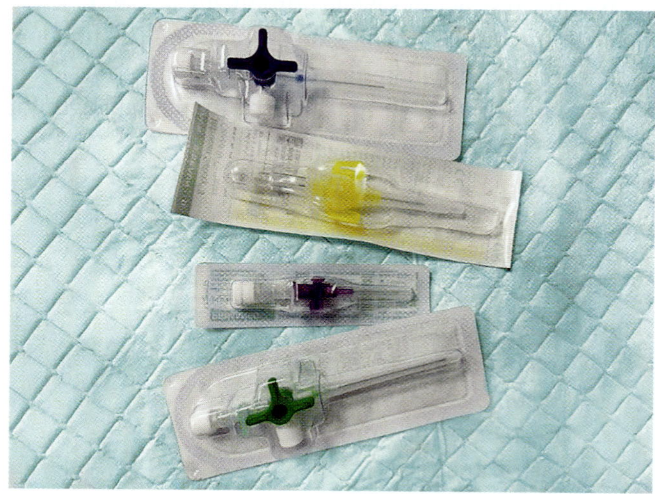

Fig. 20: Intravenous cannula of different sizes.

This contains outer plastic (polyethylene) cannula and inner metallic needle **(Fig. 20)**.

Gamma ray sterilized and disposable.

Being plastic in nature, does not damages endothelium of veins.

Plastic sheath being flexible, can be inserted into tortuous and thin vein easily.

Uses: Used for venepuncture and infusion of intravenous fluids, blood components, and drugs

Sizes and color **(Fig. 20)**:

- Violet—26 Gauze
- Yellow—24 Gauze
- Blue—22 gauze
- Pink—20 gauze
- Green—18 Gauze

In neonate, 24G and 26G are used commonly, while in pediatric age group, 22G and 24G are used commonly.

Complication:

- Extravasation—local swelling by blood or fluid or drugs. Extravasation of irritant drugs like calcium or anti-cancer drug can give rise to cellulitis, blister formation, or even gangrene of the affected limb.
- Thrombophlebitis—giving rise to fever, pain, and swelling of the area. In prolonged unnoticed cases, can give rise to cellulitis.
- Artery puncture leading to hematoma formation and prolonged bleeding

SCALP VEIN NEEDLE (BUTTERFLY NEEDLE)

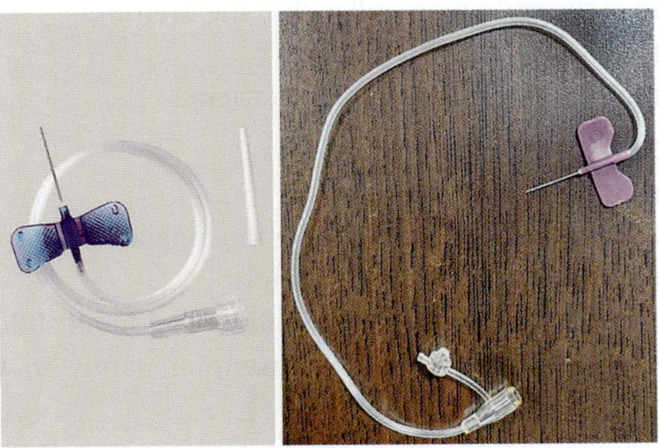

Fig. 21: Scalp vein set.

Consists of a metallic needle attached to a plastic tubing. At the junction of needle with plastic tubing, there is a butterfly shaped plastic holder which helps easy insertion of needle into the vein. This plastic holder is color coded and flexible. Commonly used sizes are 22G to 24G **(Fig. 21)**.

Uses:

- Collection of blood
- Infusion of intravenous fluids, drugs, and blood components

Infusion Set

Indication:

- Infusion of parenteral fluid
- Infusion of some drugs with larger volume like linezolid, metronidazole

Rate of infusion: Approximately 15–16 drops = 1 mL. Rate is adjusted by adjusting drops by use of the controller.

MICRODRIP SET

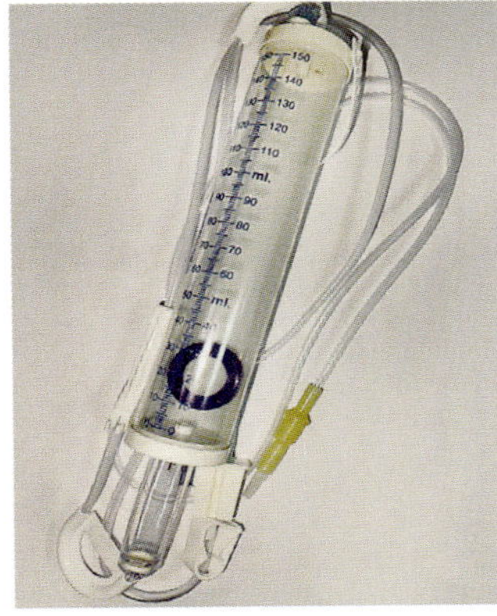

Fig. 22: Micodrip set.

It has a graduated cylinder (volume chamber) which can transfuse a given amount of fluid. Capacity usually 150 mL **(Fig. 22)**.

Indication:

- Infusion of smaller volume of fluid or drugs slowly over hours. This is particularly used in neonates who need slower transfusion. Similarly, some drugs which need more slow infusion like quinine or vancomycin or phenytoin, this microdrip set is preferred.

Rate of infusion: Approximately 60–64 drops = 1 mL. Rate is adjusted by adjusting drops in the volume chamber by use of the controller.

BLOOD TRANSFUSION SET

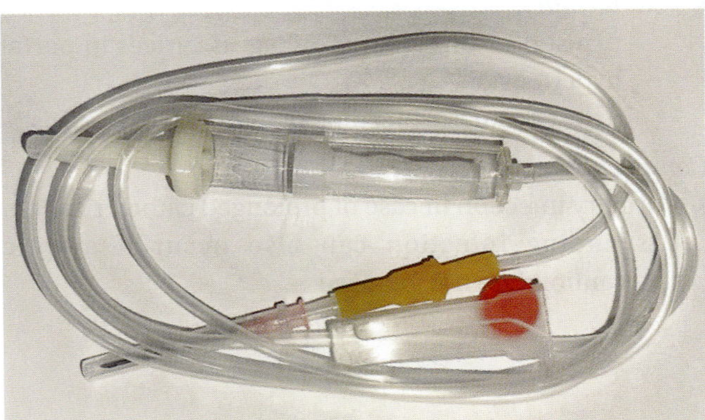

Fig. 23: Blood transfusion set.

Same as infusion set, but having an additional strainer in the chamber for straining clots and coagulated blood products **(Fig. 23)**.

Indication: For transfusion of blood and blood products.

Rate of infusion: Approximately 15–16 drops = 1 mL

Note: All the drip set and blood transfusion set usually made of polyethylene, sterilized by gamma irradiation and disposable.

FOLEY'S CATHETER (FIG. 24)

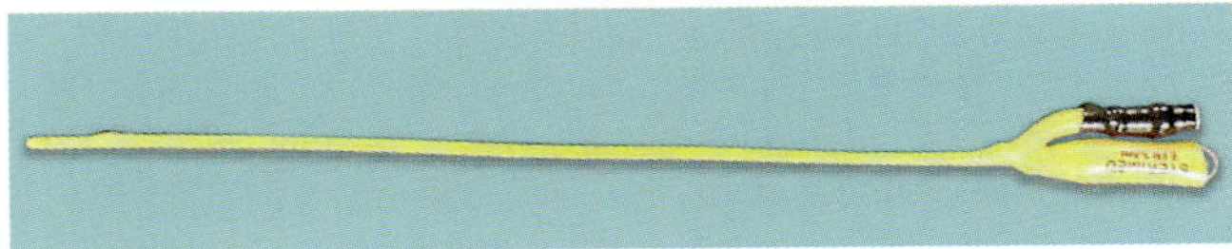

Fig. 24: Foley's catheter.

It is made up of latex and sterilized by gamma irradiation.

Self-retaining by means of a small inflatable ballon like structure at the tip of the catheter, which can be inflated with help of normal saline.

Indications:

- *Urinary:*
  - Acute retention of urine
  - Monitoring urine output in case of shock and renal failure
  - Differentiate anuria from renal failure
  - Hematuria—suspected bladder injury
  - Urinary incontinence
  - Congenital bladder diverticulum
  - Suprapubic cystostomy
  - Intravesical chemotherapy
- *Nonurinary:*
  - Arrest bleeding from esophageal varices in portal hypertension
  - Arrest postnasal bleeding in intractable epistaxis

Complication:

- Urinary infection in case of prolonged catheterization. Ascending infection can also occur if aseptic precautions are not followed.
- Urethral rupture in case when ballon is inflated while tip of the catheter is still within the urethra.
- Injury to bladder
- Inadvertent catheterization of vagina

Digital Thermometer

Temperature measurement:

- *Mouth:* Place the probe under the tongue and close the mouth. Breathe through the nose.
- *Rectum:* This method is for infants and small children. They cannot hold a thermometer safely in their mouth.
- *Armpit:* Place the thermometer in the armpit. Press the arm against the body. Less accurate
- *Tympanic membrane:* insert the thermometer within the ear cavity so that it picks up the temperature of the eardrum. This can measure the core body temperature.

A fever is an elevated body temperature with these readings: rectal, forehead or ear temperature: 100.4°F (38.0°C) or higher. Oral (mouth) temperature: 100°F (37.8°C) or higher. Under the armpit temperature: 99°F (37.2°C) or higher.

CHAPTER 17

Neonatal Resuscitation

Sanjana Samanta

Q1. What percentage of babies require neonatal resuscitation after birth?

Ans. Most newborns make the transition to extrauterine life without intervention. Within 30 seconds after birth, approximately 90% of term babies will begin breathing without any assistance. 10% babies will require resuscitation out of which 5% needs positive pressure ventilation.

Q2. What is the most important and effective step in neonatal resuscitation?

Ans. Ventilation of newborn lungs is the most important and effective step in neonatal resuscitation.

Q3. What happens during the transition from fetal to neonatal circulation?

Ans. During fetal stage, the lungs are filled with fluid not air.

After birth, a series of events take place that help the baby to breath.

- As the baby cries, the air enters the alveoli and the fluid in the lungs is absorbed.
- Air in the lungs causes the previously constricted pulmonary vessels to relax so that blood can flow to the lungs and reach the alveoli where oxygen will be absorbed and co_2 will be removed.
- Clamping the umbilical cord increases the baby's systemic blood pressure decreasing the tendency for blood to bypass the baby's lungs.

Q4. What are the equipment required for neonatal circulation?

Ans.

Warmth:

- Warmer, 2 preheated towels, plastic bag (<32 weeks)

Clear airway:

- Dilles mucous sucker, 10–12 F suction catheter attached to a wall mounted sucker machine, suction pressure set to 80–100 mm of Hg

Monitoring:

- Stethoscope, pulse oximeter

Ventilation:

- Self-inflating resuscitation bag with reservoir/T piece resuscitator
- Oxygen blender
- Oxygen tubing
- Oxygen source
- Face mask (term and preterm size)

Intubation:

- Laryngoscope with straight blade size 0, 1,00
- Stylet
- Endotracheal tube 2.5, 3, 3.5
- Waterproof tape
- Measuring tape
- CO_2 detector

Medications:

- Epinephrine (1 mg = 10 mL)
- Normal saline 100 mL bag
- Dextrose 10%
- Syringes (1 mL, 5 mL, and 10 mL)

Umbilical vein catheterization:

- Sterile gloves, sterile drape, forceps, scalpel blade
- Single lumen umbilical catheter 3.5F and 5F
- Three-way stopcock
- Heparinized syringe, clear adhesive dressing

Q5. What are the four key questions to ask the obstetric provider before the birth of the baby?

Ans.

1. What is the gestational age of the fetus?
2. Is the amniotic fluid clear?
3. Are there any additional risk factors?
4. The umbilical cord management plan is discussed.

Q6. When should the umbilical cord be clamped?

Ans. According to the current NRP guidelines, umbilical cord should be clamped after 30–60 secs.

Q7. What are the contraindications of delayed cord clamping?

Ans. Circumstances where placental circulation is deranged like placenta abruption, placenta previa, bleeding vasa previa, and cord avulsion.

Q8. What are the advantages of delayed cord clamping?

Ans. In preterms, delayed cord clamping is related with decreased need of medications to support blood pressure after birth.

In term and late preterms, delayed cord clamping improves early hematologic measurements and also there is benefit of neurodevelopmental outcomes.

Q9. How do you evaluate the newborn immediately after birth?

Ans. Rapid evaluation for every newborn after birth includes 3 questions:

1. Term?
2. Is the tone good?
3. Breathing or crying?

If answer to any of the question is *no* then the baby will need resuscitation.

Q10. What are the initial steps of resuscitation?

Ans.

1. Provide warmth: In case of vigorous babies, warmth is provided by skin to skin contact and covering the baby with warm linen.
   If the answer to any three rapid evaluation questions is no—the baby is taken to the radiant warmer and is left uncovered for good visualization of chest during resuscitation and also to permit the radiant heat to reach the baby.
2. Dry the baby: Drying is not needed in preterms less than 32 weeks because they should be covered in polyethylene plastic which reduces evaporative heat loss.
3. Stimulate the baby: Gentle rubbing the back of the baby or flicking the soles
4. Positioning the baby: Positioning should be such that the head and neck is slightly extended or neutral. The eyes are directed straight toward the ceiling. This position is called sniffing the morning air. This allows the airway to remain open and unrestricted air entry.
5. Clear the secretions: Routine clearing is not required. If the baby is not crying or gasping, the clearing of secretion to be done before starting PPV. First the mouth and then the nose should be suctioned.
   The suctioning should not be very deep and vigorous as in that case the soft tissues may be injured. Stimulation of the posterior pharynx during suction can cause vagal response leading to bradycardia.

Q11. How will you stimulate the baby during initial steps of resuscitation?

Ans.

- Gentle rubbing at the back
- Never shake the baby

Q12. What are the indications of PPV?

Ans. After completion of the initial steps of resuscitation, *positive pressure ventilation* is needed.

- If the baby is not crying
  or
- The baby is gasping
  Or
- if the baby's heart rate is <100 BPM

Q13. What do you do if the baby is breathing and the heart rate is at least 100 bpm but the baby appears persistently cyanotic?

Ans. Cyanosis limited to the extremities of the newborns is common and is termed as peripheral cyanosis. It is due to cold exposure and does not indicate low oxygen saturation.

Cyanosis of baby's lips tongue indicates central cyanosis due to low oxygen saturation. Healthy babies can also have cyanosis for initial few minutes after birth.

However persistent cyanosis needs oxygen saturation monitoring by pulse oximeter placed on baby's right hand.

Q14. What is pulse oximeter?

Ans. Pulse oximeter estimates the percentage of hemoglobin that is carrying oxygen. This is not the same as partial pressure of oxygen.

Hemoglobin that is carrying oxygen absorbs red light differently than hemoglobin that is not carrying oxygen. Pulse oximeter uses a light source and sensor to measure the absorption of red light passing through capillaries in the skin and estimates the percentage of hemoglobin that is carrying oxygen.

Q15. When is the pulse oximeter used in delivery room?

Ans. Pulse oximeter during resuscitation helps to guide us by providing oxygen saturation in the following conditions:

- In case of persistent central cyanosis
- When positive pressure ventilation is being started

Q16. Where is the pulse oximeter sensor placed?

Ans. The artery supplying the right arm branches from the aorta before the patent ductus arteriosus enters the aorta.

This is called *preductal*. It has a similar oxygen saturation as the blood perfusing the heart and the brain.

Q17. What is target oxygen saturation?

Ans. Target saturation is the saturation that is normal for the baby just after delivery **(Table 1)**.

TABLE 1: Target oxygen saturation chart according to the time of birth.

1 minute	60–65%
2 minutes	65–70%
3 minutes	70–75%
4 minutes	75–80%
5 minutes	80–85%
10 minutes	90–95%

Q18. How can we administer free flow oxygen to the baby?

Ans. Free flow oxygen can be given to a spontaneously breathing baby by holding oxygen tubing close to baby's mouth and nose.

Free flow oxygen can also be given by:

- Flow inflating bag—the bag should not inflate when used to provide free flow oxygen
- T piece resuscitator—the opening of the T piece cap should not be occluded

Q19. How is the concentration of supplemental oxygen adjusted?

Ans. For supplementation oxygen is needed it is started with 30% and then guided by the pulse oximetry, the Fio_2 is adjusted to maintain the baby's target oxygen saturation.

Q20. What to do if the baby is having labored breathing or persistently low oxygen saturation?

Ans. If the baby has labored breathing or the baby fails to maintain target oxygen saturation even after 100% oxygen then we should consider continuous positive airway pressure (CPAP).

These are the indications of delivery room CPAP.

Q21. What are the devices to provide positive pressure resuscitation?

Ans.

- Self-inflating bag
- Flow inflating bag
- T piece resuscitator

Q22. What is the disadvantage of the self-inflating bag?

Ans. Because gas does not flow out of the mask unless the bag is squeezed, the self-inflating bag cannot be used to provide free flow oxygen.

It does not provide positive end-expiratory pressure (PEEP).

Q23. How ventilatory rate is determined during PPV?

Ans. During positive pressure ventilation, rate should be 40–60 breaths per minute.

The rhythm should be *breathe two three breath two three.*

When we say breath, the bag is squeezed and breath is delivered.

Q24. What are the settings for PPV?

Ans. The settings for PPV are discussed in **Table 2**.

TABLE 2: Settings of positive pressure ventilation in NRP.

Oxygen concentration	≥35 weeks gestation >35 weeks gestation	21% 21–30%
Gas flow		10 L/min
Rate		40–60 breaths/min
PIP		20–25 cmH_2O
PEEP		5 cmH_2O

Q25. How mask is applied for PPV?

Ans. The mask is placed on the chin and the mouth and the nose is covered, taking care the eyes are not covered. A tight seal between the mask and the face is needed to ensure correct ventilation.

Q26. How can we evaluate the baby's response to PPV?

Ans. Most important indicator of successful PPV is rising heart rate.

Q27. What are MRSOPA ventilatory corrective steps?

Ans. After 15 seconds of starting bag mask ventilation, the baby's heart rate is checked.

If the heart rate is increasing, the ventilation is effective and is continued for another 15 seconds.

If the heart rate is not increasing then ventilator corrective steps are done as discussed in **Table 3**.

TABLE 3: Ventilatory corrective steps.

Corrective steps	*Actions*
Mask adjustment	Reapply the mask and lift the jaw forward
Reposition of head and neck	Place the head neutral or slightly extended

Contd...

Contd...

Corrective steps	*Actions*
Give 5 breaths and assess chest movements if no chest movements do the next step:	
Suction of mouth and nose	Use the bulb syringe or suction catheter
Open the mouth	Use the finger to gently open the mouth
Give 5 breaths and assess chest movements if no chest movements do the next step	
Increase the pressure	• Increase in 5–10 cmH_2O increments to maximum recommended pressure • Maximum 40 cmH_2O terms • Maximum 30 cmH_2O preterms
Give 5 breaths and assess chest movements if no chest movements do the next step:	
Alternative airway	Inserting an endotracheal tube or laryngeal mask airway

Q28. What is laryngeal mask airway?

Ans. A laryngeal mask is a small mask attached to an airway tube. The mask is inserted into the baby's mouth and advanced into the throat until it makes a seal over the entrance to the baby's trachea.

Laryngeal mask airway (LMA) makes a better seal than a face mask and may improve the effectiveness of ventilation.

Unlike endotracheal intubation, no instruments are required for its insertion.

Q29. When is LMA used?

Ans. LMA is considered if a baby cannot be successfully ventilated by using a bag and mask ventilation alone and intubation is unsuccessful.

Q30. What is the limitation of LMA?

Ans. LMA is used only in babies weighing 2–5 kg.

If high ventilator pressures are required air leaks through the seal between pharynx and mask resulting in insufficient pressure to inflate the lungs.

Q31. When is infant feeding tube needed?

Ans. During prolonged PPV, air enters the stomach that causes hindrance to lung ventilation. So when prolonged ventilation is anticipated, an infant feeding tube is inserted.

Q32. What are the indications of chest compression?

Ans. Chest compressions are indicated when heart rate remains <60 beats per minute despite at least 30 seconds of effective bag and mask ventilation that inflates the lungs.

Q33. What will be the position of the hands during chest compression?

Ans. During chest compressions, the pressure is applied to the lower third of sternum. An imaginary line is drawn connecting the baby's nipple. The thumbs are placed either side by side just below this imaginary line.

Q34. How deeply the chest compressions are given?

Ans. During chest compressions, the pressure applied should be such that it depresses the sternum approximately one-third of the anteroposterior diameter of the chest.

Q35. What is the compression rate of chest compression?

Ans. The compression rate is 90 compressions per minute. For this, 3 compressions and one ventilation is given in a 2 second cycle.

Q36. How are compressions coordinated with positive pressure ventilation?

Ans. For coordinated compressions and ventilation, 3 compressions and 1 ventilation are given in every 2 seconds. The goal is to give 90 compressions and 30 ventilation per minute. There are total 120 events in a minute.

Q37. What oxygen concentration should be used with positive pressure ventilation during chest compressions?

Ans. When chest compressions are started, the FiO_2 is increased to 100%.

Q38. When the baby's heart rate should be checked after starting compressions?

Ans. After 60 seconds of coordinated chest compressions and ventilation, the baby's heart rate is checked using a cardiac monitor or a pulse oximeter.

Q39. When is chest compressions stopped?

Ans. Chest compressions are stopped when heart rate is 60 beats per minute or more.

Q40. What do you do if the heart rate is not improving after 60 seconds of compressions?

Ans. After 60 seconds of coordinated compressions and ventilation if the heart rate is not improving, the following questions are asked and assessed:

Mnemonic *CARDIO:*

- Chest movement—is the chest moving with each breath
- *Airway*—is the airway secured with endotracheal tube or laryngeal mask airway

- *R*ate—are 3 compressions coordinated with 1 ventilation being delivered every 2 seconds
- *D*epth—is the depth of compressions one-third of the AP diameter of the chest
- *I*nspired oxygen—is 100% oxygen being administered

Q41. When is epinephrine used?

Ans. Epinephrine is indicated if the baby's heart rate remains <60 bpm after:

- At least 30 seconds of PPV that inflates the lungs as evidenced by chest movements
- Another 60 seconds of chest compression coordinated with PPV using 100% oxygen

Q42. What is the preparation of epinephrine that is used?

Ans. The concentration of epinephrine used for neonatal resuscitation is 1 mg/ml or 1 mg/10 mL.

Commercially available epinephrine has concentration of 1 mg/1 mL.

To prepare the recommended preparation, 1 mL of epinephrine (1 mg/1 mL) is taken in a 10-mL syringe and 9-mL normal saline is taken. Thus, 1 mg epinephrine is in 10 mL preparation making the concentration 1 mg/1 mL.

Q43. What are the routes of epinephrine administration?

Ans. The route of epinephrine for neonatal resuscitation is intravenous or intraosseous. For this, an intravenous access is made through umbilical vein catheterization. Attempting insertion of a peripheral intravenous catheter is not recommended for emergency medication administration in the setting of cardiovascular collapse.

Endotracheal route—some clinicians choose to give a dose of epinephrine into the endotracheal tube while vascular access is established. However, studies suggest that absorption is unreliable and thus not preferred.

Q44. What is the dose of epinephrine?

Ans.

- *Intravenous:* 0.01–0.03 mg/kg (0.1–0.3 mL/kg)
- *Endotracheal:* 0.05–0.1 mg/kg (0.5–1 mL/kg)

Q45. How is epinephrine administered?

Ans. Intravenous injection is given rapidly as quick as possible. The epinephrine is administered through a three way with a simultaneous flush of 3 ml normal saline.

Q46. How a preterm baby is kept warm during resuscitation?

Ans. A preterm baby is wrapped up to neck in a polyethylene plastic immediately after birth. Drying the body is not needed.

A thermal mattress is used. It contains a chemical gel. When the chemical gel is activated, it releases heat. It is activated 5 minutes before baby's birth. It takes 5 minutes to reach the target surface temperature and once activated it maintains the temperature for 1 hour **(Figs. 1 to 8)**.

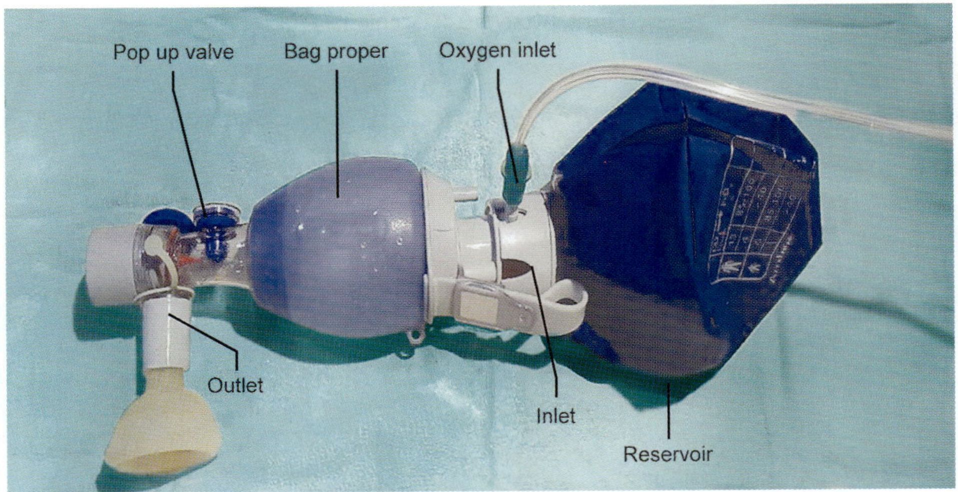

Fig. 1: Parts of self-inflating resuscitation bag and mask.

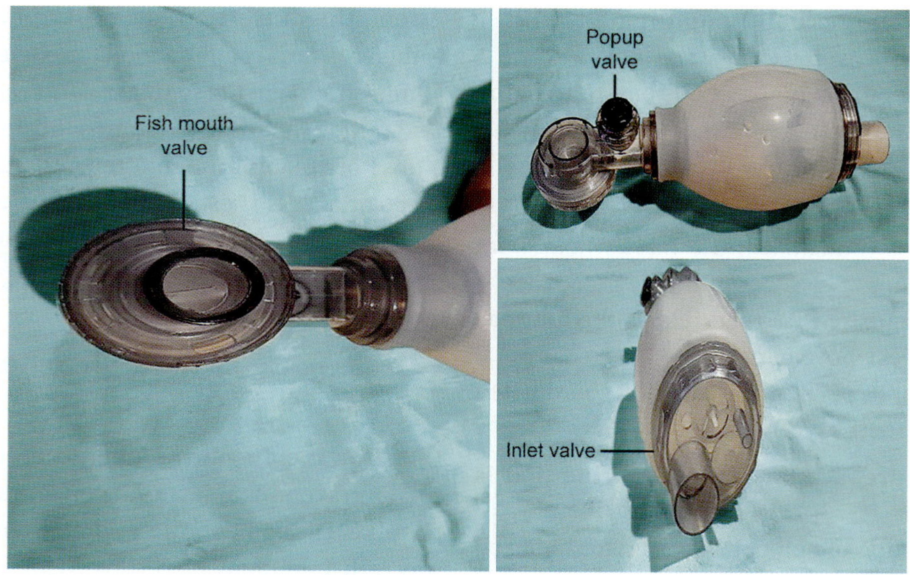

Fig. 2: Valves of bag and mask.

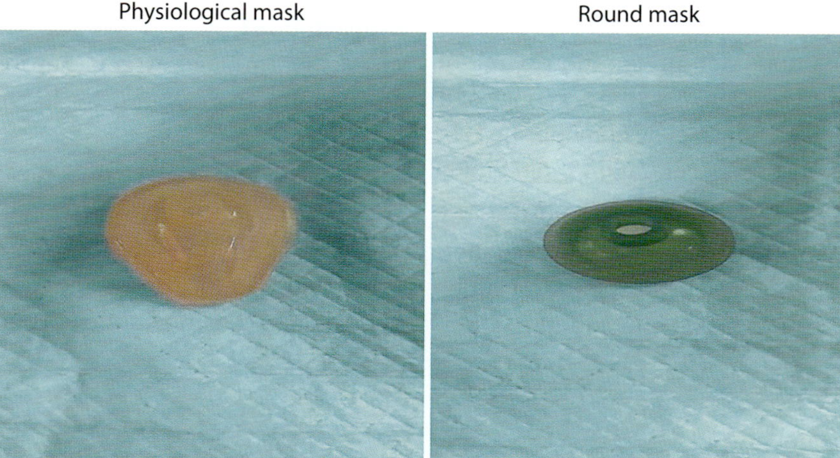

Fig. 3: Two types of facemask.

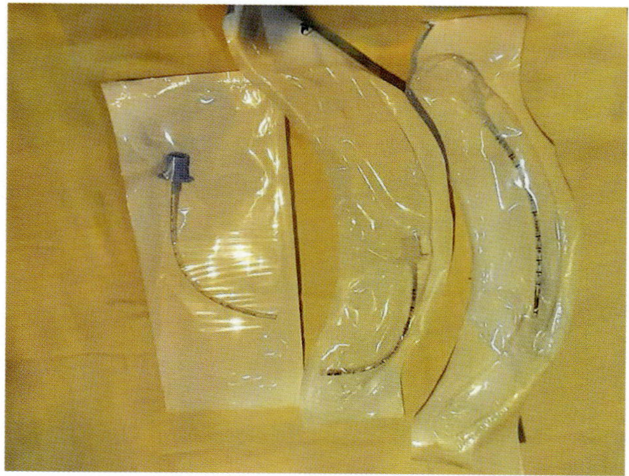

Fig. 4: Endotracheal tubes used in neonatal resuscitation.
<1 kg—2.5 mm; 1–2 kg—3 mm; 2–3 kg—3.5 mm

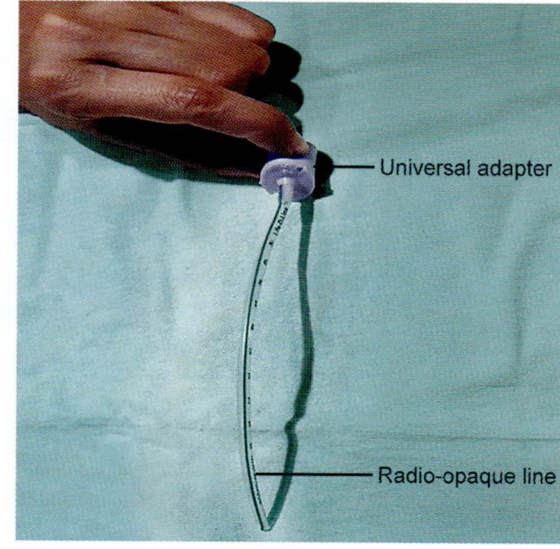

Fig. 5: Parts of endotracheal tube.

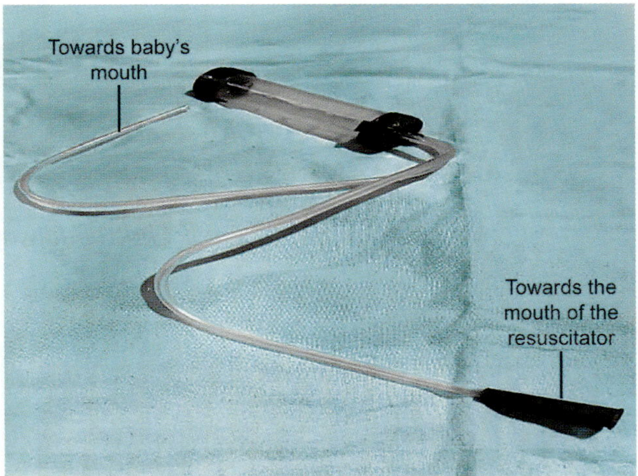

Fig. 6: Dilles mucous sucker.

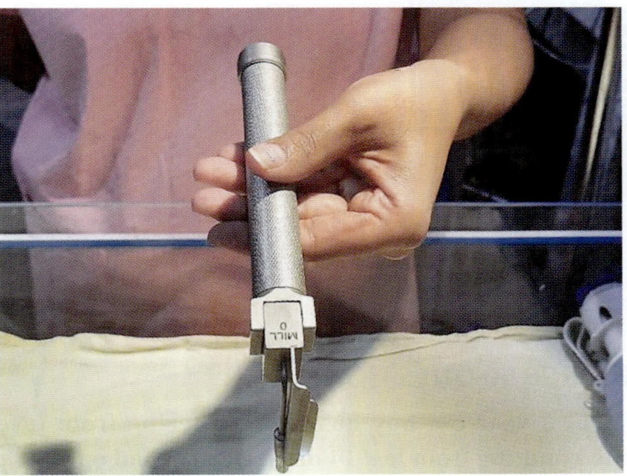

Fig. 7: Correct method of holding laryngoscope: Laryngoscope to be held in left hand universally with thumb above and two fingers below and the blade is pointed away from the body of resuscitator.

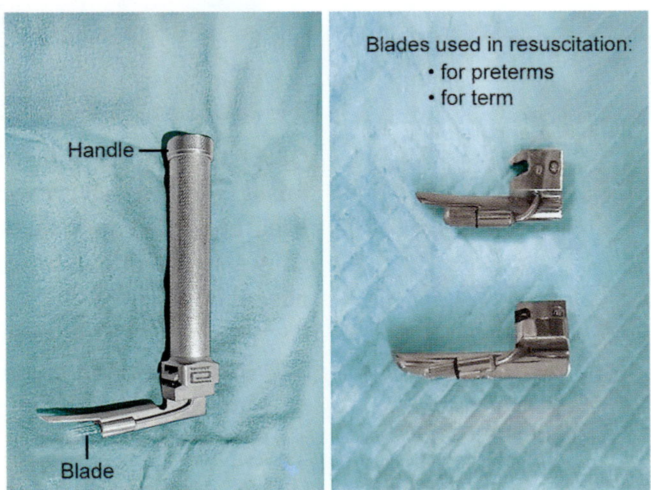

Fig. 8: Parts of laryngoscope.

SUGGESTED READING

1. American Academy of Pediatrics, American Heart Association. Textbook of Neonatal Resuscitation. 8th ed. Itasca (IL): American Academy of Pediatrics; 2021.
2. Ghai OP, Paul VK, Bagga A. Essential Pediatrics. 10th ed. New Delhi: CBS Publishers & Distributors; 2020.
3. Indian Academy of Pediatrics, National Neonatology Forum. IAP-NNF Textbook of Neonatal Resuscitation. New Delhi: Jaypee Brothers Medical Publishers; 2021.

CHAPTER 18

OSCE

Agnik Chattopadhyay

OSCE 50 QUESTIONS

Q1. A 5-year-old boy has been suffering from fever and vomiting from last 14 days. He also had episode of convulsion from last 9 days. Cerebrospinal fluid (CSF) study was done. Image is below of:

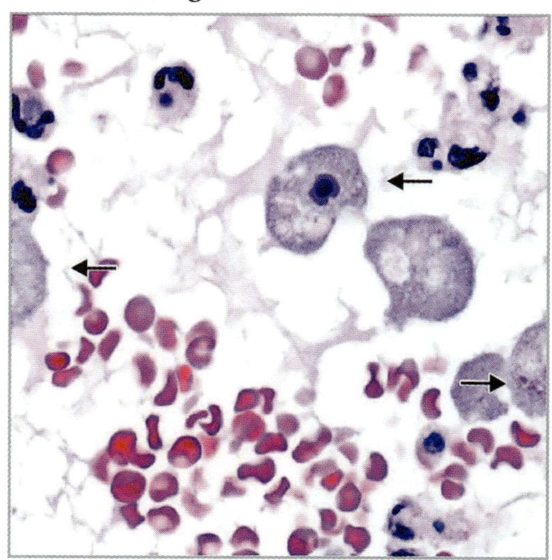

1. Identify the organism shown in the CSF picture.
2. Two routes of infection in human
3. Name two clinical condition
4. Name antimicrobial drug to treat systemic infection caused by the organism

Q2. An 11-month-old infant presented with convulsion and loss of achieved milestones since last 2 months. Physical examination shows—macrocephaly, regressed milestones, spasticity and brisk DTR, cherry red spot in retinoscopy, and exaggerated startle reflex.

1. Name the probable diagnosis.
2. What is the cause?
3. What is the inheritance?
4. Name motor milestone findings of this age.

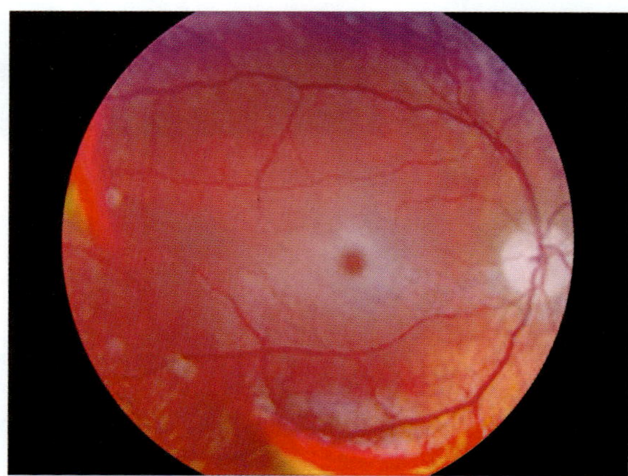

Q3. An 11-month-old infant presented with acute onset vomiting, severe diarrhea for 2 days followed by breathlessness and weak cry. Physical examination shows—tachypnea, drowsy, less limb movement, and absent DTR.

1. What is most likely diagnosis?
2. What are most common causes?
3. Name two tests to confirm the diagnosis.
4. How to treat?

Q4. A 3-month-old female baby presented with tachypnea, lethargy, and poor feeding. She appeared distressed, irritable, and diaphoretic. Temperature—36.8°C, RR—85/min, HR—180/min, SpO_2—89%, CRT = 3 s, CBG = 78 mg/dL. Examination of her chest revealed equal breath sounds. Cardiac sounds are normal, no murmur. ECG is shown below:

1. What are the abnormal findings in the ECG?
2. What is the diagnosis?
3. What is most common clinical presentation of infantile ALCAPA (anomalous left coronary artery from the pulmonary artery)?
4. What is the definitive management of this condition?

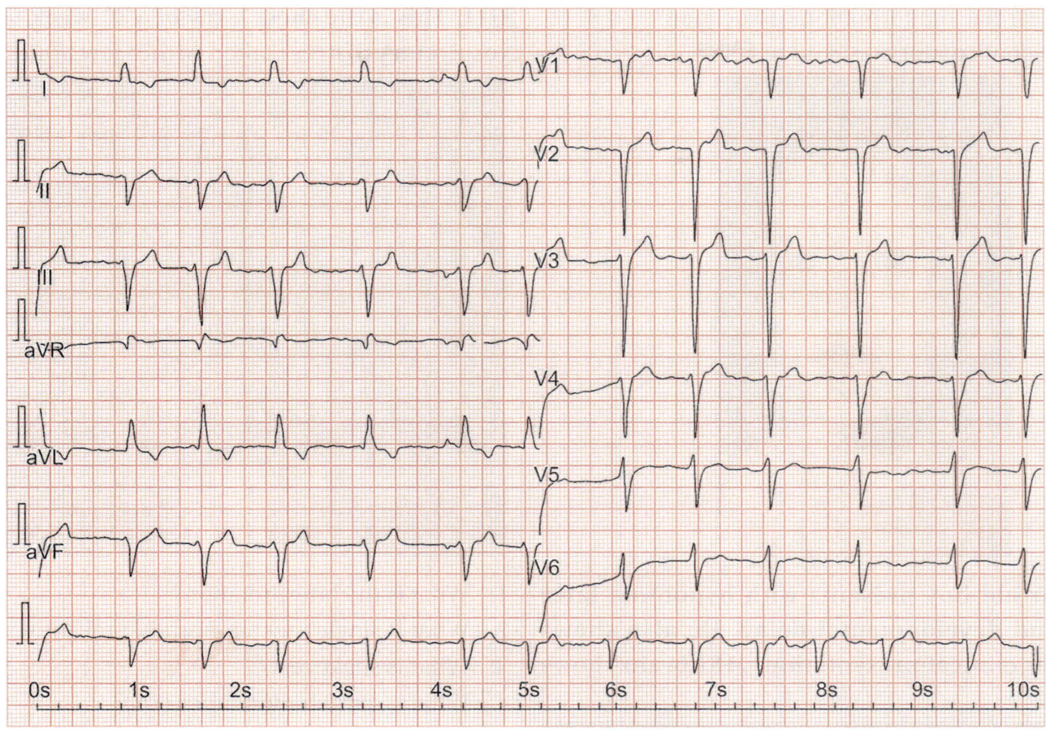

Q5. A newborn diabetic mother presented with Hb of 21% and PCV of 63 associated with red urine. Ultrasound shows bilateral enlarged kidneys.

1. What is the most probable diagnosis?
2. What is the differential diagnosis of the condition?
3. What is the most sensitive investigation modality?
4. What is the treatment?

Q6. Match the following:

	Reflexes		*Disappearing age*
i.	Stepping reflex	a.	9–11 months
ii.	Parachute reflex	b.	6 months
iii.	Moro reflex	c.	2 months
iv.	Asymmetric tonic neck reflex	d.	Never
v.	Symmetric tonic neck reflex	e.	5–6 months

Q7. A 9-month-old baby comes with bleeding per rectum for last 1 month with cry. Birth history was insignificant. USG abdomen shows such findings.

1. What is diagnosis?
2. Enumerate the USG findings interpretation?
3. What is pathophysiology behind such condition?
4. What is the treatment?

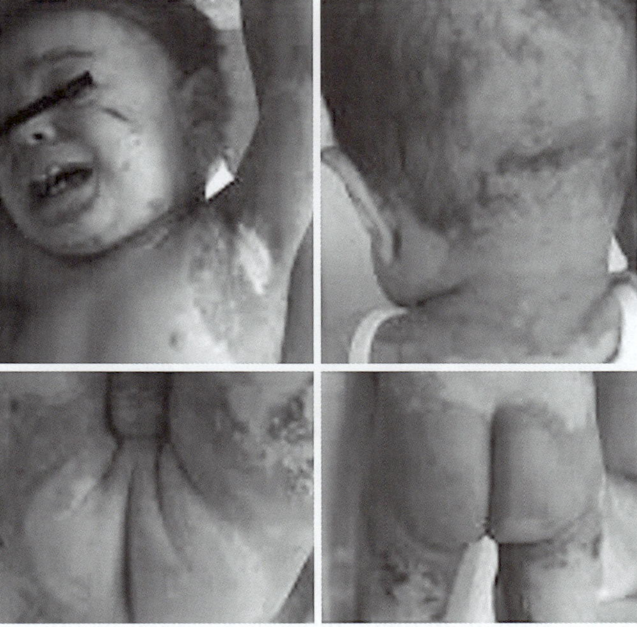

Q8. An 18-month-old usually cheerful child with mild developmental delay.

1. Write clinical diagnosis.
2. Name clinical features (any 4) associated with this syndrome.

3. What are cardiac malformations associated?
4. Name the confirmatory test and result.

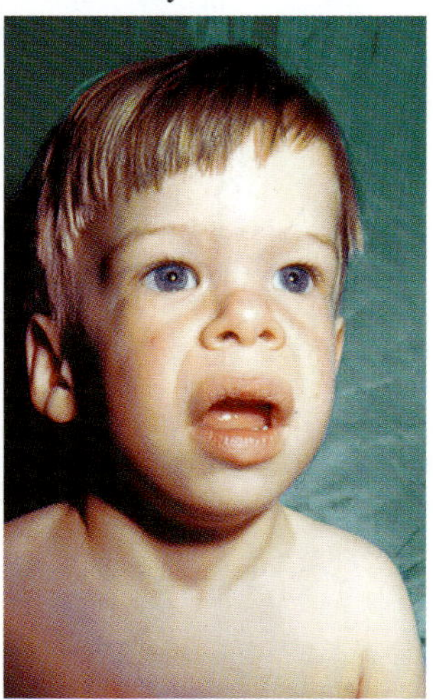

Q9. A 5-year-old boy presents with hypotonia later on ataxia and developmental delay. He also shows nystagmus in clinical presentation. MRI brain shows like this.

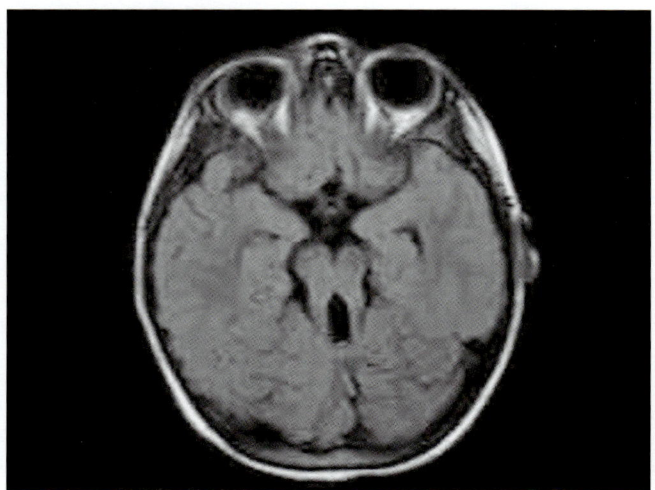

1. Name any significant findings in MRI brain.
2. What is diagnosis?
3. What is clinical presentation?
4. What are associated problems in such syndrome?

Q10. A baby of diabetic mother delivered by normal vaginal delivery. Baby presented with less movement in both arms.

1. What is the diagnosis?
2. What are etiology and complication?
3. Loss of what reflexes?
4. What is first-line maneuver to relieve this condition?

Q11. This is the chest X-ray of a 30-week-old baby with respiratory distress taken within few hours of birth.

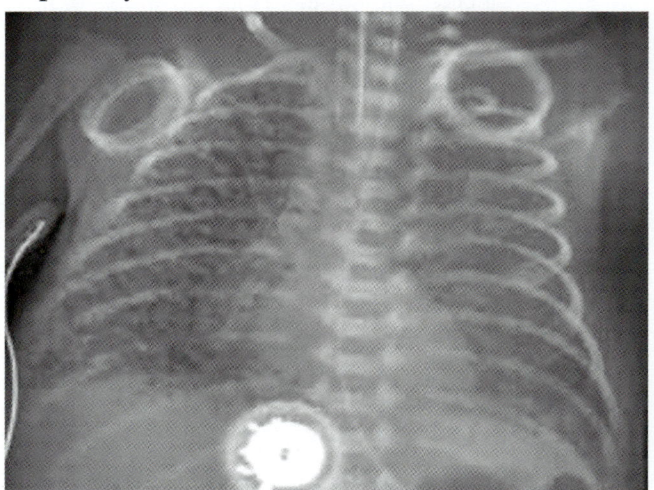

1. What is the interpretation?
2. What is single most important preventive strategy?
3. What is shake test?
4. What is oxygenation index (OI)?

Q12. A 7-year-old child presented with history of light-colored skin lesions at the time of birth which were more than 8 in number and developed small nodules over the trunk at the age of 2 and history of convulsions at 3 years of age.

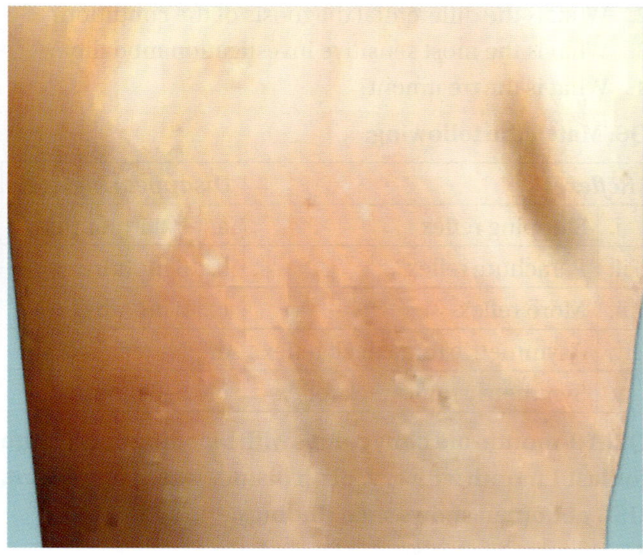

1. What is the diagnosis?
2. What is mode of inheritance?
3. Name the systems involved.
4. Name any newer drug.

Q13. A 4-month-old boy comes with convulsion and such lesion.

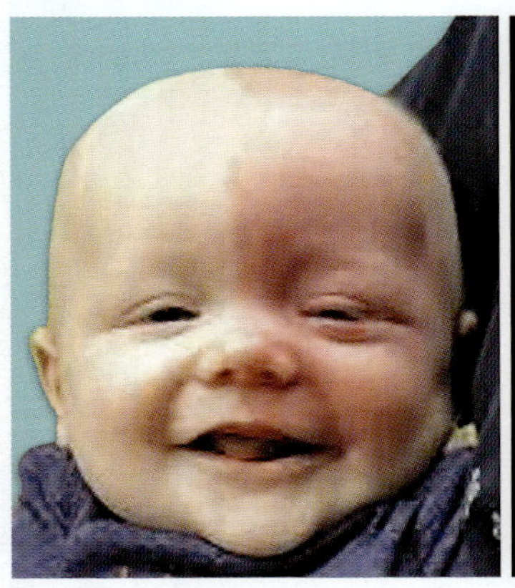

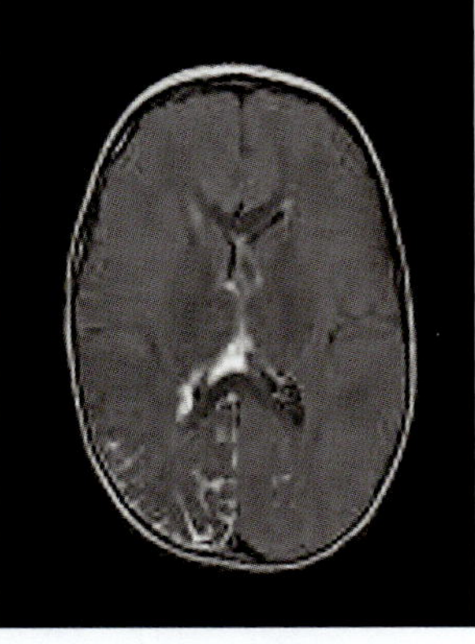

1. What is most probable diagnosis of such condition?
2. What is inheritance of the disease?
3. Name the associated clinical features with the condition.
4. What is the intracranial vascular abnormality in this disease?

Q14.

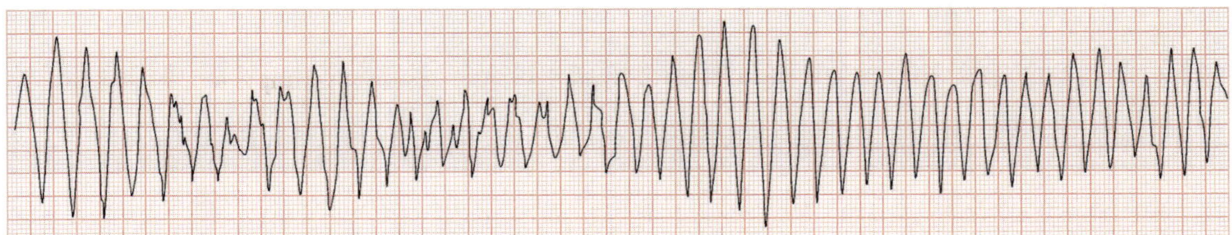

1. Interpret the ECG.
2. Name two drugs causing it.
3. Name one underlying disorder predisposing this condition.
4. Name two complications.
5. How will you manage if the condition is associated with (a) pulseless, unresponsive child and (B) with pulse?

Q15. A child who is able to momentarily stand on one foot and ride tricycle, toilet trained day time, starts group play copies a circle.

1. Identify the age of the child.
2. At which age child knows his/her gender?
3. When does bladder and bowel control develop?
4. In which age child can jump and skip a rope?

Q16.

1. What is DEIC?
2. What is the purpose of DEIC?
3. Name 4 D's in DEIC.
4. DEICs are typically established at which level?

Q17. A 5-day-old newborn developed sudden apnea, pallor, and respiratory distress. USG brain was done.

1. What is the diagnosis?
2. What is the clinical presentation?
3. How frequently should USG be repeated?
4. What is major long-term complication of such?

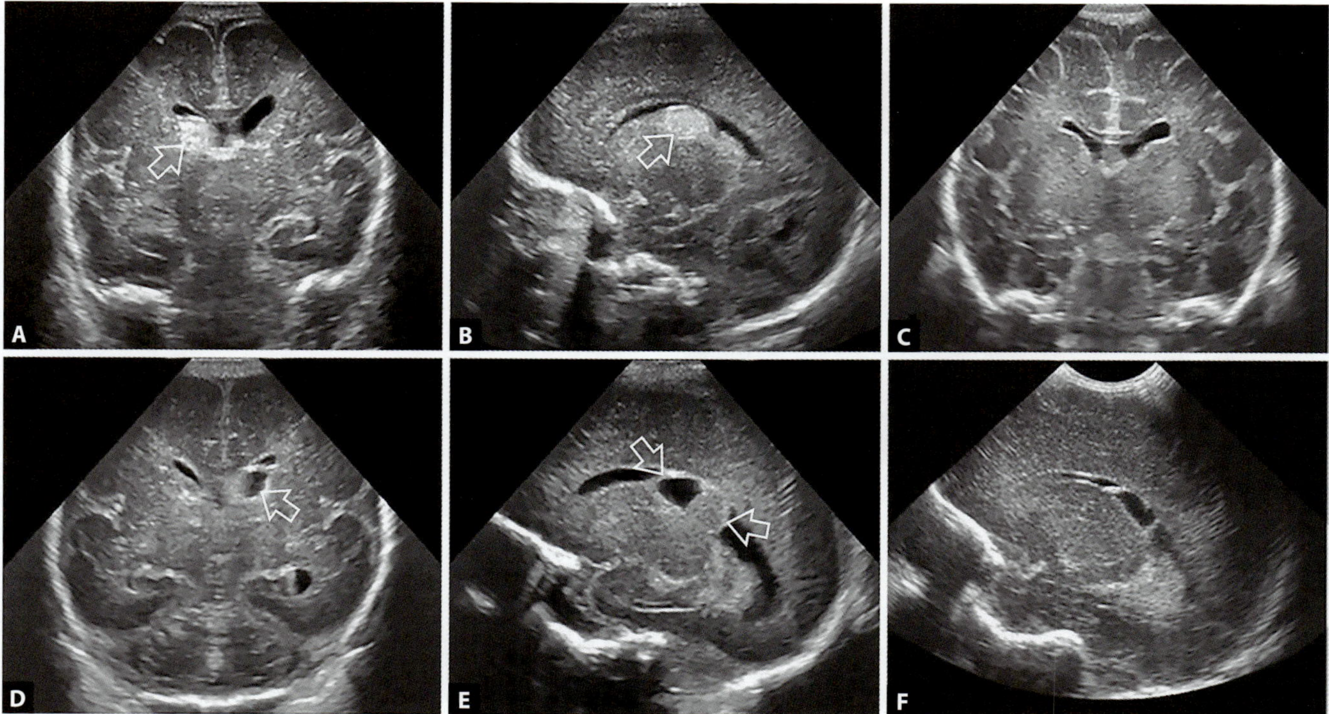

Q18. A 4-year-old girl presented with convulsion and drowsiness.

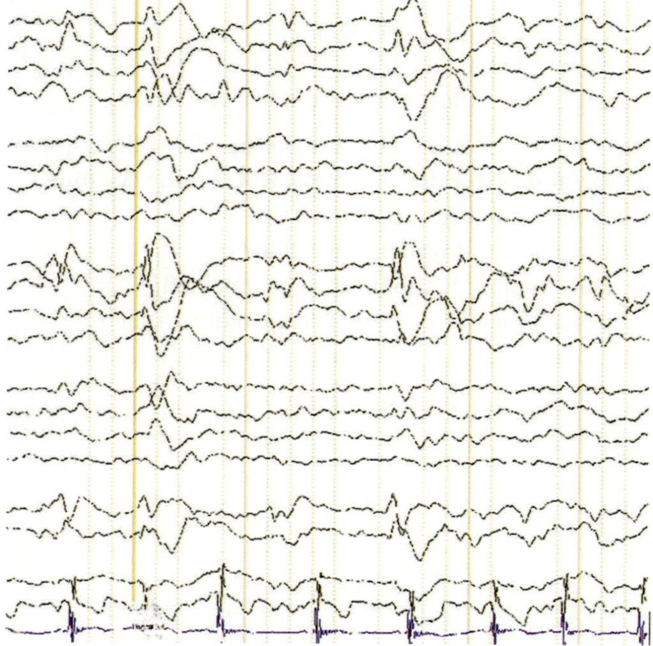

1. What are diagnosis and EEG findings of this image?
2. Name the lobe of the brain usually involved.
3. Name the drug for treatment in this case.
4. What is gold standard investigation for diagnosis?

Q19. An 8-year-old girl presents with gait abnormality and poor scholastic performance for 5 months. Eye examination shows this:

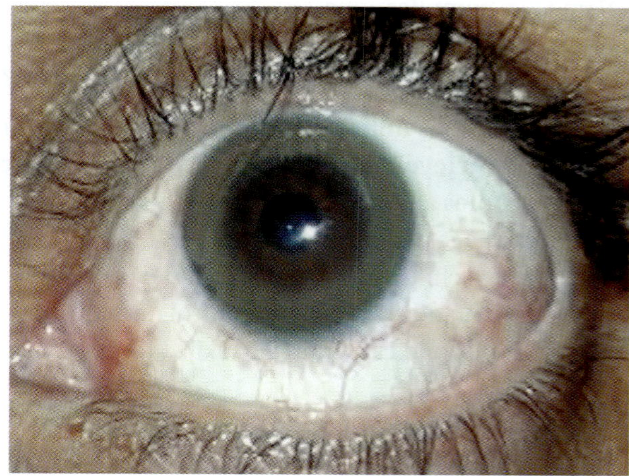

1. What are the eye findings and most probable diagnosis of such case?
2. Name the gene involved.
3. What is the inheritance?
4. Name the drugs to treat the condition.

Q20. A 5-year-old boy presents with pallor, fatigue and glositis. Peripheral smear shows like this:

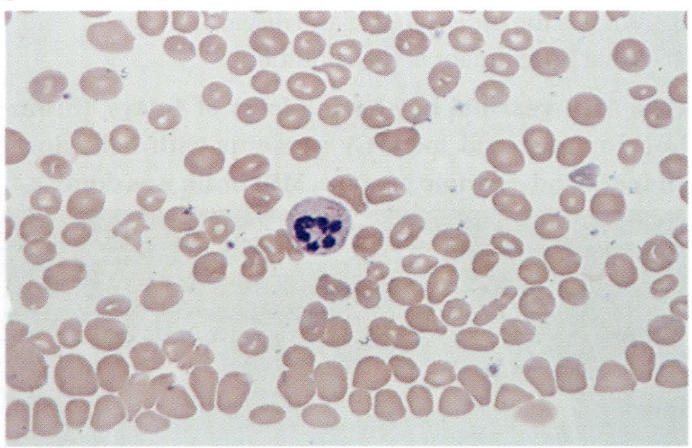

1. Name the most probable disease.
2. What is the treatment?
3. What are neurological manifestations of this disease?
4. The Schilling test was historically used to diagnose which disease?

Q21. A 5-day-old newborn presents with abdominal distension, vomiting, and fever. Straight X-ray abdomen shows like this.

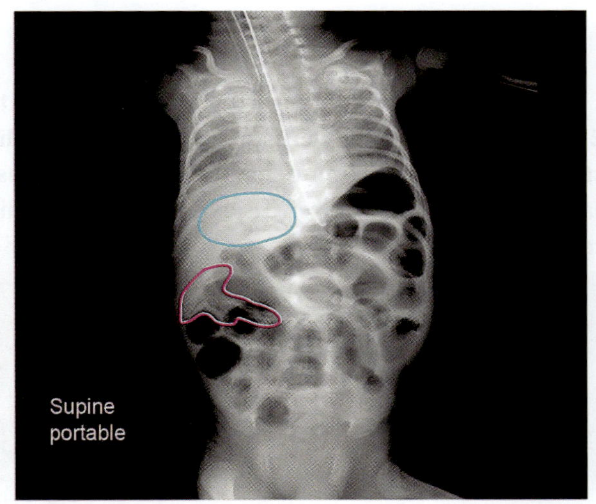

1. Identify the problem.
2. What is the stage of such disease?
3. What is classic triad?
4. What are the therapeutic modalities to treat such condition.

Q22. A 6-year-old girl has muscle weakness and delayed relaxation after contraction of hand grip from 1 year of age.

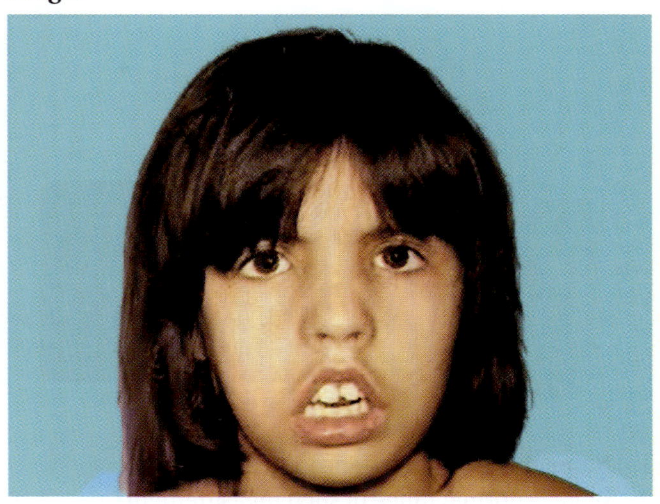

1. What is most probable diagnosis?
2. Describe the facies.
3. Name the pattern of weakness.
4. What is primary diagnosis test?

Q23. A newborn of diabetic mother, weighing 4.3 kg, had convulsion and undergone MRI.

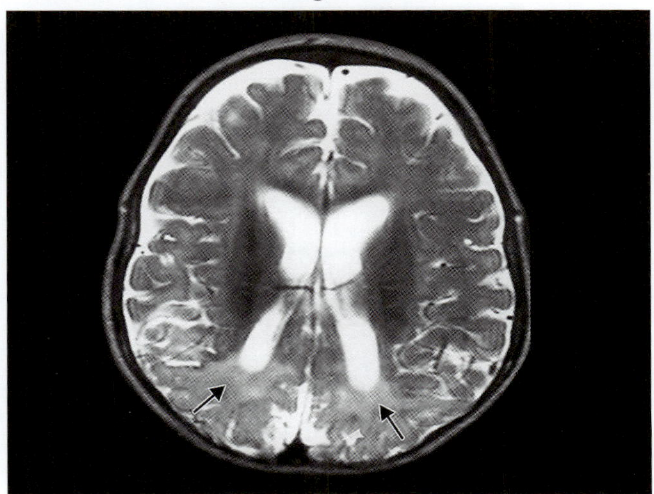

1. Describe the MRI findings.
2. What is probable etiological diagnosis?
3. What is next most probable site of lesion in brain?
4. Name few sequelae of such condition.

Q24. An 8-year-old boy having history of fall has gone through some procedure.

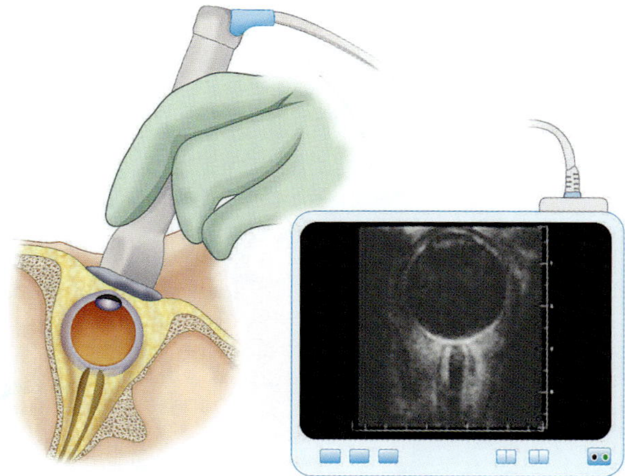

1. Name the technique done in this boy.
2. What is normal range of such measurement?
3. What is advantage of such measurement in this condition?
4. What are PECAN rules favoring risk of brain injury?

Q25. A 2-year-old boy presented with recurrent infection, rashes from 1 year. Routine blood count shows small and low platelet count.

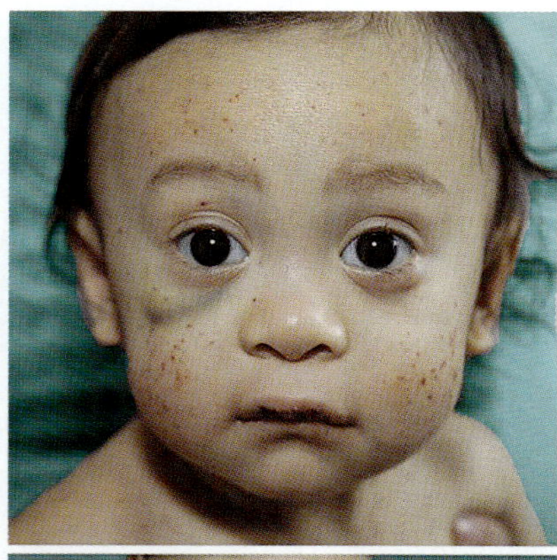

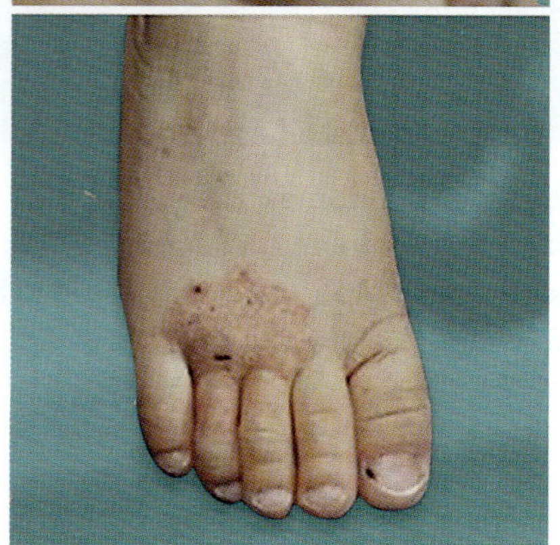

1. What is most probable diagnosis?
2. Which genetic mutation causes such?
3. What is the inheritance of the disease?
4. What is treatment of the condition?

Q26. A 10-year-old boy having fever of 4 days, thrombocytopenia, and low PCV presents with behavioral changes and dystonic posture. MRI brain was done.

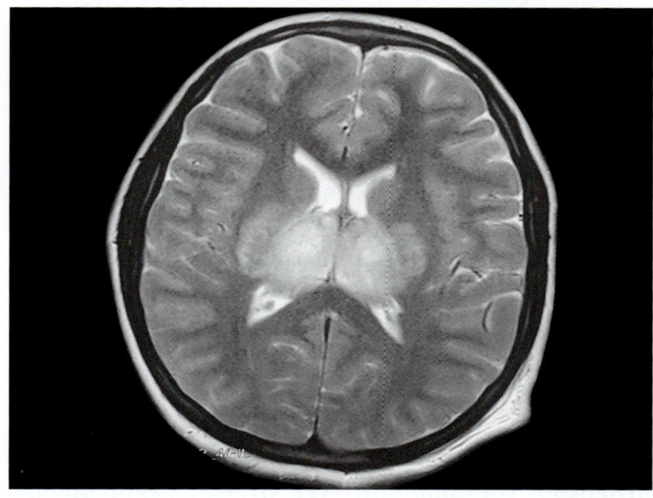

1. Name the finding in the MRI brain.
2. What are the probable diagnoses?
3. How it is transmitted?
4. What is the gold standard test to detect?

Q27. A 9-year-old boy went to Tripura to meet her sister. After returning home, he developed fever, rash, headache from last 3 days. On examination, she has vitals poor, drowsy.

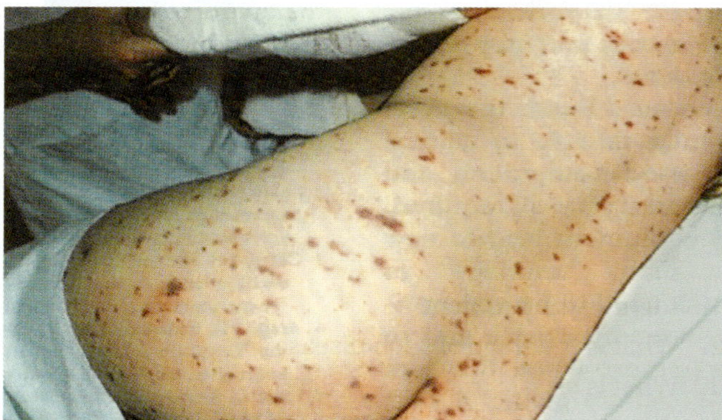

1. What is provisional diagnosis?
2. What is most significant characteristic of the rash?
3. Which complication is most specific?
4. Which of the following is used for chemoprophylaxis of close contacts?

Q28.

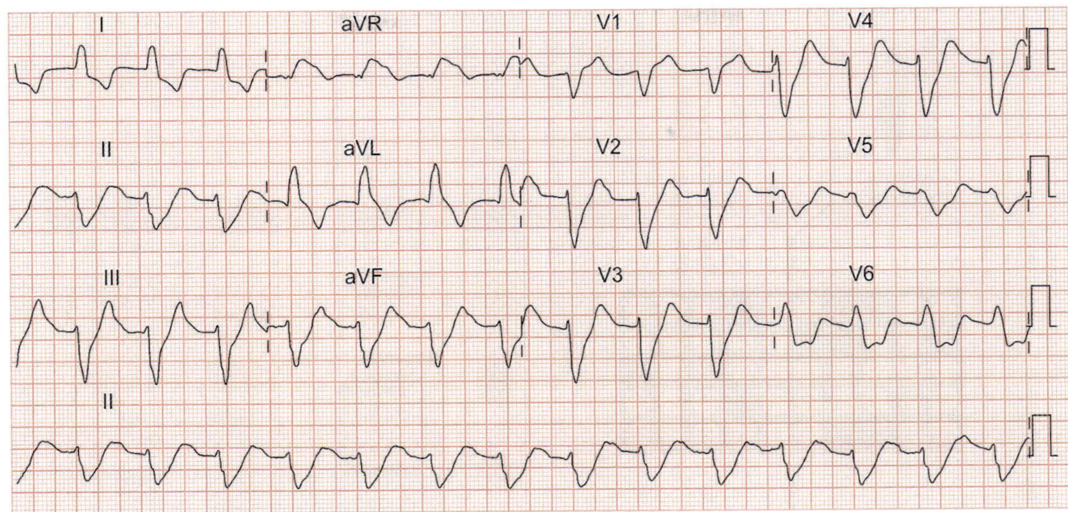

1. Identify the ECG.
2. What is the treatment?
3. Name the drugs most commonly associated with this condition.
4. Which hormone helps in reducing the condition?

Q29. A 2-year-old boy presents with painless rectal bleed for few months. The stool is maroon color. This test is performed. Following findings are shown in 20 minutes and 25 minutes.

1. Name the test.
2. What is the radioactive substance?
3. Identify the dark areas.
4. How to increase diagnostic yield?

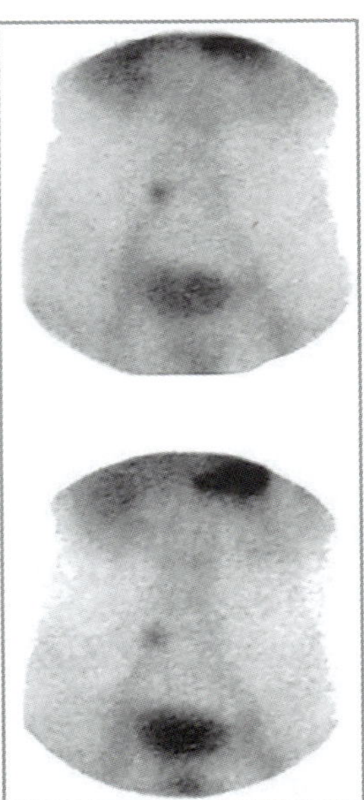

(Above image at 20 min of the study and below image at 25 min of the study)

Q30. Neonate born to a primi mother had an antenatal scan at 28 weeks of gestation which revealed lissencephaly. Baby born with microcephaly and convulsion in convulsion from day 5. This genetic test was performed.

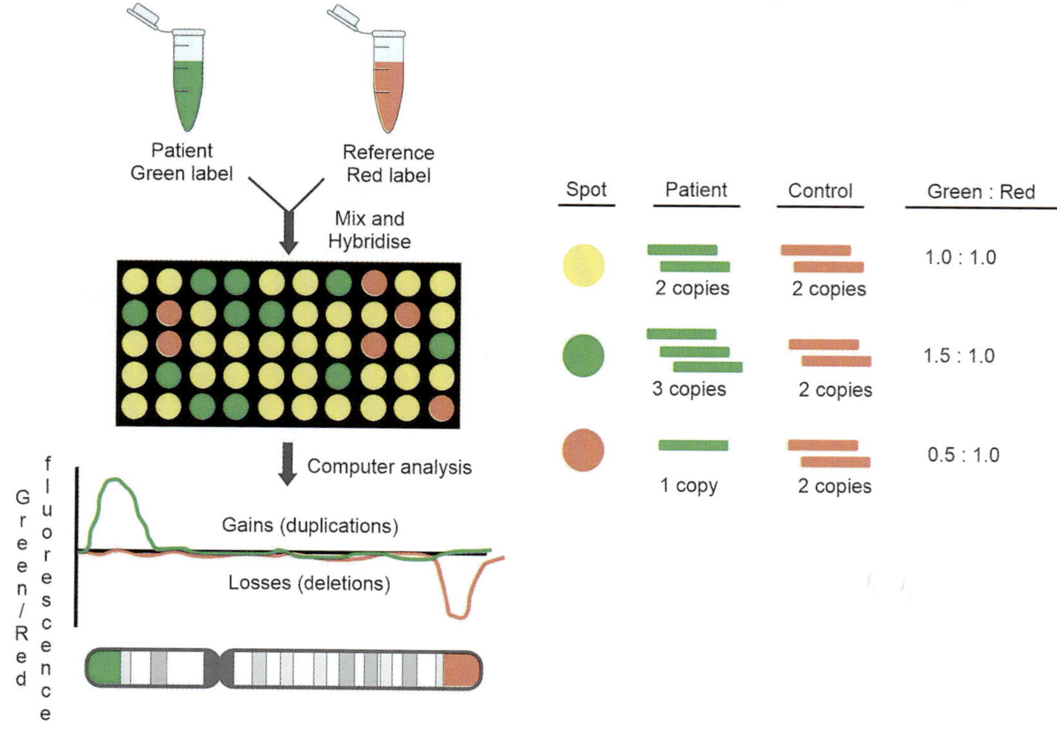

1. Write the name of the genetic testing shown in figure.
2. Name an alternate test which can be done.
3. What is the likely diagnosis detectable by above methods?
4. Write the chromosomal abnormality.

Q31.

1. What are the components of Hutchison triad?
2. Hutchinson's triad is seen in:
3. Deafness in Hutchinson's triad is due to:
4. Name the drug of choice of such condition.

Q32. An 11-month-old child presented with macrocephaly and dystonia. TMS showed elevated C5DC.

1. What is the diagnosis?
2. What is the mainstay of therapy?
3. Name a preventive strategy.
4. Name the MRI brain findings of such condition.

Q33. A 3-day-old girl with uneventful transition and antenatal period presented with refractory seizures. The neonate responded well to pyridoxine therapy.

1. What is the likely diagnosis?
2. What are the biochemical tests done for definitive diagnosis?
3. Describe the pathophysiology of the disease.
4. What is the prognosis?

Q34.

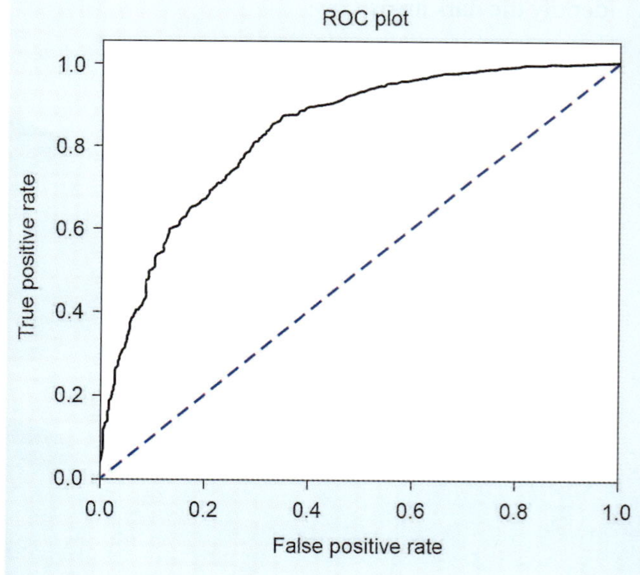

1. What does this figure show?
2. What is the purpose of this?
3. What does the X axis represent?
4. What do the dots along the curve represent?
5. How is interpretation done?

Q35.

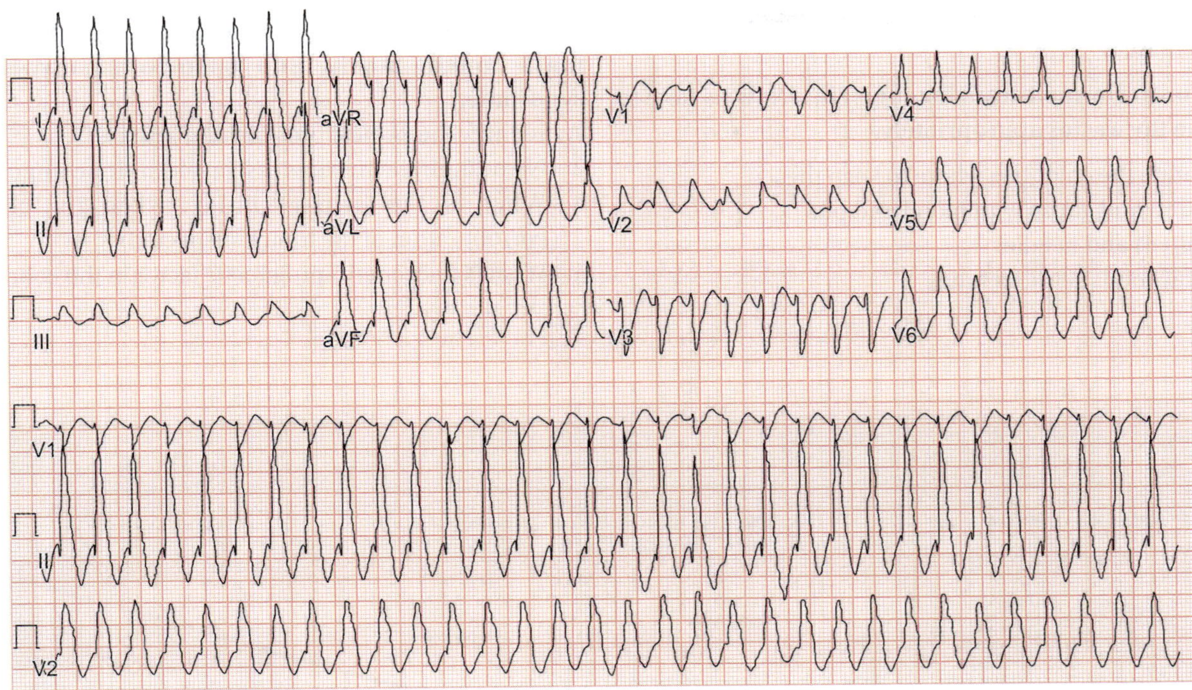

1. Identify the rhythm.
2. Write the management of a child with this ECG with palpable pulses, hypotension, and altered mental status.
3. What is the treatment if there is no cardiopulmonary compromise?
4. Name other drugs used to treat this rhythm.

Q36.

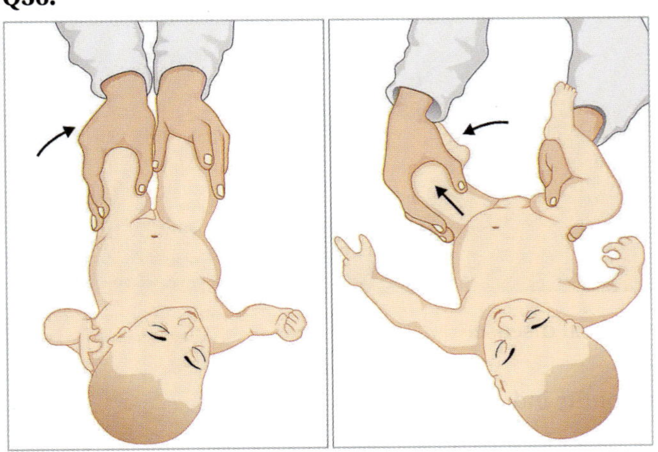

1. What is the test being performed and disease when to perform?
2. Which imaging modality is preferred for screening of this disease in infants <6 months?
3. What is used in management?
4. What is a teratologic hip?

Q37.

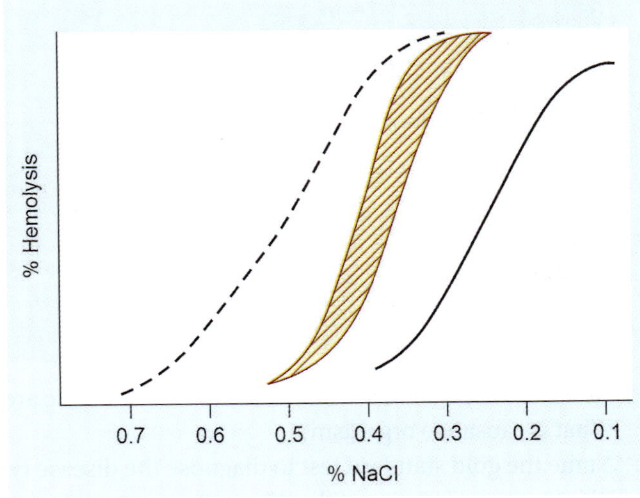

1. What is the test represented in the graph?
2. What does the test measure?

3. What are the factors affecting this test?
4. Name the conditions where it is increased and decreased.

Q38. You performed drain for empyema. Now its time to dispose the wastes appropriately.

Enumarate the color box where to keep these.

1. Cotton and gauze with blood and pus
2. Scalpels and needles
3. Intravenous sets and tubes
4. Plastic covers of the iv tubes and medicine

Q39. A 6-year-old girl presents with weight loss, neck mass cough, ptosis, and opsoclonus myoclonus syndrome.

1. Identify the clinical presentation disease.
2. Name the eye syndrome associated and its components.
3. What is the urinary index asked for clinical corroboration of the tumor suspected?
4. What is the genetic-prognostic factor in the condition?

Q40.

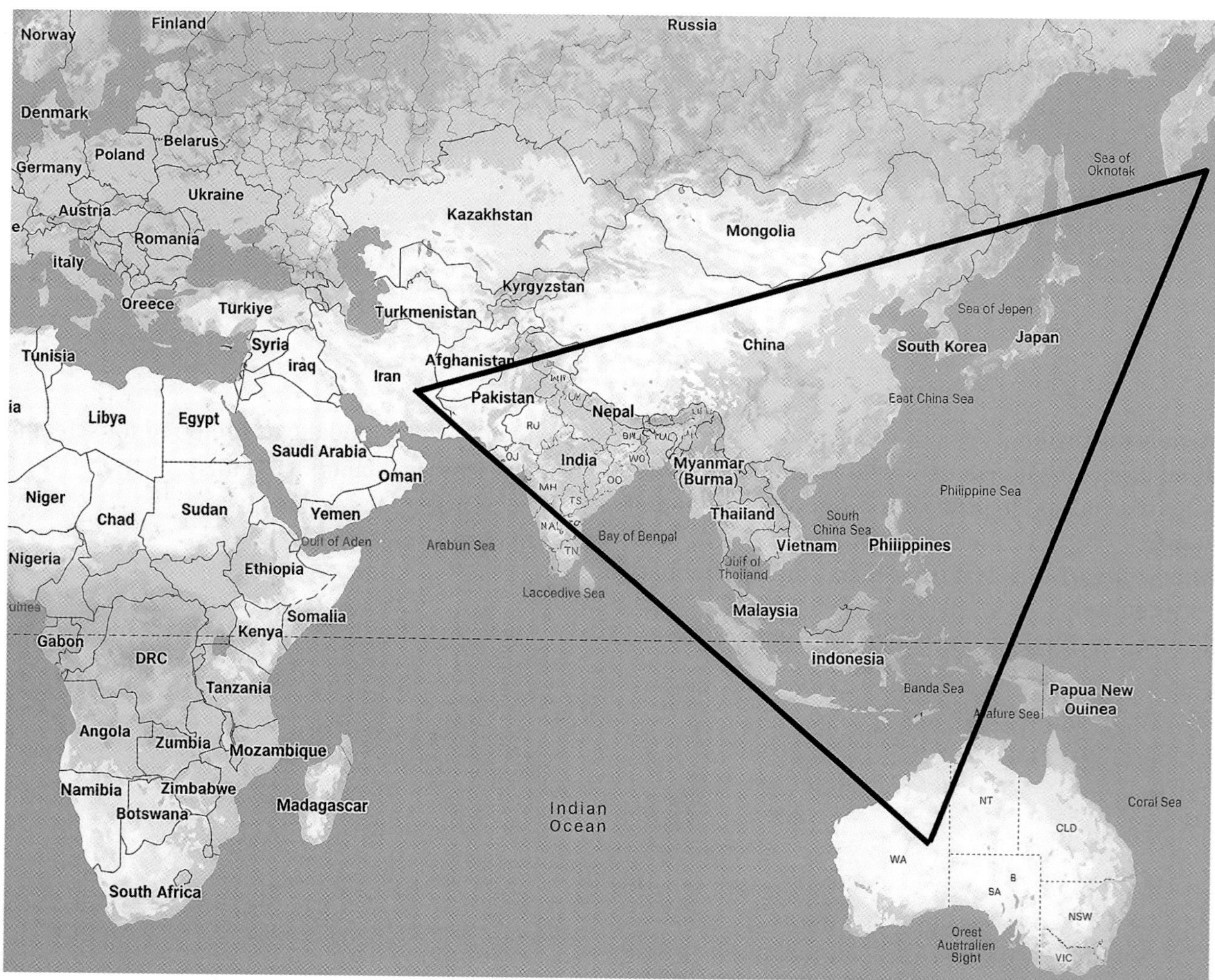

1. Name the triangle in the map which is the endemic area of typical disease.
2. What is causative organism?
3. Name the gold standard test to diagnose the disease typical for the indicated map.
4. What is drug of choice of the disease?

Q41.

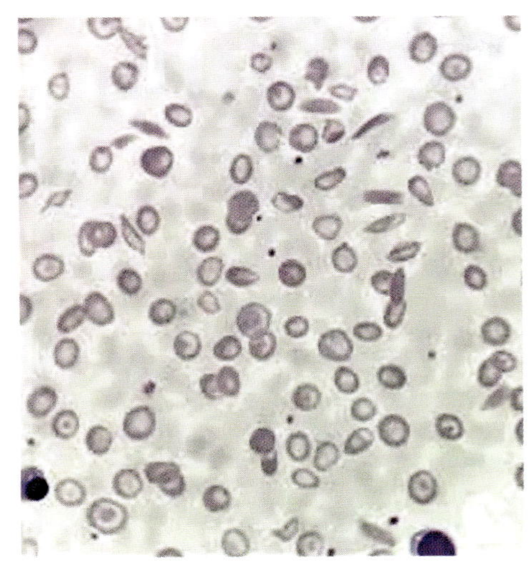

1. Identify the abnormalities in the smear.
2. Name two precipitating factors.
3. Name two complication of the disease.
4. What is the indication of starting medicine.

Q42. A 2-year-old boy was brought unresponsive to ER. You checked vital signs. You have checked pulse for at least 10 seconds, checked for respiratory efforts. There was no pluse felt and no respiratory effort.

1. What is the next step?
2. What is compression rate?
3. Name the component of high quality CPR.
4. In infants, what is the preferred site for pulse check during CPR?

Q43.

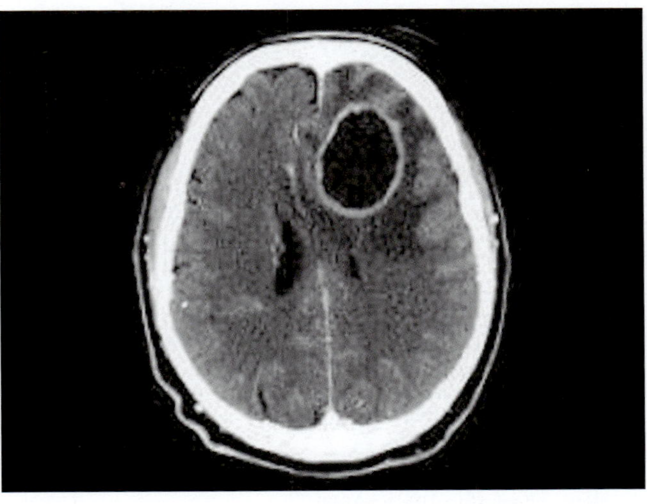

1. Enumerate finding of the neuroimaging.
2. What is most probable diagnosis?
3. Name the two predisposing conditions.
4. What is common organism of this condition.

Q44. A 7-year-old immunocompromised girl presents with painless blurring of vision from 1 month. ophthalmoscopy performed.

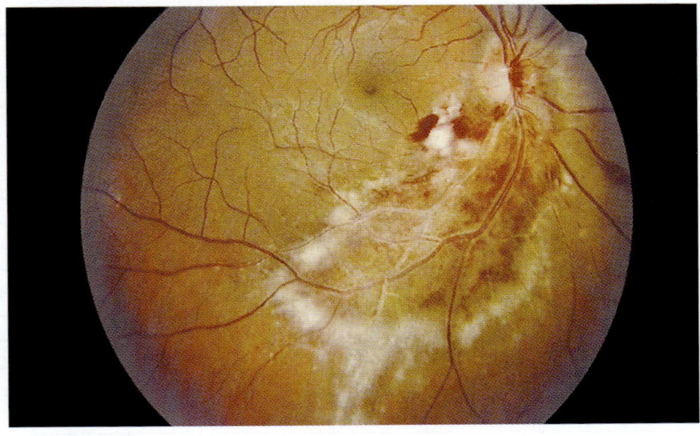

1. What is most probable diagnosis?
2. What is treatment of this condition.
3. Name one side effect of the drug used.
4. Name one dangerous complication of this condition.

Q45.

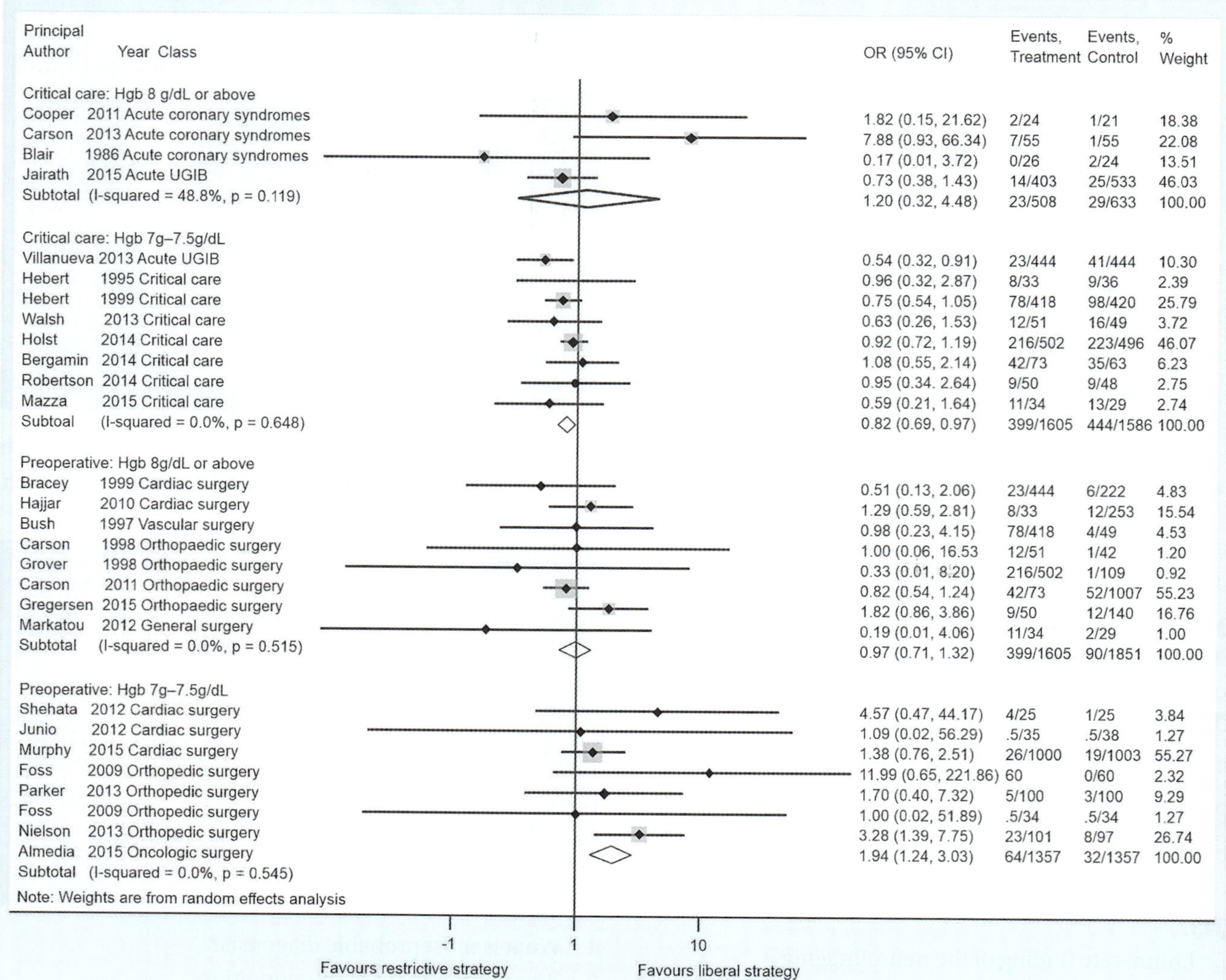

1. What is the statistical plotting?
2. What the straight line represents?
3. Why are some squares bigger than others?
4. What does the diamond represent?

Q46. A 5-year-old child presented with pallor and cutaneous markers at the back with an abnormal skeletal profile. Peripheral smear was consistent with macrocytic anemia and pancytopenia.

1. What is the most probable diagnosis of this scenario?
2. What cutaneous marker you expect?
3. What malignancies are expected in this patient?
4. Name any diagnostic test.

Q47. A 5-year-old baby presents with fever and rash on 5th day. Baby also has hepatosplenomegaly.

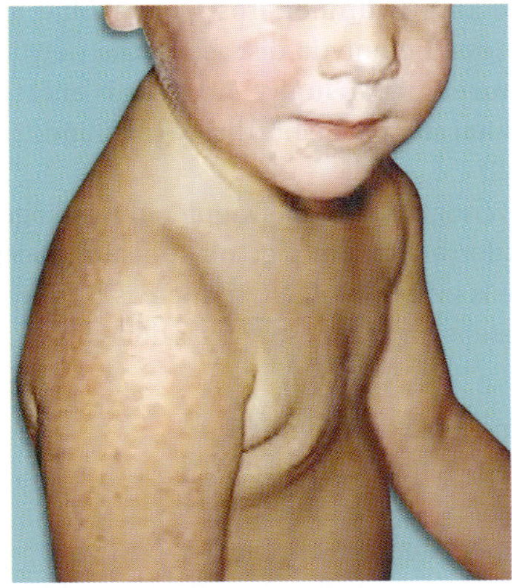

1. What is the diagnosis?
2. Identify the probable organism.
3. Name the significant hematological crisis of the disease.
4. Describe the most reliable method for diagnosis of the infection in immunocompromised baby.

Q48. This male child aged 10 months has been brought with a large tongue and hepatosplenomegaly. He was born weighing 4.2 kg and had hypoglycemia in newborn period.

1. What is most probable diagnosis?
2. Associated with increased risk of which childhood tumor?
3. The genetic basis of the disease most commonly involves:
4. What is the classic triad of the disease?

Q49.

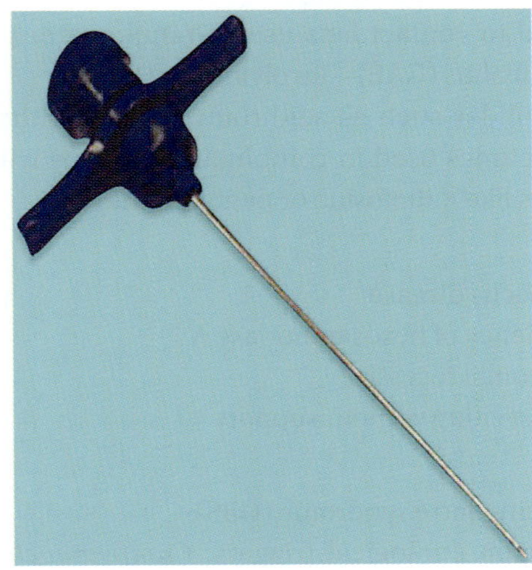

1. Identify the instrument.
2. Name two indication of such instruments.
3. What are the two contraindications to use this instrument.
4. What is most common site for bone marrow aspiration in infants.

Q50. Raju, 25 years old from Kerala comes with this type of skin lesion in leg with black grain discharge.

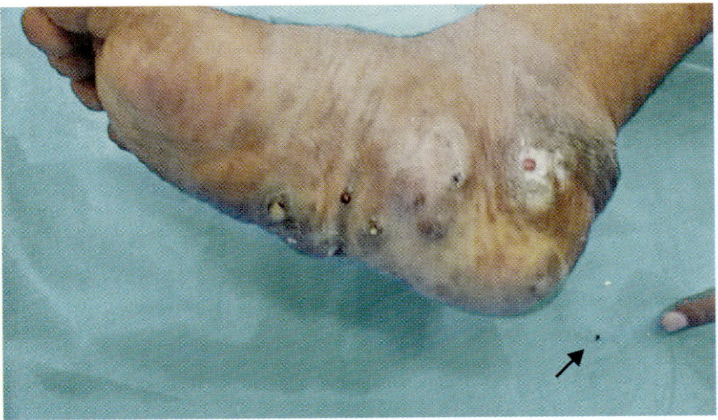

1. Identify the lesion
2. What is causative organism?
3. Name the best imaging modality to assess extent of this lesion.
4. What is the treatment of such lesion.

OSCE 50 ANSWERS

Ans. 1:

1. *Acanthamoeba* infection
2. Through the nasal passages (inhalation of cysts/trophozoites) and through the eyes (contaminated contact lenses or water exposure)
3. Acanthamoeba keratitis (corneal infection, often linked to contact lens use). Granulomatous amebic encephalitis (GAE)—involving the CNS
4. Macrolides such as azithromycin or clarithromycin (sometimes used in combination therapy with other agents like miltefosine or pentamidine)

Ans. 2:

1. Tay-Sachs disease
2. Deficiency of hexosaminidase A
3. Autosomal recessive
4. At least siting without support

Ans. 3:

1. Guillain-Barré syndrome (GBS)
2. Common etiological triggers: *Campylobacter jejuni* (most frequent), viral infections such as CMV, EBV, and influenza
3. *Confirmatory investigations*:
   - Nerve conduction studies/EMG—showing demyelination
   - Cerebrospinal fluid (CSF) analysis—albuminocytologic dissociation
   - Serum autoantibody testing (optional/supportive)
4. *Treatment:*
   - Admit to hospital (with respiratory monitoring and supportive care)
   - Intravenous immunoglobulin (IVIG) or plasma exchange (plasmapheresis)

Ans. 4:

1. Abnormal findings in the ECG—prominent Q waves in Leads I, aVL, V5, and V6. ST-T changes in V4-V5
2. *Diagnosis:* Abnormal origin of anomalous left coronary artery from pulmonary artery (ALCAPA)
3. Infants present with features of heart failure, irritability, poor feeding, and sometimes diaphoresis during feeding
4. Surgery

Ans. 5:

1. Renal vein thrombosis (polycythemia + hematuria + enlarged kidneys = classic presentation)
2. Urinary tract infection (neonatal pyelonephritis), Wilms tumor (rare in neonates, but considered with renal mass), hydronephrosis/congenital anomalies of kidneys, hemolytic disease of the newborn (with hematuria but usually no renal enlargement), congenital adrenal hemorrhage (can mimic renal mass on USG)
3. Renal venography/renal Doppler ultrasonography
4. Correction of fluid and electrolyte disturbances, LMWH if there is evidence of DIC, if there is B/L involvement with extension to IVC, surgery is done.

Ans. 6:

- Stepping reflex—2 months
- Parachute reflex—never
- Moro reflex—5–6 months
- Asymmetric tonic neck reflex—6–7 month
- Symmetric tonic neck reflex—9–11 months

Ans. 7:

1. Intussusception
2. Doughnut sign/pseudokidney sign
3. Peyer's patch hypertrophy
4. Pneumatic reduction/hydrostatic reduction/surgical reduction

Ans. 8:

1. Williams syndrome
2. Elfin facies (idiopathic hypercalcemia of infancy, nephrocalcinosis, hypothyroidism, hypermobility of joints)
3. Supravalvular aortic stenosis, narrowing of coronary ostia, branch pulmonary artery stenosis
4. FISH, deletion of elastin gene 7q11.23

Ans. 9:

1. Molar tooth sign in MRI brain
2. Joubert syndrome
3. Hypotonia, developmental delay, truncal ataxia later, episodic apnea or tachypnea, atypical eye movements. Retinal dystrophy, polydactyly
4. Retinal dystrophy, ocular colobomas, occipital encephalocele, hepatic fibrosis, nephronopathies, cystic kidney diseases (because it is a ciliopathy)

Ans. 10:

1. Shoulder dystocia, injury to upper brachial plexus C5,C6+/-C7
2. Phrenic nerve involvement, ipsilateral diaphragmatic palsy
3. Biceps, moro and grasp reflex are retained.

4. McRoberts (flexion and abduction of maternal hips) is the initial and most effective maneuver. (Fundal pressure is contraindicated as it worsens impaction.)

Ans. 11:

1. Respiratory distress syndrome—low lung volumes, homogeneous opacities, ground glass appearance, air bronchograms
2. Antenatal steroids accelerate surfactant synthesis → major preventive measure
3. Surfactant in the amniotic fluid lowers surface tension. When shaken with ethanol, stable foam/bubbles form at the air-liquid interface if sufficient surfactant is present. Absence of foam indicates immature lungs → high risk of neonatal RDS.
4. OI is calculated in ventilated babies. OI = MAP × FiO_2/PaO_2
   - OI 25–40—severe respiratory failure, mortality risk 50–60%
   - >40—mortality risk >80%

Ans. 12:

1. Neurofibromatosis 1
2. Autosomal dominant
3. Nervous system (neurofibroma, optic glioma, etc.), skin, musculoskeletal system, ocular system (lisch nodule), and cardiovascular system
4. MEK inhibitor (selumetinib)

Ans. 13:

1. Sturge-Weber syndrome
2. Sporadic in occurrence
3. Facial nevus—port-wine stain, seizures, hemiparesis, stroke like episodes, intracranial calcifications
4. Venous angioma of leptomeninges

Ans. 14:

1. Polymorphic ventricular tachycardia/torsades de pointes
2. Class IA (procainamide, quinine, disopyramide) and class III (sotalol, amiodarone) antiarrhythmics
3. Long QT syndrome
4. Ventricular fibrillation and ventricular tachycardia
5. (A) CPR and shock; (B) Rapid iv magnesium sulfate 25–50 mg/kg (within minutes) maximum 2 g

Ans. 15:

1. Around 3 years
2. By 3 years
3. 2–5 years
4. 5 years

Ans. 16:

1. District early intervention center under Rashtriya Bal Swasthya Karyakram
2. Purpose to provide referral support to children detected with health conditions (primarily up to 6 years of age), idea is to intervene early and minimize disability established at district hospital level across country.
3. Defects at birth, diseases (e.g., thalassemia, sickle cell, and rheumatic heart disease), deficiencies (e.g., anemia, vitamin deficiencies, and malnutrition), developmental delays and disabilities (e.g., CP, autism, hearing loss, and vision impairment)
4. District hospital

Ans. 17:

1. Intraventricular hemorrhage
2. Apnea, bradycardia, bulging fontanelle, seizure, anemia, and shock
3. In 1–2 week interval to check ventricular dilatation, and hydrocephalus progression
4. Cerebral palsy and neurodevelopmental delay

Ans. 18:

1. HSV encephalitis [periodic waveforms or paroxysmal lateralizing epileptiform discharges (PLED)]
2. Temporal lobe
3. Iv acyclovir 10 mg/kg 8 hourly for 21 days
4. CSF HSV-DNA PC

Ans. 19:

1. Kayser-Fleischer ring in a probable patient of Wilson disease
2. ATP7B, 13q14.3
3. Autosomal recessive
4.
   (a) Limit diet copper intake <1 mg/day
   (b) Oral D-penicillamine
   (c) Zinc therapy

Ans. 20:

1. Hypersegmented neutrophil mostly megaloblastic anemia
2. Vitamin B_{12} 1,000 μg im daily/alternate day × 1–2 weeks. Then 1,000 μg every month for life
   Folate 1–5 mg orally daily
3. Peripheral neuropathy, subacute combined degeneration of the cord
4. Pernicious anemia

Ans. 21:

1. NEC in newborn
2. IIB

3.
   (a) Pneumatosis intestinalis → gas within the bowel wall
   (b) Portal venous gas → branching lucencies over the liver
   (c) Pneumoperitoneum → free intraperitoneal air (suggests perforation)
4. NPO, TPN, IV antibiotics, and surgery

Ans. 22:

1. Myotonic muscular dystrophy
2. Enlarged facies, downturned mouth
3. Distal > proximal muscle weakness in DM1 (congenital)
4. Clinical + EMG: myotonic discharges. Genetic: CTG/CCTG repeat. CTG in DMPK gene for DM1, CCTG in CNBP gene for DM2

Ans. 23:

1. Atrophy and gliosis of parietooccipital and medial occipital region
2. Neonatal hypoglycemia
3. Temporal lobe
4. Seizure, visual impairment, global developmental delay, and ADHD

Ans. 24:

1. Optic nerve sheath diameter measurement by USG
2. Upper limits <1 year = Up to 4 mm, 1–15 years = up to 4.5 mm, >15 years = up to 5 mm
3. Rapid, bedside, noninvasive screening tool to determine increased intracranial pressure
4. Measurements above 5 mm (b/l) correspond with elevations in ICP above 20 mm Hg.

Ans. 25:

1. Wiskott–Aldrich syndrome
2. WAS gene mutation
3. X-linked recessive
4. *Curative:* Hematopoietic stem cell transplant (HSCT). *Supportive:* IVIG, prophylactic antibiotics, platelet transfusions if bleeding

Ans. 26:

1. T1 hyper- and T2 hypointensity of b/l thalamus. DWI showing thalamic swelling. Double doughnut sign
2. Dengue encephalopathy
3. *Aedes aegypti* mosquito
4. Nucleic acid amplification test (NAAT)

Ans. 27:

1. Meningococcal septicemia with purpura fulminans
2. Non-blanching petechial/purpuric rash
3. Waterhouse–Friderichsen syndrome (adrenal hemorrhage due to meningococcemia)
4. Rifampicin

Ans. 28:

1. Hyperkalemia (loss of p wave, prolonged QRS, ST elevation, tall T waves)
2. IV calcium (to stabilize cell membrane), glucose-insulin drip, sodium bicarbonate, nebulized salbutamol, sodium polystyrene sulfonate (Kayexalate) resin
3. ACE inhibitors
4. Aldosterone

Ans. 29:

1. Meckel's radionuclide scan
2. 99m technetium pertechnetate
3. Stomach, Meckel's diverticulum, urinary bladder
4. Uptake of the radioactive element can be enhanced by ranitidine, gastrin, and glucagon.

Ans. 30:

1. Chromosomal microarray
2. MLPA
3. Miller–Dieker syndrome
4. Deletion on chromosome 17p13.3

Ans. 31:

1. Interstitial keratitis, sensorineural deafness notched incisors
2. Congenital syphilis
3. Damage to CN VIII by syphilitic inflammation
4. Penicillin G (always the treatment of choice—both early and late congenital syphilis)

Ans. 32:

1. Glutaric aciduria type I (specific for TMS C5DC)
2. Dietary therapy (low-lysine, low-tryptophan diet + carnitine supplementation)
3. Newborn screening
4. Wide Sylvian fissures with frontotemporal atrophy ("bat-wing appearance")

Ans. 33:

1. Pyridoxine-dependent seizures/pyridoxine-responsive seizures
2. Plasma/urine/CSF-AASA and pipecolic acid
3. Defect in lysine metabolism → accumulation of α-aminoadipic semialdehyde (AASA) → inactivates pyridoxal-5'-phosphate (active B6 cofactor)
4. If identified and treated early, they do well. Could have breakthrough seizures.

Ans. 34:

1. Receiver operative characteristic (ROC) curve
2. Describes changes in sensitivity and specificity for a single test with many cutoffs and used to choose the optimal cutoff that minimizes the percentage of false positive and false negative results, compares the performance of different tests used to diagnose the same disease
3. 1—Specificity
4. Various cutoffs against their respective sensitivity and 1—specificity
5. Cutoff with maximum area under curve is the ideal cutoff which will have maximum possible sensitivity/ specificity and least possible false positives and false negatives

Ans. 35:

1. Ventricular tachycardia
2. ABC management and synchronized cardioversion 0.5–1 J/kg, if no improvement 2 J/kg
3. Adenosine 0.1 mg/kg rapid bolus, 2nd dose—0.2 mg/kg rapid bolus
4. Procainamide, amiodarone

Ans. 36:

1. Barlows test and Ortolani test to diagnose developmental dysplasia of hip
2. Ultrasound hip (Graf's method)
3. Pavlik's harness
4. Dislocated in utero and irreducible on neonatal examination
   - Presents with a pseudoacetabulum
   - Associated with neuromuscular conditions and genetic disorders
   - Commonly seen with arthrogryposis, myelomeningocele, Larsen's syndrome, Ehlers-Danlos syndrome

Ans. 37:

1. Osmotic fragility test
2. It measures the resistance to hemolysis of red blood cells exposed to hypotonic solutions
3. Cell membrane permeability and surface-to-volume ratio
4. Increased in hereditary spherocytosis and decreased in thalassemia and sickle cell anemia and IDA

Ans. 38:

- Cotton and gauze with blood and pus—yellow
- Scalpels and needles—blue/white—puncture proof box
- Intravenous sets and tubes—red
- Plastic covers of the iv tubes and medicine—green

Ans. 39:

1. Neck mass with ptosis: Thoracic neuroblastoma
2. Horner's syndrome: dry eyes, miosis, ptosis, and enaphthalmos
3. 24 hours urinary VMA
4. N-MYC oncogene

Ans. 40:

1. The "Tsutsugamushi Triangle" refers to the primary endemic region for scrub typhus, a disease caused by the bacterium *Orientia tsutsugamushi*, encompassing areas from the Russian far east to Pakistan in the west, Australia in the south, and Japan in the east.
2. *Orientia tsutsugamushi*
3. Indirect immunofluorescence assay (IFA)
4. *Doxycycline alternatives:* Azithromycin (safe in pregnancy and chloramphenicol)

Ans. 41:

1. Sickle cell anemia
2. Acidosis, infection
3. Vaso-occlusive crisis, acute chest syndrome
4. *Hydroxyurea:* 3 or more in 1 year, recurrent chest pain, chronic leg ulcer failed conventional therapy.

Ans. 42:

1. Call for help/activate EMS and get AED
2. Begins compressions 30:2
3.
   i. Push hard
   ii. Push fast
   iii. Allows chest recoil
   iv. Avoids hyperventilation
   v. Minimizes interruption
4. Brachial artery

Ans. 43:

1. Contrast CT, hypodense lesion left frontal region, surrounding contrast enhancement, midline shift
2. Cerebral abscess
3. Cyanotic heart disease, acute/chronic otitis media, mastoiditis
4. Streptococcus (aerobic and anaerobic) → most common, *Staphylococcus aureus*, *Bacteroides*, *Fusobacterium*

Ans. 44:

1. CMV retinitis
2. IV ganciclovir or oral valganciclovir

3. Ganciclovir/valganciclovir → Bone marrow suppression; Foscarnet → Nephrotoxicity
4. Retinal detachment

Ans. 45:

1. Forest plot, a graphical display used in meta-analysis to show results from multiple studies on the same topic
2. Line of no effect (OR = 1 or mean difference = 0)
3. Bigger squares represent studies with larger sample size/more weight in the analysis
4. Pooled effect with CI 95

Ans. 46:

1. Fanconi anemia
2. Café au lait spot
3. Acute myeloid leukemia and squamous cell carcinoma
4. Chromosomal breakage test with diepoxybutane (DEB) or mitomycin-C

Ans. 47:

1. Erythema infectiosum (fifth disease)
2. Parvovirus B19
3. Aplastic crisis in hemolytic anemia
4. PCR for viral DNA

Ans. 48:

1. Beckwith-Wiedemann syndrome
2. Wilms' tumor
3. Chromosome 11p15
4. Macroglossia, omphalocele, and hemihypertrophy

Ans. 49:

1. Jamshidi needle for bone marrow trephine biopsy
2. Bone marrow trephine biopsy—diagnosis of:
    - Myelofibrosis
    - Aplastic anemia
    - Infiltrative marrow diseases (lymphoma, metastasis)
    - Staging of leukemia
    - Bone biopsy in orthopedics
    - Vertebral body biopsy or iliac crest biopsy
3. Severe bleeding disorders (e.g., hemophilia, severe thrombocytopenia)
   Local infection at the puncture site
4. Tibial tuberosity (anteromedial surface)

Ans. 50:

1. Madura feet
2. *Madurella mycetomatis* (due to the clinical picture and black grain discharge)
3. MRI ("dot-in-circle" sign)
4. Amphotericin B or itraconazole ± surgical excision

SUGGESTED READING

1. Avery GB, MacDonald MG, Mullett MD, Seshia MMK. Avery's Neonatology: Pathophysiology and Management of the Newborn. 11th ed. Philadelphia: Lippincott Williams & Wilkins; 2023.
2. Cloherty JP, Eichenwald EC, Hansen AR, Stark AR, editors. Manual of Neonatal Care. 9th ed. Philadelphia: Wolters Kluwer; 2022.
3. Ghai OP, Paul VK, Bagga A. Essential Pediatrics. 10th ed. New Delhi: CBS Publishers & Distributors; 2025.
4. Gupta P, Menon PSN, Ramji S, Lodha R, editors. PG Textbook of Pediatrics. 3rd ed., reprint. 3 vols. New Delhi: Jaypee Brothers Medical Publishers; 2024.
5. Indian Academy of Pediatrics Committee on Immunization. IAP Guidebook on Immunization. 5th ed. New Delhi: Jaypee Brothers Medical Publishers; 2025.
6. Kliegman RM, St Geme JW, Blum NJ, Shah SS, Tasker RC, Wilson KM, editors. Nelson Textbook of Pediatrics. 22nd ed. Philadelphia: Elsevier; 2024.
7. Menon PSN, Gupta P, editors. IAP Textbook of Pediatrics. 8th ed. New Delhi: Jaypee Brothers Medical Publishers; 2025.
8. Singh M. Care of the Newborn. 9th ed. New Delhi: Sagar Publications; 2025.

Index

Page numbers followed by *b* refer to box, *f* refer to figure, *fc* refer to flowchart, and *t* refer to table.

D

E

F

J

K

L

M

N

U

V

W

X